Radiological
Sciences
Dictionary

KEYWORDS, NAMES AND DEFINITIONS

Radiological Sciences Dictionary
DAVID J DOWSETT

David J. Dowsett MSc PhD
Previously Chief Physicist at the Mater
University Hospital, University College
Dublin, Ireland
Currently Consultant Medical Physicist to
various hospitals and veterinary hospitals
in Ireland

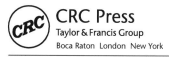

CRC Press
Taylor & Francis Group
Boca Raton London New York

CRC Press is an imprint of the
Taylor & Francis Group, an **informa** business

First published 2009 by Hodder Arnold

Published 2021 by CRC Press
Taylor & Francis Group
6000 Broken Sound Parkway NW, Suite 300
Boca Raton, FL 33487-2742

ISBN 13: 978-0-340-94167-6 (pbk)

**Visit the Taylor & Francis Web site at
http://www.taylorandfrancis.com**

**and the CRC Press Web site at
http://www.crcpress.com**

British Library Cataloguing in Publication Data
A catalogue record for this book is available from the British Library

Library of Congress Cataloging-in-Publication Data
A catalog record for this book is available from the Library of Congress

Cover Design: Helen Townson

Typeset on Boton Light 8/11 by
Macmillan Publishing Solutions

Dedication

... to George Weston and Roland Phillip who rest in a Flanders field;
may Oliver and Leo perhaps understand ...

Contents

Contents

Preface

The *Radiological Sciences Dictionary* is meant as an easy reference book for all hospital staff employed in diagnostic imaging, including established radiologists, nuclear medicine physicians, doctors in training, physicists, radiographers and technicians. Having understood the basic meaning and application of any particular keyword, then wider knowledge should be gained by consulting specialist books. Keywords in the book are linked so that a particular topic can be followed by reference to all relevant keywords. This is designed to aid revision and also act as a guide when exploring a particular subject. In many instances, keywords are further defined by showing worked examples. A particular word may be associated with a given topic (e.g. mammography, digital image filtering, radiation dose measurement, etc.). Relevant words are then either in smaller sans serif font when used in the descriptive text or identified at the end of the word's description. The author has attempted to add brief details of clinicians and scientists (alive and dead) who have, over the years, made significant contributions to diagnostic imaging. Apologies are given for unintended omissions.

Since new words are regularly being applied to the radiological sciences, recommendations and suggested additions would be gratefully received by the publishers. Errors may have made their appearance and the publishers would also welcome corrections and constructive comments. All material used will be recognized in future editions of the dictionary.

DJD
October 2008

Disclaimer: Drugs, contrast media, radiopharmaceuticals and other compounds for human use, identified in this dictionary, may not be recognized by individual countries. Relevant national drug administrations and organizations should be consulted.

Acknowledgements

When compiling this dictionary, I had many discussions with experts in the various disciplines. Amongst the doctors and scientists I wish to thank for their useful comments and advice are Greg Foley, Cari Borràs, Roger Price, Ng Kwan Hoong and Sarah Walker. I am indebted to Susie Bond and Alyson Thomas for their help and advice when editing the manuscript.

List of abbreviations

ABC	automatic brightness control	FOV	field of view
ac	alternating current	FPF	false positive fraction
ACPI	advanced configuration and power interface	FS	focal spot
		FSE	fast-spin echo
ADA	alternated delay acquisition	GFR	glomerular filtration rate
ADC	apparent diffusion coefficient; analogue to digital converter	GI	gastrointestinal
		Gy	gray
ADRF	adiabatic demagnetization in the rotating frame	HSE	Health and Safety Executive
		HU	heat unit
ADSL	asymmetric digital subscriber line	IAEA	International Atomic Energy Authority
AFP	adiabatic fast passage	IEC	International Electrotechnical Commission
AGP	accelerated or advanced graphics port		
AIUM	American Institute of Ultrasound in Medicine	IFD	image file directory
		IR	infrared
ALARA	as low as reasonably achievable	ITLC	instant thin layer chromatography
ALARP	as low as reasonably practical	IVC	intravenous cholangiography
ALI	annual limit on intake	IVC	inferior vena cava
API	application program interface	kW	kilowatt
ARP	adiabatic rapid passage	LAR	lifetime attributable risk
ASA	American Standards Association	LLE	loss of life expectancy
ASCII	American Standard Code for Information Interchange	LOR	line of response
		LUT	look up table
ASIS	aromatic solvent-induced shift	MB	megabyte
ATM	asynchronous transfer mode	MiB	mebibyte
BBB	blood–brain barrier	MIP	maximum intensity projection
BGO	bismuth germanate	MIRD	medical internal radiation dose
Bq	becquerel	MP	magnetization preparation
CBF	cerebral blood flow	MRA	magnetic resonance angiography
CFOV	central field of view	MRCP	magnetic resonance cholangiopancreaticography
Ci	curie		
CIN	contrast-induced nephropathy	ms	milliseconds
COM	component object model	MSA	multiple system atrophy
CPU	central processor unit	MTF	modulation transfer function
CR	computed radiography	NEMA	National Electrical Manufacturers Association
CSI	chemical shift imaging		
CT	computed tomography	NIC	network interface card
dB	decibels	NIST	National Institute of Standards and Technology
DGC	depth gain compensation		
DPFGSE	double pulsed field gradient spin-echo	NMR	nuclear magnetic resonance
DVT	deep vein thrombosis	NRPB	National Radiological Protection Board
ECRP	endoscopic retrograde cholangiopancreatography	ns	nanoseconds
		OD	optical density
EDTMP	ethylene-diamine-tetramethylene-phosphonate	OFD	object-to-film distance
		OLE	object linking and embedding
EIDE	enhanced integrated drive electronics	OTR	osmotoxicity ratio
ELR	excess lifetime risk	PD	Parkinson's disease
emf	electromotive force	PDA	personal digital assistants
ERC	endoscopic retrograde cholangiography	PDF	probability density function
FDA	Food and Drug Administration	POP	Post Office protocol
FFD	focus-to-film distance	PRP	pulse repetition period

PSP	progressive supranuclear palsy	SNR	signal-to-noise ratio
PTC	percutaneous transhepatic cholangiography	SPECT	single photon emission computed tomography
Rad	radians	SPGR	spoiled gradient recalled
RBC	red blood cells	SPT	selective population transfer
RBE	relative biological effectiveness	SPTA	spatial peak time averaged intensity
RCP	radiochemical purity	SSR	surface-shaded reconstructions
REID	risk of exposure-induced death	STP	standard temperature and pressure; shielded twisted pair
RF	radiofrequency		
RMS	root mean square	Sv	sievert
ROC	receiver operating characteristic	SVC	superior vena cava
ROI	region of interest	SVS	single volume spectroscopy
RPTL	reverse phase thin layer chromatography	TA	Time-averaged power
SAR	specific absorption rate	TAD	time of analogue to digital conversion
SCLC	small cell lung cancer	TGC	time gain compensation
SCSI	small computer systems interface	TMS	tetramethylsilane
SDP	slice dose profile	TPF	true positive fraction
SID	source to image distance	TSE	turbo-spin echo

Number prefix

2D display (*ct*) Visual display of a 2D distribution, e.g. the reconstructed axial image of a computed tomography (CT) scan displaying CT values as grey-scale information.

3D display (*ct*) Visual display of a 3D distribution by combining 2D axial slice data. Various methods such as shading, movement or perspective are used to create a subjective 3D impression.

2D-FFT (*mri*) Two-dimensional fast Fourier transform (FT). The standard image reconstruction for the axial plane from the phase and frequency encoding data using a fast Fourier Transform.

2π-geometry (*phys*) The geometrical efficiency of a flat surface detector (gamma camera).

3D-FFT (*mri*) The 2D-FFT can be extended to a 3D sequence by exciting the whole sample volume without using a slice gradient.

3D-MPRAGE (*mri*) 3D magnetization prepared rapid gradient echo. T1-weighted contrast from Siemens (*see* FLASF, SPGR, FSPGR, HFGR, RE spoiled, T1-FEE, STAGE-T1W).

3D GRE (*mri*) 3D gradient echo.

3D MP (*mri*) 3D magnetization prepared rapid.

3D slab (*mri*) Measurement MR volume for 3D imaging. The 3D slab is divided into partitions.

3D imaging (*mri*) An entire measurement volume using the 3D slab instead of single slices. Additional phase encoding in the *z*-axis (slice) direction provides information.

3-Phase supply (*phys*) The distributed a.c. power supply having three phases separated by 120°. The 3-phase European voltage is 440 V the US voltage 230 V. Equipment with high electrical rating (CT, MRI and most fixed x-ray generators).

3D shim (*mri*) Limits the local shim defining a 3D volume. The local magnetic field distribution is then determined in this volume. More precise than MAP shim providing better fat saturation and more precise spectroscopy.

3D Turbo SE (*mri*) TurboSE as a 3D sequence gives T2-weighted images with thin slices and almost isotropic voxels.

4π-geometry (*phys*) The geometrical efficiency of a spherical detector (*see* dose calibrator).

10BASE-T (*comp*) The IEEE 802.3I standard specification for 10-Mb ethernet transmission over UTP wiring using a star configuration with a hub at the centre (*see* 100BASE-T).

10BASE2 (*clin*) An IEEE 802.3 media standard for a 10 Mbits per second baseband, 185 m per segment ethernet LAN.

10BASE5 (*clin*) An IEEE 802.3 media standard for a 10 Mbits per second baseband, 500 m per segment ethernet LAN.

10-day rule (*dose*) An early recommendation from the ICRP for examinations involving the lower abdomen of females. Radiation exposure is least likely to pose any hazard to a developing embryo if carried out during the 10-day interval following onset of menstruation.

28-day rule (*dose*) Patients should be routinely asked if there is any chance they may be pregnant. If the answer is 'No', the radiological examination can proceed; if there is any uncertainty, the clinician or technologist is asked to check the date of the last menstrual period. If this is overdue, the examination should be delayed. This is the so-called '28-day rule'.

64-bit architecture (*comp*) This enables 64-bit computing on server, workstation, desktop and mobile platforms when combined with supporting software. Improves performance by allowing systems to address more than 4 GB (gigabytes) of both virtual memory and physical memory. Currently most processors for server and workstation platforms support 64-bit computing. With the introduction of dual core processors, most desktop and workstation processors are also 64-bit capable and provide 64-bit support for:

- address space;
- general purpose registers;
- integer size.

They also allow up to one terabyte (TB) of address space, AMD multi-core Opteron® and Athlon® 64 processors are currently available (*see* Pentium).

100BASE-T (*comp*) The IEEE 802.3u standard Ethernet specification for 100 Mbps (fast ethernet) transmission using UTP cable (*see* 10BASE-T).

100BseOT (*comp*) Also called fast ethernet, it is a 100 Mbps (megabits per second) baseband network standard. It supports different types of cabling: 100BaseTX uses twisted pair, while 100BaseFX uses fibreoptics.

180° interpolation (*ct*) A type of algorithm for z-axis interpolation which utilizes a range of $2 \times 180°$ projection angles within the measured spiral CT data (*see* z-interpolation).

360° interpolation (*ct*) A type of algorithm for z-axis interpolation which utilizes a range of $2 \times 360°$ projection angles within the measured spiral CT data (*see* z-interpolation).

510k (*legis*) *See* FDA 510k.

A

A2 (*stats*) The area under an ROC (receiver operating characteristic) curve, often used as an index of detectability or diagnostic accuracy. Strictly, A2 refers only to ROCs with binormal form, but occasionally it is used more loosely to indicate the area under any ROC curve. Perfect A2 = 1.0 and random decisions correspond to A2 = 0.5.

A_z (*stats*) The area under an ROC curve, useful as an index of detectability or diagnostic accuracy. Strictly, this refers only to ROC curves with binormal distribution (*see* **binormal ROC curve**, but more loosely can describe the area under any ROC curve. Values of A_z and the index d_a are related by the expression $A_z = \Phi(da/\sqrt{2})$, where Φ represents the cumulative standard-normal distribution function. For perfect detection $A_z = 1.0$ and for purely random decisions $A_z = 0.5$. A_z can be used as the value indicating a test **sensitivity** for a certain **specificity** ranging from 0 to 1, or, as the value of *t* specificity for a certain sensitivity ranging from 0 to 1.

A-mode (*us*) A display that gives echo strength versus time of arrival (distance). A display presentation of echo amplitude versus depth (used in ophthalmology).

ABC (*xray*) Automatic brightness control (*see* **automatic exposure control**).

α/β ratio (*dose*) The radiation dose at which the linear and quadratic components of cell killing are equal; a measure of the cell survival curve and a measure of sensitivity of a tissue or tumour to fractional radiation doses.

abdominal aortography (*clin*) Radiography of the abdominal aorta including its major branches from the diaphragm to the bifurcation. The pelvic arteries are often investigated at the same time (*see* **percutaneous abdominal aortography**).

abscissa (*math*) The horizontal *x*-axis of a graph usually holding the **independent variable**. The vertical or *y*- co-ordinate is called the ordinate.

absorbed dose (D) (*dose*) The definition given by ICRP60 is the mean energy $\bar{\varepsilon}$ imparted by ionizing radiation to matter (e.g. the body) of mass *m* in a finite volume *V*. The fundamental dose quantity given by

$$D = \frac{d\bar{\varepsilon}}{dm}$$

where $d\bar{\varepsilon}$ is the mean energy imparted by ionizing radiation to the matter in a volume

element of mass d*m*. The SI unit for absorbed dose is joule per kilogram ($J\,kg^{-1}$) and it is termed gray (Gy). The earlier definition referred to a point dose, but the ICRP60 revised definition is the average dose over the tissue volume. Conversion factor: The gray is equivalent to 100 rads; 1 rad is equivalent to 10 mGy.

absorbed fraction (*dose*) The fraction of any given radiation absorbed by a target. Used in the MIRD (medical internal radiation dose) scheme.

absorption (*phys*) The complete loss of energy in an absorbing material (*chem*) incorporated within a substance (liquid or solid) (*see* **adsorption, accretion**).

absorption coefficient (*phys*) (*see* **linear absorption coefficient**).

absorption mode (*mri*) Component of the signal that yields a symmetric, positive-valued line shape.

abundance (nuclear) (*chem*) The ratio of the number of atoms of a specific nuclide to the total number of atoms of all the natural nuclides present (sometimes expressed as a percentage). Hydrogen is a mixture of two isotopes ^{1}H (99.9852% abundant) and **deuterium** ^{2}H (0.0148% abundant); both are stable. **Potassium** has three naturally occurring isotopes: two stable ^{39}K (93.1%) and ^{41}K (6.88%) and the unstable, but long-lived, isotope ^{40}K (~0.08% abundant). (*nmed*) The fractional abundance of gamma photons actually emitted (maximum 1000) depends on a variety of secondary reactions; internal conversion being the most important.

ac (alternating current) (*phys*) An electrical power supply where magnitude of the electromotive force (emf) and current varies with time (alternates with time). A complete alternation being a cycle and the number of cycles per second (hertz) is the frequency. European frequency is 50 Hz, North America is 60 Hz. High frequency x-ray generators operate at 5–20 kHz (*see* **emf, generator**).

acceleration (angular) (α) (*phys*) Acceleration (angular) is the rate of change in angular velocity; related to **acceleration (linear)** (*a*) by $\alpha = a/r$. It is a vector quantity and has dimensions of T^{-2} given in units of degree s^{-2}, revolutions s^{-2} or rad s^{-2}.

acceleration (linear) (*phys*) Rate of change in velocity with respect to time. Acceleration (*a*) is measured in metres per second per second and is a vector quantity, where *a* = velocity

A

change/time taken. This is relevant to anode construction design; a smaller mass anode will reach operating speed faster (*see* momentum, velocity (linear)).

acceleration factor (*mri*) A factor by which faster imaging pulse sequences, such as multiple echo imaging, reduce total imaging time compared to conventional imaging sequences, such as spin echo imaging.

accelerator (*nmed*) A device that accelerates charged particles (e.g. protons, electrons) to high speed in order to produce ionization or nuclear reactions in a target; often used for the production of certain radionuclides or directly for radiation therapy. The cyclotron and the linear accelerator (LINAC) are types of accelerators.

ACCESS* (*comp*) A database program package supplied by Microsoft.

access time (*comp*) Time taken for a device to access data. Quoted in milliseconds (ms) for hard disks and nanoseconds (ns) for memory. The timing is usually an average value. Together with transfer rate, it measures the performance of hard disks.

accretion (*chem*) A surface reaction where a chemical compound unites with a surface (bone scan agent on bone surface) and does not penetrate further, so can be detached.

accuracy (*math*) Description of how a series of measured values is close to the true value. The closeness of a measured value, m, of a quantity to the true value, t. Measured as the percentage of the difference as $(m - t)/t \times 100$ and given as a percentage error.

Accuracy
Repeated dose readings from a calibrated source of 110.8 MBq give measured activities of 100.8, 100.3, 99.6, 100.1, 100.8 MBq. The average measured activity is therefore 100.3 MBq; the percentage error is then $(110.8 - 100.3)/110.8 = 9.4\%$ (an accuracy of 90.6%).

Precision does not necessarily imply accuracy since if a true reading of exactly 5.0 is measured giving a series of very high precision readings of 4.9876, 4.8631 and 5.2144, then the result, though precise, is nonetheless very inaccurate. A less precise measurement which returns: 5.0, 5.0 and 5.0 may be less precise but very accurate. (*see* diagnostic accuracy, quality control).

acetrizoic acid/acetrizoate (derivatives) (*cm*) The first water-soluble x-ray contrast medium based on triiodinated benzoic acid as 3-(acetyl-amino-2,4,6, triiodobenzoic acid. Salts: sodium or meglumine acetrizoate (*see* Urokon).

achromatic (*image*) Without colour (*see* colour scale).

acoustic absorption (*us*) The loss of sound energy by attenuation and scatter.

acoustic absorption coefficient (α_a (*us*) The overall attenuation coefficient $\alpha = \alpha_a + \alpha_s$ (the sum of absorption and scatter coefficients); the units are either m^{-1} or cm^{-1}. Also called intensity absorption coefficient. The absorption coefficient varies with frequency. The frequency where absorption is maximum is called the relaxation frequency.

acoustic amplitude (*us*) This is measured from the zero (crossover) point of the sine-wave to its peak in mV or μV.

acoustic frequency (*f*) (*us*) The compression and rarefaction events translated as a sine wave whose frequency range is 2.5–15 MHz in clinical ultrasound.

acoustic impedance (*Z*) (*us*) The product of material density and speed of sound in a medium. The unit is $kg\ m^{-2}\ s^{-1}$, also termed the rayl, and is usually calculated as:

$$Z = \rho c = \sqrt{\frac{\rho}{\kappa}}$$

where κ is compressibility ρ the material density and c the speed of sound in the medium. Some values are:

Material ($\times 10^{-6}$)	Speed of sound (m s^{-1})	α (dB cm^{-1}) at 1 MHz	Z (kg m^{-2} s^{-1})
Air	330		0.0043
Water	1492	0.002	1.48
Fat	1470	0.6	1.38
Blood	1570	0.18	1.61
Brain	1530	0.85	1.55
Soft tissue	1500	1.0	1.63
Liver	1549	0.9	1.65
Muscle	1560	1.2	1.65
Eye lens	1620	2.0	1.85
Bone	4080	20.0	6.1

(*see* compressibility).

acoustic intensity (*us*) The power per unit area as W or mW cm^{-2}.

acoustic noise (*mri*) Gradient coil vibrations creating sound waves. Caused by the interactions of the pulsed magnetic field of the gradient coil with the main magnetic field. (*us*) Sound pressure registered on a logarithmic scale as sound-pressure level in decibels (dB).

acoustic output (limits) (*us*) The Food and Drug Administration (FDA) (1976) recommended the following acoustic power limits:

Value	Heart	Opth	Fetus
I_{SPPA} (Wcm^{-2})	190	28	190
I_{SPTP} (Wcm^{-2})	310	50	310
I_{SPTA} (mWcm^{-2})	430	17	94
I_{SATA} (mWcm^{-2})	430	17	94

(*see* ultrasound intensity (pulsed)).

acoustic parameters (*us*) Pressure density, temperature, impedance.

acoustic power (*us*) The sound energy transferred per unit time through the whole cross section of the beam; measured in watts m^{-2}. Time averaged power (*TA*) equals:

$$\frac{\text{Total power per frame}}{\text{Frame duration}}$$

Potential maximum practical values:

Display mode	TA (mW)	I_{SPTA} (mWcm^{-2})
B-mode	350	1000
M-mode	350	>1000
Duplex (pulsed Doppler)	>400	>1000
CW Doppler	25–90	20–600

The spatial peak time averaged intensity (I_{SPTA}) is the time-averaged power relating peak power to pulse width and duty factor (*see* ultrasound intensity (pulsed)).

acoustic pressure (*p*) (*us*) The value of the total pressure minus the ambient pressure. The pressure difference from normal pressure induced by sound wave. Unit is the **pascal**; $1\,Pa = 1\,Nm^{-2}$ or bars, where $1\,Pa = 10\,\mu bar$; a typical range is 0.06–1.5 Mpa.

acoustic reflection coefficient (*R*) (*us*) If the incident radiation is perpendicular to the surface then:

$$R = \frac{I_r}{I_i} = \left(\frac{(Z_2 - Z_1)}{(Z_1 + Z_2)}\right)^2$$

If the incident radiation is angled (angle of incidence and **angle of reflection** <90°) then the acoustic reflection coefficient is dependent on the angle of incidence:

$$R = \left(\frac{Z_2 \cdot \cos\theta_i - Z_1 \cdot \cos\theta_t}{Z_2 \cdot \cos\theta_i + Z_1 \cdot \cos\theta_t}\right)^2$$

acoustic transmission coefficient (*T*) (*us*) The unreflected ultrasound beam passes as a transmitted beam. The efficiency of transmission of the incident beam at right angles to a smooth surface:

$$T = \frac{I_t}{I_i} = \frac{4Z_1 \cdot Z_2}{(Z_1 + Z_2)^2}$$

It is related to the reflection coefficient as: $T = (1 - R)$.

acoustic variables (*us*) These include pressure, density, temperature and particle motion; the quantities that vary with location and time in a sound wave.

ACPI (*comp*) Advanced configuration and power interface. The latest standard that specifies how computer power can be efficiently managed. Features include activating devices only when required and reducing clock speed when full processing power is not needed.

acquisition matrix (*image*) The number of independent data samples in each direction. For symmetric sampling, will roughly equal the ratio of image field of view to **spatial resolution** along corresponding directions (depending on filtering and other processing). May be asymmetric and of different size than the size of the reconstructed image or display matrix. (*mri*) The number of independent data samples in the **phase-encoding** and **frequency-encoding** directions.

acquisition time (*A*) (*mri*) The time taken to acquire image frame using the **spin echo sequence**. Depends on:

* number of **phase encoding** steps *M* (matching the matrix size);
* signal averaging *N* (usually two but can be greater);
* time to repeat, *TR*.

$$A = M \times N \times TR$$

for a 256 × 256 matrix *M* = 256, so for a signal averaging of 2 and *TR* = 500 ms, the acquisition time is 4.2 minutes.

acquisition window (*mri*) Time in pulse sequence during which the signal is recorded. This is sometimes called the TAD (time of analogue to digital conversion).

actinides/actinoids (*elem*) The group of elements in the periodic table in the atomic number range 90 (thorium) to 103 (lawrencium). It includes elements useful to radiology,

A

such as: 92 (uranium), 95 (americium) and 98 (californium).

Z	Element
89	Actinium
90	Thorium
91	Protactinium
92	Uranium
93	Neptunium
94	Plutonium
95	Americium
96	Curium
97	Berkelium
98	Californium
99–103	

activation analysis (*phys*) A method of chemical analysis used for the detection of very small concentrations of elements in a sample. Following nuclear (neutron) bombardment, certain atoms are rendered radioactive and may be detected by their characteristic gamma radiation (peaks).

active shielding (*mri*) Magnetic shielding through the use of secondary shielding coils designed to produce a magnetic field that cancels the field from primary coils in regions where it is not desired. These coils may be inside the magnet cryostat. Can be applied to the main magnet or to the gradient magnetic fields. This also applies to the gradient field system using counterwound coils to reduce eddy currents (*see* magnetic shielding, self-shielding and room shielding).

active shimming (*mri*) Shimming or adjusting the homogeneity of the main magnet by varying the currents in shim coils.

active transport (*nmed*) Passage of an agent (radiopharmaceutical) across a cell membrane by being incorporated into an energy dependent metabolic process (iodine uptake in the thyroid, ^{99m}Tc uptake in salivary glands) (*see* passive transport).

ActiveX (*comp*) A set of interactive technologies developed by Microsoft, combining OLE (object linking and embedding) and COM (component object model). Unlike Java, ActiveX is not a programming language, but a set of instructions on how an object should be used.

activity (*dose*) Average number of spontaneous nuclear transformations per unit time. Measured as the becquerel (Bq) in disintegrations per second or one radioactive transformation per second ($1\,s^{-1}$ or one disintegration per second) (ICRP60). The non-SI unit is the curie (Ci) where

1 Ci	3.7×10^{10} Bq	37 GBq
1 mCi	3.7×10^{7} Bq	37 MBq
1 μCi	3.7×10^{5} Bq	37 kBq
1 nCi	3.7×10^{2} Bq	370 Bq
1 Bq	2.703×10^{-11} Ci	27.03 pCi
1 kBq	2.703×10^{-8} Ci	27.03 nCi
1 MBq	2.703×10^{-5} Ci	27.03 μCi
1 GBq	2.703×10^{-2} Ci	27.03 mCi
1 TBq	2.703×10^{1} Ci	27.03 Ci

activity concentration (*unit*) Measured in $Bq\,m^{-3}$. A conversion factor exists for non-SI units where $1\,Ci\,L-1 = 3.7 \times 10^{13}\,Bq\,m^{-3}$.

activity-time curve (*nmed*) The plot of activity per unit time obtained from a region of interest (ROI) for a set of dynamic frames.

AcuTect* (*nmed*) Commercial preparation of apcitide (Diatide Inc).

Acutest* (*nmed*) *See* apcitide.

ADA (*mri*) Alternated delay acquisition.

adapter (*comp*) The device that connects a piece of equipment to the network and controls the electrical protocol for communication with that network; also called network interface card (NIC).

adaptive array (*ct*) Commercial detector array; those with detector elements of unequal width (the adaptive array detector), a major drawback with the adaptive array design. Narrow detector elements are close to the centre; the width of the detector rows increases with distance from the centre. The adaptive design avoids dead spaces; with the prepatient collimator a typical slice combination would be: $2 \times 0.5\,mm$, $4 \times 1\,mm$, $4 \times 2.5\,mm$, $4 \times 5\,mm$, $2 \times 8\,mm$ and $2 \times 10\,mm$.

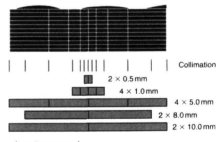

(*see* linear array).

adaptive response (*dose*) A cellular response to radiation which increases the resistance of the cell to a subsequent radiation exposure.

adaptive technology (*comp*) An Intel technology (supported in adapters and switches) that automatically and dynamically customises product performance to match network-operating conditions, thus helping to optimize network performance.

ADC (A to D conversion) (*di*) *See* analogue to digital converter.

A to D conversion (*ct*) *See* analogue-to-digital converter.

ADC map (*mri*) Apparent diffusion coefficient. Images are acquired with two or more b-values. Using equation $e^{-(bD)}$ then D is computed for each point in the image to give the ADC map, which removes artefacts in a T2-weighted image called 'T2 shine through' an emphasis which can obscure the diffusion image.

Adenoscan (*nmed*) A cardioactive drug manufactured for use as an adjunct to ^{201}Thallium myocardial perfusion scintigraphy. Its effective half-life is about 10 s.

added filtration (*ct*) Thin metal sheets (commonly aluminium or copper) used for increasing the filtration of the x-ray spectrum emitted by the x-ray source in addition to the intrinsic filtration.

adiabatic change (*phys*) Expansion or compression of a gas where no heat enters or leaves the system. Adiabatic expansion therefore cools the gas and is used as a method for gas liquefaction (helium recycling in superconducting magnets) (*see* cryogen).

adiabatic fast passage (AFP) (*mri*) Rotation of the macroscopic magnetization vector by sweeping the frequency of the radiofrequency (RF) pulse or strength of the magnetic field through resonance (Larmor frequency) in a time period which is short compared to the relaxation times. Used for spin inversion.

adiabatic rapid passage (*mri*) *See* adiabatic fast passage.

adrenal arteriography (*clin*) Selective injection of the adrenal arteries with iodine contrast material. Complete demonstration of both adrenal glands usually requires selection of the three supplying arteries on each side: the superior adrenal arteries, the middle adrenal arteries and the inferior adrenal arteries.

adrenal venography (*clin*) Radiography using selective retrograde injection of contrast material into the adrenal vein.

ADRF (*mri*) Adiabatic demagnetization in the rotating frame.

ADSL (*comp*) Asymmetric digital subscriber line. Generally referred to as DSL. Use standard telephone lines and narrow frequency bands achieving 8 Mbps for ADSL version 2+ at distances 4 km from the server.

adsorption (*phys*) The taking up of a substance on the surface of another (*see* absorption).

adverse reactions (contrast medium) (*cm*) Ionic contrast materials associated with adverse reactions in patients. Most of these reactions are mild and include sneezing, coughing, rhinitis, conjunctival edema, mild urticaria, pruritus, vomiting and light-headedness. Severe reactions occur in approximately 1 of 500 injections of ionic contrast medium. The death rate associated with ionic contrast material injection ranges from 1 in 40 000 to 1 in 100 000 injections (*see* toxicity).

■ Reference: Dawson and Clauss, 1999.

aerosol (*nmed*) An air suspension of particulate material ranging in size from 0.2 to 2.0 μm median diameter. When labelled with a radionuclide, it is used as a gas substitute in lung ventilation scintigraphy (*see* Technegas®).

a.f. (*phys*) *See* audio frequency.

a.f.c. (*phys*) *See* automatic frequency control.

AFP (*mri*) *See* adiabatic fast passage.

afterglow (*xray*) Prolonged emission of light, a feature of phosphorescence, but a degrading feature in fluorescent phosphors (detectors and intensifying screens). (*ct*) Temporal signal decay after a short radiation pulse. The sintered ceramic composite phosphor used in ceramic detectors, chosen for multislice detectors have a rapid decay time of 10^6 s. Luminescence afterglow should be <0.1% at 100 ms after x-ray cessation; too high a value results in image blurring.

a.g.c. (*us*) *See* automatic gain control.

aggregate (*stats*) The value of a single variable resulting from the combination of data for a number of variables.

AGP (*comp*) Accelerated or advanced graphics port. Most computers are provided with a number of PCI slots for adding external hardware. The AGP slot will, however, award special priority, particularly video-processing speed. An extremely fast expansion slot and bus design for high performance graphics cards. Provides hardware functions for two-dimensional and three-dimensional so the host central processor unit (CPU) has less involvement with image production. 2 × AGP has peak transfer rates of 512 MBytes/s and 4 × AGP supplies 1.1 GBps (*see* graphics card).

agreement state (USA) (*nmed*) any state which the US Nuclear Regulatory Commission or the Atomic Energy Commission has concluded an effective agreement under Section 247b of the Atomic Energy Act of 1954.

air (*material*)

Effective atomic number (Z_{eff})	7.78
Density (ρ) kg/m³	1.293 kg/m³

In addition to water vapour, the composition of air at sea level is:

Gas	Percentage
Nitrogen	78.08
Oxygen	20.95
Argon	0.93
Carbon dioxide	0.03
Neon	0.0018
Helium	0.0005
Krypton	0.0001
Xenon	0.00001

air gap (*xray*) A technique which maintains a gap between subject (patient) and image surface (film cassette). This reduces scattered radiation reaching the film surface, but increases geometrical unsharpness.

air-kerma (*dose*) The energy released from all ionizing events in a volume of air. The unit is $C\,kg^{-1}$ or Gy. The quotient of dE/dm, where dE is the sum of the initial kinetic energies of all the charge particles produced by the ionizing event in a mass of air dm. The quotient of dE_{tr}/dm, where dE_{tr} is the sum of initial kinetic energies of all the charged ionizing particles liberated by uncharged ionizing particles in a mass of air dm (ICRU, 1980). Examples of typical air kerma rates are:

90 kV x-rays at 1 m	43–52 μGy mA s^{-1}
28 kV x-rays	90 μGy mA s^{-1}
Nuclear medicine patient at 1 m (bone scintigram)	16 μGy × h^{-1}

(*see* kerma, absorbed dose).

air scan (*ct*) Test procedure with no object in the gantry; used for checking uniformity in detector channel sensitivities and also providing basic data set for calibrating the detectors.

ALARA (*dose*) As low as reasonably achievable. Making every reasonable effort to reduce radiation levels below the stated dose limits, to give adequate safety and appropriate diagnostic accuracy at reasonable cost and recognizing social factors. (*us*) For diagnostic ultrasound, combinations of thermal or mechanical indices and dwell times are considered optimum combination of acoustic output and dwell time, needed to achieve the required diagnostic information (*see* ultrasound safety, optimization).

ALARP (*dose*) As low as reasonably practical. The limiting factor being existing facilities due for update or replacement (unofficial term).

albumin (*nmed*) Serum albumin constitutes 55% of blood plasma. Soluble in water but forms insoluble coagulate when heated.

Generic name	^{125}I-RISA
Commercial names	Isojex®
Nonimaging category	Plasma volume
Generic name	^{99m}Tc-HAS
	^{99m}Tc-MAA
Commercial names	LyoMAA⁻
Imaging category	Blood pool

Albumoscint[a] (*nmed*) Bristol Myers Squibb version of **albumin** for labelling.

algebraic reconstruction (*di, ct*) Historically the oldest image reconstruction method based on data cells with scanning movements in a finite number of equally spaced angles. An iterative image reconstruction cycle corrects horizontal, diagonal and vertical estimates (*see* back projection).

algorithm (*stats*) A set of well-defined rules or statements as a result of a systems analysis forming the plan for a computer program.

ALI (*dose*) *See* Annual limit on intake.

aliasing (*di*) An artefact resulting from the violation of Shannon's equations requirements; signal contributions with higher frequencies may affect the frequency range below the Nyquist frequency in the form of aliasing artefacts. The recorded signal will appear to be at a lower frequency. The diagram shows three sampling rates (A) exceeds the Nyquist frequency, (B) is at the Nyquist frequency and (C) is sampled below the Nyquist frequency which shows aliasing.

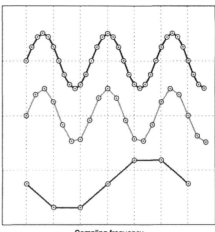

Sampling frequency

aliasing artefact (*ct*) An artefact resulting from the violation of Shannon's sampling theorem requirements; signal contributions with higher frequencies may affect the frequency range below the Nyquist frequency in the form of aliasing artefacts in the computed tomography (CT) axial image. The display artefact due to aliasing within the measured projections; appears in the reconstructed images as fine streaks and web-like patterns. There is a loss of fine detail (petrous bone) in CT images. (*mri*) Seen when the measurement object is outside the field of view (FOV), but still within the sensitive volume of the main coil. The consequence of sampling in which any components of the signal that are at a higher frequency than the Nyquist limit will be 'folded' in the spectrum so that they appear to be at a lower frequency. In Fourier transform imaging this can produce an apparent wrapping around to the opposite side of the image of a portion of the object that extends beyond the edge of the reconstructed region. (*us*) In spectral and pulsed Doppler, determines upper limit of Doppler signal frequencies. False Doppler shift information from a pulsed-Doppler or colour-flow instrument when true Doppler shift exceeds half the pulse repetition frequency.

alkali metals (*elem*) Elements of group 1 in the periodic table: lithium, sodium, potassium, rubidium, caesium and francium. All are highly reactive.

Almén, Torsten Swedish radiologist who in 1968 developed non-ionic contrast media by replacing the ionic carboxyl radical in triiodinated benzoic acid derivatives. Metrizamide (Amipaque) was the first non-ionic contrast agent. Second generation products are iopamidol, iohexol and Hexabrix (ioxaglate).

alpha (α) (*phys*) Symbol used for absorption, alpha particle, angular acceleration.

alpha-decay (*nmed*) A process of radionuclide decay, where the nucleus loses two neutrons and two protons in the form of a helium nucleus:

$$^{A}_{Z}X \rightarrow ^{A-4}_{Z-2}Y + ^{4}_{2}\alpha$$

Example: $^{226}_{88}$Ra $\rightarrow$ $^{222}_{86}$Rn $+ ^{4}_{2}\alpha$ (4.78 MeV)

alpha particle (α) (*nmed*) At the moment of emission, an alpha particle consists of the nucleus of the helium atom $^{4}_{2}$He or ^{4}He^{2+} which is a tightly bound group of two protons and two neutrons. Alphas have a mass of 4 amu and a charge of 2. As an alpha particle slows down through matter, it acquires two orbital electrons to become a neutral atom of helium $^{4}_{2}$He$_{2}$. The alpha particle forms a charged beam in cyclotron reactions.

aluminium (Al) (*elem*)

Atomic number (Z)	13
Relative atomic mass (A$_r$)	26.98
Density (ρ) kg/m^3	2710
Melting point (K)	932
Specific heat capacity J kg^{-1} × K^{-1}	913
Thermal conductivity W m^{-1} × K^{-1}	237
K-edge (keV)	1.56
Relevance to radiology: Filter material for x-ray tube	

a.m. (*phys*) *See* modulation (amplitude).

AMBER (*xray*) A technique used in chest radiography which varies exposure to each part of the chest so that the image receives optimum photon density for both the lung fields and mediastinum. The AMBER system projects 21 adjacent collimated beams in a linear array backed by its own detector. Each segment of this horizontal array is modulated by the intensity reaching the detector; in the most radio-opaque area (mediastinum) receives the most exposure and the least radio-opaque area (intercostal lung) receives only 10% of the available intensity.

ambient dose equivalent (H × d) (*dose ICRU*) The dose equivalent d in a radiation point field that would be produced by expanded and aligned fields in the ICRU sphere at a depth of 10 mm on the radius vector opposing the direction of the aligned field. The unit of ambient dose equivalent is joule per kilogram (J kg^{-1}) and its unit is the sievert (Sv) (*see* directional dose equivalent.)

AMD * (*comp*) Advanced Micro Devices Inc.

^{241}**Americium (Am)** (*elem*) Used as a marker source in scintigraphy and also as a calibration source for laboratory instruments.

Atomic number (Z)	95
Relative atomic mass (A$_r$)	243
Density (ρ) kg/m^3	13670
Melting point (K)	1267
K-edge (keV)	–
Relevance to radiology: radionuclide ^{241}Am calibration source	

Production	$^{239}_{94}Pu\,(n,\gamma)^{240}_{94}Pu\,(n,\gamma)^{241}_{94}Pu \xrightarrow{\;\beta-\;} {}^{241}_{95}Am$
Decay scheme (α)	$^{241}Am\ T\tfrac{1}{2}$ 433 yr $(\alpha, \gamma$ 60 keV) $\to {}^{239}Pu\ T\tfrac{1}{2}$ v. long
Gamma constant	$4.2 \times 10^{-3} \cdot mSv \cdot h \cdot 1\,MBq^{-1}$ ray @ 1 m
Decay constant	$0.0016\ y^{-1}$

amidotrizoate (*cm*) Ionic monomer as medrizoate sodium amidotrizoate produced commercially as Gastrografin and Urografin.

Amipaque$^{×}$ (*cm*) A non-ionic extracellular fluid contrast medium as metrizamide introduced by Nycomed in 1977. Since it is unstable in solution, it requires reconstitution in water prior to use.

Compound	Viscosity (cP)	Osmolality (mOsm/kg)	Iodine (mg I mL^{-1})
Metrizamide	2.9 at 25, 1.8 at 37	272	170
Metrizamide	12.9 at 25, 6.2 at 37	480	300

Ampère, André Marie (1775–1836) French mathematician, chemist and physicist whose name is given to the SI base unit of electric current (ampere, amp).

ampere (A or amp) (*unit*) A measure of electrical current; defined as a constant current maintained in two parallel conductors under ideal conditions 1 metre apart, in a vacuum, producing a force between the conductors of $2 \times 10^{-7}\,Nm^{-1}$. One ampere or one coulomb per second represents 6.24×10^{18} electrons s^{-1}. Smaller currents are measured in milliamps (mA; $10^{-3}A$) and microamps (μA; $10^{-6}A$). X-ray tube current is measured in mA and x-ray exposure measured as the product mA × second (mAs) so: $1\,mAs = 1 \times 10^{-3}$ coulomb (1 millicoulomb; 1 mC).

ampere second (As) (*xray*) the unit used to describe the total electron flow through an x-ray tube. It is a measure of x-ray exposure usually expressed in terms of milliampere seconds or mAs. $1\,mAs = 1\,mC$ (10^{-3} coulomb).

amplification (*us*) The process by which small voltages are increased to larger ones using an amplifier.

amplifier (*xray*) An electronic circuit for either increasing signal amplitude (e.g. ultrasound echo) or signal charge (e.g. ionization chamber).

amplifier noise (*xray*) Electronic/thermal noise given by the components of an amplifier.

amplitude (*phys*) The peak height of a waveform measured from the crossover point (zero) to the peak which is commonly a sinusoid.

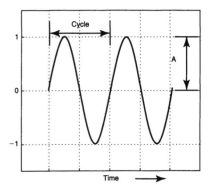

(*us*) Maximum variation of an acoustic variable or voltage (*see* a.c., RMS, sine wave).

amplitude modulation (a.m.) (*di*) Typically seen in a video signal where the carrier is VHF whose amplitude is varied in sympathy with the signal information.

amplitude resolution (*us*) The accuracy with which the smallest returning echo can be measured. Interference signals (noise) superimposed on these signals may be regarded as the limiting factor. In the near field accuracy is typically 0.0001% corresponding to 100 dB SNR at greater depths it reduces to 20 dB or 10% accuracy. (*xray*) *See* pulse height analyser.

analogue analog (*ct*) A signal type representing voltage, current or phase; the measured value of a physical quantity which can adopt arbitrary values within a certain continuous range. (*us*) The procedure or system where data are represented by proportional, continuously variable, physical quantities (varying voltage, current or phase).

analogue filter (*di*) A filter consisting of electronic components (resistors, capacitors or inductors) that can be tuned to accept or reject parts of an analogue signal.

analogue signal (*di*) Characterized by either a varying current or voltage, although frequency and phase can also be treated as analogue characteristics. Analogue signals are prone to both interference and distortion.

analogue to digital converter (ADC) (*comp*) An electronic device which samples the incoming analogue (voltage) waveform, converting the sampled amplitude to a binary value for subsequent computer processing. Conversion of an analogue input signal (usually voltage as varying amplitude) into a digital signal which can be processed by a digital computer.

analysis of variance (Anova) (*stats*) A technique for investigating how the variability in a set of measurements can be ascribed to different causes. A one way analysis of variance tests for the null hypothesis where all samples have been drawn from the same population. A two-way analysis of variance tests for two factors. Analysis of variance may also be applied to non-parametric ranked data.

anaphylactoid/idiosyncratic reactions (*cm*) Idiosyncratic reactions for contrast media are those that mimic anaphylactic responses. They range from mild, including hives and mild bronchospasm, to severe, including sudden death; proposed mechanisms include histamine release, complement cascade activation and direct central nervous system effects; these are not purely allergic reactions because no circulating IgG antibodies to contrast material can be isolated in patients with a history of idiosyncratic contrast material reaction. The most common severe anaphylactoid reactions associated with intravascular contrast media administration include tachycardia, hypotension and some element of bronchospasm. Lower incidence for non-ionic than ionic contrast media.

▪ Reference: Dawson and Clauss, 1999.

anechoic (*us*) Echo free. A region of the image that does not return echoes (e.g. large vessels).

Anger, Hal, O (1920–2005) US scientist who invented and developed a practical stationary-imaging device for nuclear medicine in 1958: the Anger or gamma camera.

angiocardiography (*clin*) Radiographic imaging of the great vessels and chambers of the heart immediately following rapid injection of contrast material. Anatomy and function of the heart chambers is revealed in left ventricular angiography together with right and left coronary angiography. Single plane or bi-plane cine-angiocardiography or real-time digital imaging equipment is used.

AngioCis (*nmed*) A commercial preparation for labelling red blood cells with ^{99m}Tc (CIS/Schering).

Angiografin (*cm*) Generic name for meglumine diatrizoate. Ionic contrast medium manufactured by Schering AG containing 65% meglumine diatrizoate.

Compound	Viscosity (cP)	Osmolality (mOsm/kg)	Iodine (mg I mL^{-1})
65% Meglumine-diatrizoate	9.3 at 20°, 5.0 at 37°;	1530	306

angiography (*clin*) X-ray examination of a blood vessel, usually done with injection of a contrast medium through a catheter inserted through an artery in the groin. Magnetic resonance angiography (MRA) uses the magnetization status or local velocity of the blood for imaging. Represents all vessels in the blood volume. Various views can be subsequently reconstructed (MIP) from three-dimensional data volumes (*see* digital subtraction angiography, DSA).

angioplasty (*clin*) Recanalization of a blood vessel using either balloon inflation or stent placement directed by fluoroscopic imaging. (*see* percutaneous transluminal angioplasty (PTA), percutaneous transluminal coronary angioplasty (PTCA)).

Angiovist282 (*cm*) Ionic x-ray contrast agent manufactured by Berlex Laboratories. The generic name is meglumine diatrizoate. Angiovist 292 has an increased iodine content with corresponding increase in osmolality and viscosity.

Compound	Viscosity (cP)	Osmolality (mOsm/kg)	Iodine (mg I mL^{-1})
Meglumine diatrizoate	6.1 at 25°, 4.1 at 37°	1400	282
Meglumine diatrizoate	5.9 at 25°, 4.0 at 37°	1500	292

angle of incidence (*us*) Angle between beam direction and the perpendicular axis.

angle of reflection (*us*) For non-perpendicular beams equals the angle of incidence (*see* reflection, Snell's law).

Angström, Anders Jonas (1814–74) Swedish physicist. The angstrom non-SI unit measures the wavelength of light.

angstrom (Å) (*unit*) Non-SI unit measuring wavelength; replaced by the SI unit, the nanometer $1nm = 10Å$.

angular acceleration (α) (*phys*) The rate of change in angular velocity; related to linear acceleration (a) where $\alpha = a/r$ or v^2/r.

angular displacement (θ) (*phys*) The angular change in angular motion defined as $\theta = x/r$ where x is the linear displacement and r the radius of angular motion. Since r (the radius) is fixed then $\theta \propto x$. Angular displacement is in radians (rad) where $360° = 2\pi$ rad and 1 rad $= 57.3° = 180°/\pi$ rad.

A

Angular parameters

Angle	θ (rad)
Angular velocity	ω (rad s^{-1})
Angular acceleration	α (rad s^{-2})
Moment of inertia	I
Torque	$\tau = I\alpha$
Angular momentum	$L = I\omega$
Work	$W = \tau\theta$
Power	$P = \tau\omega$
Kinetic energy	$\frac{1}{2}I\omega^2$

angular frequency (ω) (*mri*) Frequency of oscillation or rotation (radians s^{-1}). The symbol is ω so $\omega = 2\pi f$, where f is in Hz (*see* sine wave).

angular momentum (*phys*) A vector quantity given by the vector product of moment of inertia and angular velocity. This remains constant until an external force (torque) changes the direction of rotation causing precession. Atomic nuclei possess intrinsic angular momentum termed spin. (*mri*) In the absence of external forces, the angular momentum remains constant, with the result that any rotating body tends to maintain the same axis of rotation. In the presence of a torque applied to a rotating body in such a way as to change the direction of the rotation axis, the resulting change in angular momentum results in precession. All atomic nuclei with an odd number of nucleons possess an intrinsic angular momentum (spin) measured in multiples of Planck's constant. This is coupled with the magnetic dipole moment. Electrons and protons possess an intrinsic magnetic moment that is distinct from any 'orbital' motion, associated with and proportional to the 'spin' angular momentum of the particle.

The electron orbit of a hydrogen atom

The electron moves in a circular orbit at constant velocity. Given that the radius r of the orbit $= 0.5 \times 10^{-10}$m
Linear velocity of electron $= 2.2 \times 10^6$m s^{-1}
Since $\omega = v/r = 2.2 \times 10^6 / 0.5 \times 10^{-10}$
Angular velocity $\omega = 4.4 \times 10^{16}$rad s^{-1}
Angular acceleration $\alpha = v^2/r = 9.7 \times 10^{22}$m s^{-2} (or s^{-1}s^{-1})

Angular momentum of electron

Angular momentum (L) of orbiting electron in hydrogen atom, radius $r = 5.29 - 10^{-11}$m
Rest mass of electron m is 9.11×10^{-31}kg
Linear velocity $v = 2.2 \times 10^6$m s^{-1}
Angular momentum $L = mr^2\omega$, where ω is the angular velocity $= v/r = 4.4 \times 10^{16}$rad s^{-1} so angular momentum $= 1.054 \times 10^{-34}$kg m^{2}s^{-1}

angular sampling (*nmed*) The sampling interval for single photon emission computed tomography (SPECT) imaging.

angular velocity (ω) (*phys*) Circular motion defined from the angle through which the radius moves in radians per second (rad s^{-1}). Angular velocity is related to linear velocity v by $\omega = v/r$. For a constant speed the angular velocity (or frequency), ω, is the number of complete revolutions per second. One revolution is $2\pi r$, so angular velocity can be expressed as $\omega = 2\pi/t$ or $2\pi v$ rad s^{-1}; the time t to complete one revolution. (*mri*) The symbol ω_0 represents the angular frequency of precession.

The rotating anode of an x-ray tube.

For an anode rotating at constant angular velocity ω (or angular frequency) with radius (r) 100 mm (0.1 m), mass (m) 2.0 kg, rotating at 9000 revolutions per minute. Its angular velocity, moment of inertia, angular momentum and linear velocity are:
Angular velocity: $\omega = 9000 \times 2\pi \times 1/60 = 942.5$ rad s^{-1}
alternatively $\omega = v/r = 942.5$ rad s^{-1}
Moment of inertia: $I = \frac{1}{2}mr^2 = 0.01$kg m^2
Angular momentum: $L = I\omega = 9.425$ kg m^{2}s^{-1}
Linear velocity: $2\pi r \times$ (rpm/60)$= 94.25$ m s-1,
alternatively $v = \omega r = 942.5 \times 0.1$m $= 94.25$ m s^{-1}
(or just over 200 mph)

anisoplanasy (*xray, nmed*) Resolution varying over the image intensifier or gamma camera face.

anisotropic (*mri*) Describing a three-dimensional property of a material (crystal lattice, nerve pathways) or parameter (thermal, electrical conductivity) that varies in all directions (*see* diffusion tensor imaging).

annihilation event (*nmed*) Annihilation events are not always emitted at 180°, since the positron–electron pair is not completely at rest during annihilation. Such angular deviations may be of the order of 0.25° and can degrade the spatial resolution of the image.

annihilation radiation (*phys*) The electromagnetic radiation resulting from the mutual annihilation of two particles of opposite charge (positron and negatron or electron) giving two photons 180° opposed each of energy 511 keV (*see* positron).

annual limit on intake (ALI) (*dose*) The derived limit for amount of radioactive material taken in by the body (ingestion or inhalation) per year that would cause him/her to exceed the ICRP annual dose limit for a radiation worker. The ALI is the smaller value of intake of a given radionuclide in a year that would result in a committed effective dose equivalent currently set at 20 mSv per year. (ICRP 30 (Part 1)). Other legislation (10 CFR 20.1003.) states that the ALI is the smaller value of intake of a given radionuclide in a year by the reference man that would result in a committed effective dose equivalent to 5 rems (50 mSv) or a committed dose equivalent to 50 rems (0.5 Sv) to any individual organ or tissue. Some ALIs of isotopes in common use would be:

Nuclide	ALI (Bq)
^{32}P	3×10^7
^{51}Cr	7×10^8
^{99m}Tc	9×10^8
^{125}I	2×10^6
^{131}I	9×10^5

(*see* annual reference levels of intake (ARLI)).

annual reference levels of intake (ARLI) (*nmed*) The activity of a radionuclide that, taken into the body during a year, would provide a committed effective dose to a person represented by the reference man, equal to 20 mGy. The ARLI is expressed in becquerels (Bq).

annular array (*us*) The ultrasound transducers arranged in concentric circles.

anode (*xray*) The positive electrode of a thermionic device. Commonly applied to the x-ray tube (*see* compound anode).

anode angle (*xray*) Typically the focal track on the anode disk is at an angle to the impinging stream of electrons arriving from the cathode. It is angled with respect to the exit window that when viewed from the plane of the image in the direction of the central ray, the optically effective focal spot appears small and more or less square. In general, the smaller the anode angle, the wider the focal track which increases the loadability. Angle size also influences the field size at a given source to image distance (SID). Field size increases with anode angle as does the effective focal spot size which will degrade image resolution, so large area radiography is obtained at the expense of resolution; conversely, smaller anode angles give a smaller field size but a better resolution.

anode construction/assembly (*xray*) The construction of the x-ray tube anode uses various high refractory metals, separately and as alloys. The body of an x-ray anode is typically a disk consisting of an alloy of titanium, zirconium and molybdenum. The target is about 0.7–1.0 mm thick tungsten/rhenium alloy. Common anode constructions are:

X-ray tube	Construction (target)	Heat capacity
Mammography	Mo (Mo)	100 kJ
	Mo (Mo and Rh)	120 kJ
	W (W and Mo)	135 kJ
Conventional Fluoroscopy/CT	Mo (Re/W alloy)	160 kJ
	Mo alloy +C backing (Re/W alloy)	1.0 MJ
	Ti/Zr/Mo alloy (Re/W alloy)	1.8 MJ

anode cooling (*xray*) Measures the heat lost by the x-ray tube and determines the tube workload (loadability). Depends on anode heat storage and temperature difference between the anode t_a and the surrounding medium t_m (air, oil), since heat loss is proportional to t^4 then $t_{loss} = t_a^4 - t_m^4$. The greatest heat loss occurs at high temperature differences. Doubling the values of t_a and t_m increases heat loss by ×16. Heat loss from the anode is measured as joules per minute ($J m^{-1}$) and is most effective when the anode is operating near its maximum rating (falling load principle). Tube housing is also involved and forced convection is sometimes necessary to improve heat loss. The cooling curve shows the number of heat units (HU) remaining per minute. The heat stored in an anode mass depends on its heat capacity; expressed in heat units or joules.

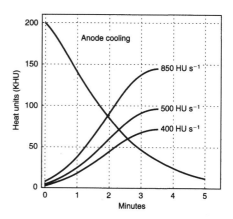

If the maximum heat capacity of the anode is 100 000 HU (from the graph shown in anode cooling) then at a rate of 850 HU s^{-1} this can be exceeded in 2.5 minutes continuous exposure. For long exposure times (fluoroscopy), thermal equilibrium occurs when the heat generated by the electron beam is balanced by factors influencing heat loss (radiation, conduction, convection). The heating curves show that equilibrium would be achieved for this tube at about 500 HU s^{-1}, levelling out at the maximum heat rating of 100 kHU (*see* heat storage, tube rating).

anode current (*xray*) Electrons emerging from the filament are accelerated towards the anode by the applied high voltage. The anode current is influenced by the space charge effect, filament current and applied high voltage.

anode heat capacity (AHC) (*xray*) May be expressed in kilowatts (kW) or heat units (HU) where 1 Ws = 1.35 HU (*see* heat capacity).

anode heating (*xray*) Considerable heat is produced by bombarding the anode with an electron beam. This heat is removed by radiation from the anode to the enclosure wall (glass or metal) and also by conduction along the bearing or by direct oil cooling. Reflector plates behind the anode prevent excessive radiant heat from reaching the rotor–bearing mechanism. Excessive heating of the anode will vaporize the target giving a rough surface so degrading focal spot geometry and reducing x-ray output by photon scatter; it will also cause bearing damage. The vaporized anode material (tungsten) deposited on the tube window will increase beam filtration (increased HVL), lowering image contrast.

anode heat storage (*xray*) For an x-ray tube, anode heat storage is the product of anode mass, specific heat and temperature rise. The maximum heat capacity of the anode may be exceeded if the rate of heat production is high. The heat energy deposited in the target limits the workload and depends on:

- exposure time;
- disk rotation;
- focal track length;
- focal spot size.

Early methods of measuring x-ray tube power used heat units which were the product of:

- tube kV × tube mA × time (single phase);
- tube kV × tube mA × 1.35 (3-phase)
- tube kV × tube mA × time × 1.4 (constant current/high frequency generator).

An increase applied to 3-phase or constant potential (or high frequency) supply allows for their improved efficiency. Conversion: HU × 0.71 = joules; joules × 1.41 = HU. A conventional anode construction would have a typical heat storage capacity of 100 kHU this would increase to a few MHU for heavily loaded tubes (fluoroscopy and CT). Current metal/ceramic tubes can have a heat storage approaching 5 MHU and a continuous load of 7 kW (*see* rating).

anode load capacity (*ct*) Maximum permitted value of the instantaneous and of the mean long-term x-ray tube power; the instantaneous maximum value for the tube current for a given tube voltage is determined by the melting point of the anode material and thus depends on the actual tube temperature, size of the focal spot (FS) and the duration of the electron beam targeting the anode's surface. For short scan times, the permitted x-ray tube loading depends mainly on the tube's heat capacity. For longer scan times, the tube capacity is limited by the rate of heat transfer from the anode away from the tube housing (*see* rotating anode).

anode size (*xray*) Anode diameter determines the heat rating of the x-ray tube and therefore its thermal loading. The disk mass and surface area also plays an important part. A larger anode diameter at the same rotational speed offers a longer track length of target and so the heat generated is spread over a greater area of metal. Larger disks therefore take higher loading (higher loadability) and are used for high power applications such as fluoroscopy and CT. A larger disk diameter increases the heat capacity and also the area radiating heat, but there is potential mechanical damage in the larger anode due to localized expansion. This is prevented by cutting radial slots into the anode; these are stress-relieved anodes.

Anode diameter and power rating
For a 100 mm diameter anode with 7 mm track width:
Mean radius: (100 − 7 mm) = 93 mm
Track length = 2π × 93/2 = 292 mm
Anode rotation speed: 3000 rpm
Complete target area exposed every 60/3000 = 0.02 s

---

antecubital vein (*clin*) Vein located in front of the elbow in each arm, commonly used for blood sampling or injection.

---

antegrade cystography (*clin*) Antegrade urography performed by introducing contrast medium into the bladder.

antegrade pyelography (*clin*) *See* **antegrade urography**.

antegrade urography (*clin*) Radiography by percutaneous injection of contrast agent with needle or catheter into renal calices or pelvis (antegrade pyelography) or into bladder (antegrade cystography).

antenna (*mri*) A coil or length of wire attached to an RF receiver as a pick-up device for RF signals. A device to send or receive electromagnetic radiation. In the NMR context, it is preferable to think of fields rather than electromagnetic radiation, as it is the magnetic vector alone that couples the spins and the coils, and the term coil should be used instead (*see* **coils (MRI)**).

anti-aliasing (*comp*) A technique used to adjust jagged diagonal lines and curves in images caused by false frequencies (aliases) to make them look smoother. Making transitions between separate pixels more gradual.

antibody (monoclonal MAbs) (*nmed*) Antibodies of uniform structure targeting a single antigenic determinant. Produced by a clone antibody population (homogenous population). Developed by Cesar Milstein and George Kohler in 1975.

antibody (polyclonal PAbs) (*nmed*) Antibodies of mixed structure targeting multiple antigenic determinants (*see* **carcinoembryonic antigen (CEA)**).

anticoagulant (*clin*) Agents preventing blood coagulation, such as heparin, ethylenediaminetetraacetic acid (EDTA).

antigen/antibody reaction (*nmed*) A mechanism in which a radiolabelled antibody binds to a surface tumour antigen to form an insoluble antigen/antibody complex, permitting imaging of the tumour.

anti-isowatt (*xray*) *See* **isowatt**.

antimony Sb (*elem*)

Atomic number (Z)	51
Relative atomic mass (A$_r$)	121.75
Density (ρ) kg/m³	6680
Melting point (K)	903.7
Specific heat capacity J kg^{-1}K^{-1}	205
Thermal conductivity W m^{-1} K^{-1}	18
K-edge (keV)	30.4

anti-neutrino (*phys*) *See* **neutrino**.

anti-reflective coating (*imaging*) A $\frac{1}{4}\lambda$ coating on video monitor screens to reduce light reflections at certain angles. Anti-reflective coatings are also found between the phosphor layer and plastic support on a variety of intensifying screens and image phosphor plates to reduce reflection of scattered light from the support surface.

anti-scatter grid (*xray*) A collimating device for reducing scattered radiation reaching the image plane (film, image intensifier). Consisting of thin lead strips (typically 36–70 µm) separated by x-ray transparent spacer material (paper, kevlar, carbon fibre, etc.). The height of the grid and spacer thickness determine grid performance.

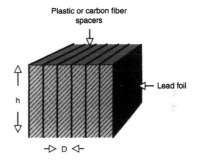

Plastic or carbon fiber spacers

Lead foil

h

D

(*ct*) A collimator system mounted in front of the detector in order to remove scattered radiation. Constructed from thin metal sheets aligned towards the focal spot and almost completely absorbs those parts of the incoming radiation which do not originate from the focal spot (*see* **grid ratio, grid factor**).

aortography (*clin*) Imaging the aorta and its branches using an iodine-based contrast medium. Percutaneous transfemoral catheterization is the usual method employed; failing this, then a percutaneous transaxilliary approach is made. The contrast material is injected via a catheter placed into the thoracic aorta (thoracic aortography) or abdominal aorta (abdominal aortography).

aortography (retrograde) (*clin*) Imaging the abdominal aorta, injecting contrast medium into the femoral artery and the visceral vessels after temporary occlusion of the artery distal to the injection site; percutaneous transfemoral catheterization is commonly employed.

apcitide (*nmed*) The preparation ^{99m}Tc-apcitide is the technetium complex of the polypeptide, apcitide, a small-molecule synthetic peptide and has a high affinity and selectivity for the GPIIb/IIIa receptor that is expressed on the

A

membrane surface of activated platelets. Plays a major role in platelet aggregation and thrombus formation. AcuTect® targets acute venous thrombosis in the lower limbs.

aperture (*optic*) The relative aperture of a lens is defined as the ratio d/f where d is the diameter of the lens and f is the focal length. The lens aperture can be controlled by an iris diaphragm behind the lens. Aperture is expressed as an f-number. An aperture of f-8 requires a $\times 16$ longer exposure time than f-2, but has a greater depth of field. (*us*) Size of the transducer or size of a number of transducer elements (*see* depth of field).

aperture (angle) (*us*) The angle between an intensity contour and the face of the transducer; a measure of the lateral resolution. It can be modified by signal delay in multi-element transducers (lateral focusing), but becomes larger in the far field.

aperture (dynamic) (*us*) Change in aperture size during transmission to maintain focus with depth (*see* focus (dynamic)).

AP file (*comp*) Also called virtual memory, this is a disk file used as a main memory supplement. Program code and data are written to it in pages and swapped into main memory when required.

Apgar score (*stats*) A scoring system used to grade neonate status.

API (*comp*) Application program interface. A common interface that allows programs to make use of services provided by the operating system or other applications. Winsock, for example, is an API that allows Windows and other programs to talk to TCP/IP for Internet access.

apodisation (*us*) Removal of sound beam side lobes by using gaussian beam profile.

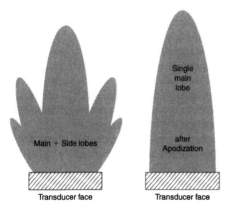

Main + Side lobes

Transducer face

Single main lobe

after Apodization

Transducer face

(*mri*) Multiplication of acquired MR data by a function reducing at higher spatial frequencies so reducing artefacts near edges, due to truncation and Gibbs phenomenon.

apoptosis (*dose*) A process of programmed cell death following radiation or other damage.

a posteriori (*stats*) Analysis suggested after the event by examination of collected data.

a priori (*stats*) Analytical predictions made before data are collected.

applet (*comp*) A small program that runs within a larger program. Cannot function as stand-alone programs. Designed to be executed from within another program. Applets are embedded in many Microsoft products, such as Windows and Excel. An applet can be a Java program which is designed to run only on a web page. Applets differ from applications in that they are governed by a strict security protocol. Applets are further restricted and can only read and write data from the same domain from which they are served.

approximation image (*di*) Original image, filtered by a smoothing scaling function at the coarsest scale.

APT (*mri*) Attached proton test.

archiving (*xray*) The medium- and long-term storage of patient details. An image data for easy retrieval, which includes paper, film and electronic methods.

Arcitumomab (*nmed*) (CEA-Scan®, Immunomedics) Murine monoclonal antibody Fab' fragment labelled with ^{99m}Tc. Targets a variety of carcinomas particularly in the gastrointestinal (GI) tract, including also Crohn's disease and inflammatory bowel disease.

area (*unit*) The SI unit is the metre squared (m^2). Conversions for non-SI units:

1 barn	$10^{-28}m^2$
1 m^2	10^4cm^2 (10^6mm^2)
1 km^2	10^6m^2
1 acre	$4.04686 \times 10^3m^2$
1 hectare	10^4m^2

The barn is the effective cross section in nuclear reactions and is equal to $10^{-28}m^2$. Dose-area-product (DAP) meters use either gray or roentgen in a more practical cm^2 area (*see* metre).

area dose product (F) (*dose*) See dose area product.

argon (Ar) (*elem*) An inert gas used as a filling for electric lamps and gas radiation detectors. Commonly found as a pressurized filling for the dose calibrator. Cheaper than xenon.

Atomic number (Z)	18
Relative atomic mass (A$_r$)	39.95
Density (ρ) kg/m^3	1.784
Melting point (K)	83.7
K-edge (keV)	3.2
Relevance to radiology: inert gas fill for ion-chamber	

Gas	Abundance (%)	Density (kg m^{-3})
Air	100	1.293
Nitrogen	78	1.25
Argon	0.93	1.784
Xenon	10^{-5}	5.88

^{41}**Argon** (*nmed*) Isotope of argon having a half-life of 110 minutes. Produced mainly from the activation of argon in the air which cools the outside surfaces of reactor vessels and their shields or present in the cyclotron room. ^{40}Ar gas molecules in the room air are activated by the reaction:

$$^{40}\text{Ar}(n,\gamma)^{41}\text{Ar} \; ; (\gamma = 1.29 \text{ MeV, T}\tfrac{1}{2} = 1.83 \text{ h}]$$

As a result, radioactive noble gas ^{41}Ar is released through a stack into the atmosphere. Being inert, it is not reconcentrated by biological systems.

ARP (*mri*) Adiabatic rapid passage.

array (*us*) A group of piezo-elements (typically several hundred) that are electronically switched to transmit and receive ultrasound signals. (*image*) A block of computer memory usually reserved for image data and treated as an image matrix.

array (adaptive) (*ct*) *See* Adaptive array.

array (linear) (*ct*) *See* linear array.

array coil (*mri*) RF coil composed of multiple separate elements that can be used individually (switchable coil) or used simultaneously. When used simultaneously, the elements can either be electrically coupled to each other ('coupled array coils') with common transmission lines ('mutual inductance') or electrically isolated from each other ('isolated array coils'), with separate transmission lines and receivers and minimum effective mutual inductance and with the signals from each transmission line processed independently or at different frequencies.

array processor (*comp*) Optional component of the computer system specially designed to speed up numerical calculations like those needed in magnetic resonance imaging; dedicated computer for reconstructing the image matrix.

ARSAC (*nmed*) Administration of Radioactive Substances Advisory Committee, which advises the UK Secretary of State for Health and authorizes doctors to administer radioactivity to patients for diagnosis, therapy and research.

arsenic (As) (*elem*)

Atomic number (Z)	33
Relative atomic mass (Ar)	74.92
Density (ρ) kg/m^3	5730
Melting point (K)	1090
K-edge (keV)	11.8
Relevance to radiology: Used as a doping agent for semiconductors.	

artefact (*xray*) An image distortion or unwanted item caused by a fault in the machine (cassette, ADC, etc.) or software (program corrupted). The random fluctuation of intensity due to noise can be considered separately from artefacts. An image distortion or unwanted item caused by a fault in the machine (cassette, ADC, etc.) or software (program corrupted).

artefact (structured noise) (*ct*) The appearance in the CT image of details not present in the scanned object. The main components of structured noise are due to a form of partial volume artefact and to beam hardening. Both effects usually result in streaking artefacts, which are observed in regions of high contrast when there is a sharp discontinuity in object density, such as at air–tissue, air–bone and metal–tissue boundaries. Streaking will also arise from mechanical misalignment within the scanner and, in clinical practice, from patient motion and the use of high-density contrast media. Image artefact can appear as false structures (aliasing artefact, beam hardening artefact, motion artefact, structured noise or partial volume artefact) or as a corruption of the CT numbers due to errors in the reconstruction algorithm.

arteriography (*clin*) Imaging an artery or arteries by using an iodine-based contrast medium using a percutaneous arterial needle puncture or placement of a percutaneous intra-arterial catheter. According to the puncture site or the organ to be visualized, different terminologies are used, such as peripheral or femoral, hepatic or renal transfemoral arteriography. Arteriography is applied for investigating adrenal arteriography, bronchial arteriography, cerebral arteriography, coeliac arteriography, pancreatic arteriography, renal arteriography, splenic arteriography, vertebral arteriography (*see* angiography).

arthrography (*clin*) The radiographic examination of skeletal joints, with specific intra-articular injection of contrast medium (gas or air) or iodine contrast material into the joint space. Displays cartilage and limits of the joint cavity. Non-ionic water-soluble contrast media are commonly used. Magnetic resonance imaging has made arthrography of the knee joint almost obsolete, and has also dramatically decreased the use of this invasive technique in other joints.

artificial intelligence (*comp*) A branch of computer science that tries to instruct a computer to learn from experiences or mistakes in order to improve its performance. Examples are chess programs and computer diagnosis using Bayes' theorem on conditional probability.

ASA (international) (*film*) Abbreviation for American Standards Association. A film speed rating taking an arithmetic scale, taking an image luminance range of 20:1 (1.3 range $\log_{10}$). The speed is based on the exposure required to give a shadow density of 0.1 above fog. DIN and BS standards also adopt this standard.

ASCII (*comp*) American Standard Code for Information Interchange. An encoding system which converts keyboard characters and instructions into binary for computer operation.

aseptic area (*nmed*) An isolated room, constructed to comply with the highest standards of air filtration (class I BS5295).

ASIS (*mri*) Aromatic Solvent-Induced Shift.

as low as reasonably achievable (*dose*) *See* ALARA.

aspect ratio (*di*) The ratio between one image plane and the other. A 35-mm slide has an aspect ratio of 3:2 and a 14-inch monitor is approximately 5:4.

assembly language (*comp*) A type of computer language which is complex but enables the most efficient way of programming the computer, particularly for speed. Assembly languages have the same structure and set of commands as machine languages, but they enable a programmer to use alpha numeric labels instead of numbers. High-level languages such as FORTRAN, Java or C. Programmers still use assembly language when speed is essential or when they need to perform an operation that is not possible in a high-level language.

assumed radiation risks (*dose*) There is mostly agreement between ICRP60 (1991a) and NCRP report 116 (1993).

Workers	4×10^{-2} Sv^{-1} for fatal cancer
	0.8×10^{-2} Sv^{-1} non-fatal cancer detriment
	0.8×10^{-2} Sv^{-1} for severe genetic effects
Public	5×10^{-2} Sv^{-1} for fatal cancer
	1.0×10^{-2} Sv^{-1} non-fatal cancer
	1.3×10^{-2} Sv^{-1} for severe genetic effects
Embryo/foetus approximately 10×10^{-2} Sv^{-1}	

astatine At (*elem*) A radioactive halogen, occurring naturally from the radioactive decay of thorium and uranium.

Atomic number (Z)	85
Relative atomic mass (A$_r$)	210
Density (ρ) kg/m^3	–
Melting point (K)	575
K-edge (keV)	95.7
Relevance to radiology: alpha emitter used for radiotherapy	

^{211} Astatine:

Nuclear data ^{211} At	
Half life	7.2 h
Decay mode	α 5.8 MeV
Decay constant	0.09625 h^{-1}
Photons (abundance)	6(γ) 96keV–1.0MeV

asymmetric sampling (*mri*) Collecting more data points on one side of *k*-space origin than on the other. With fewer *k*-space data points, a shorter echo time can be attained. Also, asymmetric acquisition in any phase encoding direction followed by partial-Fourier reconstruction gives a reduced imaging time.

asynchronous transmission (*comp*) A type of transmission in which each character is transmitted independently without reference to a standard clock. The data are commonly transmitted one character at a time to the receiving device, with intervals of varying lengths between transmissions. ADSL and most dial-up modem communications uses asynchronous communication. (*see* ATM, synchronous transmission).

ATAPI (*comp*) Advanced technology attachment packet interface. A standard for connecting a CD-ROM drive to an EIDE (enhanced integrated drive electronics) adapter. This simplifies installation of CD-ROM drives.

Athion (*comp*) The processor produced by the company AMD. A direct competitor for Intel's range of Pentium processors.

ATM (asynchronous transfer mode) (*comp*) A high-speed networking technology that transfers packets of data to transmit various kinds of information (voice, video, data). ATM provides standards for 25 Mbps and 155 Mbps transmission speeds. Current ATM cells are 53 bytes long containing a 5-byte header and a 48-byte payload packet. The header contains information for data to reach the appropriate end point for a specified priority. The payload contains any type of information, voice, video or data.

atmosphere (*unit*) A non-SI unit of pressure where $1 \text{ atm} = 1.013 \times 10^5 \text{ Pa}$ (101.3 kPa). Equivalent to 760 mmHg or 14.696 psi. Some gas detectors (CT) use xenon at 20 atmospheres equivalent to 2.0 MPa or nearly 300 psi.

atom (*phys*) The basic unit of matter consisting of a single nucleus surrounded by one or more orbital electrons. The atom is electrically neutral and can be stable or unstable.

atomic mass number A (*phys*) The total number of protons and neutrons in a nucleus $A = Z + N$. Shown below (top left) above the **atomic number** value:

$$^A_Z X_N$$

(*see* atomic weight).

atomic mass unit (*phys*) See relative atomic mass.

atomic number Z (*phys*) The proton number in the nucleus of an atom. The atomic number also equals the number of orbiting electrons in a neutral atom. This has the symbol Z in the connotation

$$^A_Z X_N$$

where A is the **atomic mass number** and N the neutron number.

Common stable isotopes are given in the example with IUPAC group numbers 13–16 showing the change of elements with different atomic numbers (bottom left) (*see* isotopes, isotones, isodiapheres, isobars).

atomic weight (*phys*) See relative atomic mass.

attenuation (*ct*) The decrease in the intensity of the x-ray beam when passing through matter; the extent of attenuation is a property of the material which is exposed to radiation and the energy of radiation. It is quantitatively described by the linear **attenuation coefficient**; (*mri*) Reduction of power by passage through an absorbing medium or electrical component. Commonly expressed in decibels. (*xray*) The process by which radiation is reduced in intensity when passing through matter. It is a combination of absorption and scattering events. (*us*) Reduction of power, e.g. due to passage through a medium. Attenuation in electrical systems is commonly expressed in dB as the product of:

* attenuation coefficient (dB cm^{-1});
* pulse length (cm);
* 0.5×frequency (MHz);
* path length in dB.

Soft tissue has an approximate attenuation of 1.0 dB cm^{-1} at 1 MHz (*see* linear attenuation coefficient, linear absorption coefficient).

attenuation coefficient (sound) α (*us*) The speed of sound is frequency independent but α is influenced strongly by frequency. The attenuation coefficient is the sum of the individual coefficients for scatter and absorption. Fractional change in intensity is given in decibels as $\mu = 4.3\,\alpha\text{dB m}^{-1}$; the decibel attenuation coefficient. The attenuation coefficient is roughly proportional to frequency as $\mu = kf$ where $k = $ dB m^{-1}MHz^{-1}. For soft tissues, this is 70 dB m^{-1} at 1 MHz or $\alpha = 0.1$ dB mm^{-1} so 3 cm of tissue will reduce the intensity by 50%; bone will give $\alpha = 1.3$ dB mm^{-1} attenuation.

13	14	15	16
$^{11}_{5}$B, boron	$^{12}_{6}$C, carbon	$^{14}_{7}$N, nitrogen	$^{16}_{8}$O, oxygen
$^{27}_{13}$Al, aluminium	$^{28}_{14}$Si, silicon	$^{31}_{15}$P, phosphorus	$^{32}_{16}$S, sulphur
$^{69}_{31}$Ga, gallium	$^{74}_{32}$Ge, germanium	$^{75}_{33}$As, arsenic	$^{80}_{34}$Se, selenium

A

attenuation coefficient (x-ray) (*xray*) *See* linear attenuation coefficient.

attenuation profile (*ct*) Spatial distribution of the total x-ray attenuation of the object to be examined measured at a certain position of the x-ray source. Intensity profiles from detected photons are converted into attenuation profiles (inverse of intensity). These are then converted to log values, so a quantity proportional to attenuation is available for back projection (*see* CT number).

attenuator (*mri*) Device which reduces a signal by a specific amount, commonly given in dB.

audio frequency (*phys*) Range of sound frequencies from 20 to 20 000 Hz. The human voice frequency is between 300 and 3500 Hz. The beat frequency in Doppler CW has a range in the audio frequency band.

Auger Pierre (1899–1993) French physicist. Demonstrated from cloud chamber photographs that the main photoelectric electron was accompanied by characteristic auger electrons. These play an important part in radiation dosimetry.

auger electron (*phys*) Electron ejected from K or L shell as an alternative to characteristic radiation emission. These electrons play an important role in estimating internal dosimetry, particularly at the cellular level (DNA damage) (*see* photoelectric effect, radiation weighting factor).

autocorrelation (*image*) Information about a signal's periodicity reveals information in the presence of noise. This is obtained by making amplitude measurements at two different times separated by a delay *t*, finding their product and averaging over the time of the recording:

$$R_x(t) = \lim_{T \to \infty} \frac{1}{T} \int_0^T x_{(t)} \cdot x_{(t+\tau)} \cdot d\tau$$

where $x_{(t)}$ and $x_{(t+\tau)}$ are the two amplitude measurements taken *t* intervals apart in a waveform of length *T*. Autocorrelation is very sensitive to the presence of periodicity in the time domain (signal) in the presence of noise. It indicates how well a shifted noise image resembles or correlates with the unshifted image. The Wiener spectrum is the Fourier transform of the autocorrelation function and vice versa. (*us*) Used in most colour-flow instruments for obtaining mean Doppler shift frequency. The Doppler signals along one image line are compared or correlated with those from the following transmit pulse (*see* Fourier analysis).

autocorrelation function (*image*) The autocorrelation function is the ensemble average of the joint second moment of any image process. The noise autocorrelation function is defined in general as:

$$C_n(x_i, x_j = \langle n(x_i) \cdot n(x_j) \rangle$$

where $n(i)$ is the noise at location *i*. For additive noise, this is equivalent to the autocovariance function, which is the autocorrelation about the mean. The autocorrelation function is the Fourier transform of the Wiener spectrum.

autocovariance (*image*) *See* autocorrelation function.

autoradiography (*xray*) A process where low energy beta emitters (^{14}C, ^{3}H) are incorporated into a living system, organ or tissue before being prepared histologically for microscopic display. A photo-emulsion is applied to the surface of the thin section specimen and, after a period of hours or days, it is developed to reveal local areas of beta activity as exposed silver grains. Resolution is subcellular. Image plate technology is now replacing film emulsion.

automatic brightness control (ABC) (*xray*) *See* automatic exposure control.

automatic exposure control (AEC) (*xray*) Also known as automatic brightness control (ABC) where the generator output is terminated when a preset radiation exposure is reached. When used for fluoroscopy, this gives a constant dose rate at the image intensifier face (typically within 0.2–0.5 μGy s^{-1}), maintaining the consistency of image quality. Either a photodiode or photo-multiplier monitors the output-screen of the image intensifier; feedback alters kV and mA (*see* iso-watt).

automatic frequency control (AFC) (*xray*) An electronic circuit that holds the frequency of a generator to within very narrow limits. This is an important component of a high frequency x-ray generator where a slight variation in frequency would give a change in voltage.

automatic gain control (*xray*) Adjusts video signal for constant display brightness in conjunction with the automatic brightness control.

autoregressive filter (*di*) An alternative to the Fourier process which is applied when only the most prominent features are to be extracted. The Fourier process is non-selective and will extract every feature.

autoscan (autoscanning) (*us*) The electronic or mechanical steering of successive ultrasonic pulses or series of pulses, through at least two dimensions.

autosomal (*dose*) Concerning chromosomes other than sex chromosomes.

auto-transformer (*xray*) This component of the x-ray generator allows fine adjustment of the a.c. supply voltage to the x-ray generator, compensating for voltage drop in the main supply.

auto-tuning (*nmed*) Automatic gain control of photomultiplier response with time by monitoring photopeak variations. Used as a method for maintaining gamma camera uniformity of response. (*mri*) Automatic tuning optimization matching the RF coils for various loading conditions. The tuning elements are typically variable capacitance diodes (varactors) and are program controlled.

average CT value (*ct*) Arithmetic mean of CT numbers within a region of interest. The mean or average CT number for an object detail can be determined with high precision, since the single values are corrupted by **quantum noise**.

average glandular dose (*mamm*) Reference term (ICRP 1987) for radiation dose estimation from x-ray mammography, i.e. the average absorbed dose in the glandular tissue (excluding skin) in a uniformly compressed breast of 50% adipose, 50% glandular tissue. The reference breast thickness and composition should be specified (*see* **mean glandular dose**).

average lifetime ($\bar{T}$) (*nmed*) A term describing radioactive decay. Average lifetime is calculated by summing all the individual lifetimes and then dividing this by the total number of nuclei involved:

$$\bar{T} = \frac{1}{\lambda} = \frac{T}{0.693} = 1.44\ T$$

Describes the time course of the number of undecayed nuclei, or the amount of the radioactive substance that is present at any time after measurements have started.

averaging (*mri*) Mean value of measured signals in a slice; improves signal-to-noise ratio.

averaging filter (spatial) (*di*) A method for reducing random noise in a signal by adding together repetitive signals. The structured signal strength will improve, while the random noise will cancel out. Applying this technique

to image noise reduction. The simplest form simply adds the pixel values in a small block (2 × 2 or 3 × 3) and constructs a new image matrix from the mean values. Resolution is lost if larger blocks are taken (*see* **frame averaging**).

averaging filter (temporal) (*di*) A recursive filter for handling image frames. The general algorithm is:

$$D_{new} = \frac{D_{old}}{k} + \frac{D_{in}}{k}$$

A version of non-recursive filtering applied to image frames *N*. A running average is performed on the image data which improves SNR by $\sqrt{N}$.

averted dose (*dose*) The radiation dose prevented or avoided by applying countermeasures; the difference between the potential dose if the countermeasure(s) had not been applied and the actual dose.

Audio video interleave (AVI) (*comp*) Designed by Microsoft to combine audio and video in a single track or frame to keep them synchronized. Files are compressed by only recording the differences between each frame.

Avogadro's constant (*unit*) The number of particles in 1 mole which is 6.022×10^{23}. The current accepted value issued by the National Institute of Standards and Technology (NIST) is 6.0221415 $(\pm 0.0000010) \times 10^{23}$. Avogadro's constant is used for calculating osmolarity, specific activity of a radionuclide and substance electron density.

axial (*us*) In the direction of the transducer axis (sound–travel direction).

axial plane (*ct*) Anatomical plane orthogonal to the longitundinal axis (*z*) of the human body and parallel to the *x/y* plane.

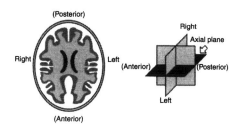

axial resolution (*us*) *See* **resolution** (axial).

axial spatial resolution (*ct*) *See* **spatial resolution**.

axis of rotation (*ct*) Axis about which the CT gantry rotates (both x-ray tube and the detector) during the measurement.

B

B_0 (*mri*) A conventional symbol for the constant magnetic (induction) field in a nuclear magnetic resonance (NMR) system. The H_0 units of magnetic field strength ampere per meter should be distinguished from B_0, unit of magnetic induction in tesla.

B_1 (*mri*) The conventional symbol for RF (radio frequency) magnetic induction field opposed to B_0 (the symbol H_1 was previously used); considered as two opposing rotating vectors in a plane transverse to B_0. At the Larmor frequency, this vector rotating in the same direction as the precessing spins will interact strongly with the spins to give the NMR signal.

B-mode (*us*) An early brightness display giving a cross-sectional (axial) image. Replaced by grey scale displays.

b-value (*mri*) This, together with the diffusion coefficient *D*, are factors describing the relative signal intensity *S* in diffusion weighted imaging (DWI). The diffusion sensitivity parameter b equals:

$$\lambda^2 G^2 \delta^2 \left(\Delta - \frac{\delta}{3} \right)$$

where λ is the gyromagnetic ratio, *G* the strength of the gradient pulse, δ the duration of the pulse and δ the time between the two pulses. The magnitude of b is measured in $mm^2 s^{-1}$ and can reach 10 000 in current magnetic resonance imaging (MRI) machines. Gradient amplitude, slew rates and duty cycles during echo planar imaging (EPI) are important in order to achieve high b values. The relative signal intensity is then given by:

$$S = e^{-bD}$$

where *D* is the diffusion coefficient.

■ Reference: Schaefer *et al.*, 2000.

backbone (*comp*) The part of the network that carries the heaviest traffic; it connects LANS, either within a building or across a city or region. It is the top level of a hierarchical network; the central connection. The main data bus for data transference. The Internet has a backbone although not existing as a virtual routing path. Also the network that joins servers to other servers, multiple concentrators or both. Smaller networks may not carry a backbone. Either fibreoptic cable or RG-6 is used for the backbone. Smaller networks using backbone technology, use RG-58 to connect between bridges, routers and concentrators.

background radiation (*phys*) Cosmic and radiation from natural radioactive sources. (*nmed*) Radiation originating in sources (environmental or artificial) other than the activity of primary concern. Measured as becquerels (Bq).

back projection (*di*) Summation or linear superposition of projections, of light or x-rays through an object, to form a simple tomographic image slice. (*ct*) A method for reconstructing a sectional display from a series of radial projections. The summation or linear superposition of projections, of light or x-rays through an object, to form a simple tomographic image slice. In computed tomography (CT) the mathematical procedure for the reconstruction of the axial image. This method suffers from serious image blurring so spatial filtration (convolution) of the raw data is necessary before back projection in order to reduce artefacts (*see* filtered back-projection).

back scatter (*xray*) Radiation scattered or deflected from its path into the sensitive volume of a detector.

back up (*comp*) Copying data from one storage medium to another, i.e. from hard disk to floppy disk. It is a protection against data destruction.

balanced gradients (*mri*) Rewinding the gradient fields so that the total time-amplitude area is zero. A gradient waveform acting on any stationary spin at resonance between two consecutive RF pulses and return it to the same phase it had before the gradients were applied.

balanced steady-state free precession (bSSFP) (*mri*) A gradient echo (GRE) sequence which produces image contrast weighted by the T2/T1 ratio; gives higher signal to noise ratio and reduced artefacts compared to SSFP. Uses balanced gradients which returns magnetization to the original phase before gradients were applied; increases the acquired signal and reduces artefacts. Typically, TR is short compared to the T2 values of the tissues of interest, TE is intermediate. The flip angle of 45° to 90° produces a T2/T1-weighted SSFP image (*see* True-Flash, True-FISP).

banding (*image*) Bands of discrete colour or tone that appear when a printer is unable to reproduce a smooth graduation from one colour to another. Instead there are noticeable jumps between one value and the next.

band-pass filter (*di*) Also called pass-band filter. A signal filter that passes a particular band of frequencies relatively strongly (*see* filtering (signal)).

band-stop (notch) filter (*di*) *See* stop-band filter, filtering (signal).

bandwidth (*image*) A general term describing range of frequencies in a signal. Usually defines as the -3 db points of a pass-band or stop-band filter. A large bandwidth signal transmits a large volume of information (video signal), while a narrow bandwidth contains a restricted volume. Large bandwidths also increase noise content. The bandwidth of a pure sine-wave is very narrow and can be represented as a pulse in the frequency domain. (*comp*) The maximum amount of data that a network cable can carry, measured in bits per second (bps). The larger the bandwidth, the more information the network can handle. General KBPS standards for modem are 14.4, 28.8, 33.6 and 56 kB. ISDN is usually 64, 128 or 256 kB. ADSL and DSL are generally faster than ISDN and sometimes faster than cable. Cable connections are usually 500 kB or 1 MB. T1 is 1.5 MB and T3 is 45 MB. Satellite uplinks are usually between 25 and 80 MB (*see* receiver bandwidth, transmission bandwidth, Q, delta (δ) pulse). (*mri*) The centre frequency of the RF transmitted pulse selects the slice location and the RF transmitter bandwidth (frequency spread) determines the slice thickness. The frequency encoding gradient depends on the field of view and the receiver bandwidth which covers the selected field of view; typically 4 to 32 kHz. (*us*) Range of frequencies contained in an ultrasound pulse; expressed as the difference between the most widely separated frequencies f_1 and f_2 at which the transmitted acoustic pressure spectrum is 0.71 of its maximum value (-3 dB).

bar (*unit*) Barometric pressure; a non-SI unit of pressure where 1 bar is 10^5 Pa, approximately 750 mmHg or 0.987 atm. 1 millibar (mbar) is 10^{-3} bar or 100 Pa (*see* atmosphere, pascal, pressure).

Baritop* (*clin*) A barium sulphate x-ray contrast medium for the gastrointestinal (GI) tract. A white suspension of barium sulphate BP 100% w/v.

barium (Ba) (*elem*) An alkali metal used as barium sulphate ($BaSO_4$) as barium contrast studies for x-ray examinations of the stomach and alimentary canal.

Atomic number (Z)	56
Relative atomic mass (A_r)	137.34
Density (ρ) kg/m^3	3600
Melting point (K)	1000
K-edge (keV)	37.4

Relevance to radiology: As barium sulphate ($BaSO_4$) as a contrast medium for x-ray examinations of the stomach and guts. Barium sulphate in this context is often called simply 'barium'.

^{133}Barium

Production	$^{235}_{92}$U(n, f)$^{133}_{56}$Ba ($+^{101}_{36}$Kr + 2n)
Decay scheme (e.c.) ^{133}Ba	^{133}Ba $T\frac{1}{2}$10.8 y (γ 81,356 keV) $\rightarrow$ ^{133}Cs stable
Photons (abundance)	81 (0.34)
	303 (0.18)
	356 (0.62)
Half-life	10.8 years
Decay constant	0.063 y^{-1}
Gamma ray constant	7.7×10^{-2} mSv h^{-1} MBq^{-1} at 1 m
Uses	Calibration isotope emulating ^{131}iodine

barium contrast studies (*clin*) Barium sulphate, being highly insoluble, is a non-toxic x-ray contrast medium as an aqueous suspension administered either orally or via the rectum in order to image the complete alimentary tract. The single-contrast barium enema is a less-preferred method to the double-contrast barium enema for the evaluation of the anatomical configuration of the colon. This technique uses barium sulphate suspensions and a less radiopaque second medium for a double-contrast or 'see-through' effect, achieved by combining the barium enema with insufflation of air (or carbon dioxide) (*see* small bowel enema).

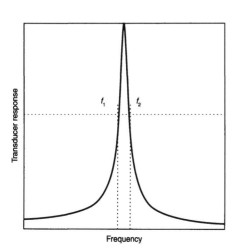

Frequency

B

barium enema (*clin*) Barium contrast study of the lower colon using a water suspension of barium sulphate as the contrast medium.

barium follow through (*clin*) Performed after the stomach and duodenum have been examined, an image is taken 1–3 h later. This provides an assessment of stomach emptying.

barium meal (*clin*) Oral administration of barium sulphate for visualizing upper gastro-intestinal tract (stomach and duodenum). The examination may be done as a single- or double-contrast examination (*see* **barium contrast studies**).

barium sulphate (*chem*) A highly insoluble compound of barium (solubility approximately 0.22 mg per 100 cm^3 water) used in a water suspension for **barium contrast studies** involving the alimentary tract. Common to all preparations is the suspension of 1 g mL^{-1}; high-density preparations of 2.5 g mL^{-1} are tailored to special requirements (*see* **Baritop**). (*dose*) In its impure state as barite (native BaSO$_4$) which is yellow/ brown and used as a plaster material for radiation (x-ray room) shielding.

barium swallow (*clin*) Oral administration of barium sulphate aqueous suspension for radiographic examination of hypopharynx and oesophagus. Both single- and double-barium contrast examinations are used.

Barkla, Charles Glover (1877–1944) English physicist. Extensive work with x-ray scattering related atomic number with the number of its electrons. Observed characteristic x-rays from K and L shells. He was awarded the Nobel prize for physics 1917.

barn (*phys*) Unit of reaction cross-section for describing particle bombardment; one barn = 10^{-24} cm^2; one millibarn = 10^{-27} cm^2.

barrel distortion (*xray*) Display distortion most commonly seen in image intensifiers due to curved input face; its converse is seen as pincushion distortion.

Bartlett window (*di*) A filter for smoothing the truncated result so that it is free of oscillations that would introduce false peaks into the resultant spectrum. A triangular window providing a sharp main peak that quickly decays to zero (*see* **Hanning filter**).

BASE (*mri*) BAsis imaging with SElective inversion-prepared.

baseband (*comp*) A network transmission technique that uses voltage to represent data. The most common type of network, data are

transmitted digitally, each wire carrying one signal at a time. A single signal, unmodulated signal of digital information over relatively short distances; the converse is **broadband, Ethernet, ARCNet** and **Token Ring** are baseband networks which use the entire bandwidth of cable to carry a single digital data signal. This limits such transmission to a single form of data transmission, since digital signals are not modulated.

base-fog (*film*) Background density film reading. Its magnitude should not exceed an optical density of 0.2. The value increases with poor film storage conditions (*see* **characteristic curve**).

baseline (*math*) A generally smooth background curve with respect to which either the integrals or peak heights of the resonance spectral lines in the spectrum are measured. (*mri*) Non-activated image, in contrast to activated image. Background signal from which the peaks rise.

baseline correction (*mri*) Processing of the spectrum to suppress baseline deviations from zero that may be superimposed on desired spectral lines. These deviations may be due to broad spectral lines.

baseline rates (*dose*) The annual disease incidence in a population in the absence of radiation exposure to the source under study.

baseline screen (*mamm*) A woman's first screening attendance (also prevalent screen), which may be part of a prevalent or incident screening round (*see* **prevalent screening round**).

baseline shift (*us*) Movement of the zero doppler-shift frequency or zero flow speed line up or down on a spectral display.

baseline value (*stats*) The value that is used for comparison when no absolute limiting value is present.

baseband (*comp*) A network transmission technique that uses voltage to represent data.

baseline value (*math*) The value that is used for comparison when no absolute limiting value is present.

BASIC (*comp*) Beginners all-purpose symbolic instruction code. A very user-friendly programming language (unlike assembler). Versions are GW Basic, Quick Basic.

basic units (phys) *See* **Systeme international (SI)**.

Bateman equation (*nmed*) Describes parent:daughter decay in a radionuclide generator.

$$A_{d(t)} = \frac{\lambda_d}{\lambda_d - \lambda_p} A_p(e^{-\lambda} p^t - e^{-\lambda} d^t) + A_d \times e^{-\lambda} d^t$$

where $A_{d(t)}$ is the daughter activity at time t; λ_p is the decay constant of parent; λ_d is the decay constant of daughter; A_p is the initial activity of parent; and A_d is the initial activity of daughter. For the ^{99}Mo/^{99m}Tc generator, the decay constant for the parent λ_p is 0.693/67 or 0.01033 h^{-1}; the daughter λ_d is 0.693/6 or 0.1155 h^{-1}.

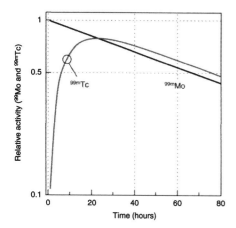

(*see* decay constant, generator).

bathtub curve (*stats*) A predictive curve descriptive of a quality assurance plan where the probability of breakdown is highest at the beginning and end of a machine's useful life.

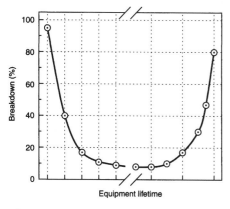

(*see* mean time between failures (MTBF), mean down time (MDT), mean time to recovery).

baud (*comp*) The speed of a modem, or other serial device, attached to and communicating with a computer. A variable unit of data transmission speed (as one baud per second). Often confused with bits per second (bps or bs^{-1}); these are

different. Only at low bit rates are they equal (300 baud = 300 bps), but at higher speeds, i.e. V22 modem 1200 bps is 600 baud. The typical speed on the network of phone company lines is 53.6 kB, though this can be increased by using various data compression techniques.

baud rate (*comp*) The number of signals that can be sent along a communications channel every second. In common usage; often confused with bits per second (bps). Modem speeds are usually quoted in bps.

Bayes' theorem (*stats*) Statistical inference drawing conclusions or diagnosis/prognosis underlying experimental or clinical data. A statistical procedure for revising and updating the prediction of some disease state in the light of new evidence. Used for suggesting the best 'next-diagnostic test', previous knowledge being available. The prevalence of the disease gives the unconditional probability P(A). The unconditional probability of a successful test is P(B). If P(A|B) represents the conditional probability of event A (disease present) conditional on event B (positive test for this disease). The sensitivity of this test gives the conditional probability of a positive test amongst patient population with the disease designated P(B|A). Then

$$P(A|B) = \frac{P(B|A) \times P(A)}{P(B)}$$

The specificity of the test gives the conditional probability of the test giving a negative result (B') in a population without the disease (A' or control group); represented by P(B'|A'). The unconditional probability of a positive test result P(B) is therefore

$\{P(B|A) \times P(A)\} + \{P(B|A') \times P(A')\}$ or

sensitivity × prevalence + (1 − specificity) × (1 − prevalence).

so the complete Bayes' theorem can be stated as:

$$\frac{\text{sensitivity} \times \text{prevalence}}{\text{sensitivity} \times \text{prevalenec} + (1 - \text{specificity}) \times (1 - \text{prevalence})}$$

predicting the probability of the test giving a positive result in a mixed population containing the disease.

beam (*us*) Region containing continuous-wave sound; region through which a sound pulse propagates.

beam area (*us*) Cross-sectional area of a sound beam.

beam axis (*us*) A straight line joining the points of maximum pulse intensity integral measured at several different distances in the far field. This line, calculated according to regression rules, is to be extended back to the transducer assembly surface.

beam cross-sectional area (*us*) The area on the surface of a plane perpendicular to the beam axis consisting of all points where the pulse intensity integral is >25% of the maximum pulse intensity integral in that plane. For situations in which the relative acoustic pressure waveform does not change significantly across the beam cross-sectional area, the beam cross-sectional area may be approximated by measuring the area on the surface of a plane perpendicular to the beam axis consisting of all points where the acoustic pressure is >50% of the maximum acoustic pressure in the plane. Unit, cm².

beam filtration (*xray*) The use of thin metal foil to remove low energy components from a poly-energetic beam.

beam former (*us*) The part of an instrument that accomplishes electronic beam scanning, apodization, steering, focusing and aperture with arrays.

beam hardening (*xray*) Filtration of a polychromatic beam by the preferential absorption of lower energy photons in tissue, with a subsequent increase in effective energy. The associated artefacts are of particular significance in computed tomography.

beam hardening artefact (*ct*) Errors in the absolute CT number values due to beam hardening; beam hardening artefacts appear when the actual object differs significantly from the assumptions made by the reconstruction beam hardening correction with respect to the x-ray attenuation. Critical regions are the base of the skull and pelvic structures.

Beam hardening (from data given under CT number)

At 100 kV the reference for water is 0.1707, but if the beam effective energy changes to 105 kV in the centre of the profile, the μ for tissue changes to 0.1750 then:

$$\text{New CT value} = \frac{0.1750 - 0.1707}{0.1707} = 25$$

and not 31 which it should be. This gives the cupping effect.

---

beam hardening correction (*ct*) Preprocessing algorithm for compensating errors due to beam hardening in the measured projection data; the beam hardening correction is based on assumptions concerning the composition of a typical object (head or abdomen).

beam homogeneity (*xray*) Comparison between poly-energetic beam and mono-energetic beam of the same effective energy (E_{eff}). A homogenous photon beam (gamma source) would be attenuated in a simple exponential fashion by increasing absorber thickness; the half value layer (HVL) reduces beam intensity to half. A second HVL will bring the intensity to 0.25. For a continuous spectrum (poly-energetic beam) of x-rays, the primary and secondary HVL are not equal since lower energy photons are preferentially removed. The simple exponential law is not obeyed.

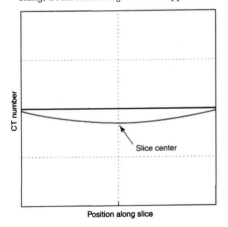

Slice center

Position along slice

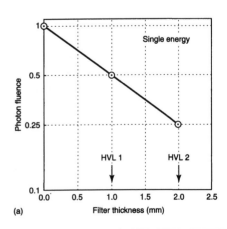

(a)

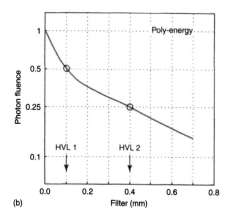

(b)

an overlaying beat frequency. The beat frequency is the difference between the two original wave frequencies. The frequency variation modulates the amplitude of the resultant wave which will have a frequency equal to the average frequency of the two waves.

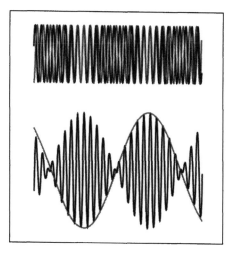

beam intensity (*phys*) The number of photons per unit area (photon fluence).

beam quality (*xray*) The penetrating power of the x-ray beam and subjectively describes the shape of the continuous spectrum. Beam quality is estimated from the half-value layer. Changing the kilovoltage changes beam quality since the penetrating power alters and the increased cut-off point (kVp) changes the spectrum shape; the effective energy also changes. Other factors: filtration and high voltage supply characteristic (single, three-phase or constant voltage supply) also changes beam quality. Tube current, although it changes the quantity of radiation has no effect on the spectrum's effective energy, so has no influence on the quality of the beam (*see* equivalent energy).

beam width (*us*) This changes with depth and images of small objects will have their width distorted close to and at a distance from the transducer face. The focal region of the transducer has the narrowest width where objects will be accurately displayed. (*ct*) The width of the x-ray beam within the scan plane measured in the direction orthogonal to the beam's direction; the beam width is determined by the scanner geometry, focal spot size and effective detector width (*see* slice width).

bearings (*xray*) Rotational support for x-ray tube anode. Either ball or sleeve bearings are used.

beat frequency (*phys*) If two waveforms have slightly different frequencies, then phase differences will change with time and wave interference alternate between constructive and destructive. These alterations of intensity cause

Beck, Robert N (1928–2008) US engineer/scientist, whose early work (1961) on the design and theory of gamma ray scintillation optimized the imaging performance of both rectilinear scanners and gamma cameras.

Becquerel, Antoine Henri (1852–1908) French physicist, discovered that Becquerel rays were a property of atoms and had by chance discovered radioactivity in 1896.

becquerel (*unit*) A measure of radionuclide activity in disintegrations per second (1 dps = 1 Bq). Multiples are kBq, MBq and GBq. 1 Ci is 3.7×10^{10} Bq (37 GBq); 1 mCi is 37 MBq; 1 μCi is 37 kBq (*see* activity, curie).

Beer's Law (*phys*) As an extension of Lambert's law. It was shown by Beer that the linear absorption coefficient for a solution is directly proportional to its concentration:

$$I = I_0 \times 10^{-abc}$$

where *a* is the linear absorption coefficient, *b* the thickness of absorber (path length) and *c* is the concentration or density of absorbing material (*see* nuclear decay).

BEIR (*dose*) Biological effects of ionizing radiation. The committee (Washington, DC: National

Academy of Sciences) has produced several reference works:

■ References: BEIR 1972, 1980, 1988, 1990, 1998, 2006.

bel (B) (*phys*) *See* decibel (dB).

Bell, Alexander Graham (1847–1922) Scottish-born American inventor. The bel (decibel) is the logarithmic comparative measure of power, intensity and amplitude or voltage gain.

bEPI (*mri*) Blipped echo planar imaging.

Bernoulli, Daniel (1700–82) Swiss mathematician who pioneered the field of hydrodynamics.

Bernoulli effect (*us*) Pressure reduction in a region of high-flow speed.

Bernoulli's principle (*phys*) The relationship between pressure and velocity in a flowing medium. Where velocity is high, pressure is low and where velocity is low, pressure is high. The principle has wide implications for vascular imaging (*see* cavitation, flow).

beryllium (Be) (*elem*)

Atomic number (Z)	4
Relative atomic mass (A_r)	9.01
Density (ρ) kg/m^3	1800
Melting point (K)	1550
Relevance to radiology: Lightest metal for x-ray tube windows	

Bessel correction (*stats*) While the mean value of a sample of n items is unbiased, the standard deviation is considerably influenced by sample size. The expected variance in a sample of n items s^2 is related to the population variance σ^2 as:

$$s^2 = \left(\frac{n-1}{n}\right) \times \sigma^2$$

The factor $(n-1)/n$ is Bessel's correction which gives the best estimate of the population variance.

Bessel function (*math*) Functions which are solutions of the second-order differential equations. They are used in heat conduction problems.

beta decay (*phys*) The unstable nucleus loses a positive or negative beta particle. Since beta decay produces a continuous spectrum and not a line spectrum, like alpha and gamma decay, it was proposed by Pauli in 1930 (*see* Pauli, Wolfgang) that another particle was emitted which shared the energy of emission. In 1932, Enrico Fermi proposed the decay process which included an anti-neutrino:

$$_0^1 n \rightarrow {}_1^1 p + {}_{-1}e + \bar{v}$$

where $\bar{v}$ is the anti-neutrino. An example is:

$$_{15}^{32} P \rightarrow {}_{16}^{32} S + \beta^-$$

The mass number of the parent and daughter is the same mass number (isobars).

$n \rightarrow p + e^- + \bar{v}$ (β^- decay with anti-neutrino)

$p \rightarrow n + e^+ + v$ (β^+ positron decay with neutrino)

$p + e^- \rightarrow n$ (electron capture, EC)

(*see* neutrino, positron, beta plus decay).

beta particle (*phys*) A negative or positive particle (*see* positron) emitted during nuclear decay. The negative particle is identical to the electron, but since the electron is not part of the nuclear construction, it is assumed that beta decay consists of 'creating' an electron from the available decay energy; this electron is then immediately ejected from the nucleus. Determination of charge e and charge to mass ration e/m confirmed them to be negative electrons. They are emitted from nuclei that have neutron excess and have a continuous energy spectrum (*see* beta decay, beta plus decay).

beta-plus decay (β+) (*nmed*) A mode of decay resulting from nuclear instability because of a neutron-deficient condition. A high-energy, positively charged electron (symbol β+) emitted by an unstable nucleus as a result of a neutron-deficient condition in the nucleus, along with a neutrino. The beta-plus particle undergoes an annihilation reaction with a free electron (*see* positron decay).

Bexxar* (*nmed*) [131]Iodine labelled antibody tositumomab, which is a murine IgG2a lambda monoclonal antibody directed against CD20 antigen found on the surface of normal and malignant B-lymphocytes.

bias (*stats*) Deviation of results from an expected conclusion.

bicisate (*nmed*) A ^{99m}Tc-ECD complex commercially available as Neurolite®.

bidirectional (*us*) Indicating Doppler instruments capable of distinguishing between positive and negative Doppler shifts (forward and reverse flow).

biexponential decay (*nmed*) Decay of a mixture of two radioisotopes with different half-lives giving a fast (biological) and slow (physical) exponential decay rate.

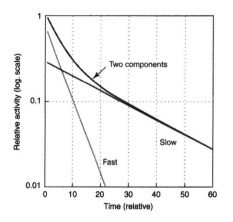

bilateral imaging (*mri*) Used for symmetric anatomic features; imaging both organs or anatomic features in the same imaging session.

biliary contrast media (oral) (*cm*) Examples of oral cholecystographic contrast media contain iocetamic acid, iopanoic acid, salts of ipodate or tyropanoate. The contrast media is absorbed intestinally, carried to the liver where it enters the hepatocytes and is conjugated with glucuronic acid, which increases its water solubility and decreases its fat solubility. It is excreted into the bile canaliculi. With intact hepatic and cystic ducts, the contrast medium flows into the gallbladder where it is concentrated by the resorption of water through the gallbladder wall (*see* cholegraphic contrast agents).

biliary contrast media (intravenous) (*cm*) Meglumine salts of iodipamide or iotroxic acids are used for intravenous cholangiography. They are transported by binding to plasma proteins competing with bilirubin for binding sites on albumin. Intravenous cholangiographic media have high water solubility, are not conjugated in the liver and are excreted unchanged in the bile, so the intrahepatic bile ducts and common bile duct are clearly imaged. No reabsorption of the cholangiograhic media occurs in the intestines (*see* cholegraphic contrast agents).

Bilibyk[x] (*cm*) *See* cholegraphic contrast agents, Biloptin, Cholebrin.

Biligrafin[x] (*clin*) A 30% concentration of meglumine iodipamide, iodine content 150 mg cm^{-3}, manufactured by Schering AG used for cholecystangiography. A 50% concentration is also available. Iodine concentration 150 mg I mL^{-1} (*see* cholegraphic contrast agents, Biliscopin).

Biligram[x] (*cm*) A 35% solution of meglumine ioglycamide manufactured by Schering AG for cholangiography and cholecystography. It is excreted in the bile with minimal enterohepatic recirculation. Biligram-Infusion® has 17% meglumine ioglycamide delivering 85 mg I mL^{-1}.

Compound	Viscosity (cP)	Osmolality (mOsm/kg)	Iodine (mg I mL^{-1})
Meglumine ioglycamide	1.57 at 20	85	1.05 at 37
Meglumine ioglycamide	2.36 at 20	176	1.86 at 37

(*see* cholegraphic contrast agents).

Bilimiro[x] (*cm*) Generic name iopronic acid. Monomeric hepatobiliary x-ray contrast for oral use (*see* Biloptin, Cholebrin, Telepaque).

Biliscopin[x] (*cm*) Generic name iotroxic acid. Low toxicity replacement for Biligrafin. Biliscopin (Schering) is a commercial preparation of meglumine iotroxate for cholecystocholangiography (infusion cholegraphy).

Compound	Viscosity (cP)	Osmolality (mOsm/kg)	Iodine (mg I L^{-1})
Meglumine iotroxate (50 mg I mL^{-1})	1.3 at 20°C	290	50

Bilopaque[x] (*cm*) *See* cholegraphic contrast agents.

Biloptin[x] (*cm*) Brand name (Schering) for sodium iopodate, a capsular contrast medium for oral cholecystography, delivering 60–68% iodine by weight. Solu-Biloptin® contains calcium ipodate (*see* cholegraphic contrast agents).

bimodal distribution (*stats*) A probability or frequency distribution with two modes.

binary (*comp*) Numbers written in base 2. The fundamental counting system used by computers where 1 is ON and 0 is OFF. (Example: 001 = 1 decimal, 111 = 7 decimal, 01010 = 10 decimal) (*see* bit, byte).

binder (*xray*) Minimum concentration of resin material with very high transparency used as a substrate for intensifying screen phosphors. Currently represents 10% of the weight of the phosphor mix.

binding energy (*phys*) The energy which is associated with an orbital electron. High for K-shell electrons and low for L, M and N. Electronic binding energies are of the order 10 to 100 keV in heavy atoms. This is the energy necessary to free an electron from its orbit.

Tungsten has a K-shell energy of 69.5 keV and an L-shell energy of 12 keV. Copper has a K-shell energy of 8.9 keV and carbon a K-shell energy of 284 eV (*see* K-edge).

binomial distribution (*stats*) The distribution of the probabilities of the various possible numbers of successes (0 to n), when n independent trials are carried out. The probability generating function is $(p + q)^n$. The mean or expectation of the distribution is given by np and the standard deviation by $\sqrt{npq}$.

binormal ROC curve (*stats*) A receiver operator characteristic (ROC) true positive fraction (TPF) where:

$$TPF = \Phi(a + b \cdot Z_{FPF}),$$

where Φ represents the cumulative standard-normal distribution function, Z_{FPF} indicates the normal deviate which corresponds to the false positive fraction (FPF), and a and b are variables. Most empirical receiver operating curves (ROCs) can be approximated to this form.

Binz, Arthur (1868–1943) German chemist who first synthesized organic iodine compounds of pyridine in 1925, later used by Räth as x-ray contrast medium Uroselectan (*see* Räth, Swick).

bioassay (*dose*) Any laboratory procedure for estimating the nature, activity, location or retention of a radionuclide/agent in the body by *in vivo/in vitro* measurement of material excreted or otherwise removed from the body.

biodistribution (*nmed*) Distribution of chemical (e.g. radionuclide or contrast agent) in a living animal. Ideally, the highest chemical concentration should be in the organ or tissue of interest.

biological half-life (*nmed*) *See* half life (biological), half life, half life (effective).

BIOS (*comp*) (Basic input/output system). A set of programs encoded on a ROM chip. Programs (stored in ROM) that handle the start-up operations on computers. It enables the computer to perform basic input/output instructions during boot-up. The BIOS advises the operating system about the presence and type of hard drives, keyboard, processor etc. (*see* boot sector).

biplanar (*xray*) A system using two C-arm fluoroscopy units which have independent positioning. Commonly used in cardiac studies.

biplane angiography (*clin*) Angiocardiography in two planes at 90° or in paired orthogonal planes or synchronous fluoroscopic acquisition in two planes. Common procedure for cardiac imaging.

biplanar transformation (*di*) Converting an analogue filter into a digital filter.

BIR British Institute of Radiology.

BIRD (*mri*) Bilinear rotation decoupling.

birdcage coil (*mri*) A volume coil designed to produce a homogeneous B_1 field with multiple parallel conductors around the surface of a cylindrical volume. These are tuned so that at resonance there is a resulting homogeneous B_1 field. When the field is circularly polarized, the structure can be used as a quadrature coil.

bismuth Bi (*elem*)

Atomic number (Z)	83
Relative atomic mass (A_r)	208.98
Density (ρ) kg/m³	9800
Melting point (K)	544.4
K-edge (keV)	90.5

bismuth germinate (BGO) (*rad*) Bismuth germinate $Bi_4Ge_3O_{12}$ has high stopping power (high efficiency), high spatial resolution and are 50% more efficient than NaI (Tl) crystals; they are not hydrophilic. However, BGO is inferior in the following areas:

Light output	15% of NaI
Decay time	300 ns
Energy resolution	>20% (poorer than NaI)
Dead time	Long

The inferior time resolution causes larger accidental detections and greater **deadtime**. BGO detectors are best suited for imaging isotopes with long half-lives, such as ^{18}F and ^{11}C (*see* PET detectors).

bistable (*us*) Having two possible states (e.g. on or off; white or black).

bistable display (*us*) Display in which all recorded spots have the same brightness.

bit (*comp*) A word coined for 'binary digit'. Each bit in a computer memory can represent 1 or 0. The fundamental computer instruction.

bit depth (*comp*) *See* display resolution.

bit range (*ct*) Number of **bits** used to store the value of a CT value numerical entity; typically using a 12-bit with sign, corresponding to the range of Hounsfield units from -1024 through zero (air) to $+3071$ (*see* byte).

bitmap (*comp*) Bitmapped (or raster) graphics are images, rather than characters, composed of bits. Each dot on the page has a one-to-one correspondence, or mapping, to a digital bit stored in computer memory. The typical file extension for a Microsoft Windows bitmap file uses the extension of .bmp. A bitmap file defines an image (such as the image of a scanned page) as a pattern of dots, or pixels.

bit specification (*comp*) The size of the computer's internal word or working register. The amount of data that can be used simultaneously. The typical size is 32-bit, but 64 and 128 are used by some mainframe computers. The computer speed increases proportionately with bit specification.

bit speed (*comp*) Bits per second (bps). The measurement of data transfer speed in communication systems.

bivariate distribution (*stats*) The combined distribution of two random variables. The normal curve is an example which shows a bivariate normal distribution (*see* normal distribution).

bleeding (*image*) A print distortion where adjacent colours run and merge into one another, sometimes caused by excess ink or over-absorbent paper.

Blackett, Patrick Maynard Stuart (1897–1974) English physicist who confirmed the existence of the positron.

Bloch, Felix (1905–1983) Swiss born American physicist who developed the technique of nuclear magnetic resonance in the 1940s. He received the Nobel prize for physics in 1952.

Bloch equations (*mri*) A set of classical equations of motion for the macroscopic magnetization vector. They describe the precession about the magnetic field (static and RF) and the T1, T2 relaxation times. Solution for the three magnetic vectors is:

$$M_x = e^{-t/T2} \cdot \cos w_o t$$

$$M_y = e^{-t/T2} \cdot \cos w_o t$$

$$M_z = e^{-t/T2} \cdot \cos w_o t$$

showing that M will exhibit a spiralling precession. Longitudinal relaxation time T1 is the time required for M_z to increase from zero to $1 - e^{-1}$ and the transverse relaxation time T2 is the time for $M_{x,y}$ to decay from e^{-1}.

blood (biochemistry) (*clin*) Normal values

Albumin	2–48 g/L
Bilirubin	3–14 pmol/L
Calcium	2.3–2.8 mmol/L
Chloride	5–105 mmol/L
Cholesterol	3.6–6.6 mmol/L
Cortisol (am)	300–800 nmol/L
Creatinine	88–133 µmol/L
Globulin	18–39 g/L

blood (biochemistry) (*Contd.*)

Glucose (fasting)	3.3–5.6 mmol/L
Iron	13–31 µmol/L
Lead	<2µmol/L
Magnesium	0.7–1.0 mmol/L
Osmolality	275–295 mmol/kg
Phosphate	0.6–1.5 mmol/L
Potassium	3.4–5.0 mmol/L
Sodium	134–146 mmol/L
Thyroxine (T4)	70–140 nmol/L
Total protein	60–80 g/L
Uric acid	0.15–0.48 mmol/L

blood (hemodynamic values) (*clin*) Normal values

Central venous pressure (CVP)/right atrium	0–8 mmHg
Right ventricle systolic	15–30 mmHg
Right ventricle end diastolic	0–8 mmHg
Pulmonary artery systolic	15–30 mmHg
Pulmonary artery end diastolic	3–12 mmHg
Pulmonary artery mean	0–15 mmHg
Cardiac output (stroke volume × heart rate)	4–6 L/min

blood–brain barrier (BBB) (*clin*) The physiological interface between the blood, at the level of the capillaries and the brain parenchyma, which is the primary site of exchange between blood and the surrounding tissues. Brain capillaries lack fenestrations, unlike other capillaries preventing free passage of materials not necessary for brain metabolism but specific carrier systems enable active transport. Some lipid-soluble (lipophiliic) compounds can diffuse across (e.g. alcohol, nicotine and certain drugs, HMPAO). Passage through the undamaged blood–brain barrier by contrast media (radiographic and MRI) has not been demonstrated.

■ Reference: Dawson and Clauss, 1999.

blood cell (*clin*) A general term covering red blood cells (erythrocytes about 7 µm) which represent 45% of the blood volume (5×10^6 per mm^3). White cells (leukocytes) are present in smaller quantities (8×10^3 per mm^3) having dimensions of 9–15 µm. White cells are further made up of different cell types.

Men	Haemoglobin (Hb)	13.5–18.0 g/dl
	Haematocrit	0.4–0.54
	Red cell count	4.5–6.5×10^{12} L
Women	Haemoglobin (Hb)	11.5–16.0 g/dL
	Haematocrit	0.37–0.47
	Red cell count	3.9–5.6×10^{12} L
Both sexes	White cell count	4.0–11.0×10^9/L
	Platelet count	150.0–400.0×10^9/L
	Mean cell volume	77–93 fl

B

blood cell labelling (*nmed*) Different labelling techniques are used for erythrocytes and leukocytes. Leukocytes may be labelled with either:

* ^{111}In as oxine or tropolone,
* ^{99m}Tc as exametazime (HMPAO).

Both ^{111}In and ^{99m}Tc leukocytes localize in sites of inflammation and infection. Differences between the two chelating agents exist; one of the most significant is that ^{111}In-oxine cannot be used to label leukocytes in the presence of plasma because of the higher affinity of ^{111}In for transferrin than for oxine. ^{111}In-tropolone is a stronger chelating agent and using it does not require the removal of plasma prior to cell labelling. ^{99m}Tc-exametazime is able to cross the cell membrane of leukocytes. Once inside the cell, its structure alters to the hydrophilic form and the ^{99m}Tc becomes trapped within the cell. ^{99m}Tc-exametazime leukocyte labelling can be performed in the presence of plasma. Erythrocytes/red blood cells are labelled *in vivo* using a prior injection of pyrophosphate by ^{99m}Tc as pertechnetate. Alternatively, they can be labelled *in vitro* by withdrawing the pyrophosphate-prepared blood and adding ^{99m}Tc or using ^{51}Cr with fresh blood.

blood coagulation (contrast medium) (*cm*) All contrast media interfere to some extent with coagulation and clotting factors. In standard doses, this interference is usually clinically insignificant. It is clear that ionic agents have a more profound effect on inhibiting blood coagulation. The lessened anticoagulant effects of nonionic contrast agents, however, do not appear to increase the risk of thrombo-embolic events associated with angiographic procedures

■ Reference: Dawson and Clauss, 1999.

blood flow (*us*) Depends on the vessel length and radius, blood viscosity and pressure difference according to Hagen–Poiseuille's equation. The SI unit is m^{-3} s^{-1} if pressure is measured in pascals, viscosity in Pa·s and radius/length in metres. Doppler volume flow (Q) can be calculated as $TAV_{mean} \times A$ where TAV_{mean} is the angle corrected time averaged amplitude weighted for **blood velocity** and A is the cross-sectional area.

blood gases (*clin*) Normal values:

	Arterial	Venous
pH	7.35–7.45	7.31–7.41
PCO_2	4.7–5.8 kPa	5.5–6.8 kPa
HCO_3	21–25 mmol/L	2–29 mmol/L
Base excess	22–+2	0–+4
PO_2	10.6–13.3 kPa	4.0–5.3 kPa
O_2 saturation	95–99%	–

blood oxygen level (*mri*) *See* BOLD.

blood pool (*clin*) The intravascular space.

blood velocity (*us*) The table lists peak and mean blood velocities. The limits of current Doppler flow velocity measurements are about 0.3 cm s^{-1}, but this depends on the ultrasound wavelength.

Vessel	Vessel diameter (mm)	Peak velocity (cm s^{-1})	Mean velocity (cm s^{-1})
Arteries	25	100	25
Arterioles	0.04–0.1	1–2	1
End arterioles	0.02–0.04	0.2–0.3	0.2
Capillaries	0.003–0.008	0.02–0.05	0.05

blood volume (*clin*) Measured in millilitres per kilogram body weight:

	Mean	Range	standard deviation
Whole blood	69.8	53.2–86.4	8.3
Erythrocytes	22.7	20.5–34.9	3.6
Plasma	42.1	30.5–53.7	5.8

Bluetooth^{x} (*comp*) A telecommunications industry specification describing how certain types of mobile phones, computers and personal digital assistants (PDAs) can be interconnected using a short-range wireless connection technology. The maximum range is 10 m; realistically, considerably less than that, but not required as line of sight. Data can be exchanged at a rate of 1 megabit per second (up to 2 Mbps in the second generation of the technology). Built-in encryption and verification give minimal security. Bluetooth is also used for wireless keyboards, mice and similar pointing and input devices. Bluetooth networks feature a dynamic topology called a piconet or PAN. Piconets contain a minimum of two and a maximum of eight Bluetooth peer devices; data are synchronized. A transceiver chip included within each device, transmits and receives in a frequency band of 2.45 GHz. There are up to three voice channels that are available. Each device has a unique 48-bit address from the IEEE 802 standard, somewhat similar to an Ethernet address.

Blu-ray⁕ disk (comp) An optical disk storage format giving high-definition video and data storage. It uses a blue-violet laser (405 nm) used to read/write. Significantly more data can be stored on the same dimension disk than on the DVD format, which uses a red (650 nm) laser. A dual layer Blu-ray disk can store 50 GB, which is almost six times the capacity of a dual layer DVD. The first mass-produced Blu-ray disk was released by Sony in 2006. It recorded both single and dual layer.

Blumgart, Herman (1896–1977) US physician. Probably performed the first medical investigation using a radionuclide (radon in solution), when he measured circulation transit time in 1927.

Blumlein, Alan Dower (1903–42) English engineer who worked with the partnership of RCA and EMI pioneering the first electronic scanning television. He also patented automatic gain control, stereophony, versions of the cathode ray tube and shielded co-axial cable.

blurring (xray) See unsharpness.

BMP (image) Microsoft Window's native bitmap format BMP supports indexing through four- and eight-bit palettes. Rather than store all three RGB values, a palette is added to the BMP format, so each pixel becomes the index to this palette avoiding the necessity for storing the much longer RGB value. This look-up table approach is more efficient for handling eight-bit images of 256 colours. Only satisfactory for images with limited numbers of colours. Indexing each colour then needs a palette of more than 16 million colours, requiring a massive built-in palette. BMP was not accepted as a universal 24-bit Truecolor standard, because it is inefficient for the most demanding tasks such as handling photographs and print output. The only compression BMP offers is run length encoding (RLE) (see TIFF etc.)

BMS (mri) Bulk magnetic susceptibility.

BNMS (nmed) British Nuclear Medicine Society.

body coil (mri) A general body coil is installed in the magnet and functions as both a transmit/receive coil. It has a large measurement field, but does not have the high signal-to-noise ratio of special coils.

body surface area (clin) This is computed for dose or GFR calculations. Combines the individual's weight and height with the formula:

$$S = W^{0.425} \times H^{0.725} \times 71.84 \text{ or}$$

$$S = \log W \times 0.425 + \log H \times 0.725 + 1.8564$$

where S is body surface area in cm², W is weight in kg and H is height in cm (see surface area).

boil off rate (mri) Rate of cryogen evaporation in superconducting magnets, usually shown as litres per hour. The boil off rate increases during ramping and with eddy currents in the cryoshields using pulsed field gradients. Typical boil off rates are 0.03–0.075 L/h. In calculating cryogen consumption, additional transfer and filling losses have to be considered.

BOLD effect (mri) Blood oxygenation level dependent contrast. Oxygenated haemoglobin has a smaller magnetic susceptibility than deoxygenated haemoglobin. Transverse magnetization in blood vessels decays more slowly. This BOLD effect extends T2 and T2*, measurable as an increase in signal in the blood volume under examination.

BOLD imaging (mri) BOLD imaging uses local changes in blood flow to indicate the current level of activity in a region of the brain. Local concentrations of oxygen associated with changes in blood flow are measured in the BOLD effect.

Boltzmann constant (phys) This is calculated as the molar gas constant divided by Avogadro's number and equals $1.38 \times 10^{-23} \, \text{JK}^{-1}$. The average thermal energy of a molecule at an absolute temperature T is $k \times (T/2)$ for each degree of freedom. This equation shows how increasing entropy corresponds to an increasing molecular randomness (see entropy).

Boltzmann distribution (phys, mri) If a system consisting of particles in thermal equilibrium exchanges energy in collision, then the relative population (number) of particles N_1 and N_2 at two particular energy levels of E_1 and E_2 is given by:

$$\frac{N_1}{N_2} = e^{-[(E_1 - E_2)/kT]}$$

where k is the Boltzmann constant and T the absolute temperature. This equation suggests that in an NMR system at room temperature, the difference in numbers of spins aligned with

B

and against the magnetic field is slightly more than one in one million. The slight excess in the lower energy state is the basis of the net magnetization and resonance phenomena.

Boltzmann, Ludwig (1844–1906) Austrian physicist who was responsible for many original ideas, extending Maxwell's theory, black body radiation and atomic theory. In 1877, he presented Boltzmann equation relating thermodynamic entropy S and statistical distribution of molecular configurations W, so that $S = k \log W$, where k is the Boltzmann constant. This formula is inscribed on his tombstone in Vienna (*see* Boltzmann distribution).

bolus (*clin*) A circumscribed small volume of fluid (*see* Oldendorf technique).

bolus examinations/tracking (*mri*) Uses a contrast agent. A small amount of contrast agent transported by blood flow whose spread is followed. A method of displaying the moving spins after tagging them (locally altering their magnetization).

bone (compact) (*mat*)

Effective atomic number (Z_{eff})	14.0
Density (ρ) kg/m^3	1650 kg/m^3

bone (spongy) (*mat*)

Effective atomic number (Z_{eff})	12.3
Density (ρ) kg/m^3	1650 kg/m^3

Bone thermal index (TIB) (*us*) The thermal index for exposure where the ultrasound beam passes through soft tissue and its focal region becomes incident on a bone surface.

boot (*comp*) The process a computer goes through when it starts up. BIOS loads the operating system from the hard or floppy disk.

boot sector (*comp*) The section of the disk (hard disk or floppy) that holds information defining the characteristics of the disk. It also hold a short assembly language program that begins the process of loading the operating system (boot-up disk).

boron B (*elem*)

Atomic number (Z)	5
Relative atomic mass (A_r)	10.81
Density (ρ) kg/m^3	2500
Melting point (K)	2600

Bose, Satyendra, Nath (1894–1974) Indian physicist, involved in the evolution of statistical quantum mechanics (Bose–Einstein statistics)

for integral spin particles. Also contributed to the work on x-ray diffraction.

BOSS (*ri*) BimOdal Slice Select RF pulse.

bound electron (*phys*) For photon electron interactions, a bound electron is defined as one having binding energies considerably higher than the photon energy (*see* binding energy, photoelectric event, Compton scatter).

boundary layer (*us*) Sound reflection and transmission occur at boundary layers between media with different acoustic impedances.

bounded-square output power (*us*) Power emitted in the non-autoscanning mode from the contiguous 1 cm^2 of the active area of the transducer through which the highest ultrasonic power is being transmitted. The symbol is $W_{o1 \times 1}$ and its unit: milliwatt, mW.

Bouwers A. Dutch engineer/physicist who in 1930 produced the first rotating anode x-ray tube.

box-and-whisker plot (boxplot) (*stats*) A method of plotting data, useful in patient dose assessment, consisting of two lines (whiskers) drawn between the extreme values (smallest dose observed and largest dose observed) and a box drawn showing upper and lower quartile and the median value.

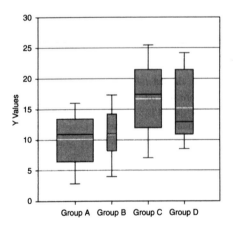

Boyle's law (*phys*) Part of the gas laws which states that pressure is inversely proportional to volume at constant temperature. Boyle's law states that gas volume is inversely proportional to pressure:

$$V \propto \frac{1}{P}$$

and as gas density is proportional to pressure, then sound velocity is independent of pressure changes (*see* Charles' law).

bow tie filter (*ct*) *See* form filter.

BP MR (*mri*) BiPhasic MR imaging.

Bq (*phys, nmed*) Symbol for **becquerel**, the unit of activity in disintegrations per second. Multiples are kBq, MBq and GBq. The non-SI unit is the curie (Ci, mCi and μCi).

braking circuit (*xray*) used to control rotating anode braking after exposure.

breakthrough (^99^Mo) (*nmed*) A **quality control** measurement for ^{99m}Tc purity. A small quantity of the parent radionuclide ^{99}Mo may be eluted with the ^{99m}Tc and can deliver an undesirable radiation burden to the patient. The National Pharmacopea limit (USA and British USP or BP) is 37 kBq/37 MBq ^{99m}Tc (0.1% of the ^{99m}Tc activity) and there should not be more than 185 kBq in any patient dose.

breakthrough (aluminium) (*nmed*) The support material in the generator column is alumina (Al$_2$O$_3$). Soluble aluminium ions can be included with the ^{99m}Tc-eluate. Freshly eluted ^{99m}Tc for radiolabelling should be used since Al concentration increases as the ^{99m}Tc decays (**specific activity** falls). The Pharmacopea limit (USP, BP) is 20 μg Al/ml ^{99m}Tc eluate for fission-produced generators.

breast compression (*mamm*) The application of pressure to the breast during mammography so as to immobilize the breast and to present a lower and more uniform breast thickness to the x-ray beam. Maximum value 130–200 N.

bremsstrahlung (*nmed*) Also called braking radiation. X-rays are produced when a charged particle undergoes deceleration as a result of the attractive or repulsive force exerted on it as it approaches an electropositive nucleus. The close passage of bombarding electrons to the target nucleus (tungsten, molybdenum) produces x-ray emission as a continuous bremsstrahlung spectrum. The intensity (*I*) of the bremsstrahlung spectrum varies with the energy of the electron (*E*) on the target and its atomic number (*Z*) as:

$$I \propto Z\,E^2 \quad \text{or} \quad I \propto Z\,kV^2$$

The complete spectrum is never available since the x-ray tube window absorbs (filters) the lowest energies. Efficiency (η) of bremsstrahlung production depends on: $\eta = k \times E \times Z$; where *k* is a constant $(1.1 \times 10^{-9}$ for tungsten). The production efficiency for tungsten and molybdenum, over a range of energies, are:

	Efficiency (η)
Tungsten (Z = 74)	
20 kV	0.162%
60 kV	0.48%
100 kV	0.814%
140 kV	1.14%
Molybdenum (Z = 42)	
20 kV	0.092%

brick (*shld*) Typical density 1800 kg m^{-3} baked clay solid building brick. Suitable for structural shielding material in diagnostic x-rays rooms. External walls mostly double brick thickness with or without cavity.

Thickness (mm)	Pb-equivalent (mm Pb)
150	1.0
260	2.0
340	3.0

■ References: Sutton and Williams, 2000; NCRP, 2004.

bridge (*comp*) Any hardware device that connects two physically distinct network segments, usually at a lower network layer than would a **router**; the two terms are often interchanged. A device that connects two networks at the OSI data link layer and passes data between them; equivalent to a two-port switch. Also a device that connects two **local-area networks** (LANs) or two segments of the same LAN. The two LANs being connected can be alike or dissimilar. A bridge can connect an **Ethernet** with a **token-ring** network. Bridges, unlike routers, are protocol independent; forwarding packets without analyzing and rerouting messages, so they are faster than routers but less versatile.

bright blood effect (*mri*) An effect of slow blood flow in MRI. Vascular spins are completely replaced by unsaturated spins during repetition time TR. In gradient echo sequences, the signal is maximum. The effect is used in bright blood imaging of the heart for dynamic display of blood flow, an effect that is similar for TOF angiography (*see* **BOLD**).

brightness (*phys*) Light intensity. The eye is sensitive to a narrow frequency range of **electromagnetic spectrum**, about 3×10^5 GHz or 400–780 nm, corresponding to the visible colour range. The amplitude of the vibration corresponds to perceived brightness, typically from 10 to 10^4 lux (*see* **contrast**, **Weber–Fechner law**).

B

brightness gain (flux gain) (*xray*) Ratio of image brightness from the output of an image intensifier to brightness at the input phosphor as:

$$\frac{\text{light photons from output phosphor}}{\text{light photons at photo-cathode}}$$

From the available x-ray flux and the total light produced by the output screen, typical values are 50–60.

broadband (*comp*) A high speed cable network transmission technique that uses radio frequencies. A broadband cable is typically shared with other networks or services, such as television or teleconferencing. Current data transmission speeds for domestic use are download at 2 Mbps and upload at 500 kbps. These can be exceeded for specific installations, i.e. medical data transmission.

broad beam (*xray*) An uncollimated radiation beam (x-ray) where scatter coincidence events can interfere with detection. Radiation shielding should take this into account. The half value layer is larger than for narrow beam measurements (*see* collimation).

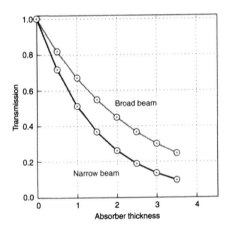

broad beam transmission factor (*shld*) An empirical model describes the broad beam attenuation (B) of x-rays through an absorber:

$$\left[\left(1+\frac{\beta}{\alpha}\right)\exp(\alpha\gamma x)-\frac{\beta}{\alpha}\right]^{-(1/\gamma)}$$

where x is the absorber thickness and α, β, γ the particular aborber fitting parameters for the polynomial.

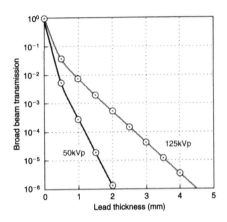

bromine Br (*elem*)

Atomic number (Z)	35
Relative atomic mass (A$_r$)	79.91
Density (ρ) kg/m³	3100
Melting point (K)	265.9
K-edge (keV)	13.4

bronchial arteriography (*clin*) Selective injection of the intercostal arteries with the contrast medium.

brachio-cephalic aortography (*clin*) Selective catheterization for subclavian artery occlusion.

bronchography (*clin*) Radiography of the tracheobronchial tree using iodinated contrast medium. Superseded by high resolution CT.

browser (*comp*) A method used for searching a database for quickly locating information; an idea extended to the Internet which approximates to a large database. The www is a hypertext-based system that uses browsers for extracting specific information. Browsers enable comprehensive program searching between documents throughout the worldwide web by clicking on highlighted keywords. Current browser packages are Mosaic (the first graphics browser and outdated), Netscape Navigator, Mozilla Firefox and Microsoft Internet Explorer.

bruit (*us*) Audible sound (using a stethoscope) originating in vessels with turbulent flow.

Bucky, Gustav (1880–1963) German engineer who in 1913 introduced a stationary metal anti-scatter grid. In 1914, he included a mechanism for moving the grid during exposure (*see* Potter).

Bucky (*xray*) Shortened expression meaning the moving anti-scatter grid.

Bucky factor (*xray*) Exposure increase factor when using an anti-scatter grid or ratio of incident to transmitted radiation.

bug (*comp*) A malfunction due to an error in the program or a defect in the equipment.

burst (*us*) A cycle or two of voltage variation.

burst-excited mode (*us*) A mode of operation by which a transducer is driven by a cycle of alternating driving voltage.

bus (*comp*) The internal pathway for signals moving inside the computer. A multi-wire connection that carries data between different parts of the computer or between computers. Buses for PCs are commonly ISA (obsolete), VESA and currently PCI which is the most efficient (*see* topology (network)).

bus master (*comp*) An intelligent device, such as a PCI adapter card, that can gain control of the bus and use it to transfer data without involving the processor.

bus network (*comp*) A decentralized local area network shared by a group of computers (nodes). The bus signals are only used by a selected computer that responds to a unique address code. Used by AppleTalk® and Ethernet. Failure of one computer does not disrupt the network.

Butterworth filter (*di*) Approximates to an ideal filter with maximally flat passband falling gradually toward the edge and passing through $1/\sqrt{2}$ (equivalent to $-3\,dB$) at the cut-off frequency. The transfer function of a Butterworth filter of order n is:

$$H_{(u,v)} = \frac{1}{1 + (D_{(u,v)}/D_o)^{2n}}$$

where D_0 is the cut-off frequency. The Butterworth filter does not have a sharp discontinuity between passed and filtered frequencies and although it has a smoothing action

this filter design passes some high frequencies so preserving edge detail.

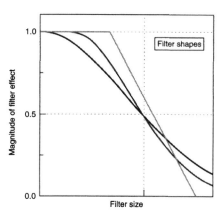

Filter shapes

The frequency response of the Butterworth filter is maximally flat (has no ripples) in the passband, and rolls off towards zero in the stopband (*see* filtering (signal), ideal filter, Chebyshev filter).

BW (*phys, mri, us*) *See* bandwidth.

by-product material (*nmed*) Radioactive material produced by nuclear fission (fission products) or by neutron activation in a nuclear reactor or similar device (*see* carrier free, radiopharmaceuticals (reactor)).

bystander effect (*dose*) The response of unirradiated cells triggered by signals received from irradiated neighbouring cells.

byte (*comp*) A unit of storage capacity made up from 8 bits (2^3). This will hold any number from 0 to 256. The byte is the composite building block common to all computers. Several bytes make up a word. Memory and disk sizes are usually quoted in kilobytes (1024 bytes), megabytes (1024 k-bytes), giga-bytes (1024 M-bytes). Byte speed in bytes per second (Bps) and bit speed in bps. However, nomenclature has become confusing and the differences between 1000 and 1024 bytes have been clarified (*see* kilobyte).

C

C/C++ (*comp*) A computer language commonly used for the creation of professional-grade applications. UNIX is primarily written in C. C is distinguished from other computer languages by using pointers (variables that point at locations in memory). Developed by Dennis Ritchie in the early 1970s, C++ is a variation based on C that uses objected-oriented programming (OOP) design principles. The language is a product of Microsoft technology and is part of the Visual Studio Development package.

C-arm (*xray*) A fluoroscopy design found both in small mobile and large fixed units. The image intensifier is fixed in-line with the x-ray tube on a C structure which is sometimes cantilevered giving oblique views.

cache memory (*comp*) An area of memory used to store a copy of information recently read from or written to a hard disk or located on the CPU chip. Temporary memory for storing information that is accessed most frequently. Typical cache memory is a small block of high-speed memory located between the CPU and the main memory. A cache memory can significantly improve data access speed. The Pentium processor has 8 k-byte of built in cache. The computer speed can be further increased by using a secondary cache formed on the DRAM or hard disk. Browsers also use a cache to store web pages so that the user may view them again without reconnecting to the web (*see* duo core, quad core).

cadmium (Cd) (*elem*)

Atomic number (Z)	48
Relative atomic mass (A$_r$)	112.40
Density (ρ) kg/m^3	8650
Melting point (K)	594.2
K-edge (keV)	26.7

cadmium telluride (CdTe) (*phys*) Semiconductor material used as a detector.

Atomic number (Z)	48, 52
K-edge(s)	26, 32
Electron/hole pair	4.4 eV
Efficiency	0.85–0.88

Uses: As a small volume room temperature photon detector probe for *in vivo* activity and also in the form of cadmium–mercury–telluride as a photon detector. Also cadmium–zinc–telluride and cadmium–mercury–telluride are used as semiconductor detectors.

caesium (*elem*) *See* cesium.

calcium (Ca) (*elem*)

Atomic number (Z)	20
Atomic weight (A$_r$)	40.08
Density (ρ)	1540 kg/m^3
Melting point (K)	1120
K-edge (keV)	4.03

^{45}Calcium

Production	^{44}Ca(n,2n) ^{45}Ca
Half-life	163 days
Decay mode	β − 0.257 MeV
Photons (abundance)	Pure beta

calcium binding (contrast medium) (*cm*) Calcium-binding characteristics inherent in ionic contrast materials and enhanced by the addition of chelating agents play a major role in the induction of adverse reactions. Sudden reductions in ionic calcium can interfere with the electrical conduction mechanisms of the cardiovascular system and lead to severe reactions.

■ Reference: Dawson and Clauss, 1999.

calcium disodium edentate (*chem*) *See* chelate.

calcium sulphate (*chem*) *See* plaster.

calcium tungstate (CaWO$_4$) (*chem*) Phosphor material used for intensifying screens. Now mostly superseded by more efficient compounds used as a detector material in conjunction with a spectrally matched photodiode, in some CT machines (*see* detectors (CT), rare earth screens, intensifying screens).

calibration (CT-scanner) (*ct*) Measurement for determining the individual detector channel sensitivity for each detector element of a CT system; the calibration is performed usually based on an air scan or an appropriate test phantom. Correction procedures are used to take account of variations in beam intensity or detector efficiency in order to achieve homogeneity within the field of view (CT number accuracy).

californium (Cf) (*elem*)

Atomic number (Z)	98
Atomic weight (A$_r$)	252
Density (ρ)	15.1 g/cm^3
Melting point	900°C

^{252}Californium

Half-life	2.6 years
Decay mode	Fission α 6.11 MeV
Decay constant	0.2665 y^{-1}
Photons (abundance)	Neutrons γ 64–590 keV

Relevance to radiology: Neutron source for activation analysis and therapy.

CAMELSPI (*mri*) Cross-relaxation appropriate for mini-molecules emulated by locked spins.

Cameron John R (1922–2005) American medical physicist. Founding member of the American Association of Physicists in Medicine (AAPM). Developed thermoluminescence for dosimetry and devices for measuring bone densitometry. Founded Radiation Measurement Inc (RMI).

Campbell-Swinton AA Scottish engineer credited with making the first radiograph following Röntgen on January 7, 1896 of inanimate objects, later published in *Nature*.

cancer (induction) (*dose*) Most information concerning the induction of cancer in humans as the result of radiation exposure comes from the Japanese atomic bomb survivor data and x- and gamma-radiation used in therapy. This has supplied information confirming the induction of malignancies due to exposure from low radiation doses. Radiation-induced cancers and the naturally occurring cancers in a population are identical, the presence of an increase due to radiation can only be achieved by statistical means on very large population groups. A considerable latency or latent period may elapse between radiation exposure and cancer appearance. It is assumed there is no threshold for the induction of malignant changes (*see* **latency period, leukaemia, dose–response curve**).

candela (cd) (*unit*) A measure of luminous intensity of a source emitting monochromatic radiation of frequency 540×10^{12} hertz in a given direction and with an intensity of 1/683 watt per steradian. Measured as candela m^{-2} (cd m^{-2}).

Object	Luminance (cd m^{-2})
White surface, sunlight	3×10^4
Viewing, light box	2×10^3
Flat panel (medical)	400–500
Flat panel (office)	350–450
White level, video screen	200
Flat panel (minimum)	170
Reading light	30
Black level, video screen	0.1
White surface, moonlight	0.03

Cannon, Walter B (1871–1945) American physiologist who pioneered the use of x-rays in 1896 to investigate the gastrointestinal tract in the dog and human oesophagus.

canonical forms (*di*) Use of expressions or equations in a form which is regarded as standard. For instance, the ellipse, parabola and quadric cone are classified by canonical form of their equations.

capacitance (*phys*) The measure of the ability of a capacitor to store charge where $C = Q/V$, where C is capacitance (farad), Q is the charge (coulomb) and V is the voltage between the conductors or plates. The unit of capacitance is the **farad**. In practice, micro-, nano- and pico-farads are used (μF, nF, pF).

capacitor (*phys*) Two conductors separated by an insulator (dielectric). The ratio of charge to potential difference is the capacitance $C = Q/V$, measured in farads. The capacitor is used to store charge (capacitor discharge mobile x-ray sets) or to give a time constant as part of a capacitor-resistor or capacitor–inductor circuit. In NMR, inductors and capacitors are used to tune the transmitter and receiver coils to the nuclear resonant frequency (*see* **farad, Geiger counter**).

capacitor charge/discharge (*phys*) This obeys the exponential law. Capacitor charging described as:

$$V_t = 1 - V_o \cdot e^{-t/RC}$$

and discharge, described by:

$$V_t = V_o \cdot e^{-t/RC}$$

where the voltage level V_t at any particular time t depends on the initial voltage level V_o and the product of resistance and capacitance termed the time constant. If R is in ohms and C in farads, then RC is in seconds. After the charge of a period equivalent to one time constant, the voltage has increased to $1 - 1/e$ of its initial value (63%) and discharged to $1/e$ of its value (37%). The process of time-constants forms the design of time base generators in most electronic circuits (timer devices, video scan rates, etc.) and critical time measurement in magnetic resonance imaging (MRI).

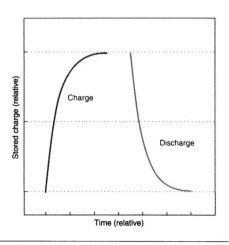

capillary blockade (*nmed*) Physical trapping of aggregated albumin particles by capillaries in the lungs, permitting performance of pulmonary perfusion imaging (*see* MAA).

capromab pendetide (*nmed*) *See* ProstaScint®.

carbon C (*elem*)

Atomic number (Z)	6
Relative atomic mass (A_r)	12.01
Density (ρ) kg/m^3	2300
Melting point (K)	>3800
Specific heat capacity J kg^{-1} K^{-1}	709
Thermal conductivity W m^{-1} K^{-1}	129

Relevance to radiology: Seen mainly as carbon fibre material in table construction and added to x-ray tube anodes to increase mass with minimum weight.

^{11}Carbon (*nmed*) A positron emitter used for positron emission tomography (PET).

Production (cyclotron)	$^{14}_{7}N(p,\alpha)^{11}_{6}C$ or $^{10}_{5}B(d,n)^{11}_{6}C$
Decay scheme (β+) ^{11}C	^{11}C $T\frac{1}{2}$ 20.4 m (β+, 2γ 511 keV) → ^{11}B stable
Half life	20 m
Decay constant	0.0693 min^{-1}
Half value layer	mm Pb
Uses	^{11}C useful for imaging drug receptor sites with PET

^{14}Carbon (*nmed*) A pure β− emitter

Production (reactor)	$^{14}_{7}N(n,p)^{14}_{6}C$
Decay scheme (β−) ^{14}C	^{14}C $T\frac{1}{2}$ 5730 y (β−, 156 keV) → ^{14}N stable
Half life 5730 y	
Decay constant	0.00012 y^{-1}
Maximum range	(water) 0.3 mm, (air) 220 mm
Uses	Sometimes used as an autoradiographic tracer and metabolic test. ^{11}C useful for imaging drug receptor sites with PET

^{14}Carbon (labelled urea) (*nmed*) As labelled urea (PyTest®). Oral test for the diagnosis of *Helicobacter pylori* (*H. pylori*).

carbon fibre (*phys*) Fine filaments of pure carbon bonded with resin to form extremely strong low attenuation material. At 70 kVp, a carbon fibre x-ray table will absorb approximately 14% fewer photons than a plastic table and a carbon fibre cassette 10–30% less depending on design. At lower energies (mammography), the attenuation figures are less (*see* Kevlar).

carcinoembryonic antigen (CEA) (*nmed*) Locally secreted antigen that may enhance uptake of labelled antibodies.

carcinogenesis (*nmed*) Induction of cancer by radiation or any other agent (a somatic effect).

Cardio-Gen$^{82®}$ (*nmed*) A ^{82}Sr/^{82}Rb generator (*see* ^{82}Rubidium).

Cardiolite® (*nmed*) In 1982, catonic ^{99m}Tc complexes containing isonitrile ligands were described. Further developments into isonitril compounds gave a commercial (DuPont Pharma, Bristol Myers Squibb) kit for the preparation of ^{99m}Tc-sestamibi, ^{99m}Tc-(MIBI)$^+$6 (Sestamibi or 2-methoxy-isobutyl-isonitrile) is taken up into the myocardium in proportion to blood flow and bound to the mitochondrial membrane. It does not distribute like thallium and remains bound for many hours (*see* thallium, Myoview).

Cardiotec® (*nmed*) *See* terboroxime.

carotid angiography (*clin*) Where selective injections are a problem in the presence of arteriosclerosis then direct puncture and catheterization of the common carotid is sometimes used. Colour Doppler sonography and magnetic resonance angiography (MRA) are largely replacing carotid angiography for diagnostic purposes and pre-operative evaluation of atherosclerotic disease.

carotid arteriography (*clin*) Arteriography using iodine contrast material for visualization of the carotid arteries usually performed from a femoral approach using percutaneous catheterization. Carotid angiography techniques are used for demonstrating the anatomy of the circle of Willis. Mostly replaced by colour Doppler ultrasonography and MRA for diagnostic purposes and pre-operative evaluation of atherosclerotic disease (*see* cerebral arteriography).

Carr–Purcell (CP) sequence (*mri*) Spin-echo sequence of 90° followed by a 180° pulse to produce a train of spin echoes; useful for measuring T2 relaxation times.

Carr–Purcell–Meiboom–Gill (CPMG) (*mri*) Modification of a Carr–Purcell sequence with a 90° phase shift in the rotating frame of reference (further 90° pulse) between the 90° pulse and the subsequent 180° pulses in order to reduce accumulating effects of imperfections. Suppression of effects of pulse error accumulation can alternatively be achieved by switching phases of the 180° pulses by 180°.

carrier free (*nmed*) Only containing the chemical of interest (e.g. radionuclide). A carrier-free state represents the highest specific activity (intrinsic).

carrier frequency (*di*) The fundamental frequency which is modulated by an input signal either by influencing amplitude or frequency (*see* amplitude modulation, frequency modulation).

Cassen, Benedict (1902–72) US scientist who developed the rectilinear scanner for nuclear medicine imaging in 1951 (*see* Mayneord).

CAT (CT) (*ct*) More commonly CT, since it now applies to any plane (coronal, saggital, oblique) (*see* computed tomography).

cataract (*dose*) A deterministic effect, the threshold dose being 2–10 Gy for acute exposure or a chronic exposure of 150 mGy y^{-1} over many years.

catheters (*clin*) These may be either radiolucent or radio-opaque. Catheters are manufactured in sterile disposable packs either straight with side holes or in predetermined shapes for selective angiography. Usually designated in French sizes.

cathode (*phys*) A negative charged nickel support for the filament.

cathode assembly (*xray*) The complete structure within the x-ray tube responsible for production and control of the electron beam. It consists of the filament(s) and surrounding precisely shaped cathode cup. A separate negative voltage can alter the beam shape in dual spot tubes or form an inertia-free switch for pulsed x-ray work (fluoroscopy and CT).

cathode cup (*xray*) A cup-shaped nickel depression in the cathode that holds the filament(s) whose sharp edges create an electrostatic field which focuses the electron beam on to the anode target.

cathode rays (*phys*) Electrons will travel through a vacuum from a cathode emitter (filament) to a positively charged electrode (anode). These electrons were given the name 'cathode rays' and could be deflected by electrostatic or magnetic fields (*see* cathode ray tube, flying spot).

cathode ray tube (*xray*) The basic vacuum tube display where an electron beam traces out a scanning motion by either electrostatic or magnetic deflection, under time base control, to give a visible signal on a phosphorescent phosphor or a raster scan image. Replaced by flat panel displays.

cavitation (*us*) Gas bubble production due to rarefaction events in a liquid. Production and dynamics of bubbles in sound (*see* ultrasound cavitation).

cavity ion dose (J_c) (*dose*) The ion dose produced by photon or electron radiation in an air-filled cavity surrounded by matter (*see* ion dose, standard ion dose).

cavography (*clin*) Angiography of the inferior vena cava usually by catheterizing the common femoral vein. Combined pelvic and caval venography may be performed by simultaneous injection of contrast medium through catheters inserted into both common femoral veins at the groin (*see* superior vena cava).

CBF (rCBF) (*clin*) Noninvasive measurement of cerebral blood flow, regional cerebral blood flow and regional cerebral blood volume (rCBV) is important clinically. Nuclear medicine techniques include ^{133}Xenon washout and PET. ^{99m}Tc labelled compounds (Ceretec™, Neurolite™) are also used for CBF studies. Major drawbacks are the poor resolution and exposure to ionizing radiation. Autoradiographic studies include ^{14}C-iodo-antipyrine. Fast MR imaging techniques now give images of tissue flow kinetics. Measured as millilitre per minute per 100 g tissue (brain); typical values being 20–30 mL/min/100 g, although this can be exceeded. Stable-xenon computed tomography is also used (*see* Kety–Schmidt technique).

CCD (*imag*) *See* charge coupled device.

CD (*comp*) Compact disk. An optical recording format on a metal foil disk (commonly 120 mm diameter), protected by plastic. Music, speech and digital data are permanently encoded in the form of pits or impressions, placed in a spiral track on one side of the disk. Information retrieval is by semiconductor laser focused on the track and modulated by the impressions. The CD-ROM is a read-only storage medium holding 650 M-bytes with a data transfer rate of 600 k-Bps and a typical seek time of 195 ms. The CD-RW (CD-Rewritable) is able to write and over-write data many times. CD-R is a one-time writing process capable of storing 550–650 M-bytes. Used for archiving and can be read by CD-ROM drives.

CD-R (*comp*) *See* CD.

CD-ROM (*comp*) *See* CD.

CD-RW (*comp*) *See* CD.

CDD (*imag*) *See* contrast detail diagram.

CDMA (*comms*) (Code division multiple access). CDMA is a digital cellular technology. Unlike GSM, CDMA does not assign a specific frequency to each user. Instead, every channel uses the full available spectrum and the frequency is divided using codes. CDMA has been implemented in 800 and 1900 MHz systems in various countries around the world. Currently three noncompatible mobile wireless protocols are vying for the wireless mobile market. They are GSM, TDMA and CDMA.

CEA (*clin*) Carcinoembryonic antigen. The expression of this tumour-associated antigen increases in a variety of carcinomas. It can be shed and detected in the serum by a variety of specific (monoclonal) and nonspecific antibodies. Labelling these antibodies enables tumour sites to be imaged (*see* carcinoembryonic antigen, arcitumomab®).

CE-FAST (*mri*) Contrast-enhanced FAST (Picker Medical Inc.); contrast-enhanced Fourier acquired steady state; commonly used for imaging cerebrospinal fluid (*see* CFAST, SSFP, DE-FGR, True-FISP, PSIF, ROAST, T2-FEE, E-SHORT, STERE).

CE-FFE-T1 (*mri*) Contrast-enhanced fast field echo gradient-spoiled GRE sequence (PhilipsT1-weighted); same pulse sequence as Siemens FLASH.

CE-FFE-T2 (*mri*) Contrast-enhanced fast field echo (T2-weighted) name of CE-FAST technique used by Philips.

CE FLASH (*mri*) Contrast-enhanced FLASH. A fast T2-weighted imaging sequence utilizing refocused transverse coherences.

cell killing (*dose*) The killing of somatic cells by radiation in a rapidly dividing cell population (e.g. blood, gut epithelium) becomes manifest in a few hours or days after exposure. In a slowly dividing cell population (e.g. nerve tissue), cell death may not be seen for months or years. If enough cells are killed, the function of the organ or tissue may be impaired (*see* deterministic effect).

cell modification (*dose*) Dose response as a result of specific DNA changes called 'neoplastic transformation'. A characteristic of this is the potential for cellular proliferation.

cell sequestration (*nmed*) The removal of damaged red blood cells from circulation by the spleen (heat-treated labelled red blood cells for spleen imaging).

cellular transformation (*dose*) Where a normal cell population is transformed into a malignant cell population by treatment with a carcinogenic chemical or radiation.

celsius (°C) (*phys*) A measure of temperature; formally degree centigrade.

Celsius	Kelvin	Fahrenheit
−273.15°C	0 K	−459.67°F
0°C	273.15 K	32°F
100°C	373.15 K	212°F

CE MRA (*mri*) Contrast-enhanced MR angiography.

centre frequency (*us*) Defined as:

$$f_c = (f_1 + f_2)/2$$

where f_1 and f_2 are bandwidth frequencies. The symbol is f_c and the unit is Hertz (Hz).

central field of view (CFOV) (*nmed*) This is 75% of the diameter of the useful field of view (UFOV). Generally, the CFOV represents the area occupied by the organ being imaged.

central processor unit (CPU) (*comp*) The central microprocessor, e.g. Pentium II, Alpha II, PowerPC.

central radiopharmacy (*nmed*) A facility that dispenses radiopharmaceuticals to a number of hospital users or institutions.

central ray (*ct*) The x-ray beam emitted from the focus and passing through the centre of the exit window of the x-ray tube that intersects the axis of rotation.

centre frequency (*di*) The frequency at which the peak gain occurs. (*us*) As: $f_c = \dfrac{f_1 + f_2}{2}$

where f_1 and f_2 are frequencies within the bandwidth. Unit: Hertz (Hz).

centre of rotation (COR) (*nmed*) The algorithm of backprojection requires accurate placement of the centre of detector rotation (e.g. gamma camera head) before data acquisition. Misplaced COR will give reconstruction artefacts. Adjusted so that 0° and 90° and 180° and 360° positions align before SPECT data acquisition.

central radiopharmacy (*nmed*) A facility that dispenses radiopharmaceuticals to a number of hospital users or institutions.

centripetal acceleration (*phys*) A mass m moving with a circular motion of radius r with uniform velocity v has an acceleration toward the centre called the centripetal acceleration (a) acting radially inward, where $a = v^2/r$. The inward force that must be applied to keep the body moving in a circle is the centripetal force (F) where $F = m(v^2/r)$. It is sometimes convenient to picture a counteracting force acting radially outward, termed the 'centrifugal force'.

CT fan beam support and x-ray tube
Centripetal/centrifugal forces on a CT x-ray tube and support of mass 100 kg and 0.6 m radius revolving at 0.5 s or 2 revolutions per second.

Force	$= ma = m(v^2/r)$
Velocity	$= 2\pi r \times 2$ m/s
Centripetal or centrifugal force is	
	$(100 \times (7.54)^2)/0.6 = 9466$ N

---

cepstrum (*di*) Whereas auto-correlation is the Fourier transform of the power spectrum, the cepstrum is the transform of the logarithm of the power spectrum. It more clearly indicates repetition of periodic signals.

ceramic scintillator (*ct*) Compounds containing yttrium, cesium, lanthanum, cadmium, tantalum, gadolinium and tungsten, are commonly used and have a high density ($>5 \, g/cm^3$). Good spectral linearity requires scintillator response to be linearly proportional to the x-ray energy changes between 90 and 140 keV. Solid scintillator materials are synthesized from transitional elements with additional doping agents used as a detector material in multislice CT scanners. Compounds used are gadolinium orthosilicate and yttrium aluminium perovskite suitably doped with cerium or europium. These have considerable detection efficiency advantages over simple scintillator compounds. Rare-earth-doped yttrium gadolinium oxide ceramic scintillators ($Y(x) \, Gd(y) \, Eu^{2+}O_3$) can be processed into a transparent cubic form with high purity >99.99% and density of $5.92 \, g \, cm^{-3}$; exhibit luminescence in the 600–900-nm range. The main europium emission peak is at 610 nm and matches the higher spectral response of the Si photodiode. Approximately 99% of the x-ray photons are stopped in a 3-mm-thick scintillator. The light output of $Y(x) \, Gd(y) \, Eu^{2+}O_3$ is 2.5 times higher than $CdWO_4$, but about 30% lower than that of CsI:Tl. High luminescent efficiency of >10.3% and a major peak emission occurs at a wavelength of about 610 nm and high light transmission in the 550–700 nm region. Doping materials are used to reduce luminescent afterglow below 0.1% at 100 ms without adversely affecting the other key scintillator properties. Important specifications for a CT ceramic detector are:

Requirements	Acceptable values
Large dynamic range	10^3–10^6
High quantum absorption efficiency	>90% (ideally 100%)
High luminescence efficiency	Ideally 100%
Good geometric efficiency	80–90%
Small afterglow	<0.01% 100 ns after end of irradiation
Good homogeneity	Purity >99.99%
Uniform response of all detector elements	<0.1% difference
High precision machineability	±10 μm

(*see* detectors).

cerebral angiography (*clin*) Radiography of vessels supplying the brain including extracranial vessels. The contrast medium is introduced percutaneously or through selected vessel by catheterization. The basic cerebral angiogram can demonstrate different parts of the cerebral vasculature depending on catheter placement. Selective cerebral angiography is divided into carotid arteriography and vertebral arteriography.

cerebral arteriography (*clin*) Demonstrates the vertebral and basilar artery and its major branches (PICA, ICA, superior cerebellar artery, posterior cerebral artery) (*see* cerebral angiography).

Ceretec® (*nmed*) A commercial preparation (Amersham) of exametazine in kit form for labelling with $^{99\,m}Tc$, also known as HMPAO. The labelled compound readily passes the intact blood–brain barrier and is retained in brain tissue probably due to intracellular conversion to a hydrophilic complex. The uptake closely matches regional cerebral blood flow (rCBF) (*see* HMPAO).

cerium (Ce) (*elem*)

Atomic number (Z)	58
Relative atomic mass (A$_r$)	140.12
Density (ρ) kg/m³	6800
Melting point (K)	1070
K-edge (keV)	40.4

^{141}**Cerium** (*nmed*) Principle gamma 145 keV and T½ 32.5d. used as a calibration source having an energy very close to 99 mTc.

^{144}**Cerium**

Half-life	284 days
Decay mode	β−
Decay constant	0.00244 d⁻¹
Photons (abundance)	134 keV (0.1)
Uses	Simulates $^{99\,m}Tc$ gamma energy and is sometimes used as a calibration source (*see* ^{57}cobalt)

Uses in radiology: Simulates $^{99\,m}Tc$ gamma energy and is sometimes used as a calibration source.

cesium/caesium iodide (Cs) (*elem*)

Atomic number (Z)	55
Relative atomic mass (Ar)	132.9
Density (ρ) kg/m³	1870
Melting point (K)	301.6
K-edge (keV)	35.9

cesium/caesium iodide (CsI) (*chem*) A phosphor compound found as the input phosphor for image intensifier tubes (CsI:Na) or, in its undoped form, as scintillation detectors attached to photodiodes.

^{137}Cesium/^{137}caesium (*nmed*) Used as a calibration source for laboratory instruments.

Production	$^{235}_{92}U(n,f)^{137}_{55}Cs\ (+^{97}_{37}Rb)$
Decay scheme (β−) ^{137}Cs	^{137}Cs $T\frac{1}{2}$ 30 y (β,γ 662 keV) → ^{137}Ba stable
Photons (abundance)	32–38 keV (0.07) 662 keV (0.851)
Decay constant	0.02296 y^{-1}
Gamma ray constant	8.7×10^{-2} mSv hr^{-1}MBq^{-1} @ 1 m
Half value layer	mm Pb
Uses	A high energy source for calibration and radiation safety tests

cesium/caesium iodide (CsI) (*chem*) A phosphor compound found as the input phosphor for image intensifier tubes (CsI:Na) or in its undoped form as scintillation detectors attached to photodiodes.

CFAST (*mri*) Cerebrospinal fluid-artefact suppression technique (Toshiba). Reduction of motion-induced phase shifts during time of the gradient spin echo (TE) (*see* GMR, GMN, FLOW-COMP, MAST, FLAG, GMC, FC, STILL, SMART, GR).

CFOV (*nmed, rad*) *See* central field of view.

CFM (*us*) Colour flow map or colour flow image (CFI) where the Doppler frequency is represented as a colour scale for each displayed pixel.

CGI (*comp*) Common gateway interface. A programming standard that permits visitors to fill out form fields on a web page and allows that information to interact with a database, possibly coming back to the user as another web page. CGI may also refer to computer-generated imaging in which computer programs create still and animated graphics.

c.g.s. (*units*) Metric measurement of centimetre, gram, second. Replaced by the m.k.s. system (metre, kilogram, second) used in SI units.

chain reaction (*phys*) A single nuclear fission initiating a series of nuclear transformations. A critical chain reaction 1:1 further transformations; a subcritical chain reaction produces 1:<1 further transformations; a supercritical chain reaction produces 1:>1 further transformations (*see* nuclear reactor).

channel (*us*) An independent element, delay and amplifier path.

characteristic curve (*film*) The graph plotting optical density against log exposure and producing a sigma plot whose position and gradient determine the characteristic of film speed

and contrast (latitude) (*see* dynamic range, film gamma).

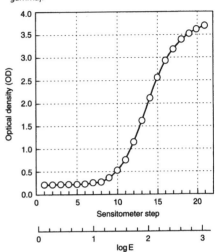

characteristic dose rate (*dose*) Defined differently according to application: (1) For x- and gamma ray studies, it is the air kerma rate K_{100} produced at the axis of the useful radiation beam without any scattering body present, at a distance of 1 m from the radiation source and a field size of 10×10 cm. (2) For x-gamma radiation, the maximum value of the water/energy dose rate D_{100} measured in water or water-equivalent phantom with the same geometry as (1). The photon equivalent dose rate for radiation protection is the value H_{X100} (*see* dose rate constant).

characteristic modulation (*image*) This is measured as the modulation transfer function value at 1 Lp/mm as is used as a guide for the overall resolution particularly for image intensifiers.

characteristic radiation (*xray*) Produced as a result of an electron vacancy in the K, L or M shell caused by either photon (photoelectric reaction) or electron (x-ray tube) bombardment. The electron vacancy in the K and L shell causes an electron cascade producing an emission spectrum (extending into the ultraviolet region) of characteristic radiation whose energy range depends on the element being bombarded. Characteristic x-ray energies for tungsten and molybdenum are seen in the continuous spectrum and characteristic x-rays are produced during electron capture decay. Characteristic K-energies:

Tungsten	69.5 and 59.3 keV
Rhenium	71.6 and 61.1 keV
Molybdenum	20.0 and 17.3 keV

For high-Z elements (e.g. lead) the photoelectric effect (PE) can be seen only as an attenuation process since the high energy characteristic radiation (88 keV) can escape taking part of the PE energy with it. Low-Z elements emit only very low energy x-rays which are entirely absorbed, so the PE effect shows complete absorption.

charge Q (electric) (*units*) The integral of the electric current with respect to time ($A s^{-1}$) and is measured in coulombs. The electron charge is $1.602 \times 10^{-19} C$.

Capacitor charge
At a voltage V the charge Q on a capacitor having a capacitance of C farads is $Q = CV$. Stored energy $J = \frac{1}{2}QV = \frac{1}{2}CV^2$. For a capacitor of $1000 \mu F$ charged to $220 V$ the stored energy is 50 joules.

---

charge (electrostatic) (*phys*) This is the integral of the electric current with respect to time and is measured in coulombs (C). The electron charge is $1.602 \times 10^{-19} C$. At a voltage V, the charge Q on a capacitor having a capacitance of C farads is $Q = CV$. Stored energy $J = \frac{1}{2}QV = \frac{1}{2}CV^2$. For a capacitor of $1000 \mu F$ charged to $220 V$ the stored energy is 50 joules.

charge coupled device (CCD) (*clin*) A semiconductor camera where a photosensitive surface is divided into many thousands of separate islands of photodiodes arranged in rows and columns. Position-sensitive array of photosensitive semiconductor material either as a linear device or as a matrix. A replacement for vacuum tube video cameras. The electron charge capacity for each pixel is 150 000. CCD cameras are commonly used with image intensifiers; their resolution depends on the image intensifier field size.

Matrix size	Pixel size (μm)
512×512	19×19
1024×1024	19×19
2048×2048	14×14

Electrons liberated by light photons are captured in a charge-coupled layer of the semiconductor. Each line of stored information is shifted electronically and read out as a direct digital signal. CCD frame area arrays:

CCD resolution: Lp/mm			
Intensifier (Lp/mm)	512^2	1024^2	2048^2
40 cm (3.6)	0.64	1.3	2.5
30 cm (4.0)	0.85	1.7	3.4
23 cm (4.6)	1.1	2.2	4.4
15 cm (5.2)	1.7	3.4	6.8

Charles' law (*phys*) Part of the gas laws and states that volume and temperature are proportional at constant pressure. From Charles' law at constant pressure $V \propto T$; since $V \propto 1/\rho$ where ρ is gas density, then $1/\rho \propto T$ so at constant pressure sound velocity is proportional to $\sqrt{T}$ (*see* Boyle's law).

Chebyshev filter (*di*) This gives a ripple effect in the passband. Its stopband performance is superior with a sharper transition. A Chebyshev filter is preferable to the Butterworth if some ripple is acceptable (*see* filtering (signal)).

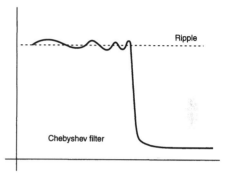

chelate (*chem*) An inorganic complex where a ligand is bonded to a metal ion at two or more points. A ligand linking at two points is bidentate; others are tridentate and tetradentate. Ethylenediamine can form two bonds with a transition metal. Common chelating agents are ethylenediamine tetra-acetic acid (EDTA) and can form four or six bonds with both transition and main group metal ions. DTPA: Chelating agents are added to iodine contrast media (EDTA) in order to inactivate heavy metals.

chelating agent (*nmed*) A chemical compound whose molecules can form several bonds to a single metal ion, so forming a chelate. Chelation combines a metal as a complex where the metal ion is part of a ring. The larger number (polydentate) of ring-closures surrounding the metal ion increases the stability.

chemical energy (*phys*) The potential energy liberated in a chemical reaction; the extent of reactivity between a functional group with a given reagent. Most commonly demonstrated by batteries both primary and secondary (*see* electron affinity).

chemical shift (*mri*) The change in Larmor frequency of a nucleus due to molecular binding;

caused by local alteration in the magnetic field. It is measured in parts per million relative to a reference compound. Chemical shifts make possible the differentiation of molecular structure in high-resolution magnetic resonance spectroscopy (MRS). The amount of shift is proportional to the magnetic field strength and is commonly specified in parts per million (PPM)

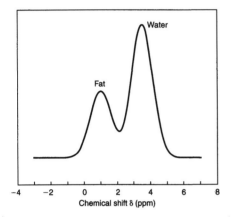

(*see* magnetic resonance spectroscopy).

chemical shift artefact (*mri*) This occurs with gradient echo sequences due to slight differences in resonant frequency between fat and water (approximately 3.5 ppm). Results in a shift in the fat images toward the water image. Visible at the tissue edges as contour artefacts (*see* chemical shift spatial offset).

chemical shift imaging (*mri*) An image of a restricted range of chemical shifts corresponding to individual line spectra. A magnetic resonance imaging technique that provides mapping of the regional distribution of chemical shifts corresponding to individual spectral lines or groups of lines. The chemical shift can be treated as an additional dimension to be reconstructed.

chemical shift reference (*mri*) A compound with respect to whose frequency the chemical shifts of other compounds can be compared. A standard compound used as a reference line in spectroscopy. Proton spectroscopy (^1H) uses tetramethylsilane (TMS). Phosphorus spectroscopy (^{31}P) uses phosphoric acid. The standard can either be internal or external to the sample; the internal is preferable since the need for possible corrections due to differential magnetic susceptibility between an external standard and the sample being measured.

chemical shift spatial offset (*mri*) Image artefact of apparent spatial offset of regions with different chemical shifts along the direction of the frequency encoding gradient, a similar effect may be found in the slice selection direction.

chemisorption (*nmed*) The surface binding of an administered radiopharmaceutical (e.g. binding of ^{99m}Tc MDP to the surface of bone tissue).

chemotoxicity (*cm*) This refers to the mechanism responsible for causing the toxic effects of contrast media that cannot be explained by other means. Chemotoxic reactions relate both to the hyperosmolality of the contrast material and to toxic effects inherent in the contrast material, including the cation. The toxicity of intravascular and intrathecal iodine contrast agents is due to chemical structure and chemotoxicity affects most organs. Chemotoxicity is expressed as high protein binding, hydrophilicity/lipophilicity, high tendency for histamine release, inhibition of biological function (enzyme damage) and coagulation effects. Toxicity of intravascular and intrathecal iodine contrast agents is due to chemical structure. Chemotoxic reactions affect virtually all organ systems. Contrast media with high chemotoxicity will have a low LD_{50} regardless of osmolality.

▪ Reference: Dawson and Clauss, 1999.

ChemSat (*mri*) Chemical saturation GE. Spectral pre-saturation to reduce MR signal intensity of fat (*see* FATSAT, SPIR).

CHESS (*mri*) CHEmical Shift Selective imaging. A pulse train used in single voxel slice selective magnetic resonance spectroscopy involving a single frequency selective excitation 90° RF pulse followed by a dephasing gradient (spoiling gradient or spoiler). This removes unwanted magnetization from the spin system. Useful in spectroscopy to selectively excite and dephase overwhelming water signals and typically precedes STEAM and PRESS pulse sequences.

chip (*comp*) *See* central processor unit.

chipset (*comp*) Provides the basic or core functionality of a device. Chipsets can be found in sound cards, graphics cards and almost every other piece of computer hardware.

chi-squared test (χ^2 test) (*stats*) A test of how well observed data fit a theoretical distribution. The chi-squared test is actually a test of the null hypothesis that the data are a sample being drawn from a parent distribution fitting the theoretical distribution being tested.

chlorine (Cl) (*elem*)

Atomic number (Z)	17
Relative atomic mass (A$_r$)	35.45
Density (ρ) kg/m^3	3.21
Melting point (K)	172.1
K-edge (keV)	2.82

cholangiography (*clin*) Radiographic examination of gall bladder and bile ducts using contrast media. Intravenous cholangiography (IVC) has been largely replaced by direct cholangiography, such as percutaneous transhepatic cholangiography (PTC) or endoscopic retrograde choledochography (ERC). MR cholangio-pancreaticography (MRCP) using T2-weighted images without any contrast material is replacing diagnostic invasive cholangiography in the majority of cases.

cholangio-pancreatography (*clin*) Radiography of the bile ducts and pancreas.

Cholebrin® (*clin*) Monomeric hepatobiliary x-ray contrast medium for oral use (Nycomed, Amersham). Generic name iocetamic acid (*see* Biloptin).

Cholecis® (*nmed*) A CIS/Schering preparation for $^{99\,m}$Tc-mebrofenin.

cholecystography/cholecystangiography (*clin*) Radiography of the gall bladder using contrast medium either through the cystic duct or intravenously, replaced in some instances by ERC or PTC. Water-soluble contrast medium can be taken orally; this remains the preferred method for gallstone detection, but its role has been diminished by high quality ultrasound imaging.

cholecystocholangiography (*clin*) Infusion cholegraphy.

cholecystostomy (*clin*) Drainage of the gall bladder, usually performed for inflammatory and obstructive biliary disease in critically ill patients; removal of gallstones.

cholegraphic contrast agents (*cm*) There are two major groups; oral cholegraphic media and intravenous cholegraphic media. In general, oral contrast media are ionic monomers and intravenous contrast media are ionic dimers. Protein binding reduces glomerular filtration in the kidneys so the major excretion pathway is the liver where the hepatocytes, combine these oral compounds with glucuronic acid and so actively excrete into the bile. Intravenous cholegraphic agents are also excreted into the bile, but are subject to different chemical pathways.

Cholegraphic media are excreted and concentrated in the bile rather than eliminated by the kidneys because of their very high degree of protein-binding. This factor causes ionic cholegraphic agents to have a higher chemotoxicity than urographic contrast media.

	Generic name	Commercial name
Oral cholegraphic media	Sodium iopodate	Biloptin®
Calcium iopodate	Biloptin®	
Iopanoic acid	Telepaque® Cistobil®	
Iocetamic acid	Cholebrin®	
Iopronic acid	Bilimiro®	
Iobenzamic acid	Bilibyk®	
Sodium tyropanoate	Bilopaque®	
Intravenous cholegraphic media	Meglumine iotroxate	Biliscopin®
Meglumine iodipamide	Biligrafin®, Cholografin®	
Meglumine ioglycamate	Biligram®	
Meglumine iodoxamate	Endobil®	

Choletec® A commercial preparation of $^{99\,m}$Tc mebrofenin (Bracco Diagnostics) and is an iminoddiacetic acid (HIDA) derivative. The structure is (2,2′-[[2-[(3-bromo-2,4,6-trimethylphenyl)-amino]-2-oxoethyl]imino) bisacetic acid. The labelled injected activity is cleared through the hepatobiliary system. Hepatic duct and gall-bladder activity occurs in about 10–15 minutes.

Cholografin® (*cm*) Intravenous preparation (Bracco) of meglumine iodipamide (52%) for intravenous cholangiography and cholecystography. Iodine concentration 257 mg I mL^{-1} (*see* cholegraphic contrast agents).

chromatic aberration (*phys*) When white light is refracted by a medium (glass), a coloured spectrum is formed due to the different velocities given by each wavelength: $c = f \times \lambda$. Red light is deflected least. Chromatic aberration is seen in some uncorrected high definition lenses.

chromatography (*chem*) A process for separating and analyzing molecules and compounds according to differences in the speed with which they travel in solution up an absorbing surface. Used for quality control techniques in radiopharmacy.

chromatography (*nmed*) High performance liquid chromatography (HPLC) formerly known as high pressure liquid chromatography, is increasingly being used for the ultimate purification of

C

radiopharmaceuticals and has found use in analysis. HPLC can separate all known and likely impurities in one analysis and is able to give chemical, as well as radiochemical, purity information.

chromatography (*nmed*) (Thin layer/paper, TLC/PC) These methods, which include reverse phase thin layer chromatography (RPTLC) and instant thin layer chromatography (ITLC) have been the main vehicle for the determination of radiochemical purity. The procedures are easy to set up and simple to use. They usually employ mixtures of commonly available solvents and chemicals, but can suffer from the inability of any one system to separate out all the likely impurities. It is the ability to quantify radiochromatograms which has made these techniques the method of choice in the analysis of radiopharmaceuticals.

Chromitope® (*nmed*) Sodium chromate preparation for labelling red blood cells (Bracco).

chromium (Cr) (*elem*)

Atomic number (Z)	24
Relative atomic mass (A_r)	52.0
Density (ρ) kg/m³	7200
Melting point (K)	2160
K-edge (keV)	5.98

^{51}Chromium (*nmed*) As sodium chromate, used for determination of red blood cell (RBC) volume or mass. RBC survival time and evaluation of blood loss.

Production	$^{50}_{24}Cr(n,\gamma)^{51}_{24}Cr$
Decay scheme (e.c.) ^{51}Cr	$^{51}Cr\ (\gamma\ 320\ keV) \rightarrow\ ^{51}V$
	stable
Gamma ray constant	$4.7 \times 10^{-3}\,mSv\,hr^{-1}GBq^{-1}$ @ 1 m
Half-life	28 days
ALI	1480 MBq (40 mCi)
Half value layer	1.7 (mm Pb)

(*see* Chromitope®).

CIDNP (*mri*) Chemically induced dynamic nuclear depolarization.

cine-camera (*xray*) A hard copy attachment to the output of an image intensifier to capture fast cardiac movement at 50–150 frames per second using 35 mm pan-chromatic film (*see* cine angiography, cine film).

cine imaging (*mri*) A set of images collected throughout the cardiac cycle where each image is acquired in a fixed portion of the cycle. When the images are replayed in a closed loop, they demonstrate cardiac pulsation, blood or cerebrospinal fluid flow.

circular polarization (CP) (*mri*) Excite or detect spins using two orthogonal transmit and/or receive channels/coils. Gives an improvement in SNR over a linearly polarized coil as a receiving coil.

CISC (*comp*) Complex instruction set computer. Processors that use a large instruction set for manipulating data. CISC computers take several clock cycles to perform a single operation.

CISS sequence (*mri*) Constructive interference in the steady state (Siemens); combines flow compensation with a DESS signal. Strong T2-weighted 3D gradient echo technique with high resolution. Two acquisitions with different excitation levels are performed internally and are then combined. Slower than balanced steady-state free precession as it uses a longer TR (repetition time). Streaking between dissimilar tissues (banding) is prevented.

Cistobil® (*cm*) *See* cholegraphic contrast agents.

class (*stats*) A group or collection (values) having a common characteristic (disease or population). One of a set of mutually exclusive, pre-established categories to which an object can be assigned.

classified person (*dose*) A worker who has been designated in accordance with local radiation safety regulations as likely to receive 3/10th of any relevant dose limit.

clean area (*nmed*) A room with a good standard of hygiene supplied with filtered air (class III BS5295) (*see* aseptic area, HESPA, laminar flow cabinet).

Clear-Pb® (*dose*) An acrylic plastic sheet produced by Victoreen Inc., containing 30% by weight of lead. Produced in the following thicknesses:

Thickness (mm)	Weight (kg m²)	Pb-equivalent (mm Pb)
7	13	0.3
12	22	0.5
18	33	0.8
22	40	1.0
35	64	1.5
46	84	2.0

This material is shatterproof and can be easily machined (*see* shielding (lead-glass)).

client (*comp*) Any computer system that requests a service of another computer system. A workstation requesting the contents of a file from a file server is a client of the file server. A client/server architecture allows many people to use the same data simultaneously. The program's main component (the data) resides on a centralized server, with smaller components (user interface) on each client (*see* server).

client/server network (*comp*) Communication structure between a client (fat client, thin client) and server in a network.

clean area (*nm*) A room with a good standard of hygiene supplied with filtered air (class III BS5295) (*see* aseptic area).

clinical trial (*stats*) A prospective or a priori clinical study designed to demonstrate the effect of a particular procedure, drug or diagnostic imaging technique on a selected group of patients. Sample size and methods of measurement play an important part, as well as a suitable control group.

clock speed (*comp*) A measure of how many times a second the processor cycles, measured in MHz. Current clock speeds can range between 500 and 1000 MHz.

clutter (*us*) Noise in the doppler signal that is generally caused by high-amplitude, doppler-shifted echoes from the heart or vessel walls.

CMOS (*comp*) The complimentary metal-oxide semiconductor is a battery-powered memory chip situated on the motherboard that maintains the clock settings and stores a record of the current system configuration.

CMYK (*image*) Cyan, magenta, yellow and black: the four basic process colours used in conventional colour printing. By overlaying or dithering combinations of these four inks in different proportions, a vast range of colours can be created.

CNR (C/R) (*image*) See contrast-to-noise ratio.

coagulation (*cm*) All contrast media interfere to some extent with coagulation and clotting factors. In standard doses, this interference is usually clinically insignificant. It is clear that ionic agents have a more profound effect on inhibiting blood coagulation. The lessened anticoagulant effects of nonionic contrast agents, however, do not appear to increase the risk of thromboembolic events associated with angiographic procedures.

coaxial cable (*comp*) A network cable with good noise immunity, also known as coax or thick-net. In coaxial cable, a single wire is surrounded by insulation and a woven copper braid that acts as shielding against electrical noise. There are two types: (1) Thick coaxial cable (also called 'thick-net'), the original Ethernet connection requires an AUI connector. Over time, thick coax proved to be expensive, difficult to install and clumsy, mostly due to its large size. (2) Thin coaxial cable (also called 'thin Ethernet' or 'thinnet') became the most popular cabling.

cobalt (Co) (*elem*)

Atomic number (Z)	27
Relative atomic mass (A_r)	58.93
Density (ρ) kg/m^3	8900
Melting point (K)	1765
Specific heat capacity $J\,kg^{-1}\,K^{-1}$	421
Thermal conductivity $W\,m^{-1}\,K^{-1}$	100
K-edge (keV)	7.7

Relevance to radiology: ^{57}Co as ^{99m}Tc calibration substitute. ^{58}Co for *in vitro* tests involving cyanocobalamine. ^{60}Co using the two close gammas for energy resolution calibration.

⁵⁷Cobalt (*nmed*)

Production	$^{56}_{26}$Fe(d,n) $^{57}_{27}$Co
Decay scheme (e.c.) ^{57}Co	^{57}Co T½ 270 d (γ 122, 136 keV) → ^{57}Fe stable
Decay constant	$0.00255\,d^{-1}$
Gamma ray constant	$1.6 \times 10^{-2}\,mSv\,hr^{-1}\,GBq^{-1}$ at 1 m
Half value layer	mm Pb

Days	Fraction remaining
10	0.975
30	0.926
60	0.858
90	0.794
150	0.681
180	0.631

Pb (mm)	Attenuation factor
0.06	0.5
0.5	10^{-1}
1.4	10^{-2}
16.0	10^{-3}
35.0	10^{-4}

⁵⁸Cobalt (*nmed*)

Production	$^{58}_{26}$Fe(p,n) $^{58}_{27}$Co
Decay scheme (β+, e.c.) ^{58}Co	^{58}Co T½ 71.3 d (γ 511, 811 keV) → ^{58}Fe stable
Decay constant	$0.00978\,d^{-1}$
Gamma ray constant	$1.5 \times 10^{-2}\,mSv\,hr^{-1}\,GBq^{-1}$ at 1 m
Half-life	71.3 days
Half value layer	mm Pb

^{60}Cobalt (*nmed*)

Production	$^{59}_{27}$Co(n,γ) $^{60}_{27}$Co
Decay scheme	^{57}Co $T\frac{1}{2}$ 70.8 d (γ 1.173, 1.333 keV)
(β−)	→ ^{60}Ni stable
Decay constant	0.13149 y^{-1}
Gamma ray	3.6 × 10^{-2} mSv h^{-1} GBq^{-1}
constant	at 1 m
Half-life	70.8 days
Half value layer	mm Pb

Cockcroft, John Douglas (Sir) (1897–1967) British physicist who with Ernest Walton in 1932 was the first to produce, artificially, a radioisotope by bombarding lithium with protons using a specially built particle accelerator, also verifying for the first time Einstein's mass-energy equivalence. Cockcroft and Walton were awarded the Nobel prize for physics in 1951. Cockcroft was director of Air Defence Research and director of the UK Atomic Research Establishment at Harwell. Elected FRS in 1936. Knighted in 1948.

Cockcroft–Walton effect (*phys*) In 1932, John Cockcroft and Ernest Walton in Cambridge, UK, bombarded ^{7}Li with artificially accelerated protons to form ^{4}He:

$$^1H_1 + {}^7Li_3 \rightarrow 2 \times {}^4He_2 + 17.3\,MeV$$

This was the first artificially induced nuclear reaction and the first demonstration of nuclear fusion. It was also the first experimental confirmation of Einstein's formula: $\Delta E = \Delta mc^2$.

code number (shielding) (*shld*) An early method of specifying lead or lead-equivalence; related to the weight per unit area in pounds per square foot (lb ft^{-2}). Examples for lead sheet are:

Thickness (mm)	Code	Weight (kg m^{-2})
1.32	3	15.00
1.80	4	20.40
2.24	5	25.40
2.65	6	30.10
3.15	7	35.70
3.55	8	40.30

coded aperture (*nmed*) Stationary collimators, usually a multi-holed design, which produce image data that need some form of decoding. The reconstruction algorithms necessary for coded aperture imaging are complex. Other coded aperture methods are applied to gamma camera imaging where the collimator is removed and an intermediate semiconductor array are used for scatter detection. The decoded image data are obtained by iterative reconstruction techniques. Sensitivity without the collimator increases camera sensitivities by up to 15 times; the resolution is degraded, however.

coefficient (*math*) A numerical constant used as a multiplier for a variable quantity when calculating the magnitude of a physical property. The coefficient μ is a linear attenuation coefficient which when multiplied by the absorber thickness gives the total attenuation.

coefficient of expansion (*phys*) See expansion.

coefficient of variation (*stats*) An absolute measure of dispersion as the standard deviation expressed as a percentage of the mean.

coeliac arteriography (*clin*) Arteriography of the arterial supply to the liver, spleen and stomach. Alternative imaging using CT, MRI and ultrasound (colour Doppler and duplex scanning) have reduced the need for coeliac arteriography.

coherence (*mri*) Maintenance of a constant phase relationship between waveforms. Loss of phase coherence in the spins result in decrease in transverse magnetization and loss of MR signal. In the quantum mechanical description of magnetic resonance, coherence refers to a transition between different states of the spin system (*see* multiple quantum coherence).

coherent (*mri*) A state of a spin sample in which all spins in a voxel are in-phase.

coherent scatter (*phys*) Also called elastic scattering. A photon interaction with the atom as a whole. The photon is scattered predominantly in the forward direction with no loss of energy. Its probability is proportional to Z^2 and inversely proportional to energy E. It is therefore reduced for soft tissues and high kV. It represents about 10% of events at diagnostic energy levels (*see* Compton scatter).

cohort labelling (*nmed*) Red blood cell (RBC) labeling using a radionuclide (i.e. ^{55}Fe), that is incorporated into the haem portion of haemoglobin by nascent RBCs during haemopoiesis, so that all cells are the same age.

coil (*mri*) Single or multiple loops of wire (or electrical conductor, such as tubing, etc.) designed either to produce a magnetic field from current flowing through the wire, or to detect a changing magnetic field by voltage induced in the wire.

coil loading (*mri*) The interaction of the patient with the RF coil due to magnetic induction and dielectric losses causing shifts in the resonant frequency and damping of the coil's resonance and hence reduction of the quality factor (Q).

coincidence counting (*nmed*) Two opposing detectors are operated in coincidence to detect simultaneous emissions of two 511-keV photons created by annihilation of electrons by positrons.

coincidence detection (*nmed*) Registering a co-incident event depends on the two 180° opposed photons being detected by the system within a specified time interval known as the 'coincidence window' (typically 10–20 ns). Opposed detectors used in PET imaging for registering the 180° dual gamma rays from a positron emitter decay. All events (*E*) that are found in coincidence can be true events (*T*), random events (*R*) or scatter events (*S*). These events are related by the formula:

$$E = T + R + S$$

True events represent good data. Random events can be estimated and corrected, and scatter events can be rejected. Location of the coincident event is assumed to be along the path between the two detectors. However, this is complicated in practice since not all events found in coincidence are true coincidence events.

coincident radiation (*nmed*) A positron β+ undergoes mutual annihilation with an electron e− yielding two 180° opposed gamma rays of 0.511 MeV; these rays are termed 'coincident radiation'.

cold spot imaging (*nmed*) Imaging a region of nonradioactivity, or relatively low radioactivity, completely surrounded by high levels of radioactivity.

collective dose (*dose*) *See* collective effective dose.

collective effective dose (*S*) (*dose*) (ICRP60) The effective dose related to exposed groups or populations. It is calculated as the product of the average effective dose $\bar{E}$ and the population number *N*: S = $N\bar{E}$. The *S* value relates to effective whole body dose. A valuable reference measure is the percentage collective dose; common diagnostic values are represented in the pie chart obtained from an exposed patient population. This indicates the relative contributions from each investigation, identifying the high-dose procedures (CT and contrast studies); the 'other' studies include chest extremities and nuclear medicine).

Collective effective dose

The mean effective dose for inhaled radon is estimated as 0.8 mSv, so for the UK population of 60 million *S* would be 48 000 man-Sv y^{-1}. The United States with 260 million *S* would be 200 000 man-Sv y^{-1}. Medical x-rays deliver a mean effective dose of about 0.5 mSv per year giving *S* values of 30 000 and 130 000 man-Sv y^{-1}, respectively.

---

collective equivalent dose (S_T) (*dose*) (ICRP60) The equivalent dose related to exposed groups or populations. It is calculated as the product of average equivalent dose $\bar{H}_T$ and population number *N*. The S_T value relates to a specific organ or tissue: $S_T = N\bar{H}_T$ The unit is the man-sievert (*see* cancer induction, equivalent dose).

Collective equivalent dose

The mean equivalent dose to the lung for inhaled radon is estimated as 6.6 mSv, so for a UK population of 60 million S_T would be 396 000 man-Sv y^{-1}. The United States with 260 million S_T would be 1 716 000 man-Sv y^{-1}

---

collimation (*xray*) Geometrical limitation of the extent of the radiation beam in the z-direction.

collimator (*xray*) Geometrical limitation of the extent of the radiation beam in the z-direction; earlier name cones. (*nmed*) The device in front of the camera crystal that accepts gamma photons only from a particular angle. Common collimators have a parallel hole design that only accept gamma photons perpendicular to the crystal face. (*ct*) CT scanners are commonly equipped with collimators between the x-ray tube and the patient (pre-patient collimation) defining the slice and dose profile according to the requested slice thickness giving geometrical limitation to the extent of the x-ray beam in the z-direction; some machines employ further collimation between the patient and the detector array (post-patient collimation) for improving the slice sensitivity profile; additional comb-shaped collimators close to the detector array in multi-slice scanners decrease the effective detector element width and so improve geometrical resolution. In conventional scanning, the slice sensitivity profile (SSP) and the dose sensitivity profile (DSP) coincide precisely. The width of this profile, measured as full width at half maximum (FWHM) is then the collimated slice thickness. Anti-scatter collimators between the individual detector elements, oriented towards the focus, have a width of typically 0.1–0.2 mm, while the separation of elements in the z-direction is approximately 0.1 mm.

colloid (nmed) A suspension of solid particles of sizes between 1 and 100 nm. There are several colloid materials, sulphur, albumin and antimony sulphide, used for imaging the reticuloendothelial system: liver, spleen and bone marrow. Tin colloid provides 80% of particle sizes between 0.05 and 0.6 μm. Sulphur colloid provides particles between 20 and 200 nm. Antimony sulphide (Sb$_2$S3) provides particles between 3 and 30 nm.

Generic name	^{99m}Tc sulphur colloid, ^{99m}Tc-albumin colloid
Commercial names	CIS-Sulphur Colloid® Nycomed SC®, Microlite®
Imaging category	RES (liver/spleen) gastric emptying, GI bleeding

(see Nanocol).

colour change (contrast medium) (cm) The main reasons for colour changes are: byproducts of manufacture and chemical decomposition. The yellow/brown discolouration is attributed to organic compounds and not free iodine.

■ Reference: Dawson and Clauss, 1999.

colour flow display/imaging (us) A 2D representation of blood flow (velocity). The Doppler signal is colour coded according to velocity and superimposed on a grey-scale ultrasound image supplied by a linear or phased array transducer. The pulsed Doppler transducer is incorporated in the array. Colour coded (blue/red) according to direction can also be displayed (see Doppler (colour)).

colour scale (di) Converting an image of count rate or signal strength into a colour-coded map usually by means of a look-up table. A rainbow scale typically represents low signal in blue and maximum as white with intermediate colours in a range from green, red, orange and yellow. A thermal scale uses an orange–yellow–white spectrum.

colour vision (clin) The human eye uses two sets of light sensitive cells: rods and cones. Rods are sensitive to low light levels, but are not colour sensitive. Cones are much less sensitive to low light levels, but have a higher resolving power and are colour sensitive.

Coltman JW American engineer who produced the first electronic fluoroscopic tube in 1948.

column (nmed) The solid matrix within a radionuclide generator where the parent radionuclide is chemically or physically bound.

columns (mri) Frequency-encoded portion of the measurement matrix (see rows).

comet tail (us) A series of closely spaced reverberation echoes.

committed dose equivalent (H_{T50}) (dose) The dose equivalent to organs or reference tissues that will be received by an individual over a 50-year period from the initial intake.

committed effective dose ($E(\tau)$) (dose) (ICRP60) If the committed organ or tissue equivalent doses are multiplied by the appropriate tissue weighting factors and then summed, the result will be the committed effective dose: $E(\tau) = \sum wT \times H_T(\tau)$ where $H_T(\tau)$ is the committed equivalent dose in tissue T, w_T is the weighting factor for tissue T, and (τ) is the integration period in years; 50 years for adults, and up to 70 years for children. The unit is the sievert (Sv).

Committed effective dose
The mean effective dose for inhaled radon is estimated as 6.6 mSv × 0.12 w_T = 0.8 mSv (whole body), giving an $E(\tau)$ value for a 50-year period of 40 mSv. A radiation worker receiving, on average, 1.5 mSv y^{-1} with a working life-time of 40 years, the $E(\tau)$ would be 60 mSv.

(see effective dose, collective effective dose).

committed effective dose equivalent (H_{E50}) (dose) The sum of the products of the weighting factors w_T to each organ or tissue and the H_T50 to these organs or tissues so:

$$H_{E50} = \sum wT \times H_{T50}.$$

committed equivalent dose ($H_T(\tau)$) (dose) (ICRP60) Committed radiation-weighted dose; subsidiary dosimetric quantity of equivalent single organ or tissue dose over a time period, where t is the integration time in years taken as 50 for adults and 70 for children following an intake of radioactive material. Defined as:

$$H_{T(\tau)} = \int H_T(t) \, dt$$

The unit is the sievert (Sv).

Committed equivalent dose
The mean equivalent dose to the lung for inhaled radon is estimated as 6.6 mSv, giving a $H_T(\tau)$ value for 50 years as 330 mSv.

(see equivalent dose, collective equivalent dose).

committed radiation-weighted dose, $H_{T(\tau)}$ (dose) See committed equivalent dose.

communications (*di*) Transfer of information between computers or computer networks. An important parts of a PAC's system (*see* **network**, PACs).

compact disk (*comp*) *See* CD.

compartmental localization (*nmed*) Placement of a radiopharmaceutical in a fluid space and then imaging that fluid space (e.g. a ventilation study with ^{133}Xe or a cisternogram with ^{111}In DTPA).

compensation (*us*) Equalization of received echo amplitude differences caused by different attenuations for different reflector depths; also called depth gain compensation (DGC) or time gain compensation (TGC).

compiler (*comp*) A special program that takes the instructions written in a programming language and turns them into machine code that a PC processor can understand.

complex numbers (*math*) There is no solution for x where $x^2 + 1 = 0$. This problem is solved by introducing an 'imaginary' number i so $i^2 = -1$. This develops as the equation $a + ib$ in physics, where a and b are 'real' numbers and i is $\sqrt{-1}$. Sometimes j and q are used instead of i (*see* **impedance, Euler's formula, Fourier analysis**).

compliance (*us*) Distensibility; nonrigid stretchability of vessels.

compliance (screening) (*stats*) The proportion of the population who present for screening amongst the total invited number.

composite (*us*) Combination of a piezoelectric ceramic and a nonpiezoelectric polymer used in the ultrasound **transducer** construction.

composite colours (*image*) Colours formed by mixing various quantities of cyan, magenta, yellow and black.

composite excitation (*mri*) Tissue excitation by a series of pulses rather than by a single radiofrequency (RF) pulse. Composite excitation provides the sum of signals to produce net excitation of a target tissue. Applications include selective excitation of water, or of tissues not subject to magnetization transfer.

compound anode (*xray*) The highest thermo-mechanical demands are placed on a rotating anode. It was originally manufactured from pure tungsten, but now has a sandwich formation of various metals including tungsten, molybdenum, rhenium and zirconium (TMZ). By alloying rhenium and tungsten, an improvement in the elastic properties of the 1–2 mm thick target is obtained, greatly increasing its wear properties. A disk base of molybdenum and zirconium increases heat capacity for the same mass.

composite colours (*image*) Colours formed by mixing various quantities of cyan, magenta, yellow and black.

composite video (*comp*) A video signal in which the luminance (brightness), chrominance (colour), blanking pulses, sync pulses and colour burst information have been combined using one of the coding standards (NTSC, PAL, SECAM).

compressibility (*us*) Ability of a material to be reduced to a smaller volume under external pressure.

compression (*phys*) The converse of expansion by heating and can only be observed in gases, since solids and liquids are incompressible. Compression increases the gas density so more molecules collide with the surface and therefore more kinetic energy is turned into heat. The heating effect by compression is the converse of expansion by heating and can only be observed in gases, since solids and liquids are incompressible. (*us*) Reduction in differences between small and large amplitudes; region of high density and pressure in a compressional wave.

compression (image) (*image*) Image compression improves both storage and transmission. Lossless and 'lossy' techniques are applied depending on acceptable image quality. Current methods employ JPEG algorithms based on a discrete cosine transform giving compression ratios of >50:1 (see Table below). Other techniques employ run-length encoding, wavelet and fractal algorithms (*see* PACS).

Image format	File size (MByte)	Property
Uncompressed TIFF	14.1	3 channels of 8 bits
Uncompressed 12-bit RAW	7.7	1 channel of 12 bits
Compressed TIFF	6.0	Lossless compression
Compressed 12-bit RAW	4.3	Nearly lossless compression
100% Quality JPEG uncompressed	2.3	Hard to distinguish from
80% Quality JPEG	1.3	Sufficient quality for 10 × 15 cm prints
60% Quality JPEG	0.7	Sufficient quality for websites
20% Quality JPEG	0.2	Very low image quality

compression (tissue) (*xray*) x-ray absorption obeys $N_x = N_0 \times e^{-\mu x}$, where N_x is the exit fluence and N_0 the incident beam intensity, μ is the linear attenuation coefficient and x the absorber (tissue) thickness. Compression reduces tissue volume, decreasing both absorption and scatter. This improves both image quality and tissue dose. Compression reduces object to film distance so reducing geometrical unsharpness and localizes the organ so reducing movement unsharpness. Compression therefore significantly influences:

- tissue dose;
- image resolution;
- image contrast;
- geometrical unsharpness;
- movement unsharpness.

compression paddle (*xray*) A rectangular transparent plastic plate parallel to the support plate carrying the imaging surface (film cassette holder) which compresses the breast using a remote control device. The maximum compression force is 200 N (approximately 20 kg).

compressibility (κ) (*us*) A factor used for calculating acoustic impedance and depends on the elastic modulus K (stress/strain) so that $\kappa = 1/K$.

Compton, Arthur H (1892–1962) US physicist who first observed and analyzed scattering of electromagnetic radiation in 1922. Awarded the Nobel prize for physics in 1927.

Compton continuum (*nmed*) The part of the gamma spectrum from the low energy region to the Compton edge which represents loss of energy in the detector material from Compton scatter events.

Compton edge (*nmed*) The edge of the Compton continuum in the gamma spectrum which represents maximum energy loss due to 180° scatter events (*see* gamma spectrum).

Compton effect (*phys*) *See* Compton scatter.

Compton plateau (*phys*) Broad, flat portion of a pulse-height spectrum corresponding to Compton scattering of photons in a scintillation detector crystal, patient and surroundings.

Compton scatter (*phys*) An interaction between an incident photon with an orbital electron in a partially elastic collision, transferring part of its energy to the electron and causing it to be ejected from its orbit. The residual gamma-ray energy is deflected at an angle opposite that of the ejected electron. The scattering of electromagnetic radiation requires that the electron absorbs energy from the photon and reradiates it as scattered radiation. The frequency of the scattered radiation is smaller than the incident frequency, so accordingly the wavelength is longer and the photon energy smaller. In order to preserve energy and momentum the wavelength before λ_1 and after λ_2 then the relationship is:

$$\lambda_2 - \lambda_1 = \frac{h}{m_e c}(1 - \cos\theta)$$

where $h/m_e c$ is the Compton wavelength for electrons. Substituting the constants gives the value 2.426×10^{-12} m. The equation demonstrates that the change in wavelength $\Delta\lambda = \lambda_2 - \lambda_1$ is not dependent on the incident wavelength. The change in energy $\Delta E = E_1 = E_2$ is given by:

$$\Delta E = \frac{E_1^2}{m_e c^2}(1 - \cos\theta)$$

$m_e c^2 = 8.19 \times 10^{-14}$ J or 0.511 MeV so rearranging gives:

$$E_2 = \frac{E_1}{1 + (E_1/0.511) \times (1 - \cos\theta)}$$

At low energies, the scattered photon retains a large fraction of the available energy as the photon energy increases, the recoil photon retains the larger fraction. For a 90° Compton event a 10 keV photon loses 1% of its energy to the Compton electron; a 100 keV photon loses 16% and a 1 MeV photon 66%.

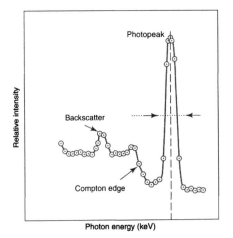

Relative intensity (vertical axis)

Photopeak

Backscatter

Compton edge

Photon energy (keV)

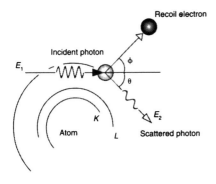

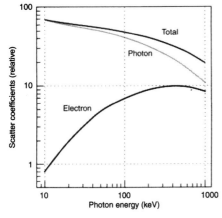

(*see* photon).

Compton wavelength (*units*) *See* Compton effect.

computed radiography (CR) (*image*) An erasable x-ray imaging device based on x-ray excitation of a phosphor layer and subsequent image data reading with an infrared (IR) laser (photostimulable luminescence); a method developed commercially by Fuji in 1983. The photostimulable phosphor plate (also known as an image plate, storage phosphor plate or computed radiography (CR)) demonstrates phosphorescence or photoluminescence so is able to store x-ray energy and later, when stimulated by an IR laser, frees the energy as emitted light. The light signal is detected by a photomultiplier tube, and the output electrical signal is digitized to form an image matrix. The final result is a digital projection radiograph (*see* Thoravision, direct radiography).

computed tomography (CT) (*ct*) A term originally applied to x-ray CT but can now be applied to other tomographic imaging techniques (nuclear medicine) where a series of ray sums are collected from a 360° sampling and then backprojected to obtain an axial section image. X-ray

computed tomography produces separate axial sectional images (transverse slices). Computed axial tomography is entirely different from linear tomography and produces radiological images as transaxial sections of the body without any intersectional interference or blurring. The method was first developed in a commercial x-ray machine in the UK by Godfrey Hounsfield in 1973.

computed tomography dose index (*ct*) *See* CTDI.

computer aided diagnosis (CAD) (*image*) A particular feature extracting algorithms used as a preliminary protocol for eliminating or detecting a specified image pattern. Used in mammography and chest radiology.

concatenation (*mri*) Distributing slices into multiple measurements. Prevents crosstalk in the case of short slice distance.

concentration (iodine) (*cm*) Both viscosity and osmolality of a contrast medium are related to the concentration or strength of the contrast medium. This is usually given in terms of concentration of iodine, indicating the concentration in milligrams of iodine per millilitre (mg/mL I).

concrete (*shld*) High density concrete 2350 kg m^{-3}. Load bearing must be at least 150-mm thick, typical density 2400 kg m^{-3}. Has a lead equivalent (Pb-eq) similar to barium plaster. Relevant details:

Lead (11340 kg m^{-3})	Concrete (2400 kg m^{-3})
0.5 mm	50 mm
1.0 mm	81 mm
2.0 mm	162 mm
2.5 mm	≈200 mm
3.0 mm	244 mm
4.0 mm	325 mm

Concrete is a cheap structural shielding material. Its density can vary between 2400 and

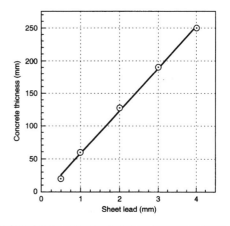

3200 kg m^{-3} and concrete blocks are typically 1750 kg m^{-3}. Modern hospital ceiling construction currently employs 200 mm prestressed concrete sections.

conditional probability (*stats*) The probability that a disease (A) exists given the positive result of a test (B). Described as P(A|B). An expression used in Bayes' theorem (*see* prevalence).

conductance (electric) (*phys*) Defined as the ratio I/V and is therefore the inverse of resistance being $1/R$. The unit of conductance is the siemens (S).

conduction (electrical) (*phys*) Depends on free electrons whose drift constitutes an electrical current. This has a slow velocity; a current density of 10 amps in 1 mm^2 cross-section wire shows an electron velocity of 6.25 mm s^{-1}.

conduction (heat) (*units*) Thermal conductivity is defined as the heat flow per second per unit area per unit temperature gradient. Thermal conductivity measured in W m^{-2} K^{-1} is called a 'U' value.

Silver	419
Copper	385
Tungsten	200
Molybdenum	150
Glass	≈1.0
Water	0.6
Air	0.02
Oil	≈0.15

Since the ratio of thermal and electrical conductivity is the same for all metals, it suggests electrons are also thermal carriers.

conduction (light) (*phys*) The phenomena of the propagation of light can be interpreted adequately by wave theory. Light is propagated by transverse waves since the vibrations are perpendicular to the direction of travel. Light interacts passively in transparent material, the main interactions being reflection and refraction.

conduction (sound) (*phys*) Sound travels through a fluid as a longitudinal wave (waves in which the particles of the transmitting medium are displaced along the direction of propagation; in solids, longitudinal, transverse and torsional waves exist. Propagation of sound into a surrounding medium involves disturbance in the medium, but because of a certain lag will have a finite speed. The speed c equals $\sqrt{E/\rho}$ where E is Young's modulus and ρ the density. For longitudinal waves, $c = \sqrt{k/\rho}$ where k is the bulk modulus. Sound waves in gas travel in longitudinal wave.

conduction (thermal) (*phys*) The speed of heat transfer. Measured in watts per metre per degree kelvin (or Celsius) W m^{-1} K^{-1} (°C^{-1}) as thermal conductivity, characteristic of the material, independent of size or shape. Generally the heat Q gained (or lost) by an object: $Q = mc\Delta T$, where m is the mass of the object, c its specific heat capacity and ΔT its temperature change. A loss of heat Q to the surroundings is $\Delta T = Q/mc$, the temperature fall ΔT of a small mass of material is greater than a large mass of material at the same temperature. The rate of cooling depends on nature and surface area, in addition to its temperature, mass and specific heat capacity. The table lists thermal conductivities of some important substances to radiology; silver has the highest value (427 J kg^{-1} K^{-1}) and air has one of the lowest 0.02 J kg^{-1} K^{-1}.

Substance	Specific heat (J kg^{-1}K^{-1})	Thermal conductivity (W m^{-1}K^{-1})
Water	4200	0.59
Oil	2130	0.15
Aluminium	910	237
Graphite	711	≈30
Titanium	523	23
Copper	386	401
Zirconium	280	22
Molybdenum	246	140
Rhenium	138	48
Tungsten	136	178
Glass	67	0.9–1.3

cones (*clin*) *See* colour vision; (*xray*) *See* collimation.

cone angle (*ct*) Aperture angle of a cone beam measured in the direction of the system axis of

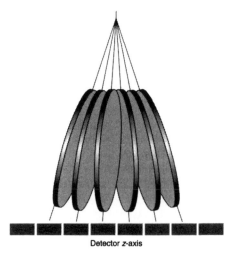

Detector z-axis

rotation. The data sets recorded by any single row in cone beam geometry will become increasingly inconsistent with increasing distance from the central plane. Artefacts will result whenever the cone angle exceeds a few degrees. Beyond four detectors, image distortion becomes pronounced and reconstruction algorithms are needed to correct for the divergent beam angles.

cone beam (*ct*) The transition from scanning one or only a few slices to data acquisition for an entire field requires the transition from fan beam to cone beam geometry. With single-detector scanners, the beam is always central to the detector and encounters the same tissue section. Increasing the number of detectors in the *z*-axis increases the angular volume and the beam dimension resembles a cone rather than a flat plane.

cone-beam artefacts (*ct*) An acquisition using cone beam geometry causes diameter decrease towards the top of the cone. These conic profiles are not treated in the same way during interpolation and this generates an artefact similar to a partial volume effect. Instead of a perfect circle, an ellipse–like reconstruction is displayed; more apparent when the cone has a large top angle, or when large pitches are used (i.e. skull).

confidence interval (*stats*) That interval within which a parameter of a parent population is calculated to have a stated probability of being positioned. The larger the sample size, the smaller the confidence interval. Commonly used for quality control charts that have confidence limits.

confidence limits (*stats*) The lowest and highest estimate of a parameter, that is statistically compatible with the data. For a 95% confidence interval, there is a 95% chance that the interval contains the measured parameter.

conformity (declaration) (*us*) A statement made by the submitter that a particular device was tested and meets the requirements of a recognized standard. It should clearly specify the following:

1 Any element of the standard that was not applicable to the device.
2 If the standard is part of a family of standards which provides collateral and/or particular parts, a statement regarding the collateral and/or particular parts that were met.
3 Any deviations from the standards that were applied.

4 What differences exist, if any, between the tested device(s) and the device to be marketed and a justification of the test results in those areas of difference.
5 Name and address of any test laboratory or certification body involved and a reference to any accreditations of those organizations.

Conray* (*cm*) Ionic monomer; a commercial preparation (Malinckrodt/Tyco Healthcare Inc) of meglumine iothalamate. Produced as Conray 30, 43, 400 also as Cysto-Conray®. Cardio-Conray has $400\,\mathrm{mg}\,\mathrm{I}\,\mathrm{ml}^{-1}$

Compound	Viscosity (cP)	Osmolality (mOsm/kg)	Iodine (mg I mL⁻¹)
Meglumine iothalamate	6 @ 25°C 4 @ 37°C	1400	282

conservation of energy (*phys*) The total energy in a closed system is always constant; this is the first law of thermodynamics. Energy may be converted into any other (mechanical into electrical in ultrasound; kinetic into electromagnetic radiation in the x-ray tube). There will always be a loss of energy in the form of heat (>95% in the case of x-ray production). This law applies to both inanimate (mechanical) objects and living organisms (*see* Compton scatter, photo-electric reaction).

conservation of momentum (*phys*) Conservation of linear momentum states that if no external forces act on a system of colliding objects. The total momentum of the objects is the same before and after the collision. Conservation of angular momentum states that the angular momentum about an axis of a given rotating body or system of bodies is constant and no external torque acts about that axis (applications in MRI) (*see* Compton scatter, photo-electric reaction).

constants (*phys*) Certain physical constants have special importance on account of their universality or place in fundamental theory. The constants commonly required in the radiological sciences are:

Speed of light, c	$2.997 \times 10^8\,\mathrm{m\,s^{-1}}$
Planck's constant, h	$6.626 \times 10^{-34}\,\mathrm{J\,s}$
Electron rest mass, m_e	$9.109 \times 10^{-31}\,\mathrm{kg}$
Compton wave length, λ_c	$2.426 \times 10^{-12}\,\mathrm{m}$
Gyromagnetic ratio, γ	$2.6752 \times 10^8\,\mathrm{s^{-1}T^{-1}}$
Avogadro constant, N	$6.022 \times 10^{23}\,\mathrm{mol^{-1}}$

constraint (*dose*) (ICRP60) A restriction on the predicted dose to persons from a defined source to ensure **dose limits** are not exceeded. The dose constraint is set at a fraction of the dose limit gained from general knowledge of exposure from the source and is seen as an **optimization**. Diagnostic radiology practice has a recommended dose constraint of 5 mSv per year (*see* **justification**).

constructive interference (*us*) Combination of positive or negative pressures.

contamination (*nmed*) Radioactive material present in undesired locations; a source of background or possible hazard requiring **decontamination**.

contingency table (*stats*) A table of observations/measurements cross-referencing a set of variable. The chi-squared test is commonly displayed this way.

continuous mode (*us*) Continuous-wave mode.

continuous spectrum (*xray*) Polyenergetic spectrum (*see* **bremsstrahlung spectrum, beta decay**).

continuous variable (*stats*) A measurement not restricted to fixed values (i.e. kidney function (glomerular filtration rate, GFR) or blood pressure).

continuous wave NMR (CW) (*mri*) Achieving nuclear magnetic resonance by continuously applying RF excitation to the sample and slowly sweeping either the RF frequency or the **magnetic field** through the resonant values; largely superseded by pulse MR techniques.

continuous wave (*us*) A wave in which cycles repeat indefinitely; not pulsed.

continuous-wave Doppler (*us*) A Doppler device or procedure that uses continuous-wave ultrasound.

contour artefact (*mri*) Chemical shift artefact.

contrast (CT) (*ct*) The absolute difference between the CT (Hounsfield) numbers of adjacent regions or structures within an image.

contrast (film) (*image*) Measured as the film **gamma**. This is not a property only of the film emulsion, it also depends on development temperature and time of the developer cycle. Contrast approaches a limiting value beyond which further development will have no effect (*see* **characteristic curve, optical density**) (*see* first figure in next column).

contrast (image) (*phys*) A measure of machine performance (e.g. CT or MRI) depending on the size and object density. Image contrast can be represented by a **contrast detail diagram** (CDD) and **contrast-to-noise ratio** (see second figure in next column).

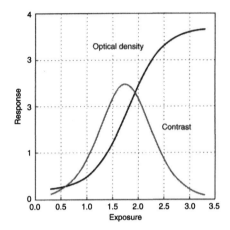

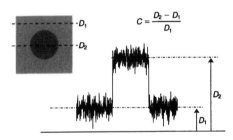

$$C = \frac{D_2 - D_1}{D_1}$$

contrast (MRI) (*mri*) The contrast behaviour in magnetic resonance imaging is complex. Contrast factors are generally divided into intrinsic and extrinsic, although they can interact and influence one another. Some of the factors are:

Intrinsic	Extrinsic
Proton density	Field strength
T1 relaxation	Gradient strength
T2 relaxation	Field homogeneity
Chemical shift	Surface coil type
Blood flow	RF pulse sequence
Tissue type	Repetition time
	Echo time
	Flip angle
	Contrast agents

contrast (radiographic) (C_r) (*phys*) A measure of image density differences by reference to the background (D_1) and object density D_2 so:

$$C_r = \frac{D_2 - D_1}{D_1}$$

This is influenced by image (film) gamma and windowing (*see* **contrast-to-noise ratio**).

contrast (subject) (C_s) (*phys*) Concerns beam intensity differences (DC) within the absorber (patient
volume, organ). If the incident beam (I_1) is attenuated when travelling through absorber (I_2); subject
contrast C_s is simply $I_1 - I_2$. The parameters
affecting subject contrast are: *kVp*, attenuation
coefficient, electron density, absorber thickness
and radiation scatter. Subject contrast should be
optimized for best radiographic contrast.

contrast (visible) (*phys*) This is measured from
the differences in the log of two intensities I_1
and I_2, so visible contrast is (log I_1 − log I_2). The
sensitivity to low contrast peaks at a brightness
level of 10–100 lux.

contrast agents (*mri*) *See* contrast (MRI), contrast
media (MRI). (*us*) These enhance blood velocity
signals, so improving vascular structures and
detecting low velocities. They are gas-filled
microbubbles (diameter < 10 μm) which respond
to pressure amplitudes of the ultrasound pulse
by expanding and contracting oscillations.
Oscillating amplitudes at low ultrasound intensities are linearly proportional to the excitation
pressure. They also allow evaluation of perfusion
textures and perfusion time courses in tissue
regions (e.g. tumour parenchyma). Contrast
agents are further used for:

- tissue differentiation in the liver;
- heart function;
- signal enhancement in transcranial applications;
- paediatric urine reflux detection from bladder to
  kidney.

Definity®, Sonovist®, Imagent®, Optison® and
SonoVue® are used for haemodynamic studies
and are various perfusion patterns associated
with specific tissue properties. Contrast harmonic
imaging shows the harmonics of the echoes from
oscillating microbubbles.

contrast detail diagram (CDD) (*image*) An example of a display threshold visibility assessment,
unlike an ROC analysis which is an assessment of
detectability. Observers see simple objects of
different sizes and contrast levels (typically circles) created by diagnostic imaging devices (CT,
nuclear medicine and digital x-ray). They are
asked to record their minimum diameter or minimum contrast that they perceive at a given
confidence level and results are plotted on a
contrast-detail diagram in which contrast (or
log-contrast) on the *y*-axis is plotted against
diameter (or log diameter) on the *x*-axis.

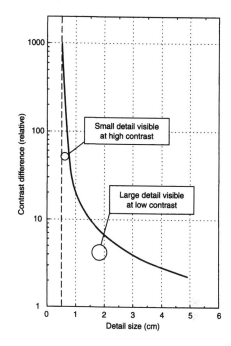

contrast-enhancement (*mri*) Contrast-enhanced
angiography utilizing the T1 reduction of moving blood through vessels.

contrast gradient (*film*) The slope of the film's
characteristic curve; measured as the gamma (*see*
sensitometry).

contrast improvement factor (*xray*) Improvement
of contrast when an anti-scatter grid is used.

contrast medium/material (*cm*) The imaging
procedure decides the most appropriate contrast medium. For x-ray imaging barium sulphate, iodinated compounds provide positive
contrast agents and gas O_2 and CO_2 provide
negative contrast; extracellular fluid contrast
media (ECF-CM) for angiography, urography, myelography, etc. Tissue specific-CM for cholangiography and macromolecular-CM confined to the
vascular space or blood pool. Water-soluble CM
is subdivided into renal excretion and biliary
excretion agents. Ionic and nonionic compounds are available. General intravascular
contrast media must have optimum osmolarity
and minimum chemotaxis including ionic
effects. Magnetic resonance imaging, paramagnetic,
diamagnetic and ferromagnetic compounds are
used, shortening T1 and T2. Ultrasound imaging (sonography) uses encapsulated microbubbles. For nuclear medicine (molecular imaging),
tissue-specific radionuclides or labelled agents

are used (*see* contrast medium, diatrizoate compounds and proprietary names).

■ Reference: Dawson and Clauss, 1999.

contrast medium (gaseous) (*cm*) Carbon dioxide is indicated intra-arterially for renal angiography. The gas displaces blood and acts as a negative contrast medium. There is an absence of nephrotoxicity and allergic reactions. Subsequently the CO_2 rapidly dissolves and is respired.

contrast medium (MRI) (*cm*) intravascular MRI contrast agents used in clinical imaging are paramagnetic compounds acting indirectly on T1 and T2 relaxation processes through alteration of the local magnetic environment, shortening both T1 and T2, the T1 shortening process dominating and produces enhancement. An MRI contrast agent has magnetic susceptibility, defined as the ratio of induced magnetism to that of the magnetic field applied. There are four categories of magnetic behaviour:

1 diamagnetic;
2 paramagnetic;
3 superparamagnetic;
4 ferromagnetic.

The most common paramagnetic substance is gadolinium and its compounds. Positive contrast agents cause a reduction in the T1 relaxation time (increased signal intensity on T1-weighted images), appearing white on the MRI display. These are compounds containing gadolinium, manganese or iron. These elements have unpaired electron spins in their outer shells and long relaxation times.

Generic name	Commercial name
Gadopentetate dimeglumine	Magnevist®
Gadoteridol	Primovist®, Prohance®
Gadoterate meglumine	Dotarem®
Gadobuterol	Gadovist®
Mangafodipir trisodium	Teslascan®
Gadodiamide	Omniscan®

Negative contrast agents are colloidal or small particle aggregates, typically superparamagnetic iron oxide (SPIO). These agents produce spin–spin relaxation effects causing local field inhomogeneities, which give shorter T1 and T2 relaxation times appearing predominantly dark on the MRI display. These compounds usually consist of a crystalline iron oxide core and a shell of dextran, polyethyleneglycol, producing a very high T2 signal. Colloids smaller than 300 nm cause strong T1 relaxation. T2-weighted effects are predominant.

Generic name	Commercial name
Ferucarbotran	Resovist®

A smaller group of negative agents are perfluorocarbons which exclude hydrogen atoms (protons).

■ Reference: Elster, 1994.

contrast medium (tolerance) (cm) A balanced addition of sodium and calcium to respect the electrophysiology of cardiac cells and improve contrast media tolerance in cardiac patients, especially during angiocardiographic procedures (*see* anaphylactic reactions, biodistribution, blood–brain barrier, distribution coefficient, excretion/elimination half-life, osmolality/osmolarity, pH value, pharmacokinetics, protein binding, tissue-specific, toxicity, viscosity).

contrast medium (ultrasound) (*cm*) These are microbubbles commonly contained in a carbohydrate envelope. These act as echo enhancers as the ultrasound beam passes from blood to gas in the microbubble. The enhanced echo signal is proportional to the magnitude in change of the acoustic impedance. Microbubbles are smaller than the capillary bed (lung and cerebral) to prevent embolization. Reflectivity is proportional to the particles diameter to the fourth power (D^4) and the concentration of microbubbles which are eventually retained by the liver. The success of ultrasound contrast material depends on its prolonged persistence in the vascular bed; however, certain targeted ultrasound contrast media are used for visualizing the liver and spleen (*see* Sonovue®).

contrast resolution (low) (*image*) A measure of the ability to discriminate between structures with slightly differing attenuation properties (CT number). It depends on the stochastic noise and is usually expressed as the minimum detectable size of detail discernable in the image, for a fixed percentage difference in contrast relative to the adjacent background.

contrast-to-noise ratio (CNR) (*image*) Ratio of the difference between two regions by reference to their signal to noise ratio: $CNR = SNR_1 - SNR_2$. Although radiographic contrast differences may be large, they may not be as visible as smaller contrast differences having lower background noise levels.

contrast ratio (*image*) A low contrast measure. Output light intensity before and after a 10% central region is shielded (*see* veiling glare).

contrast resolution (*us*) Ability of a grey-scale display to distinguish between echoes of slightly different amplitudes or intensities.

control group (*stats*) A population group not subjected to the test being applied. This is ideally a group of normals/members of the public.

controlled area (*dose*) (ICRP73) The control of occupational exposure in medicine can be simplified by the designation of workplaces into controlled and supervised areas. A controlled area is where under normal working conditions there is a possibility of exposure and workers are required to follow well-established rules and practices designed to reduce exposure. Commonly defined as a room or location, with limited access, where maximum surface exposure level is $7.5\,\mu Sv\,hr^{-1}$ or 3/10 of any maximum could be exceeded.

controlled trial (*stats*) An investigation using an agreed method of analysis on a group of patients with a matching control group (i.e. age, sex).

controller (*comp*) A circuit board that links the hard disk and the motherboard.

convection (thermal) (*phys*) The transfer of heat in air or fluid by the movement of the medium itself. There are two types:

1 Natural or free convection where the motion of the medium is due to the presence of the hot body giving rise to temperature and therefore density differences.
2 Forced convection where movement of the medium is maintained by mechanical means (e.g. a fan).

X-ray tube housing utilizes both sorts, liquid (oil and water) and air. These media can undergo free or forced convection depending on heat output.

convection (thermal: forced) (*xray*) *See* convection.

converging collimator (*nmed*) A gamma camera collimator which gives a magnified image, but also distorts with depth.

conversion efficiency (*xray*) The percentage of energy deposited in a detector that contributes to the output signal (electrical pulse or light pulse).

convex array (*us*) *See* linear array.

convolution (*ct*) A mathematical operation applied to two functions $f(x)$ and $k(x)$, where the latter is called the convolution kernel; the result $g(x)$ is defined as:

$$g(x) = f(x) * k(x) = \int f(t)\, k(x - t)\, dt$$

Commonly the * symbol is used as an abbreviation for the convolution integral. The back-projected matrix is subjected to a filter mask, or convolution kernel, whose contents are multiplied with the back-projected image. The mask is a small symmetrical matrix containing a set of numbers having positive or negative values. All the values are summed and the result placed in the central pixel of the image array. The filter mask is then shifted one column and the complete process repeated. The signal data are first logarithmically amplified to correct for transmission absorption, then beam hardening corrections are made. Each projection then undergoes the convolution process before back projection, the type of convolution filter can be chosen by the user, giving either image smoothing or edge enhancement. (*image*) For one-dimensional signals (e.g. renogram, bolus transit), convolution is the distribution of one function in accordance with a law specified by another function. If the original input signal is a delta function $f(x)$ yielding an output signal $g(x)$ influenced by the system's impulse response $h(x)$. It is assumed that the system is linear invariant. The process of deconvolution is the reverse, where $f(x)$ is extracted from $g(x)$ with a knowledge of $h(x)$. It is applied to renal transit times where a blood clearance curve undergoes deconvolution to yield the original spike injection peak.

convolution differencing (*mri*) A method of suppressing broad underlying spectral lines in order to emphasize narrower spectral lines. Strong smoothing of the spectrum (e.g. by severe negative exponential weighting of the time data) will suppress the narrow lines, but minimally affect very broad ones: subtracting such a smoothed spectrum from the original will largely remove the contributions from the broad lines. This provides a means of baseline correction. A form of spectral unsharp masking is sometimes used.

convolution kernel (*image*) A small square matrix used as an image filter. Can be small (3×3) having minimal effect or large (32×32) having maximal effect. (*ct*) A selected function for filtered backprojection, which can be varied to suit contrast detail (*see* image filter, convolution).

cookie (*comp*) A file that records information about specific details when accessing the world wide web. A message sent by a web server to a browser and stored on the client hard disk. Typically small files are downloaded to the workstation when browsing certain web pages. Cookies hold information that can be retrieved by other web pages on the site. The information usually identifies user preferences for tailoring responses.

Cooley–Tukey (*math*) The two mathematicians who developed the fast Fourier transform.

Coolidge, William David (1873–1975) American physical chemist. In 1908, he discovered how to manufacture ductile tungsten and in 1916 replaced the cold cathode in x-ray tubes with a heated cathode. The Coolidge tube was the precursor for all modern x-ray tubes.

cooling curve (*xray*) Measures the heat lost by the x-ray tube and determines the tube workload (loadability). Depends on anode heat storage and temperature t, since heat loss is proportional to t^4, measured in joules per minute. Tube housing is also involved and forced convection is sometimes necessary to improve heat loss (*see* heat storage, tube rating, anode cooling).

coordinate system (*ct*) Cartesian x, y and z-coordinate system of the CT system; the x/y-plane is the transverse or section-slice plane in anatomy (this is not the case when the gantry is tilted), the x-axis points in the lateral direction, the y-axis is oriented in the anterior-posterior or posterior–anterior direction; the z-axis is orthogonal to the scan plane and parallel to the table movement.

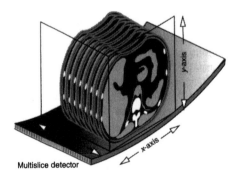

Multislice detector

COPE (*mri*) Centrally ordered phase encoding. A respiratory compensation technique.

copper (Cu) (*elem*)

Atomic number (Z)	29
Relative atomic mass (A_r)	63.54
Density (ρ) kg/m³	8930
Melting point (K)	1356
Specific heat capacity $J\,kg^{-1}K^{-1}$	385
Thermal conductivity $W\,m^{-1}K^{-1}$	401
K-edge (keV)	8.9
Relevance to radiology: Electrical conductor and x-ray beam filter	

^{64}**Copper** (*nmed*) $\beta+$ energy 656 keV

Production (cyclotron)	$^{64}_{28}Ni(p,n)^{64}_{29}Cu$
Decay scheme	^{64}Cu $T\frac{1}{2}$ 12.7 hr
($\beta+$) ^{64}Cu	($\beta+$, 2γ 511 keV) → ^{64}Ni stable
Half value layer	4.1 mm Pb (0.511 MeV γ)
Generator derived positron emission isotope for PET imaging	

CORE (*mri*) COnstrained RE-construction. Method of reconstructing artefact-free super resolution images.

Cormack, Alan MacLeod American medical physicist who pioneered the first computerized axial scanner independently of Godfrey Hounsfield, sharing the Nobel prize in 1979.

coronal plane (*ct*) Anatomical plane orthogonal to the transverse (axial) and the sagittal plane; in the CT coordinate system the coronal plane is usually oriented parallel to the z-plane.

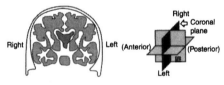

coronary angiography (*clin*) Radiography of myocardial vessels by introducing contrast medium into a selected vessel (typically femoral or brachial route or directly into aorta).

coronary arteriography (*clin*) Right heart arteriography: Using the fluoroscopic technique, a catheter is usually inserted into the median basilica or saphenous vein and advanced into the right atrium. Left heart arteriography: The catheter, under fluoroscopic control, is advanced via the femoral or axillary artery mostly using a Seldinger technique then advanced along the aorta into the chambers of the left heart and contrast medium injected.

correlation (*stats*) An interdependence between pairs of measurements/variables.

correlation coefficient (*stats*) A measure of association between two random variables. If one variable changes with the other then they are said to be correlated.

correlation time (*mri*) The characteristic time between significant fluctuations in the local magnetic field experienced by a spin due to molecular motions. For values of the correlation time, such that the magnetic field as a function of time has large Fourier components near the resonance frequency, the TI relaxation time will be shortened.

cos (*math*) Symbol used for cosine in trigonometry.

cosine transform (*di*) *See* discrete cosine transform.

couch/table increment (*ct*) Distance by which position of patient couch (table) is changed between individual slices in serial scanning or the distance the couch position is changed during one 3600 rotation of the tube during helical scanning.

coulomb C (*units*) The SI unit of charge; one coulomb is the charge carried by 6.24×10^{18} electrons and one ampere is equal to one coulomb per second $(C s^{-1})$; the charge transferred by a current of one ampere in one second; each electron has a charge Q of $1.6 \times 10^{-19} C$ so:

$$I = \frac{Q}{t} \quad \text{or} \quad Q = I \times t.$$

Radiation exposure can be measured as coulombs per kilogram $(C kg^{-1})$ where one roentgen $(1 R)$ is 2.58×10^{-4} $C kg^{-1}$ and one milligray (mGy) is 2.9452×10^{-5} $C kg^{-1}$ or $29.452 \mu C kg^{-1}$.

Radiation exposure
For an exposure 100 mA for 0.5 s (50 mAs) so since $I = 0.1 Cs^{-1}$ and $Q = 0.05 C$ or 50 mC (millicoulombs) so 1 mAs is equivalent to 1 mC.

Coulomb, Charles Augustine de (1736–1806) French physicist who measured the force of magnetic and electrical attraction. The SI unit for the quantity of charge is the coulomb (C).

coulomb field (*xray*) A force of attraction or repulsion due to an electric field interaction. The electric field surrounding a point charge or edge. Electrostatic field responsible for shaping the electron beam in an x-ray tube. Each electron has a charge (Q) of $1.6 \times 10^{-19} C$. As the force is proportional to charge $F \propto Q$ then every charge produces an electric field equal to F/Q. The magnitude of the coulomb field obeys the inverse square law (*see* cathode cup).

Council Directive 92/85/EEC (*dose*) (EEC) Directive of October 19, 1992 introducing measures to encourage improvements in the safety and health at work of pregnant workers and workers who have recently given birth or are breastfeeding.

Council Directive 96/29/Euratom (*dose*) (EEC) Directive of May 13, 1996 which lays down the Basic Safety Standards for the protection of the health of workers and the general public against the dangers arising from ionizing radiation. Repealing previous directives with effect from May 13, 2000.

Council Directive 97/43/Euratom (*dose*) (EEC) Directive on health protection of individuals against the dangers of ionizing radiation in relation to medical exposure. Referring to points: justification, optimization, responsibilities, procedures, training, equipment, special practices, special protection during pregnancy and breastfeeding potential exposure, estimates of population doses and inspection. Repealing Directive 84/466/Euratom on May 13, 2000.

count density (*image*) A term usually applied to nuclear medicine images, where 100 k, 5 M, etc. represents the total count for a particular study. The count density for a study depends on whether the organ under examination is uniform (liver, lung) or localized (bone). A larger count density would be necessary for a uniform object so that pixel values N remain high and noise low (since SNR $\propto \sqrt{N}$.

count loss (*nmed*) *See* dead time.

count rate (intrinsic) (*nmed*) Five measurements are made to characterize the count rate performance of gamma cameras (1) input count rate for a 20% count loss; (2) maximum count rate; (3) incident compared to observed count rate; (4) intrinsic spatial resolution at 75 000 cps (observed) and (5) intrinsic flood field uniformity at 75 000 cps (observed).

counts per second (cps) (*rad*) A measure of activity (*see* becquerel).

coupled array coils (*mri*) Array coils, the signals from whose elements are electrically combined before processing.

coupling (*mri*) *See* spin–spin coupling.

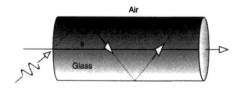

coupling constant (*mri*) Spectral lines are split by spin–spin coupling into multiplets whose frequencies are separated depending on the value of coupling constant J. The magnitude of J is independent of magnetic field strength. The unit is the Hertz (Hz). A measure of the frequency separation of spectral lines by spin–spin coupling into multiplets.

coupling gel/medium (*us*) Soft grease provides continuous interface excluding air; a gel used to provide a good sound path between a transducer and the skin by eliminating the air between the two.

CP (*mri*) *See* Carr–Purcell.

CP coil (*mri*) Circularly polarized transmission or receiver coil with two orthogonal transmission and/or receiver channels; the receiver coil gives a better signal-to-noise ratio than linearly polarized coils.

CPMG (*mri*) Carr–Purcell–Meiboom–Gill. Method used in SE imaging in which phase of RF is varied between pulses.

c.p.s. (*rad*) *See* counts per second.

CPU (*comp*) Central processing unit comprising the computer micro integrated circuit (micro-chip) and immediate ancillary circuits. Usually visible as a small block on the motherboard with its own heat sink.

critical angle (*phys*) The angle of incidence of light when proceeding from one medium to another with a different refractive index. Light incident at a greater angle suffers total internal reflection. Important consideration for fibreoptic transmission. Considering the respective velocities in the incident and refractive medium (c_i and c_t, respectively) then:

$$\frac{\sin\theta_i}{\sin\theta_t} = \frac{C_i}{C_t} = k.$$

This last statement is Snell's law and the constant k is the index of refraction of one medium with respect to the other medium. When $k < 1$, there is an angle of incidence where $\sin\theta_i = k$ then the above equation gives $\theta_t = 1$ or $90°$ and the refracted beam is parallel to the surface; θ_i is then the critical angle (θ_λ) which depends only on the velocity of ultrasound in the two media Z_1 and Z_2. If $\theta_i > \theta_\lambda$ or $\sin\theta_i > k$, then $\sin\theta_t > 1$, which is not possible, so no refracted beam exists only a reflected one. Total reflection is important to fibreoptics (*see* angle of reflection).

(*see* Snell's law).

Cranial bone thermal index (TIC) (*us*) The thermal index for ultrasound exposure, where the ultrasound beam passes through bone at the beam entrance.

Crookes, William (1832–1919) English chemist and physicist who studied cathode rays using vacuum tubes of his own design (Crookes' tubes); the forerunner of the cathode ray tube. Discovered thallium from its spectral lines.

crossed-coil (*mri*) RF coil pair arranged with their magnetic fields at right angles to each other in such a way as to minimize their mutual magnetic interaction.

cross-correlation (*us*) A rapid technique for determining time shifts in echo arrival; a technique used to determine flow speeds without using the doppler effect.

cross-over (cross talk) (*ct, mri*) Slice to slice interference in computed tomography (CT) and MRI. Cross-over between slices in CT is due to beam collimation and in MRI is due to imperfect truncation (*see* unsharpness (radiographic)).

cross talk (*mri*) Signals from close adjacent slices affect one another. Caused by a slice profile that is not ideal. Cross-talk effects T1 contrast. Cured commonly by using an interleaved slice sequence. (*us*) Leakage of strong signals in one direction channel of a doppler receiver into the other channel; can produce the doppler mirror-image artefact.

crossed-coil (*mri*) An RF coil pair arranged with their magnetic fields at right angles to each other to minimize mutual magnetic interaction.

CrossXBeam[®] **(CRI)** (*us*) A GE Healthcare technique for acquiring and combining ultrasound information in real-time to reduce speckle and clutter, and to improve the continuity of specular reflectors. This reinforces aspects of the image data and reduces noise to form a single image.

cryogen (*mri*) Liquid nitrogen or more commonly liquid helium, which enables superconductivity to occur in MRI superconducting magnets. Liquefied gas (helium or nitrogen) used to maintain superconducting magnets in a superconducting state. Helium is liquid at 4.2 K or $-268.95°C$.

cryomagnet (*mri*) *See* **superconducting magnet**.

cryo-shielding (*mri*) Cooling a metal cylinder surrounding the He-vessel in a superconducting magnet, so reducing cryogen boil-off.

cryostat (*mri*) A thermally insulated enclosure for maintaining a constant low temperature filled with liquid helium. There is commonly a recycling device for reducing helium loss.

crystallization (*phys*) Formation of crystals from a saturated solution or by evaporation. Contrast media may crystallize from concentrated solutions.

⬛ Reference: Dawson and Clauss, 1999.

CSF (*clin*) Cerebrospinal fluid.

CSF SE (*mri*) Contiguous-slice fast-acquisition spin echo. FSE/RARE variant.

CSI (*mri*) *See* **Chemical shift imaging**.

CSMEMP (*mri*) Contiguous slice MEMP.

CT (*ct*) *See* **computed axial tomography**.

CTDI (CT dose index) (*ct*) The basic measurement as defined by the US Federal Regulation 21CFR 1020.33(C) represents the dose at the centre or peripheral point on a head or body phantom from a single scan and results from absorption of the x-ray beam over a distance of approximately seven slices. The CTDI is normalized to a standard mAs product and weighted for different locations within the scan plane (CTDI$_w$). The **dose profile** from a single CT scan spreads beyond the intended section thickness. The area beyond the section thickness being the **penumbra**. The CTDI attempts to represent the dose distribution outside the section thickness, taking a representative 14 slices in air or the phantom as:

$$\text{CTDI} = \frac{1}{nT} \int_{-7}^{+7} D_{(z)} \, dz \text{ mGy}$$

This represents the dose $D_{(z)}$ for a single section at a given position z along the scan axis. This value is then divided by the intended section thickness per image (T) and the number of image slices per scan n. Measurements are taken from a plastic (PMMA tissue equivalent) phantom 16 and 32 cm in diameter (head/body). CTDI values are given in mGy per 100 mAs for 360° scan at the machines stated in kVp.

⬛ Reference: Code of Federal Regulations, 2005; European Commission's Radiation Protection Actions.

(*See* CTDI$_{100}$, CTDI$_{FDA}$, CTDI$_w$).

CTDI$_{(air)}$ (*ct*) Value of CTDI determined free in air. In practice, it is convenient to use a pencil ionization chamber with an active length of 100 mm so as to provide a measurement of CTD1$_{100}$ (mGy to air).

$$\text{CTDI} = \frac{1}{T} \int_{-\infty}^{+\infty} D_{(z)} \, dz \text{ mGy}.$$

CTDI$_{vol}$ (*ct*) The **absorbed dose** within the scanned volume. Whereas CTDI$_w$ represents the weighted absorbed dose per slice (x- and y-axis), the CTDI$_{vol}$ represents the average absorbed dose over the x-, y- and z-axes; it is similar to the **multiple scan average dose** (MSAD) and is independent of scan length. It is derived from CTDI$_w$ as:

$$\text{CTDI}_{vol} = \frac{\text{CTDI}_w}{\text{pitch}}$$

where pitch is 1, then CTDI$_{vol}$ = CTDI$_w$ and **dose length product** (DLP) = CTDI$_{vol}$ × scanned length.

CTDI$_w$ (*ct*) A weighted version of CTDI taking surface and centre dose readings of the head or body phantom, gives an adequate basis for specifying reference doses for CT. Defined by IEC 601-2-44CDV, these measurements of a weighted CTDI$_w$ represent the average dose to a single slice:

$$\text{CTDI}_w = \frac{1}{3}\text{CTDI}_{100.c} + \frac{2}{3}\text{CTDI}_{100.p}$$

where subscripts c and p denote central or peripheral measurement from the phantom. A normalized mAs value (typically 100 mAs) is used. The CTDI$_w$ will vary with slice width and is an estimate of the average dose over a single slice in a CT dosimetry phantom that is used for comparison of performance against a reference dose value set for the purpose of promoting optimization of patient protection.

Calculation of CTDI$_w$

From measurements made using a PMMA head and body phantom the following readings are obtained:

CTDI head (16 cm)		CTDI body (32 cm)	
Centre	Peripheral	Centre	Peripheral
16.2	18.1	4.9	10.9
25.2	27.7	7.8	16.4

Using the formula:

$$\text{CTDI}_w = \frac{1}{3}\text{CTDI}_{100.c} + \frac{2}{3}\text{CTDI}_{100.p}$$

The weighted dose figures are obtained

	CTDI$_w$ head (16 cm)	CTDI$_w$ body (32 cm)
110	17.2	8.8
130	26.6	13.4

CTDI$_{100}$ (ct) A more representative dose measurement than other CTDI measurements. The CTDI is measured over a fixed 100-mm length instead of the 14 arbitrary slices. The value is taken over a fixed length of integration using a pencil ionization chamber with an active length of 100 mm. Provides a measure of the basic CTDI, integrated over a standard 100-mm length expressed in terms of absorbed dose to air (mGy):

$$(mAs)\ CTDI_{(100,a/p)} = \frac{1}{S} \int_{-50\ mm}^{+50\ mm} D_{(z)}\ dz$$

where S is the slice width, the dose $D_{(z)}$ being integrated over ± 50 mm by the 100-mm pencil detector. The subscripts for the CTDI measurement include (mAs) indicating the exposure value used to normalize the result (typically doses are stated for a 100 mAs value); the subscript 100 denotes a 100-mm scan length and a or p indicate that measurements were made in air or a PMMA phantom. In addition, the phantom size 16 or 32 cm should be stated depending on either head or body values (see CTDI, CTDI$_{FDA}$, CTDI$_w$).

CTDI$_{FDA}$ (ct) A slice dose measurement allowing for scattered radiation falling outside the 100-mm detector length (CTDI$_{100}$). In order to overcome this problem, the FDA requires acquisition of 14 nominal slice widths. In multiple slice machines, it is necessary to modify the calculation of the CTDI$_{100}$ equation to take account of the number of simultaneously acquired slices (M) so:

$$_nCTDI_{(100,a/p)} = \frac{1}{S * M} \int_{-50\ mm}^{+50\ mm} D_{(z)}\ dz.$$

This formula allows comparison between machines acquiring simultaneous slices of 2, 4, 8 or more slices.

CT dosimetry (ct) Phantoms: Cylinders of polymethyl-methacrylate (PMMA) used for standard measurements of dose in CT, having a diameter of 16 cm (head phantom) or 32 cm (body phantom) and a length of at least 14 cm. The phantoms are constructed with removable inserts

parallel to the axis to allow the positioning of a dosemeter at the centre and 1 cm from the outer surface (periphery) (see CTDI, CTDI$_{(air)}$, CTDI$_w$).

CT dose index (CTDI) (ct) See CTDI.

CT dosimetry phantom (ct) Cylinders of polymethylmethacrylate (PMMA) used for standard measurements of dose in CT, having a diameter of 16 cm (head phantom) or 32 cm (body phantom) and a length of at least 14 cm. The phantoms are constructed with removable inserts parallel to the axis to allow the positioning of a dosemeter at the centre and 1 cm from the outer surface (periphery) (see CTDI, CTDI$_{(air)}$, CTDI$_w$).

CT number (ct) The comparative attenuation value that represents the mean x-ray attenuation associated with each elemental area (voxel) of the CT image. These values are expressed in terms of Hounsfield units (HU) and scaled with respect to water as:

$$CT\ number\ (Hounsfield\ unit) = \frac{\mu_{tissue} - \mu_{water}}{\mu_{water}}$$

where μ is the effective linear attenuation coefficient for the x-ray beam. The CT number scale is defined so that water has a value of 0 HU and air a value of -1000 HU; bone can exceed $+3000$ HU. Since values are scaled to water the Housfield unit is independent of beam energy (voltage).

CT number calculation

	80 kV	100 kV	150 kV
μ_{muscle}	0.1892	0.1760	0.1550
μ_{water}	0.1835	0.1707	0.1504

At 80 kev: $1000 \times \dfrac{0.1892 - 0.1835}{0.1835} = 31$

At 100 kev: $1000 \times \dfrac{0.1760 - 0.1707}{0.1707} = 31$

At 150 kev: $1000 \times \dfrac{0.1550 - 0.1504}{0.1504} = 31$

Beam hardening: At 100 kV, the reference for water is 0.1707, but if the beam effective energy changes to 105 kV in the centre of the profile, the μ for tissue changes to 0.1750 then:

New CT value $= \dfrac{0.1750 - 0.1707}{0.1707} = 25$

and not 31 which it should be (see cupping effect).

CT fluoroscopy (*ct*) This application requires rapid image reconstruction of the object currently in the scan field of view. Movement of the patient couch is under the operator's control. As the images are updated up to 12 times per second, the systems are capable of providing real-time feedback for a range of procedures, particularly during interventional procedures.

cumulated activity (*nmed*) The total number of radioactive disintegrations that occurs in the target organ. This is dependent on injected activity, biological half-life and physical half-life.

cumulative error (*di*) The gradual build up of error in an involved computation from either truncation or round-off.

curie (*nmed*) A non-SI radioactivity measurement having a disintegration rate of 3.7×10^{10} Bq as disintegrations per second, 37 GBq. Other equivalents are 1 mCi = 37 MBq and 1 μCi = 37 kBq.

Curie, Marie (née Sklodowska) (1867–1934) Polish born French scientist, stimulated by Becquerel's discovery investigated pitchblende. In 1898, she separated polonium and later the same year radium. She was awarded the Nobel prize for physics 1903 and for chemistry in 1911 (*see* Joliot-Curie).

Curie, Pierre (1859–1906) French physicist. Discovered piezo-electricity in 1880. Observed the loss and variation of magnetism with temperature (the Curie point and Curie's law) and pioneered instrumentation for measuring ionizing radiation and established that the rays from radium contained positive, negative and neutral particles. He was awarded the Nobel prize for physics 1903.

curie point (*us*) Temperature at which an element material loses its piezo-electric properties.

current (*phys*) A flow of electric charge in a substance which can be solid, liquid, gas or plasma. The charge carriers may be electrons, holes or ions. The magnitude of the current is given by the amount of charge flowing in unit time, measured in amperes. One ampere ($C s^{-1}$) represents about 6.28×10^{18} electrons per second or a rate of flow of charge of one coulomb per second. Direct current (DC) is given by batteries, dynamos and rectified power supplies and is used as the final power supply for radiology equipment whether driving high voltage x-ray tubes or low voltage semiconductor circuits. For a current (I) in amperes (A), the charge in coulombs (C) and time (t) in seconds then

$Q = I \times t$ where $1 A = 1 C s^{-1}$ (6.24×10^{18} electrons s^{-1}). X-ray tube current is measured in mA, and x-ray exposure is measured in mA per unit time mA, seconds mAs, so $1 mAs = 1 \times 10^{-3}$ coulomb or 1 milliC.

current (alternating) (*phys*) Alternating current (AC) is produced by generators/alternators and electrically oscillating circuits. It is more easily controlled than DC and is used for transmitting electrical power over long distances, eventually appearing as the domestic mains supply. Power station generators are capable of delivering many thousands of volts at a very high current. Transmission voltages sometimes exceed 500 000 volts. High voltage transmission reduces power loss, which can be reduced by either increasing the supply voltage or reducing cable resistance. Transmission uses a three-phase AC; each phase of the three-phase supply is separated by $120°$ and transmits electrical energy with much greater efficiency. Domestic supply is commonly single phase. Voltage stepdown is achieved with a transformer.

Power loss

For a cable of resistance 2 Ω supplying a 100 W lamp:

- At 110 volts, $\approx$1 amp is flowing so the power lost in the cable is $I^2R = 1 \times 2 = 2$ watts or 2% of the lamp power is lost in the cable.
- At 220 volts, $\approx$0.5 amp is flowing and the power lost in the cable is $0.25 \times 2 = 0.5$ watts or 0.5% of the available power is lost.

Power transmission

Supplying 1 MW to a small town over a cable with a resistance of 10 Ω can use:

- 500 V at 2000 amps or
- 10000 V at 100 amps or
- 500000 V at 2 amps

(all delivering the required 1 MW).

Power loss is I^2R so at:

- 500 V, there is total power lost in the cable;
- 10 000 V, 10% of the power is lost;
- 100 000 V, 0.1% of the power is lost.

Note Power transmission uses highest practical voltage to minimize power loss.

---

current density (j or J) (*phys*) The flow of electric charge or current through a conductor, either gas, metal semiconductor or tissue. The unit is ampere per square metre: A/m^2. The amount of current flowing through a given unit cross-sectional area of a current carrying medium; either a conductor or radiation beam.

curvilinear array (*us*) *See* linear array.

cut-film (*film*) 100 mm or 105 mm square film stock. Used mostly in conjunction with an image intensifier (cut-film camera).

cut-off frequency (*di*) The −3 dB point is arbitrarily called the cut-off frequency of low and high pass filters (*see* bandwidth).

CW (*mri*) *See* continuous wave.

cyanocobalamin (*nmed*) ^{57}Cobalt labelled for oral administration. Diagnosis of pernicious anaemia and defects of intestinal vitamin B_{12} absorption.

Generic name	^{57}Co-cyanocobalamine
Commercial names	Rubratope® (Bracco), Dicopac® (Amersham GE)
Non-imaging diagnostic kit	

cycle (Hz) (*phys*) Complete transition of waveform measured from identical points (zero crossing or peaks).

cycles per pulse (*us*) A typical ultrasound pulse contains one to three cycles.

cyclotron (*phys*) A charged particle accelerator where the beam travels in a circular path. Used for manufacturing short-lived positron emitters:

Nuclide	Half-life
^{15}O	2.1 m
^{38}K	7.6 m
^{11}C	10 m
^{13}N	10 m
^{18}F	110 m

(*see* ion source, Lawrence EO, positron emission tomography).

cyclotron (beam production) (*nmed*) *See* ion beam (cyclotron), hydrogen, helium, deuterium).

CYMK (*comp*) Cyan, yellow, magenta, keystone black. The four basic colours used by inkjet and laser colour printers. A huge range of colours are created by a combination of overlaying and dithering.

cystic duct cholangiography (*clin*) Radiography of the biliary system by introducing contrast medium through the cystic duct.

cystogram (*clin*) Radiographic demonstration of bladder filled with contrast medium. Micturating cystogram performed when urinating.

cystography (*xray*) Imaging the bladder by introducing contrast media through a urethral catheter. Demonstrates anatomic and pathological changes in male/female bladder or urethra and the presence of ureteric reflux (*see* urethrography).

Cystografin^x (*cm*) Commercial preparation (Bracco) meglumine diatrizoate (30%) injection containing $141 \, mg \, I \, mL^{-1}$ for retrograde cysto-urethrography.

Cysto-Conray^x (*cm*) Commercial preparation of ionic meglumine iothalamate (Malinckrodt/Tyco Healthcare Inc) containing $81 \, mg \, I \, mL^{-1}$ for retrograde cystography or cystourethrography.

cystoscopic urography (*clin*) *See* retrograde urography).

cystourethrography (*clin*) Micturating or voiding cystogram. Radiography of the bladder and urethra during voiding following filling of the bladder with contrast medium, either intravenously or by means of retrograde catheterization; performed during the phase of bladder emptying. Ascending urethrogram is where the contrast medium is instilled slowly via catheter. Descending micturating cystourethrography is where the contrast medium is instilled via catheter and the bladder adequately filled to induce micturation. Images of posterior urethra taken during voiding (*see* retrograde urography, urethrography).

d' (*image*) In signal detection theory, an effective signal-to-noise ratio (SNR) that applies only to situations in which the decision variable arises from one of two normal distributions having equal variances, but different means. In such situations, the receiver operating characteristic (ROC) curve is symmetric about the diagonal of the unit square in which it is plotted and is given by the mathematical expression:

$$TPF = \Phi(d' Z_{FPF}),$$

where Φ represents the cumulative standard-normal distribution function and Z_{FPF} represents the normal deviate that corresponds to the false-positive fraction (*see* binormal ROC curve).

d$_a$ (*image*) An effective SNR, more general than d' that applies to situations in which the decision variable arises from one of two normal distributions having different means and, generally, different variances. In such situations, the ROC curve depends on two parameters, a and b, and is given by the mathematical expression:

$$TPF = \Phi(a + b\, Z_{FPF}),$$

where Φ represents the cumulative standard-normal distribution function and Z_{FPF} represents the normal deviate that corresponds to false-positive fraction, $d_a = a\sqrt{2/(1 + b^2)}$

D (max) (*image*) *See* film sensitometry.

D (min) (*image*) *See* film sensitometry.

D$_o$ (*dose*) The dose that gives (on average) one lethal event per cell reducing survival to 37% of its previous value (*see* LD$_{50}$).

DAC (*dose*) *See* derived air concentration. (*comp*) Abbreviation for the electronic circuit digital to analogue converter.

dacryocystography (*clin*) Imaging the lacrimal ducts injecting contrast medium into the lumen. Almost entirely replaced by nuclear medicine, computed tomography (CT) and magnetic resonance imaging (MRI) techniques.

dalton (D) (*unit*) The atomic mass unit a.m.u. equal to 1/12 of the mass of an atom of 12 carbon. Equivalent to 1.66×10^{-27} kg or 931 MeV. Used principally for measuring biochemical molecules, commonly expressed as kilo- and Mega-daltons. A protein shell is of the order 13 MDa.

damped oscillation (*phys*) *See* decay (signal).

damping (us) Material attached to the rear face of a transducer element to reduce pulse duration.

damping coefficient (*mri*) Decreasing periodic function, e.g. free induction decay process.

DAP (dose–area–product) (*dose*) Values for some representative reference values (NRPB 1990).

Examination	DAP (mGy cm²)	
	Mean	Maximum
Lumbar spine (AP)	3200	5000
Lumbar spine (LAT)	3400	7000
Lumbar spine (LSI)	3600	5000
Chest (AP)	200	300
Chest (PA)	150	250
Chest (LAT)	500	1000
Abdomen (AP)	3800	7000
Pelvis (AP)	3300	7000
Skull (AP/PA)	800	1500
Skull (LAT)	500	1000
Thoracic spine (AP)	1800	3000
Thoracic spine (LAT)	3300	6000
Intravenous urography	16 000	40 000

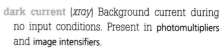

dark current (*xray*) Background current during no input conditions. Present in photomultipliers and image intensifiers.

dark fluid imaging (*mri*) A preparation pulse saturates the blood and displays cardiovascular anatomy. The TurboIR technique has a longer effective echo time and longer inversion time which suppresses fluid signals. Bright fluid signals using conventional T2 contrast are revealed by this dark fluid technique (*see* FLAIR).

DAT drive (*comp*) Digital audio tape. Large storage capacity digital tape for archiving. A helical scan magnetic tape storage with a capacity of 2–12 G-bytes uncompressed (native) data and up to 24 G-bytes compressed data. Data transfer rates are from 183 k-bytes s^{-1} to 2 M-bytes s^{-1}. It is a common back-up medium for computer-disk data (*see* storage (bulk)).

data acquisition (*comp*) Collection of electronic signals which can be analogue (voltage/amplitude varying waveform) or digital (nuclear medicine or x-ray photon events), processed (e.g. intensification or amplification) and perhaps preprocessed (voltage compression or pulse clipping) before being used to form the image (film or digital matrix). Losses occur at all stages of data acquisition and handling.

data acquisition system (DAS) (*ct*) Electronic systems of the CT machine responsible for detector signal amplification, integration and analogue to digital conversion.

database (*comp*) A program that stores information so that it can be easily retrieved by searching

D

and sorting facilities. A collection of similar information stored in a file, such as a database of addresses. This information may be created and stored in a database management system (DBMS).

data compression (*di*) *See* compression (image).

data interpolation (*ct*) For sequential CT, slice sensitivity profiles (SSPs) are approximately rectangular with widths equal to the section width; however, in spiral/helical acquisition they are extended and more peaked. The SSP represents the resolution element along the *z*-axis and significantly influences 3D resolution reconstruction. Since the patient is moved during data acquisition, the information obtained is distorted over the body volume depending on the slice thickness and table increment per rotation. This data inconsistency causes artefacts, but can mostly be compensated by data interpolation. The interpolation methods most commonly employed work from either the full data set (360°) or a half data set (180°) (*see* 180° interpolation, 360° interpolation).

data matrix (*ct*) These CT numbers are stored in computer memory and represent a volume slice element or voxel. The matrix store must hold a range of voxel values from −1000 to +4000. This requires a memory location of 16 bits including a 'sign' bit positive or negative.

data set (*stats*) A collection of numbers that usually have one common property.

DaTSCAN™ (*nmed*) A radio-iodinated cocaine analogue ^{123}I-ioflupane (Amersham/GE Healthcare Inc).

daughter (*phys, nmed*) Decay product of a 'parent' radionuclide (*see* radionuclide production (generator)).

dB (*phys*) Abbreviation for decibel.

dB/dt (*mri*) Time derivative rate of change of magnetic field with respect to time. Using alternating magnetic fields/electrical fields produced in conductive material (soft tissue); related to MR safety limits.

d.c. (*phys*) Direct current, as supplied by batteries and rectified power supplies to drive electrical or electronic circuits.

DCE (*comp*) Data circuit terminating equipment. A device used to connect two DTEs over a network.

DCL (*comp*) Data circuit terminating equipment. A device used to connect two DTEs over a network. A modem is a DCE.

DDR1/DD1 RAM (*comp*) Double data rate RAM is used in some graphics cards, having 184 pins; replaced by DDR2.

DDR2/DD2 RAM (*comp*) Currently the most common computer memory; significant improvements over the DDR1 RAM specification doubling the transfer rate. It has 240 pins and so is not a replacement for DDR1 unless the motherboard is changed.

DREF (*dose*) *See* dose and dose-rate effectiveness factor.

de Broglie, Louis-Victor Pierre Raymond 7th Duke (1892–1987) French physicist interpreted Einstein's work on the photoelectric effect into wave theory suggesting that the electron can exhibit wave-like properties. He was awarded the Nobel prize for physics in 1929.

de Broglie's equation (*phys*) A photon or particle (electron) of mass *m* moving with a velocity *v* will exhibit wave-like properties, having a wavelength $\lambda = h/mv$, where *h* is Planck's constant (*see* photon).

DE FGR (*mri*) Driven equilibrium fast gradient recalled acquisition in the steady state.

dead time (*nmed*) The time required for a detector system to process (count or reject) the signal from a single photon interaction, during which additional photon interactions will be missed. The count rate capability of a detector system (gamma camera) is limited by the decay time of the scintillator, about 240 nS for NaI(Tl), along with its charge amplifier and associated converter electronics. The measured count rates from a gamma camera fall short of expected count rate. It is therefore expressed as a figure representing a 10, 20 or 30% count loss. The common value is taken at 20%. If N_i is the incident number of gamma photons and N_a is the photon counts recorded, then the dead time τ is given as:

$$\tau = \frac{\ln\frac{N_i}{N_a}}{N_a}$$

The dead time calculated from this equation for a 20% loss at 200 000 cps typically giving a value of just over 1 μs. Two types of detector dead time are distinguished:

1 Paralyzable, where further photon events serve to increase the total dead time.

2 Non-paralyzable where further events are ignored, the detector operating again after a set time.

Most gamma cameras behave as paralyzable detectors over the clinical count range.

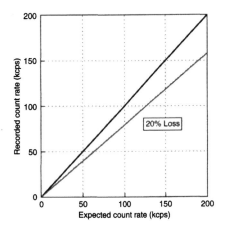

decay (*nmed*) The rearrangement of a nucleus resulting in emission of one or more different particles, thereby returning the nucleus to stability and resulting in formation of an atom (the daughter) different from the original atom (the parent).

decay (signal) (*phys*) In a simple harmonic motion $\sin(x)$, the amplitude A of the vibration does not remain constant, but decreases exponentially with time t due to loss of energy (damping) following the expression $A = \sin(x) \cdot e^{-t}$. This decay signal is shown by all electrical and mechanical signals whose energy input is not constant. Examples are seen in the ultrasound transducer, free induction decay (MRI) and the damped response of an electronic oscillator.

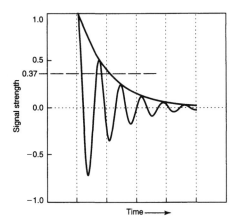

decay constant (λ) (*nmed*) For an unstable nucleus (radionuclide), the number of atoms N disintegrating per second is dN/dT which is directly proportional to the number of atoms at any one time so $dN/dT = -\lambda N$, where λ is the decay constant characteristic for the atom. If N_0 represents atoms present at time zero then the number at time t is: $N_t = N_0 \times e^{-\lambda t}$. Half-life is $T_{\frac{1}{2}} = 1/\lambda \ln 2$ or $0.693/\lambda$. It follows that $N_t = N_0 \times e^{-0.693} \times t/T_{\frac{1}{2}}$. So the decay constant of any radionuclide $\lambda = 0.693/T_{\frac{1}{2}}$. It is common to express decay constants as 'per second' so that comparisons can be made easily.

decibel (dB) (*units*) The comparative measure of power, intensity and amplitude or voltage gain; a ratio of relative powers or intensities. It uses a logarithmic scale as:

$$dB = 10 \log_{10} \frac{I}{I_0}$$

where I_0 is the reference sound level commonly fixed at $10^{-12} \, W \, m^{-2}$ at 1 kHz at audible levels. A 3-dB change halves or doubles the sound intensity. A sound level of 20 dB is ten times more intense than a 10-dB sound level. Comparisons of amplitude or pressure differences uses a factor of 20 as:

$$dB = 20 \log_{10} \frac{A}{A_0}.$$

Here, a change of 6 dB halves or doubles the amplitude or pressure. The attenuation given by a material is quoted as dB mm^{-1}; this is the attenuation coefficient α (*see* Bell, Alexander Graham).

decimal place (*math*) The figures to the right of the decimal point giving a specified degree of accuracy (*see* significant figures).

decision criterion (*stats*) In signal detection theory, the critical value that separates the range of decision-variable outcomes associated with 'negative' decisions from the range associated with 'positive' decisions.

decision variable (*stats*) In signal detection theory, a statistical quantity that is assumed to underlie decisions made under uncertainty. For 'detection' tasks that involve two mutually exclusive ('positive' and 'negative') alternatives, the decision is assumed to be made by comparing the value of the decision variable to a critical value (i.e. decision criterion).

decontamination (*nmed*) The reduction of surface activity after an accidental spill of radionuclide, by either physical means or isolation, allowing physical decay for short-lived nuclides. The minimum surface activity varies and local rules

D

should be consulted for acceptable thresholds which usually relate to fractions of maximum doses (typically 0.1).

deconvolution (*math*) *See* convolution.

decoupling (*mri*) Decoupling involves (1) removing the multiplet structure in a particular resonance due to spin–spin coupling; (2) preventing mutual inductive coupling between coils by detuning. Decoupling can take the form of active decoupling where an externally controlled switching circuit is used to detune the nonselected coils or passive decoupling where RF energy from the transmitter pulse is used to switch diodes to detune the appropriate coil.

decubitus view (*clin*) Imaging performed with the x-ray beam horizontal 'across the table'. Named according to the patient side viewed: Right or left lateral decubitus.

deep dose equivalent (H_d) (*dose*) External whole body dose equivalent at 1 cm depth. The dose equivalent to any organ, except the eye. Some authorities still retain the recommendations given by ICRP26 of 500 mSv, but modifications have been made to this.

DEFAISE (*mri*) Dual-echo fast-acquisition interleaved spin echo. A double-echo variant of RARE.

default (*comp*) The predefined configuration of a system or an application. In most programs, the defaults can be changed to reflect personal preferences, such as font or paragraph indents.

DE FGR (*mri*) Driven equilibrium fast gradient recalled acquisition in the steady state. Commonly used for imaging cerebrospinal fluid (*see* SSFP, CE-FAST, True-FISP, PSIF, ROAST, T2-FEE, E-SHORT, STERE).

defocussing (*mri*) *See* dephasing.

degree (*unit*) Defined as a plane angle which the central area of a circles cuts from 1/360th part of the circumference. $1° = \pi/180$ rad or approximately 0.01745 rad (*see* radian).

degrees of freedom (*stats*) The number of free variables in a system. Commonly given as $n - 2$, where n is the number of points. For the t-test, the number of degrees of freedom is $n - 1$. (*phys*) One of the separate ways in which a molecule can have energy. A gas will have three degrees of freedom: kinetic energy from motion from motion in three directions 90° to one another.

delta (Δ) pulse (*di*) An infinitely narrow (spike) input. The ideal requirement to measure point spread or line spread function of a system (*see* Dirac function).

delay time (*mri*) *See* trigger delay (TD).

demodulation (*phys*) The reverse of modulation, where the signal is separated from its carrier wave by a demodulator, RF-detector or ultrasound detector circuit.

demodulator (*phys*) Another term for detector, by analogy to broadcast radio receivers. An electronic circuit which separates a single signal from a mixed signal. (*us*) An electronic circuit which separates a single signal from a mixed signal. Frequently a phase detector (quadrature phase detector). The echo signal is more easily processed by mixing with a reference signal (frequency, f) obtained by an inbuilt oscillator. After processing, rectification separates the signal and a fast Fourier transform (FFT) calculates the Doppler frequencies from the demodulated Doppler signal sampled at intervals where $T = 1/PRF$ (pulse repetition frequency). Maximum frequency detectable is the Nyquist limit as ½ PRF. (*mri*) Electronically separating mixed signals. A part of the nuclear magnetic resonance (NMR) signal receiver that converts the raw signal to a lower frequency for analysis. This is also phase sensitive (quadrature demodulator) and will give phase information (detecting phase encoded RF signals).

densitometer (*film*) Measures film density in optical density units (*see* optical density).

density (ρ) (*units*) The physical density of a material (ρ) is:

$$\rho = \frac{\text{mass}}{\text{volume}}$$

The SI unit is kg m^3, although non-SI g cm^3 is often used. A conversion factor of 10^3 is used.

Density

50 g of aluminium displaces 18.5 cm^3 of water so its density is:

$$\rho = \frac{50}{18.5} = 2.70 \text{g cm}^3 \quad \text{or} \quad 2700 \text{ kg m}^3$$

The density of elements important to radiology usually follow their atomic number (Z), but there are exceptions as shown in the table.

Z	Material	Density kg m^{-3}
	Air	1.225
	Water	1000
	Muscle	1000
	Fat	900
	Bone	1650–1800

(Contd.)

---

density (ρ) *(Contd.)*

Z	Material	Density kg m^{-3}
13	Aluminum	2700
26	Iron	7870
29	Copper	8900
42	Molybdenum	10 200
73	Tantalum	16 600
74	Tungsten	19 320
76	Osmium	22 480
79	Gold	19 300
82	Lead	11 340

density (optical) (OD) *(image)* The logarithm of the ratio of the intensity of perpendicularly incident light (I_0) on a film to the light intensity (I) transmitted by the film:

$$OD = \log_{10} \frac{I_0}{I}.$$

Optical density differences are always measured in a line perpendicular to the light source axis.

density (relative) *(units)* Water has a density of $1000\,kg\,m^{-3}$ ($1\,g\,cm^{-3}$) and this liquid is used as a reference for density measurements. The relative density for aluminium is therefore just 2700. The density of a substance divided by the density of water is the specific gravity or relative density; for a gas the relative substance is usually air.

density resolution *(ct)* The capability to display small differences in tissue densities (*see* low contrast resolution).

depletion (barrier) layer *(elec)* A region between a p–n junction (*see* depletion junction).

dephasing *(mri)* Phase differences occurring between precessing spins after RF excitation, causing a decay in transverse magnetization. Caused primarily by spin–spin interaction and inhomogeneity in the magnetic field. Can also be caused by switching specific gradient fields (flow dephasing).

dephasing gradient *(mri)* Magnetic field gradient pulse used to create spatial variation of phase of transverse magnetization. It may be applied prior to signal detection in the presence of a magnetic field gradient with opposite polarity (or of the same polarity if separated by a refocusing RF pulse) so the resulting gradient echo signal will represent a more complete sampling of the Fourier transform of the desired image (*see* spoiler gradient pulse).

depletion junction *(elec)* About $10^{-3}\,mm$ wide which exists without a biasing voltage. When the junction is reversed biased (positive pole

to n and negative to p), the depletion width increases preventing current conduction. Ionizing radiation causes electrons and holes to form and a small current signal is obtained. This is the semiconductor version of the gas ionization chamber (*see* semiconductor).

Depreotide *(nmed)* ^{99m}Tc depreotide is an amino acid peptide binding for somatostatin receptors type 2, 3 and 5. It has a high affinity to lung cancer.

Generic name	^{99m}Tc depreotide
Commercial names	Neotect®
Imaging category	Somatostatin receptor lung masses

depth of field *(image)* A circle of 0.25 mm viewed from 250 mm is just visible as a point source. This is termed 'the circle of least confusion' and is used as a standard of reference in photographic images. It corresponds to an angle of ~0.001 radians subtended by the eye. This reference is used to determine the 'in focus' distance covered by a lens and is dependent on the lens f-number. Smaller f-numbers produce larger depths of field. An important factor with cameras in cine-fluoroscopy and film recording.

depth of image *(us)* *See* image depth.

depth of response *(us)* The point from the transducer face where echoes are $-50\,dB$.

depth gain compensation *(us)* *See* time gain compensation.

depth pulses *(mri)* Multiple RF pulses with an inhomogeneous RF field, so acquiring data from only selected regions within the field. Provides a one-dimensional localization along isocontours of the magnetic field.

derating (derating factor, derated) *(us)* A factor applied to acoustic output parameters intended to account for ultrasonic attenuation of tissue between the source and a particular location in the tissue. As referred to in this document, the average ultrasonic attenuation is assumed to be $0.3\,dB\,cm^{-1}\,MHz^{-1}$ along the beam axis in the body. Derated parameters are denoted with a subscript '3'. Unit is decibel per centimetre per megahertz, $dB\,cm^{-1}\,MHz^{-1}$ (*see* mechanical index).

derated spatial peak time average intensity *(us)* The largest value in an ultrasound beam of any derated time averaged intensity.

derived air concentration (DAC) *(dose)* The annual limit on intake (ALI) of a radionuclide divided by the volume of air inhaled by a reference person in a working year estimated as $2.4 \times 10^3\,\text{m}^3$. The unit of DAC is $\text{Bq}\,\text{m}^{-3}$.

Derived air concentration
^{131}Iodine has an ALI of 9×10^5. The DAC value is:

$$\frac{9 \times 10^5}{2.4 \times 10^3} = 375\,\text{Bq}\,\text{m}^{-3}.$$

---

derived reference air concentration (DRAC) (*nmed*) The annual reference limit on intake (ARLI) of a radionuclide divided by the volume of air inhaled by reference man in a working year. The unit of DRAC is $\text{Bq}\,\text{m}^3$.

derived units (*phys*) *See* Systeme International (SI).

designated standard mode (*us*) Consist of the following specific operating modes: A-mode, B-mode, M-mode, PW Doppler, CW Doppler and colour Doppler.

des Plantes, Bernard George Ziedses (1902–93) Dutch radiologist who produced first subtraction images in 1930, displaying only the contrast filled vessels. He also introduced radiographic tomography. The idea of producing subtraction images dates back to the 1930s, when this Dutch radiologist produced subtraction images using plain films. From the 'mask' image, i.e. the image of the object just before the contrast medium is injected, he produced a positive copy, on to which the images with contrast medium were overlaid to coincide, thus producing a subtraction image only displaying the contrast-filled vessels.

DESS (*mri*) Double-echo steady state (Siemens) combining FISP and PSIF. A 3D gradient echo during which two different gradient echoes (FISP and PSIF) are acquired during TR. During image reconstruction, the strongly T2-weighted PSIF image is added to the FISP image. Applied to joint imaging giving good contrast for cartilage.

destructive interference (*us*) Combination of positive and negative pressures.

detail resolution (*us*) Ability to image fine detail and to distinguish closely spaced reflectors (*see* axial resolution, lateral resolution).

detail transfer function (*math*) A descriptor for how the imaging system averages, displaces or blurs the input signals before they are detected in the output signal. For linear, shift invariant systems, the detail transfer function is the point spread function (PSF) or, in frequency space, the optical transfer function (OTF).

detective quantum efficiency (DQE) (*image*) Comparison of input and output signal to noise ratios. Signal to noise ratios vary at every stage of image production. The SNR_{in} represents subject contrast. The SNR_{out} represents the detection process then:

$$DQE = \left(\frac{SNR_{out}}{SNR_{in}}\right)^2$$

The SNR of the incident photon flux N is $\sqrt{N}$ due to quantum noise. The SNR of the detector is dependent on photon absorption, which is influenced by μ thickness and conversion efficiency.

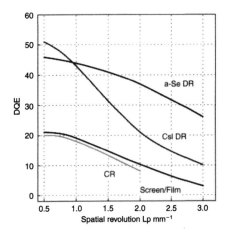

(*see* signal to noise ratio, noise equivalent quanta).

detector (*phys*) A gas, solid or liquid which yields a signal (electrical or light) when radiation interacts within its volume. (*ct*) A single element of a detector array, which produces an electrical or light signal in response to stimulation by x-rays. Current detectors are pressurized xenon ion chambers and solid scintillators of either cadmium tungstate or rare earth oxide ceramic, optically bound to photodiodes spectrally matched to the scintillator. Conversion efficiency and photon capture for the solid detector approaches 99%. (*mri*) A circuit of the receiver that demodulates the RF signal converting it to a lower frequency signal. Most detectors now used are phase sensitive (e.g. quadrature demodulators) giving phase information about the RF signal. (*us*) A demodulator or circuit for separating the original sound signal from the carrier wave (*see* ceramic detector).

detector array (*ct*) The entire assembly of detectors, including their interspace material, arranged along an arc or circumference (depending on scanner technology) of a circle centred on the axis of rotation.

detector channel (*ct*) A single detector element (*see* detector spacing, detector width).

detector channel sensitivity (*ct*) The sensitivity of a specific single detector element; the channel sensitivity as measured is crucial for machine calibration; slight variations in the detector sensitivity will lead to ring artefacts without.

detector dead-time (*nmed*) A gas detector has a dead time measured in fractions of a second. The dead time of a scintillation detector is measured in nanoseconds. A typical value for NaI(Tl) is 250 ns. The dead time of a gamma camera includes crystal and electronics and can be measured by using two activities A_a and A_b, the combined activity A_{ab} exceeding the count rate of the detector. The dead time t is:

$$t = \frac{A_{ab}}{(A_a + A_b)^2} \ln \frac{A_a + A_b}{A_{ab}}.$$

The count rate for 20% loss is $1/t \ln (1.25) = 0.223/t$. For a 2 µs dead time, the count rate for a 20% loss is about 110 000 cps (*see* dead time).

detector efficiency (*phys*) The factors that influence detector efficiency are:

- geometry;
- absorption;
- background radiation;
- collimation;
- dead time;
- conversion efficiency.

Geometry depends on 4π or 2π design. The absorption depends on both density and detector thickness. Background radiation must be low for distinguishing small activities. Collimation shields the useful detector surface. A poor dead time will render the detector inefficient at high count rates. Conversion efficiency measures signal output for energy deposited. (*ct*) The ratio between the number of events recorded by the detector and the number of x-ray photons incident on the detector. The detector efficiency is the product of the absorption efficiency for the photon energy used and conversion efficiency (x-ray photon to light photon conversion). Approximately 98%

for a 120 kVp x-ray spectrum. The ratio between the number of pulses recorded and the number of x-ray photons incident on the detector (*see* 4π geometry, 2π geometry).

detector element (*ct*) The section of a detector element orthogonal to the direction of the incident radiation which has a rectangular shape; the length of the side of the rectangle which is parallel to the scan plane determines the effective detector width and so determines the beam width; the other side of the rectangle, oriented in the *z*-direction, defines the maximum available slice width.

detector material (*ct*) Solid detectors should have a high relative light output (luminescent efficiency) giving high signal-to-noise ratios, and have low values for afterglow. Early CT detectors were thallium-activated CsI and self-activated CdWO$_4$. They had a high luminescent efficiency, but they exhibited high values of afterglow (>0.3%).

detector (ceramic) (*ct*) *See* ceramic scintillator.

detector offset/quarter shift (*ct*) The x-ray tube focal spot can be shifted in order to double detector resolution. Sample spacing in the scan plane can also be improved by quarter ray offset to improve ray sampling within the projection; opposing projections will be offset by one-half the detector width. If the central ray is offset by one fourth of the sampling distance from the centre of rotation then this ray will again be shifted by one fourth of the sampling distance in the opposite direction after 180° rotation. This allows interlacing of opposing projections and so doubling sampling frequency which improves resolution and reduces aliasing artefacts.

detector sensitivity (*phys*) The sensitivity of a detector is commonly related to the absorption properties of soft tissue. Air and certain phosphors (LiF) have almost an identical photon energy response as soft tissue; these detector material are deemed tissue equivalent (*see* detector efficiency).

detector spacing (*ct*) Distance between the centres of two adjacent detector elements; the detector spacing determines the sampling distance for a single projection (*see* detector offset/quarter shift).

detector width (*ct*) In a detector array, the distance between the two opposite faces of any single detector.

deterministic (*dose*) A model where all events are inevitable consequences of antecedent causes. An effect seen at a defined point (count rate, dose, etc.) resulting in a loss of organ function due to cell damage. Deterministic effect has a threshold below which no effect is seen.

deterministic effect (tissue reactions) (*dose*) (ICRP60) A type of radiobiological effect displayed by a group of cells which is characterized by a severity that increases with dose, above a certain threshold. Below that threshold, the effect is not observed. Examples are visual impairment due to cataract formation, temporary or permanent loss of fertility, loss of glandular excretion (salivary, thyroid), skin erythema and fetal damage. Deterministic effects are also called 'tissue reactions' (*see* sterility, cataract, hemopoiesis).

deterministic threshold (*dose*) Threshold doses (acute and chronic) for some deterministic effects (ICRP 92 2003c 2005(draft)):

Tissue and effect	Single dose (Sv)	Annual dose (Sv y^{-1})
Testes		
Temporary sterility	0.15	0.4
Permanent sterility	3.5–6.0	2.0
Ovaries		
Sterility	2.5–6.0	>0.2
Lens		
Detectable opacities	0.5–2.0	>0.1
Cataract	5.0	>0.15
Bone marrow		
Haemopoiesis, depression	0.5	>.4

detriment (*dose*) (ICRP73) A measure of the total harm that would eventually be experienced by an exposed group and its descendants from a radiation source. The combination of probability and severity of harm or health detriment. The probability of causing a level of total harm judged to be equivalent to one death that causes a loss of 15 years lifetime. Tissue-weighting factors are derived from this definition (*see* weighting factors (tissue)).

detriment coefficients (*dose*) (ICRP73) The nominal coefficients are average values for the whole population of equal numbers of males and females of all ages (except for breast and ovary). They apply to moderately low doses and dose rates associated with diagnostic procedures. The remainder tissue is 0.59 and the hereditary detriment figure for gonads is 1.33.

Organ or tissue	Nominal detriment coefficient (% per Sv)
Bone marrow	1.04
Colon	1.03
Stomach	1.00
Lung	0.80
Breast (female)	0.73
Ovary	0.29
Bladder	0.29
Oesophagus	0.24
Liver	0.16
Thyroid	0.15
Bone surface	0.07
Skin	0.04

deuterium (^{2}H) (*chem*) Symbol D. A naturally occurring stable isotope of hydrogen having a nucleus consisting of one proton and one neutron (^{2}H; heavy hydrogen). It has 0.015% abundance and is obtained from water by electrolysis. D_2O or heavy water has a density, boiling point and freezing point greater than H_2O. D_2O is used as a moderator in nuclear reactors and clinically to estimate body water content (*see* hydrogen, tritium).

developer (film) (*image*) A reducing compound of hydroquinone or metol (commonly hydroquinone and phenidone) variety which magnifies the latent film image. The action of the developer on exposed and unexposed silver halide grains is distinguished by rate. Exposed grains develop more rapidly than unexposed grains. The latent image acts as a catalyst. Density resulting from development of unexposed grains is fog. Commercial developer commonly consists of:

- a reducing/developing agent;
- a preservative/antioxidant (usually sodium sulphite);
- an alkali to keep the pH >10;
- a restrainer; commonly potassium bromide.

Hardeners are also present (gluteraldehyde) and anti-fogging agents.

deviation (*stats*) The percentage difference between measured value and prescribed value. (*maths*) The percentage of difference between measured value (*m*) and prescribed value (*p*) according to $(m/p - 1) \times 100\%$ (*see* accuracy).

device driver (*comp*) A small software package that will let the operating system (and programs running with it) control a particular output hardware device (e.g. keyboard, monitor, printer, modem, monitor, graphics card or CD–ROM drive).

DFSE (*mri*) Double fast spin echo.

DFT (*mri*) Discrete Fourier transform.

DGC (*us*) Depth gain compensation (*see* time gain compensation).

diagnostic accuracy (imaging) (*stats*) The ability to detect disease in members of a chosen population (from a hospital clinic or screening group). It depends on (1) the incidence of disease in the population and (2) the sensitivity of the test. The confidence in any assessment of diagnostic accuracy depends on the gold standard used to judge the results; whether they are abnormal (true positive (TP)) or negative (true normal (TN)). The most reliable gold standard is the autopsy, but other references are acceptable with certain provisos (laboratory findings, biopsy or phantom test object). Results from the imaging process are tabulated as positive (*I*+) or negative (*I*−) findings, comparing these with the known positive and negative values from the gold standard (*G*+ and *G*−). False-negative (FN) and false-positive (FP) are then discovered.

	G+	G−	Totals
I+	TP	FP	TP + FP
I−	FN	TN	FN + TN
Totals	TP + FN	FP + TN	Total

Breast screening

A screening population of 60 000 gives 3000 suspect images of which 300 are true-positives, 2700 false-positives and 50 false-negatives. So,

	G+	G−	Totals
I++	300	2700	3000
I−	50	56950	57 000
Totals	350	59 650	60 000

From this table calculations can be made for sensitivity, specificity, general accuracy, predictive positive accuracy (PPA), predictive negative accuracy (PPN).

These basic results can be used for receiver operator curves (ROC analysis) and an estimate of improvement in diagnostic accuracy due to integrated imaging or double reading of mammograms. Diagnostic accuracy has also been used in a different way to indicate the proportion of medical diagnoses that prove to be correct, thereby depending not only upon the detectability of the disease, but also upon its prevalence and the particular decision criterion that is adopted (*see* Bayes' theorem).

diagnostic reference levels (*dose*) (ICRP73) These are recommended by the ICRP and are usually the absorbed dose in air or in a tissue equivalent sample. In nuclear medicine, it will be the administered activity. The diagnostic reference level is intended to reduce unusually high patient doses. It is inappropriate to use them for regulatory or commercial purposes. They are obtained from a percentile point on an observed distribution of doses to patients. Advisory dose levels set by professional bodies to prompt local reviews of practice if consistently exceeded.

diamagnetism (*mri*) A material with a small negative magnetic permeability which decreases the local magnetic field and has negative magnetic susceptibility. Water and oxygen rich compounds are examples (*see* contrast medium).

diatrizoic acid/diatrizoate compounds (*cm*) The first fully substituted tri-iodobenzene contrast medium developed in the 1950s. Water-soluble ionic contrast medium, monomeric salts of tri-iodinated benzoic acid. Joining a set of almost identical analogous compounds iothalamate, metrizoate, iodamide and ioxithalamate. Mixtures of meglumine and sodium salts of diatrizoic acid have been used.

Compound	Viscosity (cP)	Osmolality (mOsm/kg)	Iodine (mg I ml⁻¹)
Diatrizoate	4.2 at 37°C	1570	300

The proportions of the two salts are adjusted to give the most suitable medium for the required clinical examination. The anion is the radio-opaque portion, but both anion and cation are osmotically active; therefore, the solution will be hypertonic to plasma leading to toxicity. Diatrizoate may be used as an intravascular contrast agent or as an oral contrast medium for the gastrointestinal tract (*see* Angiografin®, Hypaque®, Renografin®, Urografin®, Urovison®, Gastrografin®, Gastrovist®, Gastrovision®).

DICOM (*comp*) Digital imaging and communications in medicine is a standard for handling imaging data, developed by the American College of Radiologists (ACR) and National Electrical Manufacturers Association (NEMA). The DICOM standard enables the transfer of digital medical images and corresponding information, independent of device and manufacturer. It also provides an interface between hospital

D

systems (HIS) and radiological systems (RIS) based on other standards. DICOM deals with imaging equipment, printers, picture archival and communication systems (PACS), and also offers other functions such as film printing or CD burning. DICOM Version 3 (2007) provides program protocols for integrating various image data formats between imaging and nonimaging modalities, devices and systems (*see* HL7, IHE).

Dicopac" (*nmed*) ^{57}Co/^{58}Co-labelled cyanocobalamine preparation for Schilling test (Amersahm/GE Healthcare).

dielectric (*phys*) A substance commonly found in capacitors that can sustain an electric field and act as an insulator. Substances have different dielectric constants or permeability.

diethylene triamine pentaacetic acid (DTPA) (*nmed*) *See* DTPA.

differential uniformity (*nmed*) The intrinsic differential non-uniformity of sensitivity U_d for a gamma camera is $U_d = \Delta C/M \times 100\%$ where ΔC is the maximum difference in counts between two adjacent pixels and M is the larger of the two counts. Typical current values, for nonuniformity in central regions, are $\leqslant 2.5\%$ and for useful field of view 2.8% (*see* integral uniformity, uniformity (intrinsic)).

differentiation (*dose*) Stem cells entering a pathway of cell division where the daughter cells acquire specialized functions.

diffraction (*phys*) Bending of a beam at the edge of an absorbing surface into the shadow area of the surface.

diffusion (*image*) *See* unsharpness (radiographic). (*mri*) The process by which molecules or other particles migrate due to their continuous random thermal motion (Brownian molecular movement). Particles/molecules move from areas of higher concentration to areas of lower concentration. The diffusion in a homogeneous medium shows a Gaussian distribution. The variance (σ^2) of this distribution depends on the diffusion coefficient and time interval t so $\sigma^2 = 2(D \times t)$ where D is the diffusion coefficient characterized by the medium viscosity ($3 \times 10^{-9} \mathrm{m^2\,s^{-1}}$ for water at 37°C). The effect is exponential: so e^{-bD}. Diffusion of water molecules along a field gradient reduces the MR signal. With equal concentrations there is a statistical balance, but in areas of lower diffusion (diseased tissue), signal loss is less intense, and the display from these areas is brighter. The diffusion image provides a sensitive

technique for measuring diffusion of small molecules in specific tissue types; the diffusion may be directed (i.e. along myelin sheaths). This preferential diffusion is anisotropic diffusion.

diffusion coefficient (*mri*) *See* diffusion.

diffusion image (*mri*) Random diffusion of small molecules (i.e. water) in tissue due to thermal processes. Diffusion imaging can be presented as diffusion weighted imaging (DWI) or diffusion tensor imaging (DTI).

■ Reference: Elster, 1994; Hagmann *et al.*, 2006.

diffusion sensitivity (*mri*) *See* b-value.

diffusion tensor imaging (DTI) (*mri*) Uses diffusion-weighted images of the brain and tensor field mathematics to produce maps of individual fibre tracts, determining their direction and course from their origin in the white matter to their connection in the cortical grey matter. Isotropic diffusion (i.e. cerebrospinal fluid) can be described simply by the diffusion coefficient. Anisotropic diffusion (i.e. fibre direction) requires tensor mathematics in order to describe the direction of dominant diffusion pathways. The direction of greatest diffusion is given by the eigenvector of the diffusion tensor. If diffusion gradients are applied in six or more directions then a tensor can be calculated that gives a three-dimensional picture of dominant diffusion pathways. This can identify cerebral white matter lesions.

■ Reference: DaSilva *et al.*, 2003.

diffusion weighted imaging (DWI) (*mri*) Provides information on the viability of brain tissue. In any tissue sample undergoing a 90°/180° selected gradient pulse sequence, the echo signal is not received from water proton spins that are moving (the normal state in healthy tissue); this results in darker areas in the image. If the proton spins are relatively stationary, the dephasing effect of the gradient pulses cancels giving a stronger echo and brighter areas in the image. Image contrast therefore depends on the motion of water protons, which may be substantially altered by disease. DWI uses fast (echoplanar) imaging technology so is resistant to patient motion. Imaging time ranges from a few seconds to 2 minutes. It requires highperformance magnetic field gradients for its operation. The primary application of DWI has been in brain imaging where it can differentiate acute stroke from other processes that are associated with neurological deficit. DWI has also assumed an essential role in the detection of acute brain infarction.

■ Reference: Schaefer *et al.*, 2000.

DIGGEST (*mri*) Direct imaging of local gradients by group echo selection tomography.

digital circuit (*elec*) An electronic circuit using semiconductor devices (transistors, diodes) as logical switches. The basis of all computers and logic devices.

digital filter (*image*) In a general sense, a device for selecting any particular frequency or set of frequencies. Usually confined to a system which transmits a certain range of frequencies rejecting all others. It acts on a sampled version of a signal using a discrete logical hardware or software elements. Digital filtering can take place in either the time domain or frequency domain. The ideal filter would have a rectangular shape; unity transmission in the passband and zero transmission in the stopband, but this is not achieved in practice (*see* Butterworth filter, Chebyshev filter).

digital radiography (*di*) An imaging procedure where the intensity of the x-ray beam or single photon events are recorded on an image matrix either from an image intensifier, image phosphor plate or CT detector array (*see* direct radiography).

digital scan converter (*us*) Computer memory that stores echo information.

digital subtraction angiography (DSA) (*xray*) An imaging technique where digital x-ray images before and after iodine contrast injection are subtracted using computer procedures yielding a difference image of the vascular structure alone. DSA systems use digital fluoroscopy/fluorography systems. A reference mask image is first collected followed by serial images containing contrast material. A DSA processing unit is designed in such a way that two separate image memories hold the mask and the image with contrast medium, respectively. The mask image is stored in memory and the subtraction of the mask image from the contrast images made in an arithmetic unit, from which the result is passed on to an image processing and display unit.

digital to analogue converter (DAC) (*image*) An electronic circuit which converts digital signals into a matching voltage waveform. This can also be part of a digital to video converter responsible for the video display on a computer system. The bit size of a DAC determines the accuracy of high-resolution displays.

digital versatile disk (*phys*) *See* DVD.

digitization (*image*) Process of conversion of continuous analogue signals, such as the detected MR signal (voltage) into numbers. This is carried out with an analogue to digital converter. Typically, the voltage is measured (sampled) at particular discrete times and only voltages within a particular range and separated by a certain time can be distinguished. Voltages beyond these ranges are said to exceed the dynamic range of the digitizer.

digitization noise (*image*) Noise introduced into signals by the analogue to digital converter (ADC) either by electronic noise or by the limitation of digital resolution (bit depth). Also called quantization noise.

digitizer (*comp*) *See* analogue to digital converter.

dimeric (*cm*) Linking two monomer rings gives a compound with more iodine per unit, resulting in a larger molecule with up to six iodine atoms attached. The increased iodine improves x-ray absorption and consequently the contrast effect in the image. The more effective dimeric contrast agents reduce chemotoxicity and other adverse reactions.

dimeric ionic contrast agents (*cm*) *See* ionic dimer.

DIMM (*comp*) Dual inline memory module. A memory board that is effectively a double single in-line memory module (SIMM). Its 64 bit-wide bus allows single modules to be installed in Pentium systems.

diode (*phys*) An electronic device (thermionic or semiconductor) which passes current in one direction only.

diopter (*phys*) A method of quoting focal length of a lens system as the reciprocal of a meter. One diopter has a focal length of 100 cm, four diopters 25 cm, etc. Higher diopter figures have shorter focal lengths. Sometimes used for specifying camera performance.

diploid (*dose*) Relates to cells having a double set of chromosomes, usually relates to all mammalian cells except gametes.

dipole (*phys*) A system of two equal and opposite charges or poles influencing a very small distance. The product of charge and distance is the dipole moment. Electric and magnetic dipole moments exist. (*mri*) *See* magnetic dipole.

dipole–dipole interaction (*mri*) The interaction due to their magnetic dipole moments, between a nuclear spin and its neighbours.

D

An interaction contributing to relaxation times, which in solids and viscous liquids results in broadening of the spectral lines.

dipole field (*mri*) The field pattern produced by a closely spaced positive and negative electric charge or a north and south magnetic pole. At distances, it is large compared to the dipole length. The field falls off as the third power of the distance away from the charges or poles producing it.

dipyridamole (*clin*) Indirect vasodilator used in cardiac stress imaging. Increases serum adenosine levels.

Dirac, Paul Adrien (1902–1984) British mathematical physicist. Produced relativistic wave equations to explain electron spin and discovered the possibility of negative energy states, which he interpreted as antimatter, anticipating electron/positron pair formation. He also predicted the existence of the magnetic monopole. Awarded Nobel prize for physics in 1933 with Schrödinger for work in quantum theory.

Dirac function (*image*) Theoretically a perfect impulse signal, where x is defined as zero for all values except for a central point where x has an infinitely high value, $\Delta(x - x_0)$ located at x_0.

direct radiography (*image*) A multilayer digital x-ray detector consisting of a thin film transistor (TFT) array behind either a 500-μm amorphous selenium x-ray detector or phosphor material. A pixel size of $140 \times 140 \, \mu m$ is currently available. A full field $35 \times 43 \, cm$ has a matrix 2560×3072. The selenium detector requires a bias voltage and incident x-rays generate electron-hole pairs in the selenium. These charges are collected by the storage capacitors connected to the thin-film transistors. The phosphor material requires a photodiode array connected to the TFT. The digital image can be directly viewed, unlike image plate devices (*see* fill-in factor).

directional dose equivalent ($H'd$, Ω) (*dose*) (ICRU) The **dose equivalent** at a point that would be produced by an expanding field in the ICRU sphere at depth d on a radius Ω. For weakly penetrating radiation, a depth of 0.07 mm for the skin and 3 mm for the eye are employed; for strongly penetrating radiation a depth of 10 mm is employed. The unit is joule per kilogram ($J \, kg^{-1}$). Unit of measurement is the sievert (Sv).

directory (*comp*) A list of files stored in the computer.

direct splenoportography (*clin*) *See* splenoportography.

discrete cosine transform (*di*) Selecting the real coefficients of a Fourier series (cosine terms) for use in a fast Fourier transform.

discrete Fourier transform (DFT) (*image*) Since Fourier transformation is carried out by computer, the summing is over a finite or discrete number of data points rather than the integral described by the Fourier transform. The discrete Fourier transform is:

$$F(u) = \frac{1}{N} \sum_{x=0}^{N-1} f(x) \times e^{-jwx/N}$$

and the inverse, which gives the original signal is:

$$f(x) = \sum_{u=0}^{N-1} F(u) \times e^{jwx/N}$$

Euler's formula allows this to be expressed as the complex sum of cosine and sine transforms.

discrete variable (*stats*) Data points, measurements having only integer values, i.e. number of patients, births, number of lesions.

DISE (*mri*) Driven inversion spin echo.

DISIDA (*nmed*) *See* disofenin.

disk (*comp*) A general term covering various types of media used to store program and data files on a permanent basis (*see* bulk storage, CD-ROM)

disk (floppy) (*comp*) *See* bulk storage.

disk (hard) (*comp*) *See* bulk storage.

disk spindle speed (*comp*) The speed of the disk medium. Hard drives are restricted to one speed which can be 3600–3880, 4500, 5400 and 7200 r.p.m. Disk speed directly influences transfer rates (*see* disk transfer rate).

disk transfer rate (*comp*) The speed at which data is moved to and from the disk media. Hard disk transfer rates increase from the inner diameter to the outer diameter of the disk surface.

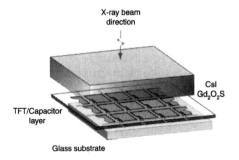

X-ray beam direction

CsI
Gd$_2$O$_2$S

TFT/Capacitor layer

Glass substrate

The disk transfer rate is dependent on the disk speed (r.p.m.) and the data density on the disk in bits per inch (b.p.i.).

disofenin (*nmed*) Diisopropyl iminodiacetic acid. Diisopropyl-IDA kit for the preparation of ^{99m}Tc-disofenin for injection, A radiopharmaceutical for cholescintigraphy.

Generic name	^{99m}Tc disofenin (DISIDA)
Commercial names	Hepatolite®-CIS
Imaging category	Hepatobiliary

dispersion (*us*) An ultrasound pulse spreads out as it passes through medium losing high frequencies. Pulse height decreases as pulse width increases. Depends on the property of the medium. The spread of a distribution. *See* standard deviation, quartile).

displacement (angular) (θ) The angular change in angular motion defined as $\theta = x/r$, where x is the linear displacement and r the radius of angular motion. Since r (the radius) is fixed then $\theta \propto x$. Angular displacement is in radians (rad) where $360° = 2\pi$ rad and 1 rad $= 57.3° = 180°/\pi$ rad.

display resolution (LCD) (*comp*) *See* flat panel display.

display matrix (*ct, image*) The array of rows and columns of pixels in the displayed image, typically between 512×512 and 1024×1024. It may be equal to or larger than the size of the reconstruction matrix due to interpolation procedures.

display window (*ct*) Selectable range, by the operator, within the CT number scale displayed on the screen and using the full range of brightness levels. The display window is usually defined according to the window width and window centre (off-set). Pixels outside the defined values are displayed as either white (above) or black (below the chosen window).

distortion artefact (*mri*) Image distortions caused by inhomogeneity of the magnetic field, gradient nonlinearity, or ferromagnetic materials in proximity to the examination.

distribution coefficient (*cm*) *See* partition/distribution coefficient.

disturbed flow (*phys*) Flow that cannot be described by straight, parallel stream lines.

dithering (*image*) A half-toning method where several dots of the primary colours are printed in various patterns to give the impression of a larger colour spectrum. The printing process of simulating additional colours or shades by mixing available colours and varying dot sizes and spacing. A half-toning method where several dots of the primary colours are printed in various patterns to give the impression of a larger colour spectrum; the printing process of simulating additional colours or shades by mixing available colours and varying dot sizes and spacing.

diverging collimator (*nmed*) A multiple-hole collimator whose holes diverge with a focal point behind the camera crystal. The diverging collimator reduces patient images, permitting imaging of patients whose width is greater than the diameter of the camera crystal.

divergent angle (θ) (*us*) The angle describing far field divergence (*see* Fraunhofer zone).

DLL (*comp*) Dynamic link library. A small program that can be shared between several tasks simultaneously. An essential component of a device driver. A program module that contains instructions common to different applications. Instead of including these in a program, the DLL can be called as required, loaded into memory and run. As the link is dynamic, the majority of DLLs can be unloaded when no longer needed, so saving memory resources.

DMA (*comp*) Direct memory access. A process for fast data retrieval from a device such as a hard disk that writes it into main memory without involving the processor, thus freeing it up for other tasks.

DMF (*dose*) *See* dose-modifying factor.

D_{min} D_{max} (*image*) *See* film sensitometry.

DMSA (*nmed*) Meso-2,3-dimercapto-succinic acid reconstituted with ^{99m}Tc. Localization and evaluation of various kidney diseases. Because of binding to plasma proteins, clearance is mainly through tubular absorption, showing a specific affinity for the renal cortex. Renal accumulation increases for 6 hours when 20–35% of the injected activity resides in each kidney. DMSA(V) targets tumour sites.

Generic name	DMSA (III)
	DMSA (V)
Commercial names	Succimer® (MediPhysics Inc)
	Amersham DMSA
Imaging category	Static renal function

DMSA(V) (*nmed*) Labelling DMSA with ^{99m}Tc under moderate reduction conditions, i.e. alkaline pH and low concentration of Sn(II), leads to the formation of a ^{99m}Tc(V) – DMSA complex which has proved suitable for tumour imaging.

DMSSFP (*mri*) Double-mode steady state free precession.

DNA (*clin*) Desoxyribonucleic acid. A type of nucleic acid found in the nucleus of the cell. The other nucleic acid RNA or ribonucleic acid is found in the cytoplasm and in small amounts in the nucleus. Radiation damage to this structure causes cellular malfunction, but there are elaborate systems of repair processes that have evolved for correcting DNA damage.

domain (*comp*) Represents an IP (internet protocol) address or set of IP addresses that comprise a domain. The domain name appears in URLs to identify web pages or in email addresses. For example, john.doe@centralhospital.com, where 'centralhospital.com' is the domain name. Each domain name ends with a suffix that indicates what top level domain it belongs to. These are: .com for commercial, .gov for government, .org for organization, .edu for educational institution, .biz for business, .info for information, .tv for television, .ws for website. Domain suffixes may also indicate the country in which the domain is registered: .ie for Ireland, .de for Germany, etc. No two parties can ever hold the same domain name.

dominant (*xray*) Applied mainly to fluoroscopy where the region of the object (patient anatomy) which is of diagnostic interest is selected in the field of view of the image intensifier. The automatic exposure device (dose limiting) coincides with this area. In a radiograph, this region should maintain a specific average optical density (including mammography).

door (shielded) (*xray*) A fire-rated lead-lined door set which should comply with BS476 Part 8 (1972) and Part 22 (1987) (*see* lead shielding).

DOPING (*mri*) Double pulse interlaced echo imaging.

doping (*phys*) The addition of a known quantity of impurity to either a semiconductor to alter its electrical characteristics or to a phosphor to improve its efficiency or alter its emission spectrum. For scintillator compounds used in the construction of x-ray detectors, appropriate doping improves the detector performance: signal decay and absorption efficiency.

doping agents (*phys*) Elemental impurities added to phosphor crystal structures in order to introduce traps in the forbidden energy band.

Application	Phosphor	Doping element
Intensifying screens	LaOBr	Tb, Tm
	GdOS	Tb
	YTaO	Nb
Image intensifier phosphor	CsI	Na
Nuclear medicine	NaI	Tl
Computed radiography	BaFX (X = Cl, Br or I)	Eu
Thermoluminescent dosimetry	LiF	Mg, Ti
	CaSO4	Dy

Doppler, Christian Johann (1803–1853) Austrian mathematician and physicist. Noticed the apparent difference between the frequency at which sound waves leave a source and that at which they reach an observer caused by the relative motion of the observer and source.

Doppler (colour) (*us*) This display uses echo location and Doppler shift to give a display of blood flow on a grey scale anatomical background. Time-shift colour flow imaging the Doppler effect is not used, but echo arrival time shifts are used for determining reflector motion. In each case, the Doppler shift or time shift variation is colour coded to give a blood flow display either towards or away from the transducer. Imaging frame rates are decreased due to the added computational time (*see* Doppler (power)).

Doppler (continuous) (*us*) *See* Doppler (CW).

Doppler (CW) (*us*) Continuous wave Doppler. A transducer having separate transmitter and receiver transducer crystals active continuously. No depth sensitivity but able to give audible Doppler velocity signals in a portable machine (*see* pulsed Doppler).

Doppler (power) (*us*) The difference between colour and power Doppler is that power Doppler maps colour to power value rather than the mean frequency. The machine uses autocorrelation detectors to produce a colour power map. The main advantage is that noise is restricted to a uniform low level and so the colour signal strength is increased with an overall gain of 10–15 dB over the conventional colour Doppler showing increased sensitivity to small flow differences. Noise reduction is obtained mainly by frame averaging which tends to affect the persistence of the image and introduce movement artefacts due to low frame rates.

Doppler (pulsed PW) (*us*) Measuring the Doppler frequency by pulsing the ultrasound beam (pulsed wave Doppler). A single transmit/receive transducer is depth sensitive and the user can select a region of interest (sensitive area). A sample gate is opened to accept echo signals from a specified depth. The **pulse repetition frequency** (PRF) is critical for accurate depth selection.

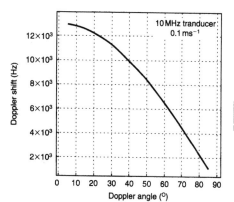

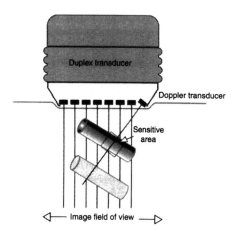

D

Doppler (reflector speed) (*us*) Commonly refers to flowing blood cells. The reflector speed of blood cells ($20–200\,\mathrm{cm\,s^{-1}}$) is much less than the speed of sound in soft tissue ($1540\,\mathrm{m\,s^{-1}}$).

$$\frac{\text{Propogation speed} \times \text{Doppler shift}}{2f \times \cos(\theta)}$$

Doppler–reflector speed

For a 5 MHz ($f = 5000\,\mathrm{kHz}$) transducer used at an angle of 45° ($\cos(\theta) = 0.707$) gives a Doppler shift frequency of 900 Hz (0.9 kHz); the reflector speed is:

$$\frac{15400 \times 0.9}{2 \times 5000 \times 0.707} = 19.6\,\mathrm{cm\,s^{-1}}$$

Since distance to reflector surface is 154 000/2 the equation can be simplified to:

$$\frac{77000 \times 0.9}{5000 \times 0.707} = 19.6\,\mathrm{cm\,s^{-1}}$$

Doppler angle (*us*) The angle between the sound beam and the flow direction. If the angle between the transducer and vessel is zero (parallel) the Doppler shift is maximum; at 90° it is zero (graph).

Doppler effect (*us*) Frequency change of a reflected sound wave as a result of reflector motion relative to the transducer. The frequency shift between transmitted and reflected ultrasound wave $f2 - f1$ as Δf, described by:

$$\Delta f = 2\frac{f}{c}(v\cos\theta)$$

where c is the propagation velocity of sound in blood and v is the blood velocity. The angle (θ) between the transducer and skin surface is the angle of insonation. The value 2 represents the double Doppler effect, once from the moving blood cells and again when the transducer receives the echo.

Doppler sample volume (*us*) The sensitive volume from which the Doppler signal is obtained. The position within the beam is dependent on pulse repetition frequency (PRF) (*see* sample volume).

Doppler shift (*us*) This is calculated as the difference between echo frequency and incident frequency. Both are measured in MHz. It can also be calculated from the transducer incident frequency f (MHz), the reflector speed (v) in $\mathrm{cm\,s^{-1}}$ and propagation speed (c). Also in $\mathrm{cm\,s^{-1}}$ as:

$$\frac{2f \times v \times \cos\theta}{c}$$

Doppler shift

A 5 MHz Doppler signal from a transducer placed at an angle of 60° (0.5). It measures a blood velocity of $50\,\mathrm{cm\,s^{-1}}$ (speed of sound in soft tissue = $154\,000$ $\mathrm{cm\,s^{-1}}$). The Doppler shift frequency is:

$$\frac{2 \times (5 \times 10^{6}) \times 50 \times 0.5}{154\,000} = 1623\,\mathrm{Hz}.$$

Doppler (spectral) (*us*) A time (*x*-axis) versus velocity magnitude display calculated from the Doppler shift on the *y*-axis. The common velocity spread is intensity coded by pixel brightness. Spectral Doppler assesses organ perfusion identifying stenoses and occlusion. It also evaluates heart function. Volume blood flow can be assessed directly or indirectly from the Doppler spectrum as:

$$Q = TAV_{mean}A.$$

TAV_{mean} is the amplitude-weighted averaging over all instantaneous flow velocities registered in the sample volume. *A* is the cross-section of the vessel at the sampling site obtained from the vessel diameter measured in the B-mode image.

DOS (*comp*) Disk operating system. An operating system designed for early IBM-compatible PCs.

dosage (*nmed*) The amount of radiopharmaceutical administered to a patient, measured in becquerels (Bq).

dose (entrance) (*dose*) The dose or dose rate at the surface of the patient or absorber. Any dose level measured at the surface will include a fraction back-scattered from deeper tissue layers: the back scatter fraction (BSF). Entrance exposure and entrance surface dose (ESD) distinguish with and without BSF correction, respectively. ESD is a measure for individual radiographs (*see* dose area product).

dose (exit) (*dose*) The air kerma measured at the absorber surface opposite the beam. Typically this is maintained at a constant level in order to provide a mean image density or optimum input rate at the image intensifier face (*see* entrance dose).

dose (organ) (*dose*) *See* mean glandular dose.

dose (patient) (*dose*) Measured as:

- absorbed dose in air (air-kerma); as a dose-area product;
- surface dose using tissue equivalent dosimeters;
- depth dose (CTDI);
- patient activity levels (nuclear medicine).

(*see* diagnostic reference levels).

dose (x-ray) (*xray*) From an exposure giving a photon fluence of 3×10^{10} photons cm^{-2} at 60 keV$_{eff}$ delivers an approximate dose of 10 mGy (1 R).

Dose, x-ray
From the data given in photon exposure. The photon fluence for a chest radiograph is 8.3×10^{8} photons cm^{-2}. Then the equivalent dose is $8.3 \times 10^{8}/3 \times 10^{10} = 0.2$ mGy (0.027 R).

(*see* dose – area product, diagnostic reference levels, photon fluence, photon flux).

dose and dose-rate effectiveness factor (DDREF) (*dose*) (ICRP60) A factor that generalizes the usually lower biological effectiveness (per unit of dose) of radiation exposures at low doses and low dose rates as compared with exposures at high doses and high dose rates.

dose area product (DAP) (F_a) (*dose*) Used in x-ray examinations to control radiation exposure to patients. It is the dose integral of the air-kerma K_a over the intersecting surface *S* of the useful radiation beam:

$$F_a = \int_S K_a \cdot dS.$$

The SI unit for the dose area product is Gy m^2, replacing R cm^2 where 1 R cm^2 is approximately 0.87 cGy cm^2 or 0.87 µGy m^2. The DAP is a measure of the complete study. National protocols give recommended dose quantities for entrance surface dose (ESD) for individual radiographs and dose – area-product (DAP) for complete examinations. The doses are reference levels intended to trigger department investigations if they are routinely exceeded.

Entrance surface dose (UK)	
Study	ESD (mGy)
Lumbar spine, AP	10
Lat	30
LSJ	40
Abdomen, AP	10
Pelvis, AP	10
Chest, PA	0.3
Lat	1.5
Skull, AP	5

Dose area product (UK)	
Study	DAP (Gy cm^{-2})
Lumbar spine	15
Barium enema	60
Barium meal	25
Intravenous urography	40
Abdomen	8
Pelvis	5

- Reference: IPSM/NRPB/CoR, 1992.

(*see* dose (entrance)).

dose calibrator (*nmed*) A device (ionization chamber) for measuring the amount of radioactive material within a container. Used to verify dosage prior to administration. It is commercially available as a 'dose calibrator'.

Having a cylindrical 4π construction used for measuring radionuclide activity levels in nuclear medicine. The activity range covered is commonly a few MBq to many GBq.

dose coefficient (*dose*) Alternative for dose per unit intake, can describe other coefficients linking quantities or concentrations of activity to doses or dose rates.

dose constraint (*dose*) An agreed restriction on the individual dose from a radiation source, which serves as an upper limit on the dose in optimization of protection for that source. For occupational exposures, the dose constraint reduces the individual **dose** limits considered in the process of optimization. For public exposure, the dose constraint is an upper limit on the annual doses that members of the public should receive from the planned operation of any controlled source.

dose descriptor (*ct*) Measurable parameter, such as $CTDI_{air}$, $CTDI_w$, etc. or DLP, from which the effective dose or the organ dose delivered to a patient in a CT examination can be estimated, or the performances of different CT scanners can be compared.

dose distribution (*ct*) The spatial distribution of dose as a function of the position within the scan plane ($CTDI_w$). For CT, the ratio of surface dose and the dose at the centre is closer to one than for projection/conventional radiography because of the rotating x-ray source around the patient during the examination.

dose–effect curve (*dose*) See **dose – response curve**.

dose efficiency (*ct*) Number that quantifies the amount of dose absorbed by the detectors as a fraction of the total dose reaching the detector; overall dose efficiency of a CT scanner is described as the product of three factors:

1 **geometric efficiency** of the detector array;
2 **detector efficiency**;
3 x-ray beam **z-axis efficiency**.

The results given in the table show an improvement in the overall dose efficiency for thin slices when progressing from the 2-slice, 4-slice and 16-slice scanner. This improvement is mainly due to the wider beam width used to acquire the thin slices in the 4- and 16-slice scanners. (*See* Table below)

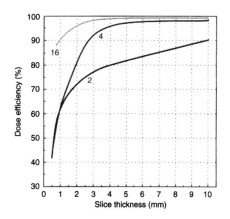

dose equivalent (H) (*dose*) (ICRP26) The product of the **absorbed dose** at a point in tissue and **radiation quality factor** Q. So the product: grays $(Gy) \times Q = H$, where H is measured in sieverts (Sv). The previous unit the **rem** (non-SI) is replaced by the **sievert** (SI). This term has been replaced by the **equivalent dose** which measures absorbed dose over a specified area.

dose length product (DLP) (*ct*) Dose measurement used as an indicator of overall exposure for a complete CT examination. Allows performance comparisons. The associated dose – length product (DLP) for a complete examination, can be derived as:

$$DLP = \sum_i CTDI_w \cdot T \cdot N \cdot C \,(\text{mGy cm})$$

where i represents each scan sequence forming part of an examination, and $CTDI_w$ is the weighted CTDI for each of the N slices of thickness T (cm) in the sequence and C the exposure in mAs (as fractions of 100 if the $CTDI_w$ was standardized to 100 mAs). For spiral acquisition the formula changes to:

$$DLP = \sum_i CTDI_w \cdot T \cdot A \cdot t \,(\text{mGy cm})$$

For each study or scan sequence, A is the tube current (mA) and t the study acquisition time. It is also convenient to modify this formula to accommodate multislice scanners using $CTDI_{100}$. The scattered radiation component increases slightly with multislice machines increasing the

Scanner	Slice number	Geometric efficiency (%)	z-axis efficiency (%)	Overall dose efficiency (%)
Dual	2 × mm	80	63	50
Quad	4 × mm	78	72	54
Sixteen	16 × 1mm	75	93	65

overall dose. European guidelines for CTDI$_w$ and DLP values are obtained as 75th percentile figures from a European wide CT survey.

Organ	CTDI$_w$ (mGy)	DLP (mGy/cm)
Head	60	1050
Face and sinuses	35	360
Vertebral trauma	70	460
Chest	30	650
HRCT of lung	35	280
Liver	35	900
Abdomen	35	800
Pelvis	35	600

■ Reference: Tsapaki *et al.*, 2001.

dose limitation (ICRP) (*dose*) A controlling factor regulating radiation practices which ensures an equitable distribution of individual benefits and detriment.

dose limits (environmental) (shld) The US Environmental Protection Agency's generally applicable environmental radiation standards in 40 CFR Part 190 shall comply with those standards. Environmental Conservation Law: Subpart 380.5: Radiation dose limits for individual members of the public; 380-5.1: Dose limits for individual members of the public; 380-5.2: Compliance with dose limits for individual members of the public. The total effective dose equivalent to individual members of the public does not exceed 0.1 rem (1 mSv) in a year. Unrestricted area in the environment from external sources does not exceed 0.002 rem (0.02 mSv) in any one hour; in an unrestricted area, the dose from external sources would not exceed 0.002 rem (0.02 mSv) in an hour and 0.05 rem (0.5 mSv) in a year. The principal European limit for radiation exposure was 0.5 mSv yr^{-1} (1977 ICRP values). This is based on a mortality risk of 5×10^{-6} per annum. This has been reduced to 0.3 mSv yr^{-1}.

dose limits (staff) (*dose*) (ICRP73) These apply to workers and members of the public who require to be in an area where radiation is being used. Dose limits do not apply to patients, provided that these doses have been justified.

Application	Occupational	Public
Effective dose	20 mSv per year, averaged over 5 years	1 mSv y^{-1}
Equivalent dose		
Eye lens	150 mSv	15 mSv
Skin	500 mSv	50 mSv
Extremities	500 mSv	–

The use of optimization in the work place and the ALARA principle now makes these dose limits less important.

dose-modifying factor (DMF) (*dose*) The ratio of radiation doses with and without modifying agents, causing the same level of biological effect.

dose modulation (*ct*) Currently the two methods are chosen by manufacturers for modulating the x-ray beam are essentially:

● A prior scoutview of the scanned area to alter a look-up table for modulating the x-ray beam during the intended scan: Whole body-dose modulation uses a scoutview to vary mA along the patient and during rotation. Prior to the axial scan a look at attenuation along one or two scout views is made this mapping made to vary the mA in each slice accordingly.

● A continuous slice by slice sampling and modulation of the x-ray beam: This uses feedback during the scan study to vary x-ray tube mA along the patient and during rotation, according to the attenuation seen in the previous rotation. The tube mA gradually changes in response to anatomy in real time.

dose-mortality curve (*dose*) The exposure of a population to a whole body dose of radiation can be plotted as dose versus mortality. This generally gives a sigmoid shape curve where the upper and lower portions of the curve are poorly defined. The midpoint of the curve at the 50% survival mark is the median lethal dose (LD$_{50}$).

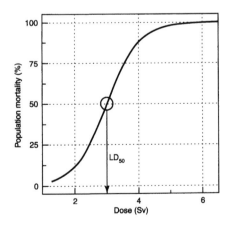

dose profile/slice dose profile (SDP) (*ct*) Representation of dose as a function of position along a line perpendicular to the tomographic plane. The dose as a function of the position along the z-axis resulting; due to x-ray scatter, the slice dose profile (SDP) is always broader than the slice sensitivity profile (SSP) in spite of detector collimation.

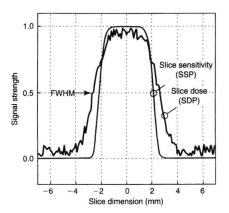

dose rate (*dose*) Amount of energy absorbed per gram per unit time. Unit is sievert per unit time per gram of tissue (*see* kerma).

dose rate constant (*nmed*) This replaces the specific gamma ray constant (Γ) according to ICRU33, although the two terms are not identical. For radiation therapy, the dose rate constant G_d of a radionuclide, emitting photons is the quotient $K_d \times r^2$ and the activity A. The symbol K_d is the air kerma rate which would be produced by all the photons of energy $E \geqslant d$ at a distance r from a point radiation source of activity A, if the radiation were neither absorbed nor scattered at the source or in any other matter:

$$G_d = \frac{K_d \times r^2}{A}$$

The SI unit being $Gy\, m^2 s^{-1} Bq^{-1}$. The selection of the lower energy limit d expressed in keV, depends on the application. The dose rate constant G_H is defined for radiation protection, where H_x is used in place of the air kerma rate K_d. The energy threshold is 20 keV for all nuclides:

$$G_H = \frac{H_x \times r^2}{A}$$

The practical exposure rate constant of a radionuclide is given as $mGy\, cm^2 MBq^{-1} h^{-1}$ (SI units) or $mrad\, cm^2 mCi^{-1} h^{-1}$ (non-SI units). A variation is $cGy^{-1} U^{-1}$ where U represents the unit of air

kerma strength $1\, \mu Gy\, m^2 h^{-1}$. Conversion factors to convert exposure dose rate constants ($mGy\, cm^2 MBq^{-1} h^{-1}$) to specific gamma ray constants ($mGy\, h^{-1} MBq^{-1}$ at 1 m) are available.

Nuclide	$mSv\, hr^{-1} m^{-1} GBq^{-1}$
[57]Cobalt	1.6×10^{-2}
[60]Cobalt	3.6×10^{-1}
[111]Indium	8.4×10^{-2}
[131]Iodine	5.7×10^{-2}
[99]Molybdenum	4.1×10^{-2}
[99m]Technetium	1.7×10^{-2}

- Reference: Siegel *et al.*, 2002.

dose-rate-effectiveness factor (DREF) (*dose*) A correction factor which allows for the low-dose nonlinear response for low linear energy transfer (LET) radiation when interpreting low-dose effects from high-dose observations. This is used to project cancer risk determined at high doses and high dose rates to the risks that would apply at low doses and low dose rates (ICRP 60, 1991). In general, cancer risk at these low doses and low dose rates is judged, from a combination of epidemiological, animal and cellular data to be reduced by the value of the factor ascribed to DDREF. It reduces by a factor of 2 (current ICRP value) the probability coefficients seen at high dose rates. Used for dose estimations below 200 mGy or $<100\, mGy\, h^{-1}$.

dose-response curve (*dose*) Also called dose-effect curve. Generally there are three specific responses at low doses:

1 linear response;
2 quadratic;
3 linear-quadratic.

The general form includes both linear and quadratic terms for defect (cancer) induction (α_1 and α_2), as well as β_1 and β_2 coefficients for exponential cell killing. The product of the polynomial component:

$$(\alpha_0 + \alpha_1 D + \alpha_2 D^2 + \alpha_n D^n)$$

and the exponential form, $e^{(-\beta_1 D - \beta_2 D^2)}$, combine. Coefficients α (determining the curvature of the slope) are selected to give the best fit to the data. At low doses, the exponential effect is small and cell killing is not present (due to cellular repair mechanisms). The polynomial component then dominates in its simpler forms of linear, quadratic or linear-quadratic depending on cell type. None of the curves shows a threshold below which no effect is seen.

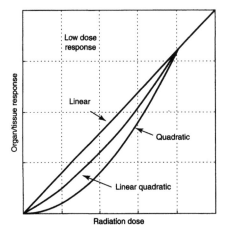

Low dose response

Linear

Quadratic

Linear quadratic

Organ/tissue response

Radiation dose

(*see* linear non-threshold hypothesis).

■ Reference: Brill, 1982.

dose–survival curve (bacteria) (*dose*) The loss of proliferation in a single cell organism (bacterial colony) is related as a simple exponential to dose over a very wide range of exposure. A typical LD_{50} is 200 Sv.

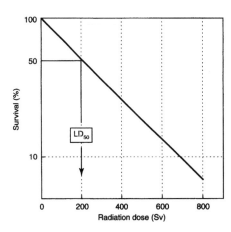

100

50

LD_{50}

10

0   200   400   600   800
Radiation dose (Sv)

Survival (%)

dose–survival curve (mammalian) (*dose*) Cell survival to a single dose of radiation. The curve characteristics are described by two parameters D_o which describes the slope of the exponential portion of the curve after the shoulder. The size of the shoulder (which represents cellular repair effectiveness) is measured by extrapolating the straight portion of the curve (plotted on log/linear scales) upwards to the vertical axis where

it intersects at N. The curve for sparsely ionizing radiation (low LET) is given by:

$$S = 1 - (1 - e^{-D/D_o})^N$$

where N is the extrapolation number at zero dose. D_o is the dose at 37% survival or the reciprocal of the slope, typically 1–2 Gy. D_q is the 100% survival shoulder.

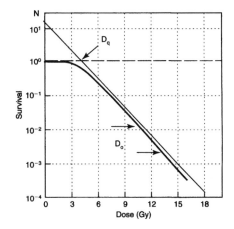

N

10^1

D_q

10^0

10^{-1}

10^{-2}

D_o

10^{-3}

10^{-4}

0   3   6   9   12   15   18
Dose (Gy)

Survival

(*see* dose – response curve).

dose–threshold hypothesis (*dose*) A specified dose above background below which it is hypothesized that the risk of excess cancer and/or heritable disease is zero.

dosimetric terms (individual) (*dose*) The table gives the complete updated family introduced in ICRP60. Separate detailed descriptions are given under the headings identified in 1–5.

Measure	Unit	Derivation
1. Absorbed dose, D	gray (Gy)	$E/m\,J\,kg^{-1}$
2. Equivalent dose, H_T	Sievert (Sv)	$H_T = \sum D_T \times w_R$
3. Effective dose, E (effective dose equivalent, EDE)	Sievert (Sv)	$E = \sum H_T \times w_T$
4. Committed equivalent dose, $H_{T(\tau)}$	Sievert (Sv)	$H_{T(\tau)} = H_T \times \tau$
5. Committed effective dose, E_τ	Sievert (Sv)	$E_\tau = E \times \tau$

dosimetric terms (population) (*dose*) *See* collective equivalent dose, collective effective dose.

dosimetry (*dose*) Calculation of dose received by an organ or tissue or whole body from ionizing radiation. For x-ray studies, this determines the energy dose in body tissue which cannot be directly measured in the body cavity, but can be calculated from the energy dose produced in a small air probe (thimble dosimeter). The ion dose is measured from which the dose in air and thus the energy dose can be calculated. The ion dose is frequently measured using tissue equivalent thermoluminescent detectors. The energy dose is calculated from the measurement and conversion factors (f-factor) listed in tables (*see* absorbed dose, equivalent dose, effective dose, MIRD).

dosimetry phantom (*dose*) Cylinders of polymethylmethacrylate (PMMA) used for standard measurements of dose in CT, having a diameter of 16 cm (head phantom) or 32 cm (body phantom) and a length of at least 14 cm. The phantoms are constructed with removable inserts parallel to the axis to allow the positioning of a dosemeter at the centre and 1 cm from the outer surface (periphery).

dot-matrix (*comp*) A printer where the characters and graphics are formed from a grid of dots produced by wire pins striking the paper through a fabric ink-ribbon. A common design uses 24 pins as found in line printers producing continuous documentation (patient documents and labels) where very fast printing is essential and top quality is less important (*see* laser printer, ink jet printer, bubble jet printer).

dot pitch (display monitor) (*image*) Monitor dot pitch is measured as the distance between dots of the same colour (red, green or blue) and therefore refers to pixel dimensions; typical values are 0.28, 0.25 or 0.22 mm. Colour monitors are rated as pixels per inch (ppi) which is typically 72 to 96 ppi (*see* flat panel display).

dot pitch (printer) (*image*) Dot pitch on a printer refers to dot density as dots per inch (dpi) typically 300, 600 or a commercial printers quality of 1200 dpi (*see* display resolution).

Dotarem® (*cm*) Commercial preparation (Guerbet) of gadoteric acid, a paramagnetic ionic MRI contrast agent. (*See* Table below)

double blind (*stats*) A method for avoiding bias in clinical trials. Single-blind trial has only one group (scientist or patient) knowing the treatment. In double-blind trials, neither group know the distribution of drug or treatment protocol.

double contrast enema (*clin*) Removal of barium enema and introducing air into the rectum, showing fine detail of the rectal and colon mucosa.

double contrast sequence (*mri*) Turbo spin echo (SE) counterpart to double echo sequences. For short pulse trains only echoes for PD and T2-weighted images having the phase-encoding gradient are measured. The echoes that determine resolution are used in both raw data matrices (echo sharing), reducing the number of echoes required. More slices can be acquired for the TR period; giving a lower specific absorption rate (SAR).

double echo sequence (*mri*) Spin echo (SE) sequence with two echoes; obtained without increasing the measurement time since they are produced from the first echo of a T2-weighted double echo sequence.

double-oblique slice (*mri*) Rotating an oblique slice about one axis in the image plane.

double reading (mammography) (*clin*) Two clinicians reviewing the same mammograms can improve both sensitivity and specificity. If a single reading yields a sensitivity of 80% and a specificity of 70%, then double reading using the statistics described in integrated imaging, condition (1) yields sensitivity 96% and specificity 91%, and for condition (2) yields sensitivity 99% and specificity 97%.

downscatter (*nmed*) Scattered photons of lesser energy resulting from Compton scattering of primary gamma emissions of a radionuclide.

downtime (*comp, xray*) The percentage of time during which a piece of equipment is routinely not working or broken; a measure of equipment reliability. Zero downtime implies 100% reliability. An annual reliability of 90% means a downtime of 10% or 36.5 days. A 99% reliability means a downtime of 3.6 days and 99.99% gives a downtime of 1 hour per year and 99.999% just over 5 minutes. Mission critical

Compound	Concentration (mg mL⁻¹)	Viscosity (cP)	Osmolality (mosm/kg)
Gadoterate meglumine Gd-DOTA	279.32	3.2 at 20°C 2.0 at 37°C	1350

applications demand very small downtime values (*see* MTBF).

DPD (*nmed*) A preparation as ^{99m}Tc-labelled 2,3 dicarboxypropane-1,1-diphosphonate produced from diphosphonopropane-dicarboxylic acid. Used as a diagnostic bone imaging agent. Reported to show higher normal/abnormal bone ratios than MDP or HMDP.

dpi/DPI (*comp*) Dots per inch. A common measure of dot pitch, the resolution on a printer, scanner or display.

DPSF (*mri*) Diffusion/perfusion snapshot flash.

DQE (*image*) *See* detective quantum efficiency.

DRAM (*comp*) Dynamic random access memory. The most common and cheapest form of computer memory which uses one capacitor and transistor to store one bit of information. Being dynamic, the capacitor needs refreshing every few milliseconds or it will lose its charge (losing information).

Draximage^R (*nmed*) *See* gluceptate.

DREF (*dose*) *See* dose rate effectiveness factor.

drip infusion cholangiography (*clin*) Commonly used when oral techniques have failed. Contrast material introduced by intravenous infusion.

drip infusion urography (*clin*) For demonstrating space-occupying lesions within the kidney and outlining the whole extent of the ureters. Direct intravenous injection using drip infusion over an extended period.

driver (*comp*) *See* device driver.

DSA (*xray*) *See* digital subtraction angiography.

DSL (*comp*) Digital subscriber line. A method of connecting to the Internet via a phone line. A DSL connection uses copper telephone lines, but is able to relay data at much higher speeds than modems and does not interfere with telephone use (*see* ADSL).

DSO2 (*dose*) A revised dose system developed for estimating gamma and neutron exposure under a large variety of situations and which allows the calculation of absorbed dose to specific organs. DSO2 improved on the DS86 system.

DS86 (*dose*) An early dose system developed for estimating gamma and neutron exposure under a large variety of situations which allowed the calculation of absorbed dose to specific organs for members of the Life Span Study.

D$_T$ (*dose*) *See* absorbed dose.

DTE (*comp*) Data terminal equipment. An end device on a communications circuit – a computer terminal or PC.

DTI (*mri*) *See* diffusion tensor imaging.

DTPA (*nmed*) Diethylene-triamine-penta acetic acid usually present as a calcium or sodium salt complex as monocalcium trisodium diethylene-triamine penta-acetic acid, a chelating substance containing five acetate groups which forms a stable complex with metallic ions, typically ^{99m}Tc or ^{111}In. It is a strong chelating agent more commonly found as a radiopharmaceutical for ^{99m}Tc labelling when it forms a glomerular filtration rate (GFR) agent for renography. DTPA also forms complexes with ^{111}In for cerebrospinal fluid (CSF) studies or as a method for labelling antibodies with ^{111}In-DTPA as an intermediate.

Generic name	^{99m}Tc-DTPA
Commercial names	Techeplex Bracco®
	DTPA-CIS®
	Draximage DTPA®
	Mallinckrodt DTPA®
	Amersham DTPA®
Imaging category	Renal, ventilation V/Q

(*mri*) Gd-DTPA and Mn-DTPA are used as paramagnetic contrast agents (*see* EDTA).

DTR (*comp*) Data terminal ready. An RS232C circuit that is activated to let a DCE know when a DTE is ready to send or receive data.

dual-energy CT (DECT) (*ct*) A machine design (Siemens) that exposes the same slice simultaneously with two different x-ray beam energies: 140 kVp, then 84 kVp. Dual-energy CT promises additional diagnostic information including bone mineral content, improved beam hardening correction and display quality.

dual energy subtraction (*xray, image, ct*) A method for removing hard and soft tissue contributing to a subtracted image. X-ray energies of 60 and 110 kVp are commonly employed.

dual focal spots (*xray*) A target (x-ray) carrying a single focal spot is restrictive since many applications require two focal spot sizes; for general applications and a second smaller focal spot for higher resolution or magnified radiographs (i.e. mammography or spot imaging). Two methods are used for providing two focal spot sizes on the same anode. (1) A single filament refocuses the electron beam electrostatically varying the negative voltage on the cathode cup, so bombarding a smaller area on the anode track. (2) A double filament, each one directed to a different angled target, which requires a dual track anode to give two focal spot sizes.

dumb terminal (*comp*) A monitor and keyboard that displays information only (as opposed to the processing capability of a PC); usually connected to a mainframe or local area network (LAN).

duo core processors (*comp*) Two independent processors (CPUs) in one package run at the same frequency and share 4 MB of L2 cache. It has a 1.066 MHz bus performing parallel processing.

duplex (*comp*) A method of data transmission. Full-duplex allows a packet of information to be transmitted and received at the same time. Half-duplex allows packets to be either transmitted or received, but not at the same time.

duplex imaging (*us*) Combining a grey-scale image with a colour Doppler image.

duplex instrument (*us*) An ultrasound instrument that combines gray-scale sonography with pulsed Doppler and, possibly, continuous-wave Doppler.

duty cycle (*us*) The percentage of time the pulse occupies in the operational cycle:

$$\text{Duty cycle} = \frac{PD}{PRP \times 1000} = \frac{PD \times PRF}{1000}/1000\ ms.$$

The percentage or fractional measure of the time that the pulse occupies in the transmit receive cycle. It increases with increasing PRF. Time fraction that the pulse is on. Typical value 5 ms, range 1–10 ms. Both PD and PRP are measured in microseconds (μs) to give the DF as a unitless fraction (*see* ultrasound (safety)). (*mri*) The time during which gradient switching can be run at maximum power. Based on the total time (as a percentage), including the cool-down phase (*see* SAR).

duty factor (DF) (*us*) The product of the pulse duration and the pulse repetition frequency for a pulsed waveform. A typical pulsed sequence consists of an 'on-time' or mark (m) and an 'off-time' or space (s). The duty factor is then:

$$DF = \frac{m}{m + s} \times 100\%.$$

DVD (*comp*) Originally meaning digital video disk then digital versatile disk. A DVD disk is the same size as a CD but offers enlarged storage due to its double-sided storage capacity and double-layer design. Capacities of 17 G-Bytes are possible, each layer holding 4.7 G-bytes. Smaller indentations and shorter wavelength lasers are used. Using MPEG2 compression, extensive audio and video information can be stored. DVD-ROM is a read-only device similar to the CD-ROM, but DVD-RAM is a read/write version, which is completely reusable. Regional coding (currently six regions are recognized) is introduced to protect DVD data content (e.g. film videos, regional variations of software), so that American disks will not play in Europe or Japan, etc. The various storage capacities for DVD are:

- 2.6 GB single sided;
- 3 GB single sided;
- 4.7 GB single side/single layer;
- 5.2 GB doubled sided for DVD-RAM;
- 6 GB double sided for DVD RW;
- 8.5 GB single sided/double layer;
- 9.4 GB double sided/single layered;
- 17 GB double sided/double layered.

The latest disks have two layers and DVD drives use a laser with two focal points to read each one. Each layer holds 4.7 GB, so a dual-layer, dual-sided disk will store 17 GB of data (*see* Blu-ray® disk).

dwell time (*us*) The amount of time that the transducer is actively transmitting ultrasound power.

DWI (*mri*) *See* Diffusion-weighted imaging.

dynamic aperture (*us*) The beam width at the focus point is limited by the size of the transducer or groups of transducers (elements), their focal length and wavelength. The beam width is controlled by the aperture increasing the aperture (number of apertures) with increasing focal length, so maintaining constant focal width during transmission.

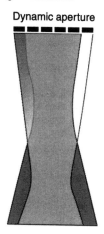

Dynamic aperture

dynamic focusing (*us*) When a transducer array receives echoes, the receiving focus depth may be continuously increased by altering receiver delay as the transmitted pulse travels forward. The continuously changing echo receiver window used for dynamic focusing increases image resolution with depth.

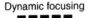

Dynamic focusing

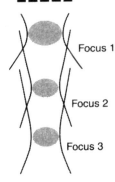

Focus 1

Focus 2

Focus 3

dynamic imaging (*us*) Rapid-frame-sequence imaging; real-time imaging.

dynamic range (*xray*) The dynamic range carried by the beam when considering subject contrast is the ratio of intensity with no attenuation to the maximum tissue attenuation. Overall attenuation obeys the general equation $I_{out} = I_{in} e^{-\mu x}$. The dynamic range to register all the attenuation information is I_{in}/I_{out}, where I_{in} is unity. Typical film dynamic range (latitude) ranges from 1:10 to 1:100. Image plate and direct radiography detectors have dynamic ranges approaching 1:10 000.

Dynamic range

Mammography, where E_{eff} is 20 keV, $x = 5$ cm and $\mu = 0.76$. The dynamic range is:

$$\frac{1}{e} - (0.76 \times 5) = 1{:}45$$

Chest x-ray, where E_{eff} is 100 keV, $x = 20$ cm and $\mu = 0.17$. The dynamic range is:

$$\frac{1}{e} - (0.17 \times 30) = 1{:}164.$$

(*ct*) For an acceptable wide dynamic range, the ADC must be capable of responding to a large variation in tissue attenuation values; the ADC which must be capable of registering 10^6 steps. The dynamic range represents the largest signal (no attenuation) to the smallest signal (maximum attenuation) that can be detected.

Dynamic range, CT

For a 20-bit ADC, the dynamic range is 1:10⁶ ($2^{20} = 1\,048\,576$) the uncertainty in voltage measurement is $\sqrt{10^6}$ or 1000 representing 0.1%. The attenuation coefficient for soft tissue (μ) at 150 kev is 0.155 and water is 0.1504. A variation of 0.1% in μ is 0.000155:

$$(0.155155 - 0.1504)/0.1504 = 32$$

$$(0.154845 - 0.1504)/0.1504 = 30$$

A variation exceeding 0.1% will significantly affect CT number calculation.

(*us*) The range of echo intensities. This can be up to 100 dB at the input amplifier, 60–80 dB at the time gain compensation (TGC) and 50 dB after compression. Dynamic range. Ratio (in decibels) of the largest power to the smallest power that a system can handle; ratio of the largest to the smallest intensity of a group of echoes. (*mri*) Range of signal intensities distinguished in an image or spectrum. If the signal dynamic range is too great, the need to keep the highest intensities from overloading the digitizer may result in the weaker features being lost in the digitization noise. This can be dealt with by using an analogue to digital converter with a larger range of sensitivity or by using techniques to reduce the dynamic range, e.g. suppressing the signal from water in order to detect the signal from less abundant compounds.

dynamic scanning (*ct*) A method of obtaining CT scans in rapid sequence so as, for example, to follow the passage of contrast material through vessels or tissue, or to decrease examination time.

dynamic study (*xray, nmed*) A study where a certain number of time frames are collected (*see* renogram).

dyne (dyn) (*phys*) a centimetre – gram – second (cgs) unit of force. 1 dyn = 10^{-5} N.

dynode (*elec*) An electrode in a vacuum tube device whose function is to excite secondary electron emission (*see* photomultiplier).

dysprosium (Dy) (*elem*)

Atomic number (Z)	66
Relative atomic mass (A$_r$)	162.50
Density (ρ) kg/m³	8500
Melting point (K)	1680
K-edge (keV)	53.7

Relevance to radiology: Doping agent for glass and phosphors.

e (*math*) Symbol for the transcendental number 2.718282 used as the base for the natural logarithm (*see* exponential).

e-mail (*comp*) Electronic mail. An important facility offered by the Internet giving the ability to send/receive messages, pictures and computer data (files). The email address has the form myname@company.com or myname@server.xx, where country xx has a two letter identifier (*see* domain).

ECD (*nmed*) ^{99m}Tc-labelled ethyl-cycteinate diethylester or ^{99m}Tc-bicicisate. Has similar uptake kinetics to HMPAO, but remains stable *in vitro* for up to 6 hours after reconstitution.

ECG-gated image reconstruction (*ct*) A method for cardiac imaging freezing cardiac motion by retrospectively reconstructing CT images for selected heart phases. Correlating each measured projection with the recorded electrocardiogram (ECG) signal.

ECG triggering (*ct*) Triggering computed tomography (CT) scan data collection using the ECG signal.

echo (*mri*) The point where spins (transverses magnetization) come back in phase and produce an MR signal. An echo can be produced by a gradient reversal (gradient echo) or by the use of a 180° refocusing pulse. (*us*) The returning ultrasound signal reflected from a surface within the body of the patient. The time of arrival of these echoes is used to calculate the depth of tissue interface.

echo amplitude (*us*) This is determined by the structure and composition (acoustic impedance) of the reflecting surface used to determine the brightness (grey-scale) of the ultrasound display.

Echogen^x (*cm*) Ultrasound contrast agent using perfluorocarbons instead of air, produced by Sonus Pharmaceuticals (*see* Echovist®, Levovist®).

echo offset (*mri*) Adjustment of radio frequency (RF) spin echo and gradient echo to be non-coincident in time, so as to create phase differences between the signals from different spectra (e.g. fat and water). The magnitude of the resulting phase difference will be equal to the product of the difference in frequency of the spectral lines and the difference in the echo times (TE).

echo planar imaging (EPI) (*mri*) Extremely rapid imaging sequence where the complete image is obtained using a single selective excitation pulse. Field gradients are switched periodically to generate a series of gradient echoes. The FID is detected while switching the *y*-gradient magnet with a constant *x*-gradient. The Fourier transform of the spin-echo sequence then supplies the image of the selected plane. Several artefacts are generated, the resolution is limited and it is sensitive to magnet in-homogeneities (*see* TurboFLASH, ultrafast gradient echo).

echo sharing (*mri*) Used in double contrast sequences. Echoes that determine the image resolution are used in both raw data matrices.

echo spacing (*mri*) The distance between two echoes (e.g. turbo-spin echo (turbo-SE) or EPI sequences). A short echo space produces short sequence timing and fewer image artefacts.

echo time (*us*) The arrival time of echoes is used for locating the depth of objects. One ultrasound pulse yields one scan line along which returns echoes from objects at various depths. Axial resolution determines the ability to separate close echoes.

Echo time

If the speed of sound in soft tissue is $\sim 7\,\mu s\,cm^{-1}$ ($1500\,m\,s^{-1}$) then echo-times from objects 12 and 20 cm from the transducer (allowing double distances for transmission and reception) are:

$2 \times 12 \times 7 = 168\,\mu s$ and $2 \times 20 \times 7 = 280\,\mu s$.

(*mri*) (TE) Time between the excitation pulse of a sequence and the resulting echo used as the MR signal. Determines image contrast. The time between the 90° pulse and the echo peak is the echo time TE. Additional 180° pulses can create additional echoes. Gradient field reversal can take the place of the 180° pulse to yield gradient echoes.

echo train (*mri*) Applied to multi-echo sequences, where two or more echoes are acquired, each of which obtains a different phase-encoding direction.

Echovist^x (*clin*) Saccharide-based ultrasound contrast agent containing microbubbles of air, manufactured by Schering AG and introduced in 1991. Due to limited *in vivo* stability after injection, the microbubbles dissolve during lung transit so it is particularly useful for right ventricle imaging (*see* Levovist®).

ED$_{50}$ (*stats*) Median effective dose.

eddies (*us*) Regions of circular flow patterns present in turbulence.

eddy currents (*mri*) Electric currents induced in a conductor by a changing magnetic field (e.g. gradient fields) or by motion of the conductor through a magnetic field. A source of image artefacts and concern for safety in rapidly switched gradients used in superconducting magnets. A source of concern about potential hazard to subjects in very high magnetic fields or rapidly varying gradient or main magnetic fields. A problem in the cryostat of superconducting magnets. The influence of eddy currents on gradient fields can be reduced by eddy current compensation and shielded gradient coils.

eddy current compensation (*mri*) A means of reducing the incidence of eddy currents on pulsed gradient fields by employing an electrical pre-emphasis in the gradient amplifiers. Multiple time constants are commonly used to correct for eddy current effects in various structures of the MR system (cryoshields and RF-shields).

edentate (calcium/disodium) (*cm*) A chelating agent used as a stabilizer in some contrast media preparations.

edge (*image*) A set of pixels with values significantly different from pixels on the opposite side of the edge resulting in different grey levels (*see* penumbra).

EDGE (*comp*) (Enhanced data rate for global system for mobile (GSM) communications evolution). EDGE refers to five technologies in development that are aimed at GSM networks. There are disagreements about whether Edge should be described as a 2.5G or a 3G technology. Edge promises a maximum theoretical rate of 384 Kbps (kilobits per second).

edge enhancement (*di*) Applying a differentiating filter to an image which will exaggerate any sharp changes in count density difference.

edge-packing (*nmed*) High-count density artefact that appears at the periphery of all Anger-type gamma camera images.

edge oscillation (*mri*) Truncation artefact (*see* Gibbs artefact).

edge response function (ERF) (*ct*) *See* edge spread function.

edge spread function (ESF) (*ct*) The image of a high-contrast edge positioned orthogonal to the imaged plane. Objects made from polymethyl-methacrylate (PMMA) or aluminium within a water bath can be used in order to measure the ESF of a CT system if the object provides at least one even boundary plane oriented orthogonal to the scan plane.

Edison, Thomas A (1847–1931) American inventor. After testing 8000 substances, discovered calcium tungstate as a fluorescent material for x-ray inten-sifying screens in 1896.

EDMP (*nmed*) *See* samarium.

EDO (*comp*) Extended data out RAM. The current memory used for computers offering improved performance. To read a word of computer memory it must be pre-charged first. EDO memory speeds up this sequence by pre-charging the nest word while still reading the current word.

EDTA (*nmed, mri*) Ethylenediamine-tetra-acetic acid having a formula:

$$(CH_2COOH)_2 \cdot N \cdot (CH_2)_2 \cdot N \cdot (CH_2COOH)_2.$$

A chelating agent widely used for sequestering di- and trivalent metal ions (M), such as ^{99m}Tc, ^{111}In or gadolinium.

EFAST (*mri*) Blood flow artefact suppression and motion artefact reduction technique (Toshiba) motion artefact reduction techniques. Spatial pre-saturation to reduce MR signal intensity in specific locations (*see* SAT, REST, PRE-SAT, PRESAT, SATURATION).

effectance (*dose*) (ICRP60) *See* effective dose.

effective detector width (*ct*) Width of a single detector element within the scan plane projected on to the isocenter according to the scanner geometry (*see* detector element).

effective dose (*E*) (*dose*) Also termed effective dose equivalent (EDE). It is the product of the equivalent dose and a tissue weighting factor (ICRP60). It is therefore a doubly weighted absorbed dose for all the irradiated tissues:

$$E = \sum (D_T \times w_R \times w_T) \quad \text{or}$$

$$E = \sum w_T \times H_T.$$

where D_T is the absorbed dose; w_R and w_T are the weighting factors for radiation and tissue, respectively; H_T the equivalent dose. The effective dose is a whole body dose equivalent allowing comparisons to be made between different radiological procedures. This calculation indicates that the risk of fatal cancer associated with this pattern of irradiation corresponds to the risk of fatal malignancy and serious hereditary harm from a dose equivalent of 0.825 mSv received uniformly throughout the body. In comparison, a high voltage chest radiograph delivers an equivalent dose of about 0.2 mSv to the lung and rib cage giving an effective dose of 0.05 mSv (*see* weighting factor (tissue)).

Effective dose

A routine nuclear medicine lung scan using ^{99m}Tc-MAA returns the following equivalent organ doses:

- lung tissue: 5 mSv
- liver: 1.5 mSv
- ribs: 1 mSv
- ovaries: 0.15 mSv.

The weighting factors (ICRP60) for these tissues are 0.12, 0.05, 0.12 and 0.20, respectively, so the effective dose (E) is:

$(5 \times 0.12) + (1.5 \times 0.05) + (1 \times 0.12) + (0.15 \times 0.2)$

$E = 0.825$ mSv.

This serves as an estimate of the whole body dose from a ^{99m}Tc-MAA perfusion lung scan.

---

effective dose (CT) (*ct*) This is a useful indicator of patient radiation risk, although it is also not particularly suitable as a reference dose quantity since it cannot be measured directly and its definition may be subject to further changes. Broad estimates of the effective dose (H_e) may be derived from the DLP as:

$$H_e = E_{DLP} \times DLP$$

where E_{DLP} is the region or tissue specific normalized effective dose in $mSv\,mGy^{-1}cm^{-1}$. Multiplying factors for obtaining the effective dose H_e from the DLP values.

Organ	DLP	E_{DLP}	H_e (mSv)
Head	1050	2.3×10^{-3}	2.4
Chest	650	1.7×10^{-3}	1.1
Abdomen	800	1.5×10^{-3}	1.2
Pelvis	600	1.9×10^{-3}	1.1

- Reference: Hidajat *et al.*, 1999.

effective dose equivalent (EDE) (*nmed*) *See* effective dose.

effective echo time (*TE*$_{eff}$) (*mri*) The period between the excitation pulse and the echo. Both the contrast and signal-to-noise ratio of the image are determined mostly by the timing of the echo at which the phase-encoding gradient has the smallest amplitude. The echo signal in this case undergoes minimal dephasing and has the strongest signal.

effective energy (*E*$_{eff}$) (*xray*) The modal point on the continuous x-ray spectrum, identified on the curves as E_{eff}. The beam's effective energy can be influenced by changing kVp and filtration. The intensity Q of the beam is seen to increase as $Q \propto kV^2$; a 30% increase in kilovoltage

roughly doubles x-ray beam intensity along with an increase in effective energy. The effective energy of a moderately filtered x-ray spectrum is approximately $\frac{2}{3}$ kVp, so 100 kVp would translate as 70 kV$_{eff}$.

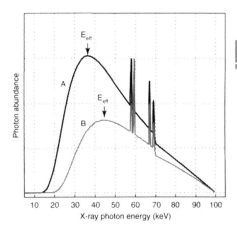

effective focal spot (*xray*) The projected dimensions from.the angled anode target as calculated from the line-focus principle. The effective focal spot for general radiography is 0.6–1.2 mm and for mammography 0.4 mm. The dimensions of the effective focal spot differs over the image plane.

effective half-life (*nmed*) The time required for the amount of a radionuclide deposited in a living organism to be diminished 50% as a result of the combined action of radioactive decay and biological elimination.

effective repetition time (TR$_{eff}$) (*mri*) Repetition time (TR) is not fixed during cardiac triggering so it is determined by the time interval for the trigger. The effective repetition time TR$_{eff}$ established by the trigger interval fluctuates with the cardiac rhythm.

effective slice thickness (*ct*) The total effect of the collimation, pitch and interpolation as described by the slice sensitivity profile (SSP). The FWHM of this profile is commonly used as a measure for the effective slice thickness. With the 180° interpolation, the FWHM of a pitch 1 acquisition is similar to that of a conventional scan with the same collimation. For larger pitches, the FWHM increases linearly. While the SSP of the conventional scan has very steep edges, the SSP of the spiral multi-slice scan is more bell shaped, so the area of anatomy that contributes to the image is wider.

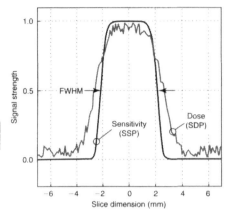

efficiency (conversion) (*xray*) The efficiency of signal (e.g. light) production in a detector.

efficiency (geometrical) (*phys*) The fraction of the isotropic emission collected by the detector surface.

efficiency (quantum) (*phys*) A measure of photon absorption.

EFG (*mri*) Electric field gradient.

EFOMP (*phys*) European Federation of Medical Physics.

EFR (*mri*) *See* electron spin resonance.

EHIDA (*nmed*) A radiopharmaceutical from the family of HIDA complexes (N-[N'-(2,6 dimethyl-phenyl) carbamoyl-methyl] iminodiacetic acid). The diethyl variant is EHIDA used for investigating hepatic function and for scintigraphic imaging of the hepatobiliary system.

EIDE (enhanced IDE) (*comp*) An improved version of IDE that supports large hard disks, faster access speeds and DMA. It is two controllers providing primary and secondary channels which handle two devices each and can also talk to CD-ROMs and tape drives.

eigen value (*image*) Literally 'characteristic value'. A set of values associated with a square matrix whose columns are called eigen vectors. It is common to use the symbol λ for eigen values.

eigenvector (*math*) Characteristic vector (German *eigen*, characteristic). A vector *x* corresponding to a given eigenvalue of a square matrix (*see* tensor, diffusion image).

▪ Reference: Nelson, 2003.

Einstein, Albert (1879–1955) Albert Einstein was born in Ulm, Germany and died in Princeton, USA. In 1905, he published papers on light quanta, Brownian motion and special theory of relativity ($E = mc^2$). He published papers on general relativity in 1913 and 1916. He was awarded the 1921 Nobel prize for physics for his work on the photo-electric effect (*see* Cockroft-Walton, pair production, positron).

EISA (*comp*) Extended industrial standard architecture. A non-IBM design of PC more advanced than AT and XT machines. It is a competitor to microchannel and ISA.

elastic collision (*phys*) In which the kinetic energy of the colliding bodies is the same after collision as before. No energy change.

elastic scattering (*phys*) An interaction between an incident photon and the atomic field. There is no loss of energy.

elasticity (*phys*) The property of a body which tends to resume its original size and shape after being deformed. The modulus of elasticity is the ratio of stress to strain. Young's modulus is defined as:

$$\frac{\text{applied load per unit area}}{\text{increase in length}}.$$

Other definitions apply to bulk modulus and shear modulus.

ELD (*mri*) Energy level diagram.

electric charge (*units*) Electric charge (Q) coulomb (C), where $1\,C = 6.24 \times 10^{18}$ electrons; the charge/electron 1.6×10^{-19} C (*see* charge).

electric field intensity (E) (*phys*) The fundamental quantity for describing electric field, it is defined in terms of the force exerted by the field on a stationary charge. The unit is newton per coulomb $N\,C^{-1}$. An important factor playing a part in electron beam focusing in x-ray tubes and gas multiplication in Geiger tubes (*see* electric field strength).

electric potential or electromotive force (emf) (*phys*) Defined in terms of the electric potential energy difference or work done in moving a unit charge between two points. The NMR signal is measured as an emf across the terminals of the receiver coil. Unit, the volt (V) (*see* electrical energy).

electrical conductivity (*phys*) The reciprocal of resistivity. It is also defined as current density divided by electrical field strength. Measured in siemens (S) m^{-1}.

electrical energy (*phys*) A form of potential energy, obtained when a quantity of electricity (electrons) moves between two points (positive and negative) which have a potential difference. A potential difference of 1 volt exists when 1 joule is generated when 1 coulomb moves between two terminals so $1\,\text{volt} = 1\,\text{JC}^{-1}$. Energy $W = QV$ joules. If 5 coulombs moves between points having a potential difference of 2 volts then $10\,\text{J}$ is generated.

Energy for x-ray unit 50 kV at 50 mAs
Since $Q = I \times t$ then $W = IVt$ joules, 50 000 volts (50 kV) at 50 mAs (50 mA for 1 s), energy consumed:

$0.1 \times 50\,\text{kV} \times 0.5\,\text{J} = 2500\,\text{J}$.

---

electrical field strength (E) (*units*) The intensity of an electric field at a given point exerted by the field at that point. Measured in volts m^{-1} (V m^{-1}). The electrical field strength increases at sharp edges or projections; a factor used in the x-ray tube cathode cup.

electrical heating (*phys*) The heating effect of electric current depends on:

- the electric current being passed, I;
- the resistance of the circuit, R;
- the time spent, t.

The following relationships can be established:

1 For a constant current, I, and fixed resistance, the heat produced is proportional to time spent.
2 For a constant resistance and fixed time, the heat produced is proportional to I^2. Joules' laws of electrical heating summarize these findings. The heat developed in a wire is proportional to:
- the time spent;
- the current squared, I^2;
- resistance of the conductor (wire), $P = I^2 R t$ J.

electrical interaction (*phys*) A repulsive force acting between electric charges of like sign and force of attraction between dissimilar electric charges.

electrical power (AC) (*phys*) The measurement in alternating current circuits is only valid when current and voltage waveforms are in phase; the case with purely resistive circuits (heaters and lighting). Electrical loads that include inductors (motors, transformers) the voltage and current waveforms are not in phase. The degree of phase-shift is expressed by the power factor (cos φ) or phase angle. The relationship between true power P measured in kW and apparent power S measured in kVA is: $P = S \times \cos \varphi$.

When comparing electrical energy, W, produced by a direct current with an alternating current flowing through the same load requires a measure of the root mean square for the alternating current.

electrical power (DC) (*phys*) Electrical power P relationships are derived as:

$$\frac{\text{Energy delivered}}{\text{Time taken}} \quad \text{so} \quad P = \frac{IVt}{t} = IV \; \text{J s}^{-1}$$

where $1\,\text{J s}^{-1}\,1 = 1$ watt. Power loss is calculated by restating Ohm's law as $V = IR$. Then $P = I \times (IR)$ or $P = I^2 R$. Similarly, since $I = V/R$ then $P = V \times (V/R)$ or $P = V_2/R$, which gives three standard formulas relating power with voltage, current and resistance. Since all conductors have some electrical resistance, power is always lost during transmission.

Electrical energy
Energy gain
Energy W (1 volt = $1\,\text{JC}^{-1}$)
Since $Q = I \times t$, then $W = IVt$ J
For 50 000 volts (50 kV) at 50 mAs (50 mA for 1 s), energy consumed $0.1 \times 50\,\text{kV} \times 0.5\,\text{J} = 2500\,\text{J}$.
Electric power
A 100 W electric light bulb at 220 volts consumes: $w/v = 0.45$ amp and 110 volts consumes 0.9 amp. Commercial electric power is measured in kilowatts (kW). Electrical energy consumed is expressed as kW × time which is the kW × hour. So 4 × 100 W lamps burning for 8 hours consume: $100 \times 4 \times 8 = 3.2\,\text{kW}$ hour independent of supply voltage (1 kWh = 3.6×10^6 J).

Electrical power	$1\,\text{J} = 1\,\text{W s}$
watt (W)	$W = EQ = I^2 R t = V^{2t}/R = VIt$
kilowatt (kW)	$1\,\text{W} = 1\,\text{J s}^{-1}$
	$1\,\text{kWh} = 3.6 \times 10^6\,\text{J}$.

(*see* electrical units).

electrical resistance (Ω) (*phys*) One ohm (Ω) maintains a current of one amp at one volt so that: $R = V/I$. Variations of this basic formula are: $I = V/R$ and $V = IR$. If a is the cross-sectional area of a conductor, then providing the length L is constant, its resistance is proportional to cross-sectional area. So that,

$$R \propto \frac{L}{a^2}.$$

If the diameter of the wire is doubled then resistance decreases by a quarter.

Electrical resistance (ohm, Ω)	$I = V/R$
	$R = V/I$
	$V = IR$
	$P = V^2/R$

electrical units (*phys*) The basic SI units and their relationships are:

Measure	Parameter	Relationships
Charge (Q)	Coulomb (C)	$1\,C = 6.24 \times 10^{18}\,e$
	Electron charge	$1.6 \times 10^{-19}\,C$
Potential difference (PD)	Volt (V)	$1\,V = 1\,J\,C^{-1}$
		$1\,V = 1\,W\,A^{-1}$
Energy (E)	Joule (J)	$J = QV$
		$E = W/Q$
	Electron volt (eV)	$1\,J = 6.24 \times 10^{18}\,eV$
		$1\,eV = 1.6 \times 10^{-19}\,J$
Current (I)	Ampere (A)	$Q = I \times t$
		$1\,A = 1\,C\,s^{-1}(6.24 \times 10^{18}\,es^{-1})$
		$P = IV$
		$P = I^2R$

electrolyte (*phys*) A substance that conducts electricity in solution or in the molten state due to the presence of ions. Sodium chloride dissociates into ions when dissolved in water or in a molten state:

$NaCl \rightarrow Na^+ + Cl^-$.

electromagnetic field (*phys*) The influence that electromagnetic radiation exerts on another object in close proximity or at a distance.

electromagnetic induction (*phys*) When a magnet is moved within a coil a current is induced in the coil. The coil can be moved producing the same effect. This is the principle behind the dynamo and alternator, producing electric energy from mechanical energy. Conversely in induction by current, if two coils are placed closely together and one energized by switching a battery in circuit causing a growth of a magnetic field then this induces a current in the second coil. The current in one must be changing to induce a current in the second coil. This is the principle behind the transformer.

electromagnetic radiation (*phys*) Radiation propagated through space or material in which electric and magnetic fields are vectors which are 90° opposed. Unaffected by external electrical or magnetic fields and absorption follows an exponential law. Speed in vacuum *c* is a constant: $2.99792\ 5 \times 10^8\,m\,s^{-1}$ or approximately $3 \times 10^8\,m\,s^{-1}$. Each frequency band has unique properties, but the wave character is identical having an electrical and magnetic component. Wavelength can range from several kilometres to $10^{-14}\,m$. The energy content of an electromagnetic wave is a multiple of the basic quantum: the photon, where:

$E = hf$

f is frequency in Herz ($Hz \equiv$ cycles s^{-1}) and *h* is Planck's constant. Wave energy increases with frequency. The frequencies *f* of some electromagnetic radiations are:

Red light	$3.7 \times 10^{14}\,Hz$
Blue light	$7.5 \times 10^{14}\,Hz$
Ultraviolet	$4 \times 10^{15}\,Hz$
X-rays	$5 \times 10^{17}\,Hz$
Gamma radiation	$5 \times 10^{19}\,Hz$

In comparison, radio and television waves (FM and UHF) are much lower down the scale and have frequencies between 80 MHz and 1 GHz (80×10^6 to $1 \times 10^9\,Hz$).

Measure	Equation	Values
Velocity, c	$c = f\lambda$	$c = 3.0 \times 10^8\,m\,s^{-1}$
Wavelength, λ	$\lambda = c/f$	λ in m or nm
Frequency, f	$f = c/\lambda$	f in Hz
Energy, E	$E = hc/\lambda$	$hc = 1.24 \times 10^{-6}\,eV$

electromagnetic spectrum (*phys*) A spectrum of electromagnetic radiation represented either as increasing frequency or decreasing wavelength. Electromagnetic radiation exhibits the following approximate values of wavelength and frequency:

	Wavelength (m)	Frequency (Hz)
Radio	10^5 to $10^{-3}\,m$	5×10^5 to 10^{11}
Infrared	10^{-3} to $10^{-6}\,m$	10^{12} to 5×10^{15}
Visible	4 to $7 \times 10^{-7}\,m$	5×10^{15} to 10^{16}
UV	10^{-7} to $10^{-9}\,m$	10^{16} to 10^{18}
X-rays	10^{-9} to $10^{-11}\,m$	10^{18} to 5×10^{19}
Gamma	10^{-11} to $10^{-14}\,m$	$>10^{19}$

Radiation energy as electron volt

Ultra violet frequency = $4 \times 10^{15}\,Hz$

$$\lambda = \frac{3.0 \times 10^8}{4} \times 10^{15} = 75\,nm$$

$E = 16\,eV$.

Red and Blue light have wavelengths of 700 and 400 nm, with energies of 1.77 and 3.1 eV, respectively. X-rays have a continuous spectrum from 60 to 120 keV, their wavelength ranges from 0.02 to 0.0099 nm and a frequency range from 1.5 to $3.0 \times 10^{19}\,Hz$.

---

electromotive force (E) (*phys*) Electromotive force of an electrical source (battery, dynamo or generator), measured in volts. A device with an e.m.f. E passing a charge, Q, through a circuit liberates electrical energy, QE. Basic electrical definitions derive from this as charge, Q, is a steady current, I, for time, t. Then energy $W = QE = IEt$. Total power $P = W/t = EI$ (*see* power).

electron (*phys*) Negative charged elementary particle, e^-. The fundamental charge on the electron is 1.6×10^{-19} C. and electron rest mass is 9.1×10^{-31} kg. Since $E = mc^2$, the rest mass is equivalent to 8.19×10^{-14} J or 0.511 MeV (*see* electron volt).

electron (bound) (*phys*) For photon–electron interactions (photoelectric effect, Compton scatter), a bound electron is one having a binding energy higher than the incident photon. In higher Z materials (calcium, barium, iodine) the K and L shells are treated as 'bound' and the orbitals above M are 'free' with respect to the x-ray photon energy (*see* electron (free)).

electron (free) (*phys*) Those obital electrons whose binding energies are low compared to the photon energy. In low Z materials (e.g. soft tissue), any electron outside the K-shell can be treated as 'free' in C, N and O for the diagnostic x-ray range (*see* electron (bound)).

electron (rest mass) (*phys*) This is also a fundamental constant being 9.1×10^{-31} kg.

electron affinity (*phys*) Either the energy required to remove an electron from a negative ion to form a neutral atom or the ability of oxidizing agents to capture electrons.

electron beam (*phys*) The stream of electrons generated by thermionic emission from a hot metal or metal oxide. The beam produced is usually narrow and consists of high-velocity electrons whose intensity is controlled by the filament temperature.

electron beam CT (EBT, EBCT) (*ct*) Alternative design for a CT scanner which functions without any moving mechanical parts. The electron beam is deflected and steered at high speed around the patient. The beam strikes an anode ring and produces a fan of x-rays.

electron capture (*phys*) A decay process seen in 'neutron-poor' nuclides (cyclotron produced) where a proton is converted into a neutron by capturing an electron from the K-shell and liberating a neutrino.

$$^1_1 p_0 + e^- \rightarrow {}^1_0 n_1.$$

This has a similar end result as positron emission. $^{201}_{81}$Tl (e.c) α $^{201}_{80}$Hg with the emission of Hg x-rays (68–82 keV).

electron cascade (*phys*) Filling vacancies in electron orbits (normally K- or L-shell vacancies) by electrons in higher (less energetic) orbits. Accompanied by characteristic radiation and Auger electrons.

electron charge (e) (*units*) This is the charge on the electron 1.602×10^{-19} C so one coulomb represents 6.24×10^{18} electrons.

The energy gained by electron beam in a x-ray tube

If 3×10^{17} electrons representing 50 mA (1.6×10^{-19} C each electron) move along an x-ray tube at 120 keV, then energy gained is

$E = QV$ Joules
$= (3 \times 10^{17}) \times (1.6 \times 10^{-19}) \times (120 \times 10^3)$
$= 5760$ joules

The charge of an electron beam

If Q coulombs flows during t seconds then:

$Q = I \times t$ coulombs.

X-ray exposure for 100 mA at $t = 0.5$ s (50 mAs), then $I = 0.1$ coulombs s^{-1} and $Q = 0.05$ coulombs or 50 milliCoulombs (mC). So x-ray exposure in mAs is equivalent to mC.

---

electron density (*phys*) The number of electrons per gram shows a difference between dense materials (bone, lead, etc.) and less dense materials (water, soft tissues, etc.). Hydrogen has the highest electron density, so substances containing more hydrogen (water) cause greater scatter. The number of electrons per gram is: ($N \times Z)/A$, where Z is the atomic number, N is Avogadro's number and A the atomic mass. The probability of a Compton event can be estimated from the number of electrons per cm^3 which is:

Density (g cm^3) $\times$ electrons g^{-1}.

Material	Density (kg m^{-3})	Electrons (g$^{-1} \times 10^{23}$)	Electrons (cm$^{-3} \times 10^{23}$)
Hydrogen	0.09	6	5.4×10^4
Air	1.225	3.01	3.8×10^{20}
Water	1000	3.34	3.34
Muscle	1000	3.36	3.36
Fat	910	3.48	3.16
Bone	1650–1850	3.00	5.55

electron emission (*phys*) The liberation of electrons from a surface. They can be liberated by (1) thermionic emission resulting from the high temperature of the surface; (2) photoelectric emission resulting from photon bombardment; (3) field emission resulting from intense electric fields; and (4) electron emission due to nuclear decay.

electron paramagnetic resonance (EPRI) (*mri*) *See* Electron spin resonance.

electron spin resonance (ESR) (*mri*) magnetic resonance phenomenon involving unpaired electrons, e.g. in free radicals. The frequencies are much higher than corresponding NMR frequencies in the same static magnetic field.

electron traps (*phys*) Locations within the forbidden band introduced by impurities that either hold electrons falling from the conduction zone or provide further electron events after a particular event has finished (*see* energy bands).

electron volt (eV) (*units*) A measure of radiation energy, since the joule is too large a quantity being 6.24×10^{18} eV or conversely 1 eV is equal to 1.6×10^{-19} J. Wavelength and energy can be converted since $c = \lambda f$. This function can then be substituted for f to give:

$$E = \frac{hc}{\lambda}$$

Then $hc = (6.62 \times 10^{-34}) \times (3.0 \times 10^8) = 1.98 \times 10^{-25}$ Jm. Expressed in electron volts (eV) providing the wavelength is given in metres (m); alternatively, the answer can be given in kiloelectron volts (keV), if the wavelength is in nanometres:

$$E = \frac{1.2375 \times 10^{-6}}{\lambda} \text{ eV or}$$

$$E = \frac{1.2375}{\lambda \text{ (nm)}} \text{ keV.}$$

Equivalent values of the electron volt are:

$1 \text{ eV} = 1.6 \times 10^{-19} \text{ J}$

$h = 4.13 \times 10^{-15} \text{ eV.}$

Units of work and energy

SI joule (J)	$1 \text{ J} = 1 \text{ Ws} = 1 \text{ Nm} = 1 \text{ m}^2\text{kg s}^{-2}$
eV	1.60218×10^{-19} J
keV	1.60218×10^{-16} J
MeV	1.60218×10^{-13} J

The energy equivalence of an electron volt

The electron velocity v at 1 volt is $6 \times 10^5 \text{ m s}^{-1}$
The rest mass, m, is 9.1×10^{-31} kg so:

$$\frac{1}{2}mv^2 = 0.5 \times (9.1 \times 10^{-31})$$
$$\times (6 \times 10^5)^2 \text{ or } 1.6 \times 10^{-19} \text{ J.}$$

This is the energy equivalent of 1 eV.

Electron velocity at 100 kV is:

$1.6 \times 10^{-19} \times (1 \times 10^5) = 1.6 \times 10^{-14}$ J so $\frac{1}{2}mv^2$
$= 1.6 \times 10^{-14}$.

Velocity v is $1.88 \times 10^8 \text{ m s}^{-1}$ at 100 kV which is about two-thirds the speed of light. Relativistic effects (mass–velocity) play a small part in electron velocity.

---

electronic focal spot (*ct*) Targeted area of intersection of the electron beam from the cathode and the surface of the x-ray tube anode (*see* focal spot).

electronic noise (*ct*) Contribution of the electronic devices (thermal) of the data acquisition system to the sampling noise or error of the attenuation CT measurements.

electrophoresis (*nmed*) Utilizes the property of ions to move under the influence of an electric charge. Components of a sample will move at different rates along a strip of paper or gel medium according to their charge and ionic mobility. This procedure is used in a number of applications and the electrophoretograms are measured in the same manner as thin layer and paper chromatograms.

electrostatics (*phys*) A branch of physics that deals with static or very high voltages (relevant to x-ray generators and x-ray tubes). The static electric charge arises when electrons are transferred from one object to another. An object with excess electrons has a negative charge and conversely an object having lost electrons has a positive charge. The basic measurement of charge is the coulomb (*C*), where one coulomb represents 6.24×10^{18} electrons.

element (ultrasound) (*us*) The piezoelectric component of a transducer assembly.

elliptic filter (*di*) Alternative type of Chebyshev filter with equal ripples in the stopband and passband. Digital elliptical filters offer the sharpest possible passband/stopband transitions.

elongation velocity (*us*) Velocity of a particle about its equilibrium position. Typical value is $35\,\mathrm{mm\,s^{-1}}$.

eluate (*nmed*) The solvent carrying the decay product when a generator is eluted. Removing the daughter radionuclide from a generator using a suitable solvent. Partial elution will improve the specific activity per unit volume.

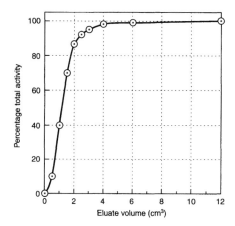

emergency reference level (*rad*) Radiation doses to the general public from ionizing radiation likely to be averted by introducing countermeasures after accidental exposure.

e.m.f. (*phys*) *See* electromotive force.

emission (field) (*phys*) Emission resulting from intense electric fields at the surface of a material. If the metal has a high negative potential with respect to an external electrode, electrons can escape, particularly from sharp points. Application to radiology is seen in x-ray tubes and charging equipment for selenium image plates (*see* direct radiography).

emission (photoelectric) (*phys*) Emission resulting from the irradiation of a material by electromagnetic radiation: light, x- and gamma radiation. For certain solids (semiconductors), electrons are liberated when the photon energy exceeds a certain photoelectric threshold. Selenium, silicon and germanium exhibit this effect and are used as photodetectors. Higher energy photons (x-rays, gamma rays) cause a photoelectric effect in all materials.

emission (secondary) (*phys, xray*) Resulting from bombardment of material by electrons responsible for secondary electron emission in x-ray tubes and the broadening of the focal spot.

emission (thermionic) (*phys, xray*) As a substance is heated, the thermal energy gained increases the excitation of the atoms. At a certain temperature, the outermost electrons gain sufficient energy to escape from the atom. The amount of heat energy required is the work function. The electrons emitted are inversely related to the work function:

Tungsten	4.53
Sodium	1.8
Oxide coating	1.0–1.3

The filaments of x-ray tubes are therefore oxide coated (*see* space charge).

emission temperature (*phys*) The available electron density from a heated filament (emission current density) depends on the filament temperature and work function of the filament material. The graph shows that small changes in filament temperature induce large changes in emission current.

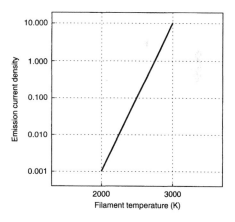

emulsion (*film*) A complex of silver halides. Silver chloride, bromide and iodide are used in various mixtures to alter the sensitivity of the film. They have cuboid crystal structure. Photosensitivity increases with added silver iodide, but rarely exceeds 8%. Emulsion formation involves:

- silver nitrate reaction with alkali halides in gelatine;
- emulsion ripening, influencing grain size;

- sensitive centre formation;
- optical sensitizers added, extending spectral sensitivity.

emulsion ripening (*film*) After silver halide grain formation, the suspension in gelatine undergoes a series of ripening processes which introduces a small proportion of silver sulphide; these act as sensitivity centres influencing the speed of the film.

encryption (*comp*) The process of transmitting scrambled data so that only authorized recipients can unscramble it. Commonly used to encrypt, and so scramble, credit card information when purchases are made over the Internet.

Endobil" (*cm*) A contrast medium for intravenous cholangiography containing meglumine iodoxamate (Bracco) (*see* cholegraphic contrast agents).

Endografin" (*cm*) Commercial preparation (Schering Inc) of 70% meglumine iodipamide.

Compound	Viscosity (cP)	Osmolality (mOsm/kg)	Iodine (mg I mL^{-1})
70% meglumine iodipamide	55 at 20°, 18 at 37°C	– 840	350

Endomirabil" (*clin*) Generic name iodoxamic acid.

Endorem" (*clin*) Magnetic resonance imaging (MRI) contrast agent manufactured by Guerbet.

endoscopic retrograde choledochography (ERC) (*clin*) The nonsurgical removal of biliary calculi using papillotomy followed by stone retrieval.

endoscopic retrograde cholangiopancreatography (ERCP) (*clin*) A procedure using an endoscope for evaluating the biliary tree and pancreatic ducts by endoscopic retrograde cannulation of the papilla of Vater. Water-soluble contrast medium injected via a catheter under fluoroscopic control; opacified ducts are imaged in multiple projections. More invasive than MRI techniques (*see* magnetic resonance cholangiopancreatography (MRCP)).

endoscopy (*clin*) Study of internal organs by means of fibreoptic instruments.

energy (*physics*) The capacity to do work and in so doing to create heat. Work and the amount of heat are physical quantities having the same dimensions and measured in a common unit, the joule (J); the units of energy are also measured in joules. Energy may take the form of either potential energy (the capacity to do work due to position) or kinetic energy (the capacity to

do work due to motion). Joule equivalents and conversions are:

SI units		
1 joule (J)		1 Ws
		1 Nm
		1 m^{2}kg s^{-2}
1 eV		1.602 × 10^{-19} J

Non-SI units	SI equivalent	
1 erg	1 cm^{2}g s^{-2}	10^{-7} J
1 kWh	kW × h	3.6 × 10^6 J
1 Btu		1.05 × 10^3 J

energy (effective) (E_{eff}) (*xray*) Defined as the modal energy of a polyenergetic beam (*see* x-ray (spectrum), energy (equivalent)).

energy (equivalent) (E_{eq}) (*xray*) *See* equivalent energy.

energy (fluence) (Ψ) (*xray*) Measured in MeV cm^{-2}. For a monoenergetic beam this is:

$$\Psi = \frac{\text{Number of photons} \times \text{energy (MeV)}}{\text{Unit area}}.$$

For an exposure of 60 kV at 5 mAs (about 1.5×10^{14} available photons) over 1000 cm^2 this would be $(1.5 \times 10^{11}) \times 0.06 = 9 \times 10^9$ MeV cm^{-2}.

energy (flux) (Ψ) (*xray*) Measured in MeV cm^{-2} s^{-1}. For a monoenergetic beam, this is photon flux × enery (MeV). For a polyenergetic x-ray beam, the proportion of each energy (E_i) per unit time must be considered giving the sum:

$$\Psi = \sum (\Psi \times E_i) \text{ MeV cm}^{-2} \text{s}^{-1}.$$

(*see* photon fluence, photon flux, energy fluence).

energy absorption coefficient (μ_{en}) (*phys*) The linear attenuation coefficient combines the total attenuation due to absorption (μ_{en}) and scatter (μ_{tr}). The energy absorption coefficient describes the energy absorbed by a material, omitting that lost by scatter. It is defined as:

$$\mu_{en} = \mu \times \frac{E_a}{h\nu}$$

where E_a is the average energy absorbed (*see* energy transfer coefficient, mass energy absorption coefficient).

energy bands (*phys*) Ranges of energies that electrons can have in a solid (crystal or metal).

The sharply defined levels of electrons become bands of allowed energy. In solid compounds or crystals, the energies of the orbitals change slightly so single energy levels become ranges of energy called 'energy bands'. Electrons move across into empty bands by changing from one quantum state to another. The bands are:

- The 'valence band', where the valence electrons are found.
- The 'conduction band', where there are both electrons and spaces for more electrons. The electrons are mobile and materials which have a conduction band are the only ones which can conduct electricity at room temperature.
- The 'forbidden band' is the range of energies between two energy bands which is not occupied by electrons. The electron must cross this band gap to occupy a higher electron band. The band gap is large in insulator materials, very narrow in semiconductors and does not exist at all in conductors.

These bands are relevant to radiology since they play a significant role in semiconductor electronics and scintillator radiation detector operation.

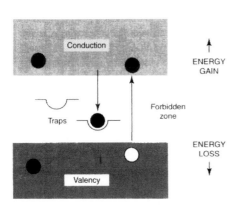

energy conversion (*phys*) In a given system, the total amount of energy is always constant although the energy may change from one form to another (i.e. electrical energy into light and heat energy). The total amount of energy is obtained by adding the kinetic and potential energies. From the equation $E = mc^2$ a mass/energy relationship can be calculated so that 1 kg mass is equivalent to 9×10^{16} J and 1 gram is equivalent to 9×10^{13} J.

Energy/mass conversion: nuclear power station

Fuel consumption (*m*) of a commercial 600 MW nuclear reactor per day (8.64×10^4 seconds).

$$E \text{ (joules)} = (600 \times 104) \times (8.64 \times 104)$$
$$= 5.184 \times 10.13\,J.$$

$$m = \frac{E}{c^2} = \frac{5.184 \times 10^{13}}{(3 \times 10^8)^2} = 5.76 \times 10^{-4}\,kg$$

or just over 0.5 g of fuel per day! Compared with many thousand kilograms of coal or oil consumed by conventional power stations.

---

energy level (*mri*) In a magnetic field, each spin can exist in one of a number of distinct states having different energies. This number is determined by the spin quantum number.

energy (photon) (*phys*) *See* photon energy.

energy resolution (*nm*) The detector's ability to differentiate photon energy. Measured as full width at half maximum (FWHM) of the energy photopeak. Energy resolution differs depending on detector type, proportional counter, scintillation detector or semi-conductor detector. A typical value for a gamma camera would be 10%, for a single 7.5×7.5 cm NaI(Tl) detector crystal 5% and for a HpGe semiconductor detector <1%.

energy transfer coefficient (μ_{tr}) (*phys*) The linear attenuation coefficient combines the total attenuation due to absorption (μ_{en}) and scatter (μ_{tr}). The energy transfer coefficient is a measure of the energy transferred from primary photons to charged particles in a scatter interaction. A related quantity kerma (K) is the energy transferred per unit mass of the material. For monoenergetic photons of energy, hν:

$$K = \left(\frac{\mu_{tr}}{\rho}\right)\Psi$$

where Ψ is the energy fluence (*see* energy absorption coefficient, mass energy transfer coefficient).

enhanced IDE (EIDE) (*comp*) An improved version of IDE that supports large hard disks, faster access speeds and DMA. It is actually two controllers providing primary and secondary channels which handle two devices each and can also talk to CD-ROMs and tape drives.

enhancement (*us*) Increase in echo amplitude from reflectors that lie behind a weakly attenuating structure.

enriched uranium (*phys*) 238-Uranium where the content of 235-uranium has been increased above the natural occurrence of 0.7% by weight.

ensemble length (*us*) Number of pulses used to generate one colour-flow image scan line.

enteroclysis (*clin*) Introduction of dilute barium sulphate contrast into the small bowel following passage of a nasojejunal tube (*see* small bowel enema).

enthalpy (H) (*phys*) This is a thermodynamic function of a system involving energy U, pressure p and volume V, so that: $H = U + pV$. The heat absorbed in a system equals the increase in enthalpy.

entrance beam dimensions (EBD) (*us*) The dimensions of the $-12\,dB$ beam width where the beam enters the patient. For contact transducers, these dimensions can be taken as the dimensions of the radiating element, if so stated. Unit, centimetre (cm).

entrance dimensions of the scan (EDS) (*us*) For autoscan systems, the dimensions of the area of the surface through which the scanned ultrasound beams enter the patient, consisting of all points located within the $-12\,dB$ beam width of any beam passing through that surface during the scan. Unit, centimetre, (cm).

entrance exposure rate (EER) (*dose*) A measure of the fluoroscopy patient dose rate at the surface. Routinely performed by using tissue equivalent absorbers.

entrance surface air kerma (ESAK) (*dose*) Air kerma value measured in free air, without back-scatter, at a point in a plane corresponding to the entrance surface of a specified object, e.g. patient skin or phantom.

entrance surface dose (*dose*) Absorbed dose in air including back-scatter, measured at a point on the entrance surface of the patient or phantom (*see* air-kerma, dose (entrance), dose area product).

entrance window (*ct*) The metallic front covering of a detector on the side of the incident radiation. The entrance window protects the detector surface from mechanical or chemical (oxidation) damage, but inevitably causes a decrease in the detector dose efficiency.

entropy (*phys*) A thermodynamic concept following from the second law of thermodynamics. All changes in a closed system result in an increase in entropy which can be seen simply as an increase in disorder.

envelope (*us*) A smooth curve tangent to and connecting the peaks of successive cycles of a waveform.

environmental exposure (man-made) (*dose*) Originating from artificial sources, such as medical exposure and nuclear power, but almost entirely of medical exposure to x-rays. A smaller proportion is due to nuclear medicine and therapy radionuclides and <1% to discharges from nuclear power or fall-out from nuclear weapon testing.

Man-made	Dose (mSv)	%
Medical	500	21.00
Nuclear	13	0.55
Occupational	9	0.36
Air travel	8	0.34
Total	530	22.25

environmental exposure (natural) (*dose*) Caused by all radiation of natural origin: alpha, beta, gamma, x-ray, cosmic ray, etc. The total of natural and man-made is typically 2.5 mSv, although this has a wide range. The largest exposure to respiratory tissue comes from radon, produced by the decay of ^{238}U series. ^{226}Radium decays by alpha decay to ^{222}Radon, which then decays to ^{218}Polonium.

Natural	Dose (mSv)	%
Cosmic	310	13
Terrestrial	380	16
Radon	800	33
Internal	370	15
Total	1860	77

Eovist[x] (*clin*) A liver-specific MRI agent manufactured by Schering.

EPC (*mri*) Echo phase correction.

EPI (*mri*) Echo planar imaging. A rapid acquisition of a train of separately phase-encoded gradient echoes to produce a fully resolved image after a single excitation.

EPI factor (*mri*) The number of gradient echoes of an echo planar imaging (EPI) sequence, acquired after a single excitation pulse (typically 64–128). An EPI factor of 128 means a measurement time 128 times faster than a normal gradient echo sequence.

epoch (*mri*) In functional magnetic resonance imaging (fMRI), a portion of the MR signal measurement during which the stimulus presentation or response task is similar or unchanged.

EPP/ECP (*comp*) Enhanced parallel port/extended capabilities port. Improved parallel port which provides transfer rates of over 2 MB (megabytes per second) and bidirectional operation. The latter is mainly used by printer monitoring software as it can receive status information from the printer while sending it data. EPP mode is designed for other devices, such as zip drives.

equations of state (*phys*) Characteristic equations showing the relationship between pressure, volume and thermodynamic temperature in a system. Many equations of state have been proposed (van der Waals equation, Clausius equation, Debye equation).

equivalent dose (H_T) (*dose*) Also the equivalent organ dose. The absorbed dose averaged over a tissue or organ (rather than at a point as in the previous **dose equivalent**) and weighted for radiation quality by a radiation weighting factor (ICRP60). The equivalent dose in tissue, T, for a single radiation type, R, having a weighting factor w_R, is then given by $H_T = w_R \times D_T$, where D_T is the absorbed dose averaged over the tissue or organ. Since w_R is dimensionless, the unit for the equivalent dose is the same as for **absorbed dose**, $J\,kg^{-1}$; the sievert (Sv).

Equivalent dose
An absorbed dose of 100 mGy is measured in tissue for gamma ($w_R = 1$) and alpha ($w_R = 20$) radiation. The equivalent doses are then 100 mSv and 2 Sv, respectively.

(*see* weighting factor (radiation), effective dose).

(*xray*) Defined as the energy of the mono-energetic beam which gives the same half-value layer (HVL) as the x-ray spectrum. The single energy whose photons would be attenuated to the same extent as those of the mixed energies of the x-ray beam continuous spectrum.

Equivalent energy
A 100 kVp x-ray spectrum having an HVL of 5 mm Al gives an attenuation coefficient of:

$$\mu = \frac{0.693}{HVL} = 1.38\ \mu\,cm^{-1}.$$

The graph shows an equivalent energy of 40 keV. This should not be confused with the **effective** energy which is the x-ray spectrum modal point.

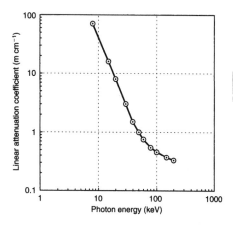

erbium (Er) (*elem*)

Atomic number (Z)	68
Relative atomic mass (A_r)	167.26
Density (ρ) kg/m³	9000
Melting point, (K)	1770
K-edge (keV)	57.4
Relevance to radiology: x-ray beam K-edge filter	

[169]**Erbium** (*nmed*) A radionuclide as citrate for synovectomy.

Half life	9.3 days
Decay mode	β+ 0.34 MeV
Decay constant	0.0745 day⁻¹
Photons (abundance)	116 keV(weak)

ERCP (*clin*) Endoscopic retrograde cholangiopancreatography. Using an endoscope to investigate and cannulate the ampulla of Vater and radiographically visualize the pancreatic, hepatic and common bile ducts using contrast medium (*see* relevant contrast medium).

erg (*phys*) A non-SI unit of energy, where 1 erg equals 10^{-7} joules (*see* energy).

Ernst angle (*mri*) The flip angle (<90°) of a gradient echo sequence which generates the maximum signal for a given tissue. The Ernst angle:

$$\alpha_E = e^{-(TR/T1)}.$$

The optimum flip angle is 90° only when TR is much greater than T1.

error correction protocol (*comp*) A technique used in modems to cancel out extraneous electrical noise and repeat unsuccessful online transmissions.

erythema (*dose*) A few days after exposure to about 8 Gy, the skin may redden. This is early erythema which increases during the first week, but starts fading at the end of about the tenth day. The main erythematous reaction then becomes maximal on the 15th day after exposure and lasts 20–30 days. The main erythema reaction involves the epidermis, the underlying skin strata and blood vessels. On regeneration, the erythema disappears leaving dry or moist desquamation.

ESE (*phys*) *See* **entrance skin exposure.**

ESD (*phys*) *See* **entrance surface dose.**

ESP (*mri*) Echo spacing: time between echoes in a FSE sequence.

ESR (*phys*) *See* **electron spin resonance.**

E-SHORT (*mri*) Short repetition technique based on echo steady-state free precession commonly used for imaging of cerebrospinal fluid (*see* SSFP, DE-FGR, CE-FAST, True-FISP, PSIF, ROAST, T2-FEE, STERE).

Ethernet (*comp*) A decentralized tree or bus topology for computer networking developed by Xerox PARC, using a specific protocol for transmitting data. Collisions are detected and retransmitted. A shared media technology, Ethernet broadcasts packets to as many as 1024 nodes on a network segment via twisted pair, coaxial or fibreoptic cabling. The general classification of Ethernet encompasses 10 Mbps Ethernet networks and 100 Mbps fast Ethernet networks, promising to include 1000 Mbps (gigabit Ethernet) networks. Currently, Ethernet is by far the most widely deployed local area network (LAN) access method, followed by token ring. ARCNET and FDDI are other network designs (*see* fast Ethernet, gigabyte Ethernet).

ETL (*mri*) Echo train length. Number of echoes per TR in FSE sequence.

Euler's formula (*math*) Enables the Fourier transform to be expressed in complex form, extracting real and imaginary roots (phase and amplitude) so:

$$e^{-j\omega x} = \cos(\omega x) - j\sin(\omega x)$$

where j is $\sqrt{-1}$ (sometimes represented by i) and ω is $2\pi f$: f being frequency, $\cos\theta + j\sin\theta$ is referred to as cis θ (*see* complex numbers).

EURATOM Formed from the signing of the Euratom Treaty in 1957 laying down uniform safety standards and issuing directives and guidelines for radiation safety in the workplace. The major directives (recent and historical) relevant to medical applications of ionizing radiation are:

- 97/43/EURATOM (Patient Protection); Medical Exposure Directive;
- 96/29/EURATOM (Basic Safety Standards);
- 84/467 EURATOM (Revised Basic Safety Standards);
- 84/466/EURATOM (Patient Protection);
- 80/836 EURATOM (Basic Safety Standards).

These were the foundation for the legislation adopted by European member states (*see* Ionising Radiation Regulations).

europium (Eu) (*elem*)

Atomic number (Z)	63
Relative atomic mass (A_r)	151.96
Density (\rho;) kg/m^3	5200
Melting point (K)	1100
K-edge (keV)	48.5

Relevance to radiology: doping agent for phosphors. This is a rare earth element used as a dopant in some intensifying screens (BaSrSO$_4$:Eu) and image plate thermoluminescent materials (BaXF:Eu).

evaporation (*phys*) The change of liquid to vapour. Liquids vary in the ease with which they change. Liquids which evaporate easily have a low boiling point, e.g. volatile liquids. Latent heat (LH) is needed for the change from liquid to vapour and this heat is absorbed (taken) from the surface (cooling). Liquids with large latent heats (water) remove heat more effectively.

Substance	LH (vaporization) (MJ kg^{-1})
Water	2.260
Alcohol	0.850

even echo rephasing (*mri*) Rephasing occurring when constant velocity spins return to the same starting phase they had after the initial RF excitation, as a result of the application of an even number of gradient pulses. This may also result from the application of multiple gradient echo pulses following the RF pulse.

even–odd rules (*nmed*) Rules that are used to predict nuclear stability based on whether the numbers of neutrons and protons are even or odd. These rules are not very reliable.

event location (PET) (*nmed*) The distance travelled by the positrons before annihilation; the path distance increases with the positron energy, leading to a degradation in spatial resolution. This distance is limited by the maximal positron energy of the radionuclide and the density of the tissue. A radionuclide that emits lower energy positrons yields superior resolution. Activity in bone yields higher resolution than activity in soft tissue, which in turn yields higher resolution than activity in lung tissue. Approximate values are shown in the table.

Positron nuclide	β+ Energy (MeV)	Range (mm)
^{18}F	0.24	1.0
^{11}C	0.38	1.6
^{13}N	0.49	2.1
^{15}O	0.73	2.8
^{82}Rb	1.4	5.6

(*see* time of flight (TOF)).

exact framing (*di*) Recording the entire circular image of an image intensifier or gamma camera (*see* over-framing).

exametazine (*nmed*) *See* HMPAO.

EXCEL$^{\circledR}$ (*comp*) A versatile spreadsheet program produced by Microsoft.

excess absolute risk (*dose*) The rate of disease or mortality incidence seen in an exposed population compared to the control data in an unexposed population. Commonly expressed as the additive excess per Gy or per Sv.

excess relative risk (*dose*) The rate of disease in an exposed population divided by the rate of disease in a control unexposed population, expressed as a fraction (unit = 100%). Commonly expressed as the excess relative risk per Gy or per Sv.

exchange diffusion (*nmed*) Diffusion of a radiopharmaceutical into a tissue and then exchange of a chemical group on the radiopharmaceutical for a different chemical group on the tissue; one SF-fluoride ion exchanges with the hydroxide group on hydroxyapatite in bone tissue to form fluoroapatite.

excitation (*mri*) Putting energy into the spin system: if a net transverse magnetization is produced. A magnetic resonance signal can be observed.

excitation energy (*phys*) Energy required to change an atom or molecule from its ground state to a specified excited state, without ionization.

excitation pulse (*mri*) The spin equilibrium in the magnetic field distorted by a brief RF pulse. The higher the energy of the excitation RF pulse,

the higher the expansion of magnetization. The final expansion of the magnetic field after the RF pulse is the flip angle.

excited state (*phys*) The state of an atom or molecule having a higher energy state than its ground value. Electromagnetic radiation has sufficient energy to cause excitation states in biological materials which may rupture chemical bonds.

exclusion (*dose*) Excluding a particular category of exposure from measurement on the grounds that it is not considered amenable to control through the regulatory instrument in question.

excretion/elimination half-life (contrast medium) (*clin*) Glomerular filtration is the major excretory route a typical half-life value being 1.5 hours, increasing to 10 hours or more in cases of renal failure.

exemption (*dose*) Decision by a regulatory body that a source or practice can be exempt from some or all aspects of regulatory control on the basis that the exposure (including potential exposure) due to the source or practice is too small to warrant the application of those aspects or that this is the optimum option for protection irrespective of the actual level of the doses or risks.

exit dose (*dose*) *See* dose (exit).

expansion (*phys*) Expansion in metals is measured as a coefficient of linear expansion defined as the increase in length, per unit length, for a temperature change of 1 K. The coefficient of expansion is a percentage so has no units.

Solid	Expansion (10^{-6} K^{-1})
Lead	29.0
Aluminium	25.0
Steel	12.0
Copper	17.0
Molybdenum	5.0
Tungsten	4.0
Glass	9.0–12.0
Glass (pyrex)	3.0
Invar	0.9

The small expansion shown by molybdenum, tungsten, pyrex glass and Invar make these ideal metals for x-ray tube construction.

Expansion of metal
1 metre of steel increases its length to 1.10 m when the temperature rises by 90 K, the linear coefficient of expansion is:

$$\frac{1.10}{1.000 \times 90} = 1.22 \times 10^{-5} \text{K}^{-1}$$

---

exponent (*math*) Indicator for decimal point shift (left or right) in scientific notation, or in an exponential function x^n, then n is the exponent.

exponential (*math*) Most commonly used when the exponent is the power of e; the exponential of x is e^x.

exponential distribution (*math*) A continuous distribution with probability density function given by $f(x) = e^{-\lambda x}$, where the mean is $1/\lambda$ and the variance $1/\lambda^2$.

exponential weighting (*mri*) Used in spectroscopy, multiplication of the time-dependent signal data by an exponential function, $e^{-(t/t_c)}$, where t is time and t_c is the time constant, chosen to either improve the signal-to-noise ratio (with a negative t_c) or decrease the effective spectral line width in the resulting spectrum (with a positive t_c). The use of a negative t_c to improve signal to noise ratio (SNR) is equivalent to line broadening by convolving the spectrum with a Lorentzian function.

exposure (*dose*) Measured in roentgen (R) or air-kerma, where $1 \text{ mR} = 8.7 \, \mu\text{Gy}$. Exposure is also a timed exposure to x-rays measured in milliampere-seconds. The exposure in mGy from an x-ray exposure can be approximately estimated from the formula:

$$0.5 \times \frac{kV^2 \times mAs}{D^2}.$$

A 1 R incident x-ray exposure (8.7 mGy) with an effective energy of 30 keV has a fluence of 1.3×10^{10} photons cm^{-2} (*see* **equivalent dose, effective dose**).

Radiation exposure

Illustrating the benefits of high kV imaging. A high energy radiograph having a focus film distance (FFD) of 200 cm, at 110 kVp 2 mAs gives a surface dose of:

$$0.5 \times \frac{110^2 \times 2}{200^2} = 0.30 \, \text{mGy}.$$

A low energy radiograph using 70 kVp requires an increase in mAs estimated by $(70/110)^4$ or $\times 6$. The equation for the same FFD is now:

$$0.5 \times \frac{70^2 \times 12}{200^2} = 0.73 \, \text{mGy}$$

which is a $\times 2.5$ increase in surface dose.

---

exposure (*nmed*) The incidence of ionizing radiation on living or inanimate material. Also, a measure of the ionization produced in a specified mass of air by x- or gamma radiation, which may be used as a measure of the ionizing radiation to which one is exposed. When using SI units, air kerma is often used in place of exposure. Air kerma has the units of J kg^{-1} (Gy). In conventional units, the special unit of exposure is the roentgen (R). An exposure of 1 R corresponds to an air kerma of 8.7 mGy (*see* **kerma, gray, roentgen**).

exposure factors (*xray*) These are the parameters altered either manually or by the automatic exposure control to achieve the optimum image density for a particular imaging medium. The image surface can be film-screen, **image intensifier** or image plate. Four factors are usually considered: **kilovoltage, tube current, exposure time** and **distance (FFD)**. These factors are interdependent, e.g. to maintain the same **exit dose** when the kV is increased from 60 to 70 kV, the mA should be reduced by $(60/70)^4$ or 0.54; an increase by 10 kV requires the tube current to be halved or the exposure time halved for the same current. High kV studies can therefore be performed at faster exposure times (*see* **isowatt**).

exposure time (*xray*) Duration of emission of radiation by the x-ray tube (seconds) for an individual slice in axial scanning or total acquisition time for helical scanning.

external focus (*us*) A focus produced by a lens attached to a transducer element.

extracellular (*clin*) External to the cells of an organ or tissue.

extra corporeal shock lithotripsy (*clin*) Focused shock waves, for the fragmentation of renal calculi, were first applied by Chaussy and Brendel in 1980. The shock waves employed in clinical practice are produced by lithotriptors which generate acoustical pulses with very fast pressure rise times and duration (nanoseconds). The maximum pressures attained are between 500 and 1500 bar. Three types of lithotripster are available commercially:

- *High pressure* (1200 bar), with a small focal area using ultrasound (piezoelectric transducers) as manufactured by Wolf, EDAP, Diasonics.
- *High pressure* (500–1000 bar), having a large focal area generated by spark gaps as manufactured by Dornier, Direx, Technomed and Medstone.

- *Low pressure* (<500 bar), with a medium-sized focal area using electromagnetic principles as manufactured by Siemens.
  - Reference: Chaussy *et al.*, 1980.

extrafocal radiation (*xray*) The greatest source of radiation from the x-ray tube comes from the optically effective focal spot; radiation also originates from other regions within the tube, outside the focus. This radiation component is referred to as extrafocal radiation. A fraction of the electrons are reflected back from the landing position on the target, falling back towards the anode and landing outside the focus, giving rise to extrafocal radiation. The strongly emitting focus of the x-ray tube is surrounded by a weak but extensive source of extrafocal radiation. Radiation originating from the optical focus provides a sharply defined projection image of the object, but the extrafocal radiation superimposes an unsharp projection of the object, so degrading image contrast. The intensity ratio of sharp image to superimposed unsharp image depends on the relative intensities of the focal and extrafocal radiation. The use of an antiscatter grid does not reduce the amount of contributing extrafocal radiation.
  - Reference: Buchmann, 1994.

extrametazine (*nmed*) See HMPAO, Ceretec.

extrapolation (*math*) Estimation of a value of a variable beyond known values.

extrinsic efficiency (*nmed*) The ratio of gamma photons traversing the volume of a scintillation detector to the total number emitted by a radionuclide.

extrinsic resolution (*nmed*) See resolution (extrinsic).

eye (resolution) (*image*) Visual resolution.

eye (response) (*image*) See visual response.

eye dose equivalent (*dose*) External exposure of the lens of the eye. The dose equivalent at 0.3 cm depth.

F

f-factor (*dose*) A factor used for converting exposure in air to exposure in tissue. The mass absorption coefficient ($\mu a/\rho$) only concerns photoelectric absorption, which is responsible for tissue radiation dose:

$$\text{Grays kg}^{-1}\text{ tissue} = \text{beam energy} \times \frac{\mu a}{\rho}.$$

The *f*-conversion factor is then:

$$\frac{\text{Absorbed energy kg}^{-1}\text{ tissue}}{\text{Absorbed energy kg}^{-1}\text{ air}}$$

Using a conversion factor expresses *f*- in terms of grays:

$$f_{\text{(grays)}}34 \times \left[\frac{\mu_a/\rho_{\text{tissue}}}{\mu_a/\rho_{\text{air}}}\right]$$

This converts $C\,\text{kg}^{-1}$ exposure in air to exposure in tissue as Gy.

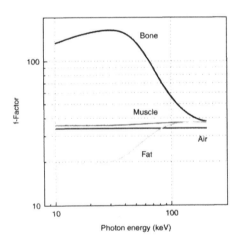

Photon energy (keV)

FA (*mri*) Flip angle.

FacE (*mri*) Free induction decay (FID) acquired echoes.

factorial (*stats*) The product of all the integers from 1 up to and including a given integer. Symbol *n*! Thus 5! is $5 \times 4 \times 3 \times 2 \times 1 = 120$.

FADE (*mri*) FASE acquisition double echo. True FISP technique sampling both FID and SE/STE.

fahrenheit (*phys*) A temperature scale invented by GD Fahrenheit (1686–1736) who took the lowest temperature of ice/salt as zero and the highest temperature of ice/salt as zero and the highest

(body temperature) as 96°F; on this scale water freezes at 32°F and water boils at 212°F. The celsius scale, $C = 5(F - 32)/9$ (*see* kelvin).

fall out (*dose*) The nuclear weapons tests carried out in the 1950s and 1960s have deposited about 3 tonnes of ^{239}Pu globally. Other nuclides are ^{14}C, ^{90}Sr, ^{137}Cs and with some ^{99m}Tc added from nuclear reprocessing effluent. The average effective dose from fallout is $10\,\mu\text{Sv}\,\text{y}^{-1}$ ($80\,\mu\text{Sv}\,\text{y}^{-1}$ in the 1960s). The collective effective dose is about $560\,\text{man-Sv}$ (UK) and $2600\,\text{man-Sv}$ (USA).

falling load (*xray*) Using the maximum electrical rating to give a shorter exposure time. The diagram shows that by running the tube at maximum output: 500 mA at 0.06 s followed by 300 mA at 0.15 s, followed by 200 mA at 0.125 s achieves a 100 mAs exposure time of 0.33 s; a fixed 100 mA tube current would have taken 1.0 s. Very fast exposure times (<0.5 s) do not lend themselves to falling load exposures.

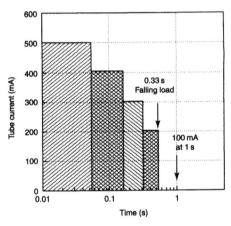

false-negative fraction (FNF) (*stats*) The conditional probability of deciding that in an observed data set the fraction of patients where a diagnostic test suggests the disease is absent is in fact present (*see* ROC analysis).

false-positive fraction (FPF) (*stats*) The conditional probability of deciding that an observed data set (e.g. image) was generated by a specified state (e.g. that a specified disease was present) when, in fact, that state was absent. False-positive fraction is equal to one minus the 'specificity' index often used in the medical literature to indicate the ability of a diagnostic test to produce 'negative' results when the disease of interest is absent (*see* ROC analysis).

FAME (*mri*) Fast-acquisition multi echo acronym for FSE/RARE technique used by Picker Medical Inc.

fan angle (*ct*) Angle covered by the fan of x-rays within the scan plane (*see* **fan beam system**).

fan-beam system/fan beam (*ct*) The geometry of a third-generation machine describing the fixed assembly between x-ray tube and detector array which rotates together. The geometry of the fan beam is determined by collimation. Two types of fan beam designs: third-generation scanners, in which the x-ray tube and detector arc rotate simultaneously; fourth generation scanners or ring detector (now discontinued), where the x-ray tube rotates only.

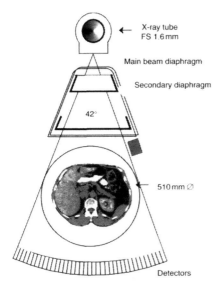

(*see* **fan angle, cone beam**).

fanolesomab (*nmed*) Murine IgM monoclonal antibody directed against the CD15 antigen expressed on the surface of polymorphonuclear neutrophils (PMNs), eosinophils and monocytes; ^{99m}Tc-fanolesomab (**NeutroSpec®**) indicates infection sites.

FAQ (*comp*) Frequently asked question(s). This term generally refers to a document posted on the Internet or elsewhere for the specific purpose of assisting new users.

far field (*us*) *See* **Fraunhofer zone**.

farad (*units*) Storage capacity of a capacitor is equal to the ratio of charge (coulombs) to the rise in potential (volts) as $A s V^{-1}$ ($C = A s$); equivalent to $C V^{-1}$. Capacitance is typically expressed in microfarads (μF).

Faraday shield (*mri*) Electrical conductor, typically a copper mesh, interposed between transmitter and/or receiver coil and patient to block out electric fields. A Faraday cage, constructed from copper mesh, surrounds a magnetic resonance (MR) imaging machine in order to shield the feint nuclear magnetic resonance (NMR) signals from radio interference.

Farmer FT (1912–2004) British medical physicist who developed an accurate ion-chamber dosimeter for measuring dose in x-ray exposure; the Farmer dosimeter.

far zone (*us*) The region of a sound beam in which the beam diameter increases as the distance from the transducer increases; also called far field.

FASE (*mri*) Fast spin echo. FSE/RARE variant.

FAST (*mri*) Fourier acquired steady state. A pulse sequence used by Picker Medical Inc. similar to GRASS and FISP. Enhanced intensity; rewinding of phase–encoding and no intentional spoiling (*see* **FGR, GFEC, F-SHORT, SSFP**).

fast Ethernet (*comp*) A high-bandwidth networking technology based on the IEEE802.3 Ethernet standard (100BASE-7); supports 100 Mbps performance, a 10-fold increase over original 10 Mbps Ethernet (10BASE-7).

fast Fourier transform (FFT) (*math*) The number of complex multiplications and additions required to complete the **Fourier transform** is proportional to N^2. The number of multiply and add operations can be made proportional to $N \log_2 N$ representing a considerable saving in computational time. This is the fast Fourier transform proposed by Cooley and Tukey. (*ct*) The preferred method for the reconstruction algorithm for filtered back projection. The data in each profile are treated as a mixed frequency, and the entire image reconstruction then takes place as a series of amplitudes in the frequency domain. After filtering, each modified projection is added to the sum of the previous filtered back projections (*see* **Fourier analysis**).

▪ Reference: Cooley and Tukey, 1965.

fast neutrons (*phys*) Neutrons with energies greater than 0.1 MeV having velocities of approximately 4×10^6 m s^{-1}.

fast spin-echo (*mri*) Increasing the acquisition of the basic spin-echo acquisition by acquiring only part of the data and synthesizing the remainder by half-Fourier matrix techniques. Only the positive phase-encoding steps are acquired and a mirror image copy of the positive data is created. A complete image can then reconstructed. Scan time is halved.

fat (mat) A component, with muscle, of soft tissue.

Effective atomic number (Z_{eff})	6.46
Density (ρ) kg/m^3	916

FAT (comp) File allocation table. A table held on a floppy or hard disk that tells the operating system the location of data and the order in which it is stored. Using 16-bit addresses it can only support disk sizes of 2 G-byte, whereas FAT32 uses 32-bit addresses and supports hard disk sizes up to 278 (terabytes) (see FAT16, NTFS, Windows).

FAT16 (comp) File allocation table. This is the map that Windows maintains on each disk volume. FAT16 uses 32 k-byte clusters on 2 G-byte drives from 1966 onwards, keeping the cluster count below 65 536 imposed by 16 bits. This inefficient storage protocol means that even small files occupied this full 32 k disk space (see FAT32, NTFS, Windows).

FAT32 (comp) This file allocation table uses 4 k-byte clusters on drives up to 8 G-bytes and 8 k on drives up to 16 G-bytes. FAT32 is incompatible with Win95 disk compression (see FAT16, NTFS, Windows).

fat client (comp) A client station that performs most of the application (image) processing and very little or none performed by the server.

fatal exception (comp) An error message generated by the processor when it detects invalid code, invalid data or illegal instructions being accessed by a program. It frequently causes 'blue screen of death' and generally requires a computer reboot.

fat saturation (FatSat) (mri) Suppressing the fat component in an MR signal. The protons in the fat are saturated by frequency-selective RF pulses. The saturation affected by magnet homogeneity. Chemical shift values are 3.5 ppm (see presaturation).

fat suppression (mri) The signal comprises the sum of water protons and fat protons. Various techniques are used for suppressing the fat signal (see fat saturation, FATSAT).

FATE (mri) A spin-echo version of FLASH with two 180° pulses.

FATSAT (mri) FAT SATuration. The mixed water/lipid spectrum has a separation of only 3–4 ppm causing a chemical shift artefact in gradient echo pulse sequences. Spin echo pulse sequences do not produce these phase errors. Gradient echo pulse sequences which lack the 180° rephasing pulse show fat and water resonance alternating in phase (approximately 6.6 ms for a 1T magnet) cancelling signals from pixels containing both water and fat. Visible as a black border in tissue interfaces, such as muscle. A presaturation signal is applied causing a reduction in the MR signal intensity from fat; very narrow bandwidth RF pulses can selectively saturate the fat peak and remove its influence. Requires very high magnetic field homogeneity. Examples of FATSAT pulse sequences use short inversion recovery (STIR). Higher field strengths have greater bandwidths which cover the chemical shift 62–189 Hz due to fat/water (see SPIR, ChemSat).

Fat/water separation

The 3–3.5 ppm fat/water separation in a 1T field represents:

$$(3 \times 10^{-6})42.576\,MHz = 127.7\,Hz.$$

0.5 T would give separations of 62 Hz; 1.5 T would give separations of 189 Hz. A gradient field of 0.1 mT cm^{-1} for a 0.5 T field has a bandwidth of 120 Hz (256^2 matrix). A gradient field of 0.15 mT cm^{-1} for a 1.0 T field has a bandwidth of 374 Hz (256^2 matrix).

FC (mri) Flow compensation.

FDD (xray) Focus to diaphragm distance which influences the field of view (FOV) and the penumbra magnitude, p, as:

$$FOV = D \times \frac{FFD}{FDD}; \quad p = FS \times \frac{FFD - FDD}{FFD}$$

where FDD is focus to diaphragm distance and D the diaphragm setting (see FFD).

FDA (gov) The United States Food and Drug Administration. An agency within the Department of Health and Human Services. The FDA promotes and protects the public health by helping safe and effective products to reach the market. It also monitors products for continued safety after they are in use.

The FDA consists of:

- Center for Biologics Evaluation and Research (CBER)
- Center for Devices and Radiological Health (CDRH)
- Center for Drug Evaluation and Research (CDER)
- Center for Food Safety and Applied Nutrition (CFSAN)

- Center for Veterinary Medicine (CVM)
- National Center for Toxicological Research (NCTR)
- Office of Chief Counsel
- Office of the Commissioner (OC)
- Office of Regulatory Affairs (ORA).

FDA 510(k) (*us*) A guidance document which provides information for manufacturers seeking US marketing clearance of diagnostic ultrasound systems and transducers. It provides guidance in the preparation of a regulatory submission to the US FDA.

FDDI (*comp*) The acronym for fibre distributed data interface, a standard for fibreoptic cable. Category 7 fibre, supports 100+ Mbps data. Data transmission speeds greater than 1 Gbps per second, or 100 million bits per second, with this type of cable. The network uses one fibre cable for transmitting and another for receiving to minimize interface problems. Connecting into a fibre cable is difficult, making fibre a very secure network technology (*see* fibreoptics).

FDG (*nmed*) Fluoro-deoxyglucose; ^{18}F-fluoro-2-deoxyglucose (^{18}F-FDG). A glucose analogue labelled with ^{18}F that becomes trapped in the cell glucose cycle enabling metabolic activity to be imaged with positron emission tomography (PET). This can detect active metabolic processes and the morphologic features associated with them in a single examination. The role of ^{18}F-FDG PET has been proven in a variety of cancers.

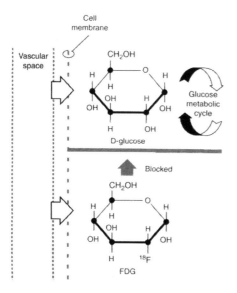

FE (*mri*) Field Echo, general sequence, Picker Medical Inc., Toshiba (*see* FFE, GRE, MPGR, GRECO, PFI, GE, Turbo-FLASH, TFF, SMASH, SHORT, STAGE).

feathering (*image*) A term used to describe printed text quality. Feathering occurs when deposited ink follows the contours of the paper. Depending on the viscosity of the ink, the rougher the grain of the paper the more pronounced the feathering.

feature (*image*) A characteristic of an object; something that can be measured and that assists in classification of the object (e.g. size, texture, shape).

feature space (*image*) In pattern recognition, a dimensional vector space containing all possible feature vectors (patterns).

FEDIF (*mri*) Field echo difference (Picker Medical Inc.) for GRE sequence with water and fat signals out of phase.

feedback (*elec*) Applied to electronic circuitry where a fraction of the output signal is returned to the input. If the phase of the feedback augments the input signal, this is positive feedback and causes possible instability and oscillation. If the feedback phase decreases the input signal, this is negative feedback which stabilizes the device (amplifier).

FEER (*mri*) Field even echo by reversal.

femto (*phys*) Prefix of unit measurement 10^{-15} (femtoamps sometimes encountered in detectors).

Feridex (*cm*) An aqueous colloid of superparamagnetic iron oxide as injectable ferumoxides taken up by the reticuloendothelial system. Gives a reduced signal on normal liver in T2-weighted images. Consists of 11.2 mg Fe/mL and 61.3 mg of manitol. Osmolality 340 mosm/kg.

Fermi, Enrico (1901–54) Italian physicist. Performed fundamental work with Dirac, established the theory of neutrino production during beta decay which causes the continuous beta spectrum and lifetimes of the nuclei. Responsible for the first controlled nuclear assembly in Chicago in 1942. He studied induced radioactivity using neutrons that formed the foundation for the production of artificial radioisotopes in nuclear reactors. He was awarded the Nobel prize for physics in 1938.

ferromagnetic (*mri*) A substance, such as iron, that has a large positive magnetic susceptibility. Outer orbital shells have unpaired electrons, which give them magnetic susceptibility. When placed in an applied magnetic field, these compounds show an induced positive magnetic moment resulting in an attractive force (*see* contrast agents (MRI)).

FESUM (*mri*) Field echo with echo time set for water and fat signals.

FFD (*xray*) The film to focal spot distance. An important parameter in geometrical unsharpness and field size. Now replaced by the term 'focus to image distance (FID)' in order to encompass digital imaging (*see* unsharpness, FDD).

FFE (*mri*) Fast field echo, general sequence, Philips. Fast field echo steady-state GRE sequence acronym used by Philips (*see* GRE, MPGR, GRECO, FE, PFI, GE, Turbo-FLASH, TFF, SMASH, SHORT, STAGE).

FFF (*mri*) Fast Fourier flow.

FFP (*mri*) Fast Fourier projection.

FFT (*math*) *See* fast Fourier transform.

FGR (*mri*) Fast gradient recalled acquisition in the steady state. Fast GRASS, GE, enhanced intensity; rewinding of phase–encoding and no intentional spoiling (*see* GRASS, FISP, FAST, GFEC, F-SHORT, SSFP).

fibreoptics (*phys*) Transmission of light along a small transparent fibre. The speed of light in a vacuum is $3 \times 10^5 \, \text{km s}^{-1}$. However, when it enters a transparent medium (glass), the speed of light is less by a factor of about 1.5 ($2 \times 10^5 \, \text{km s}^{-1}$). This factor is the refractive index of the material. Light passing from one medium to another changes in speed and causes the light to bend (refraction). Under certain conditions, the light ray will be reflected back into the denser medium: this is total internal reflection. Light rays in glass are totally internally reflected if their angle of incidence is increased beyond a critical angle (42°). Coherent fibres where the position of the fibres is identical at the start and the end of the bundle length (endoscopes, image intensifier output). Tapering the fibre bundle can either minify or magnify the image. Signal losses are about $0.5 \, \text{dB km}^{-1}$ resulting in a small signal loss of about 10% per km. Signals can be transmitted over about 50 km without amplification (*see* FDDI, Ethernet).

Fick principle (*clin*) Establishes that the cardiac output can be calculated as:

$$\frac{\text{Total body oxygen consumption}}{\text{Arterial O}_2 - \text{venous O}_2}$$

By extension, this principle can be applied to cardiac output or organ perfusion measurement using any indicator (radionuclide) providing the

indicator substance is inert (*see* Kety–Schmidt principle).

FID (*mri*) *See* free induction decay. (*image*) *See* focus–image–distance.

field echo (*mri*) *See* gradient echo.

field emission (*phys*) *See* emission (field).

field gradient (*mri*) The magnitude of the gradient winding in mT m^{-1}. Typical current values are $20–40 \, \text{mT m}^{-1}$ (*see* slew rate, magnetic field gradient).

field inhomogeneity (*mri*) *See* homogeneity.

field lock (*mri*) A feedback control used to maintain the static magnetic field at a constant strength, usually by monitoring the resonance frequency of a reference sample or line in the spectrum.

field of measurement (FOM) (*ct*) Region or volume for which complete data sets can be acquired; the size depends on scanner geometry (gantry tilt) and the fan angle; the object to be scanned has to be within the FOM to avoid artefacts due to data inconsistencies (*see* truncation error).

field of view (FOV) (*image*) The extent of the area visible on the film or display. The FOV alters in fluoroscopy with zoom setting and in nuclear medicine with collimator types and in radiography with diaphragm setting. (*ct*) The maximum diameter of the reconstructed image.

field strength (*mri*) The main magnet strength measured in tesla (T) (*see* magnet).

field size (*xray*) In general, the smaller the anode angle the wider the focal track which increases the power rating; however, angle size also influences the field size of the x-ray beam at a given source to image distance (SID). Field size increases with anode angle, as does the effective focal spot size which will degrade image resolution, so a large area radiograph would be obtained at the expense of resolution. Conversely, a smaller anode angle would give a

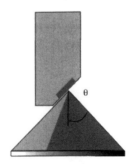
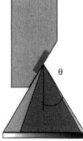

smaller field size, but a better resolution. The choice of anode angle depends on the application required and the SID. Larger focal spots have higher heat rating or loadability (*see* heel effect).

field uniformity (*nmed*) Acceptable planar imaging nonuniformity in the central field of view is about 3%, but SPECT requires uniformity <1%.

filament (*xray*) The electron emissive surface in an x-ray tube. It is manufactured from drawn tungsten wire and is part of the cathode assembly. The filament is heated by a low voltage supply derived from the a.c. (when it has a low frequency ripple) or from the constant potential generator (zero ripple). Single- and dual-filament designs are used according to x-ray tube type and focal spot requirements (*see* emission (thermionic)).

filament cup (*xray*) Part of the cathode assembly surrounding the filament which concentrates the negative charge so shaping the beam.

filament current (*xray*) The x-ray tube filament current is supplied by a low voltage transformer. Controlling factors are maximum operating filament temperature and filament size. Filament current is increased for low kVp work (mammography) to maintain tube current and compensate for the space charge effect. In practice, filament current is kept in a standby mode between exposures (about 5 mA) and increased to operating currents (4.5–5.5 A) for exposures.

file (*comp*) A section of information stored on disk and given a name.

file extension (*comp*) A DOS three letter code which identifies file characteristics, e.g. .doc, .txt, .tif, .exe.

file server (*comp*) *See* server.

fill-in factor (*image*) Direct radiography thin film transistor (TFT) image capture. The potential image artefact caused by gaps between TFT detectors are corrected by bending the field lines (*see* direct radiography).

filling factor (*mri*) A measure of the geometrical relationship of the RF coil and the object being studied, affects the efficiency and signal detection, thereby affecting the signal-to-noise

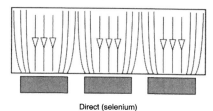

Direct (selenium)

ratio. Achieving a high filling factor requires fitting the coil closely to the patient.

film (*xray*) The first recording medium used in radiography. Three film types exist: monochromatic (blue light sensitive), orthochromatic (blue/green light sensitive) and panchromatic (sensitive to the complete visible spectrum).

film badge (*dose*) A double emulsion dental film used as a personal dosimeter. Placed in a holder complete with metal filters it can indicate radiation type (soft x-ray, gamma, beta, neutrons) and approximate energy. It is a permanent record of personal dose; an assembly containing unexposed photographic film and one or more absorbers, worn by those working with radiation sources. When the film is developed, an estimate of the dose and type of radiation can be made. Film dosimeters are not tissue equivalent (*see* TLD, dosimeter).

film base (*film*) A polyester material supporting the emulsion, sometimes coloured blue.

film contrast (*film*) An indication of latitude or dynamic range. Obtained from the film or image detector gamma (*see* film gamma).

film emulsion (*film*) *See* emulsion.

film formatter (laser) (*film*) A method for recording image data on film using a scanning laser beam. Typically, a 14×17 in (350×430 mm) film is digitized to 4260×5182 pixels; each pixel dimension being 0.082 mm (82 μm).

film gamma (*image*) A measure of film contrast; the rate of change of density with exposure or $\Delta D / \Delta \log E$. This is expressed as the slope of the characteristic curve, taken as the straight middle portion of the curve. If two pairs of density D and exposure $\log E$ values are taken in this range then:

$$\text{Gamma } (\gamma) \frac{D_2 - D_1}{\log E_2 - \log E_1}$$

This ratio is the film gamma, which is also the tangent of the angle between the straight part of the curve and the $\log E$ axis. If $\gamma = 1$, then there is a proportionality between exposure and density (1:1); if $\gamma = <1$, then doubling $\log E$ increases density by a factor <2 (increased latitude, poorer contrast); if $\gamma = >1$, then density changes increase faster (good contrast, poor latitude). The steeper the curve, the higher the contrast and the smaller the latitude or **dynamic range**. Film contrast depends on emulsion type and also on development conditions (temperature) and the period of time spent in the **developer** (film processor speed).

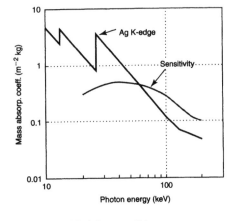

film screen (*film*) *See* intensifying screen.

film sensitometry (*film*) A laboratory procedure for exposing a film to a standard grey scale using a **sensitometer** and measuring its response by means of a **densitometer**.

film speed (*image*) Film sensitivity to exposure, measured for an optical density $= 1$. In the following diagram, film A is the faster:

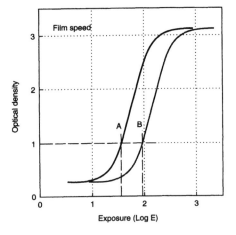

(*see* optical density).

film viewer (*film*) A uniform light source for viewing transparent x-ray film images. Usually $2000\,\mathrm{cd\,m^{-2}}$ for conventional film and higher for mammography.

filter (*image*) Any process which alters the relative frequency content. Can be achieved with an analogue (conventional electrical) filter; remove higher frequency components to prevent aliasing in digitizing. Filtering can also be carried out numerically on the digitized data. (*cf*

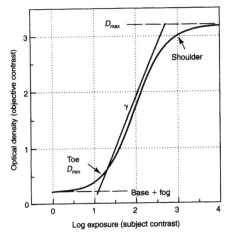

(*see* characteristic curve, contrast (film)).

film grains (*film*) The crystals of silver halide which separate from the silver salt solution and are mixed with the gelatine base. Conventional (mixed grain size), T-grain (flattened profile to the grains) and cubic grain geometry are currently used in radiography emulsions.

film processor (*film*) A method for the daylight processing of x-ray film accepting the unopened cassette and after a fixed period of time (typically 90 s or 3 minutes) providing a fully processed and dried film (*see* film formatter).

film response (*film*) The film response to x-rays as its mass absorption coefficient is shown in the graph. The film sensitivity to x-rays is superimposed against an arbitrary scale showing maximum sensitivity over the diagnostic energy range (*see* film badge).

Mathematical procedure used for the convolution of the attenuation profiles and the consequent reconstruction of the CT image.

filter (K-edge) (*xray*) A high atomic number (Z) metal foil having a K-edge absorption in the diagnostic energy range. Common materials for conventional K-edge filtering are erbium, which reduces patient dose but reduces beam intensity. Mammography uses molybdenum, palladium and rhodium.

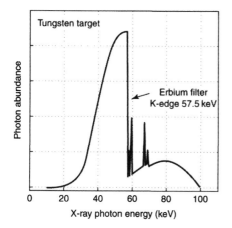

filter (kernel) (*di, ct*) mathematical procedure used for the convolution of the attenuation profiles and the consequent reconstruction of the CT image (*see* kernel).

filtered back projection (*comp*) An image reconstruction technique applied to axial tomography to create images from a set of multiple projection profiles. The projection profiles are backprojected to produce a 2D or 3D image. The projection profiles are processed by convolving them with a suitable filter kernel in order to remove high frequency reconstruction noise. (*ct*) Method for image reconstruction, which can be divided into two steps: backprojection of the measured attenuation profiles and then convolution (*see* algebraic reconstruction).

filtering (signal) (*di*) An ideal filter provides a step response to signal frequencies. Four types are commonly employed: a low pass filter where all frequencies from 0 to a certain point are transmitted unchanged, a high pass filter where all frequencies from 0 to a certain point are blocked, a pass-band filter where a frequency window is preferentially transmitted and a stop-band filter where frequencies within a chosen window are blocked. (*image*)

Signal noise is removed by restricting frequency components. Filters are usually specified in terms of its frequency response. Filters allow frequency components of the input signal lying within a certain band (the passband), and stop, or at least attenuate, components within the stopband(s). The three filter types are:

- a low pass filter, where the passband extends from zero frequency to some chosen 'cutoff' value;
- a high pass filter, where the passband extends from the chosen cutoff frequency up to the maximum frequency dictated by the sampling rate (the applet assumes a sampling rate of 8000 samples/s, so the maximum frequency is 4000 Hz);
- a band pass filter, where the lower and upper passband limits can have any values between 0 and 4000 Hz, although obviously the upper limit should be greater than the lower. The stopband attenuation is the minimum acceptable attenuation, in dB, within the stopband. The transition bandwidth is the maximum acceptable frequency width of the transition band, in hertz, separating the passband from the stopband. The choice of window function is determined mainly by the stopband attenuation requirement.

Window function	Minimum stopband attenuation (dB)
Rectangular	21
Hanning	44
Hamming	54

A Hamming filter function would give an attenuation of at least 50 dB throughout the stopband.

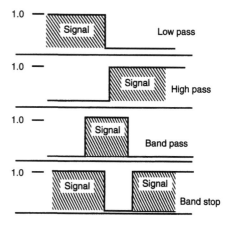

The filter order mainly determines the width of the transition bandwidth; the higher the order, the narrower the transition between the passband and stopband which gives a sharper cutoff in the frequency response. The transition bandwidth (the filter cutoff sharpness) can be improved by increasing the order of the filter.

filtering (spatial) (*di*) Applying a function to an image matrix (kernel) which will affect all the pixels in a linear, nonlinear or weighted fashion. Simple filters are smoothing or edge enhancement.

filtering (temporal) (*di*) Frame averaging or recursive filtering takes the average value from a small series of images (typically four) which reduces image noise.

filtration (*ct*) Application of metal sheet foil on the exit port of the x-ray tube; filtration removes the lower-energy of the polychromatic x-ray spectrum and increases the effective energy. Thus the surface radiation exposure of the patient is reduced without significant decrease of the measured signal. The remaining x-ray distribution is less prone to beam hardening, so that the beam hardening correction is less complicated and beam hardening artefacts are less frequent.

filtration (added) (*xray*) Additional filter material (aluminium or copper) added in order to remove low energy x-rays. This can be up to 2.5 mm aluminium for conventional tubes with an added 0.25 Cu for chest x-ray, fluoroscopy and CT x-ray tubes (*see* half value layer).

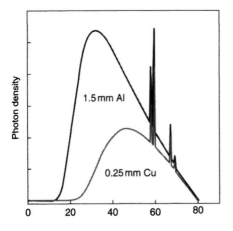

filtration (inherent) (*xray*) The filtration offered by the x-ray tube glass envelope, the insulating oil and any glass insert material. It is expressed as an equivalent thickness of aluminium and is typically 0.5–1 mm Al for conventional tubes

and <0.1 mm Al for mammography tubes with beryllium windows.

filtration (total) (*xray*) This is the sum of inherent + fixed filtration. Total filtration should be at least 1.5 mm aluminium for a 80 kVp beam energy.

firewall (*comp*) A system designed to prevent unauthorized access to a network. All information entering or leaving the network is interrogated and rejected if it fails to meet established criteria. A firewall can also be used by a company to control what resources outside the network can be accessed by employees.

FireWire[*] (*comp*) A very fast serial interface for connecting external devices. Also known as 1394 or iLink, it supports up to 63 devices and speeds of 400 Mbps (megabits per second). First implemented on the Apple Macintosh, it is more complex than a universal serial bus (USB) and suites devices that require high-speed transfer rates.

FIRFT (*mri*) Fast inversion-recovery Fourier transform.

firmware (*comp*) Software that is permanently stored on read-only memory (ROM). It provides many devices, such as printers, modems and tape drives, with basic instructions and, where Flash-ROM is used, the code can be changed by downloading a new set of instructions.

first pass (*nmed*) A fast dynamic study (i.e. heart/lungs), which follows transit of a bolus of activity (labelled blood cells); involves collecting fast dynamic frames while a bolus is in transit through the major heart chambers (*see* blood cell labelling).

FISP (*mri*) Fast imaging with steady-state precession; a steady-state GRE sequence. Siemen's name for GRASS (GE). The generic name being Steady State GRE with free induction decay (FID) sampling, where the remaining transverse coherence is preserved. The sequence has the phase-encoding gradient balanced after the readout period prior to the next RF pulse. True FISP has all three gradients balanced. Dephasing the transverse magnetization due to the phase-encoding gradient is resolved by a negative gradient after data acquisition and before the next RF pulse. The net effect is the same from one TR interval to the next and both the longitudinal and transverse magnetization reach equilibrium, contributing to a steady state signal. The advantages with FISP are:

- short imaging time;
- high signal to noise ratio (SNR);

- 3D imaging possible;
- strong T1 or T2* contrast.

A fast imaging sequence sensitive to the effects of magnetic field inhomogeneities and imperfections in the gradient waveforms (*see* FLASH, GRASS, FGR, FAST, GFEC, F-SHORT, SSFP PSIF).

fission (*phys*) *See* nuclear fission.

fission products (*phys*) Stable and unstable nuclides from a fission reaction. Some examples are:

Nuclide	Emission	Half-life	Fission yield (%)
^{90}Sr	Beta	28 years	6
^{99}Mo	740 keV-γ	66 hours	6
^{131}I	364 keV-γ	8 days	3
^{133}Xe	81 keV-γ	5 days	6.5
^{137}Cs	662 keV-γ	30 years	6

fixer (*image*) A thiosulphate compound which removes unexposed silver halide; this is typically ammonium thiosulphate $(NH_4)_2S_2O_3$.

$$Ag + Br' + S_2O_3'' \rightarrow Ag(S_2O_3)'(\text{insoluble}) + Br'$$
$$\rightarrow Ag(S_2O_3)' + S_2O_3''$$
$$\rightarrow Ag(S_2O_3)_2'''(\text{soluble and removed})$$

The development process is stopped by acidifying the thiosulphate fixer with acetic acid (pH 4.0–6.0). Unfortunately, this causes instability in the thiosulphate ion which breaks down to yield sulphite ion and sulphur:

$$2S_2O_3'' + 4H^+ \rightarrow 2H_2S_2O_3$$
$$\rightarrow 4H^+ + 2O_3'' + S_2$$

The sulphite ion breaks down further to yield sulphur dioxide.

FLAG (*mri*) Flow-adjustable gradients (Philips). Reduction of motion-induced phase shifts during TE (*see* GMR, GMN, FLOW-COMP, CFAST, MAST, GMC, FC, STILL, SMART, GR).

FLAIR (*mri*) Fluid attenuated inversion recovery. IR technique using long TI value to null signal from liquids. It requires a long TR so has long imaging times (*see* dark fluid imaging, RARE).

FLARE(mri) Fast low-angle recalled echoes. *FSE/RARE* variant using low flip angles.

flare (*xray*) Light dispersion at the input phosphor surface (*see* image intensifier).

FLASH (*mri*) Fast low angle shot. Rapid gradient-echo imaging sequence. Siemen's name for spoiled gradient. Contains a spoiler gradient after the readout period to disperse residual transverse magnetization; T1-weighted image contrast. As transverse magnetization is dephased prior to each RF pulse, only the longitudinal magnetization reaches a steady state. FLASH and SE contrast are very similar. T1 weighting increases with flip angle. Equivalent to SPGR or spoiled GRASS (GE Medical), where the coherence of the transverse magnetization is spoiled or disrupted (*see* FISP, GRASS, SPGR, FSPGR, HFGR, RE spoiled, 3D-ME-RAGE, STAGE-T1W).

flash memory (*comp*) A non-volatile computer memory that can be electrically erased and reprogrammed; it is non-volatile so does not lose stored data when the power supply is removed. Primarily used for memory cards and USB flash drives (memory stick, flash stick, etc.) for data storage/transfer between computers and digital devices (cameras, MP3 players, etc.). It is a specific type of EEPROM (electrically erasable programmable read-only memory) that is erased and programmed in large blocks. Currently available up to 8 GB capacity.

flat-panel display (*comp*) A low voltage replacement for cathode ray tube (CRT) displays, consisting of a TFT array, backlight and colour dot matrix. Clinical quality displays have higher resolution than conventional computer displays. Typical specifications for 2–6 million pixel displays are:

	2 M	3 M	6 M
Matrix size	1600 × 1200	2048 × 1536	3280 × 2048
Pixel size	0.270 mm	0.207 mm	0.1995 mm
Bit depth	12	30 colour	12
Luminance	900 cd m^{-2}	1000 cd m^{-2}	800 cd m^{-2}
Contrast ratio	700:1	900:1	800:1

Flexiled" (*shld*) Flexible lead/PVC sheeting.

flicker (*di*) Video displays can cause visible flickering if their scan times are too short. Scan times below 20 have serious visible flicker interference.

flip angle (*mri*) Amount of magnetization vector rotation produced by RF pulse. Flip angles of 15–30° used in fast acquisition sequences.

Only a part of the longitudinal magnetization is converted to transverse magnetization reducing the recovery period. A net signal advantage is achieved with short TR intervals.

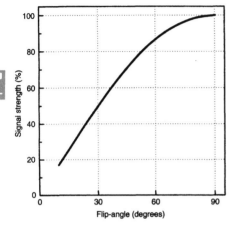

floating point (*comp*) A method of writing real numbers as $a \times 10^n$ or aEn, where $a > 1$, but $\geqslant 0.1$ and n is the integer exponent directing decimal point position −, left; +, right. For example 0.564E$2 = 56.4$, but 0.564E$1 = 0.0564$. Floating point format is a common notation used in computing.

flood image (*nmed*) Image of gamma camera detector flooded with a uniform source of photons.

floppy disk (*comp*) A small disk either 5.25 in (obsolete) or 3.5 in, which can be removed and used on other machines (*see* storage (bulk), hard disk, jazz disk, super disk, zip disk).

flops or FLOPS (*comp*) Floating point operations per second. Mega-flops and giga-flops are used.

flow (*mri*) Nuclei from liquids moving into an excited slice-region can be distinguished from static tissues. (*phys*) In a steady laminar flow of liquid, a pressure difference exists and so must contain energy by virtue of the work done:

$$P + \frac{1}{2}\rho v^2 + \rho gy = \text{constant}$$

where v is the velocity and y the fluid height difference. This is Bernoulli's principle which relates kinetic energy density ($\frac{1}{2}\rho v^2$) with the bulk motion of the liquid, a potential-energy density (ρgy) and pressure energy density (P) arising from the moving liquid. The net energy density contained in a flowing system (blood) is therefore constant throughout the vessel. Poiseuille flow is concerned with steady laminar flow of a liquid of viscosity η, through a vessel of circular cross-section with radius r, length l and a pressure difference $p_1 - p_2$. The quantity of liquid Q flowing per second is:

$$Q = \frac{\pi(p_1 - p_2)r^4}{8\eta l}.$$

The flow varies as the fourth power of the radius: a slight increase produces a large change in flow rate.

flow artefact (*mri*) A motion artefact generated by local signal changes during measurement. Examples would be the inflow intensity of a vessel perpendicular to the image plane whose movement changes periodically due to pulsatile blood flow. In sectional body imaging, ghosting appears in the aorta. Turbulent blood flow in the heart results in smearing of the image.

FLOW COMP (*mri*) Flow compensation GE, Toshiba. Reduction of motion-induced phase shifts during TE (*see* GMR, GMN, CFAST, MAST, FLAG, GMC, FC, STILL, SMART, GR).

flow compensation (*mri*) Means of reducing flow effects, such as gradient moment nulling. For overriding the (GMR) signal loss caused by spin movement, both moved and unmoved spins are rephased. Additional gradient pulses of a suitable size and duration are applied.

flow dephasing (*mri*) Nulling the signal from flowing blood by the application of specifically applied gradient fields (*see* dephasing).

flow effects (*mri*) Motion of material being imaged, particularly flowing blood, can result in signal increase (flow-related enhancement) or decrease or displacement (image misregistration). Caused by time-of-flight effects (wash-out or wash-in due to motion of nuclei between two consecutive spatially selective RF excitations). The inconsistency of the signal resulting from pulsatile flow can lead to artefacts in the image, which can be reduced by:

• synchronization of the imaging sequence (cardiac gating);

- suppression of the blood signal with saturation pulses;
- reduction of phase shifts with gradient moment nulling.

flow encoding (*mri*) Phase encoding obtains information regarding the direction and velocity of moving fluid material (blood, cerebrospinal fluid (CSF) etc.). Provides quantitative information on the velocity of blood flow by:

- bright blood effect;
- inflow amplification;
- jet effect;
- signal elimination;
- washout effect.

  (*see* flow quantification).

flow enhancement (*mri*) The increased intensity that may be seen due to flowing blood as a result of loss of saturated spins from the imaged slice; signal increase given by flowing blood due to washout of saturated spins (*see* saturation).

flow quantification (*mri*) Flow measurements using phase contrast to examine large vessels or as part of an extensive cardiovascular study. Flow measurements enable noninvasive evaluation of blood flow.

flow-related enhancement (*mri*) The increase in intensity that may be seen for flowing blood or other liquids with some MR imaging techniques, due to the washout of saturated spins from the imaging region (*see* saturation).

flow rephasing (*mri*) A phenomenon commonly seen in blood vessels whose flow is within an imaging plane and having a component of their flow in the frequency encoding direction. The increase in flow signal on even echoes (second and fourth) is even echo rephasing; the loss of signal on the odd echoes (first and third) is called 'odd echo dephasing'. These echo signal effects are seen during the frequency encoding gradient.

flow sensitivity (*mri*) Phase contrast angiography. The blood velocity at which the phase difference between flow compensating and flow encoding scans is 180°.

flow void (*mri*) Low signal in regions of flow. The lack of refocusing a spin echo sequence in blood which is excited by the 90° pulse, but not by the 180° pulse. For a gradient echo sequence, this is caused by the dephasing of blood signal.

fluence (*phys*) Radiation intensity per unit area (*see* photon fluence, photon fluence (energy)).

fluorescence (*phys*) A luminescence phenomenon, as seen in radiology and clinical applications, first named by George Stokes after the mineral fluorite, a strongly fluorescent mineral. Caused by absorption of some form of radiant energy, such as ultraviolet radiation or gamma or x-rays ceasing immediately, or very shortly after, the radiation causing it ceases. The simplest model for an inorganic scintillator involves crystal impurities and lattice defects providing energy levels in normally forbidden region. The process is:

1 The traps in the forbidden energy band are full before irradiation.
2 Photons dislodge electrons from the valency band with sufficient energy to displace them into the conduction band.
3 The holes created in the valency band attract electrons from the traps and light with short emission times (100–200 ns) is emitted.
4 Equilibrium in the phosphor material is established when displaced electrons in the conduction band fill the empty traps.

Electron de-excitation occurs almost spontaneously, and emission from a luminescent substance ceases when the exciting source is removed. The quantum yield ϕ of a fluorescent substance is defined by:

$$\frac{\text{Number of photons emitted}}{\text{Number of photons absorbed}}$$

Light in the U/V visible wavelength is emitted from a substance under stimulation or excitation by other forms of electromagnetic radiation of shorter wavelength. Photons are emitted only while the stimulation continues or for a very short time after cessation (dead-time), differing from phosphorescence, where photon emission continues for a time after the excitation has ceased. Organic and inorganic fluorescent substances are found in radiology as α, β, γ and x-ray detectors, as well as coatings for video displays (flat panel displays, as well as CRT), intensifying screens, gamma cameras) (*see* energy bands).

fluorine (F) (*elem*)

Atomic number (Z)	9
Relative atomic mass (A_r)	19.0
Density (ρ) kg/m^3	1.7
Melting point (K)	53.5

Relevance to radiology: Element of the halide family (Z = 9), useful in radiology as the positron radionuclide ^{18}F which labels deoxyglucose, without distorting the molecule, forming fluoro-deoxyglucose, used for imaging metabolic sites (heart and various tumours).

^{18}Fluorine (*nmed*)

Production (cyclotron)	$^{20}_{10}Ne(d,\alpha)^{18}_{9}F$ or $^{16}_{8}O\ (p,n)^{18}_{9}F$
Decay scheme ($\beta+$)	$^{18}F\ (\beta+, 2\gamma\ 511\ keV) \rightarrow\ ^{18}O$ stable ^{18}F
Half-life	110 minutes
Dose rate constant	$0.143\ \mu Sv\,m^2 MBq^{-1}hr^{-1}$
Half value layer	4.1 mm Pb

96.73% positron emission and electron capture 3.27%. The positron energy is 635 keV. A major radionuclide in positron emission tomography (PET).

^{18}Fluorine tracers (*nmed*) The production of ^{18}F tracers is typically by substitution with ^{18}F. Fluoride trapped from ^{18}O water and purification by high performance liquid chromatography; currently available compounds from automated cyclotron analyzers are:

Tracer	Application
^{18}F long chain fatty acids, ^{18}F FTHA	Anaerobic metabolism
^{18}F fluoromisonidazole	Hypoxia
^{18}F methylbenperidol	Dopaminergic D_2 receptor
^{18}F methylspiperone	Dopaminergic D_2 receptor
^{18}F fluorostradiol	Steroid metabolism
^{18}F altanserine	Seratonergic S_2 receptor
^{18}F FLT fluoro-L-thymidine	DNA sysnthesis
^{18}F fluoro-deoxyglucose (FDG)	Glucose metabolism

fluoro-deoxyglucose (*nmed*) *See* FDG.

fluoroscopic CT (*ct*) Continuous imaging by CT to control or to guide a diagnostic or therapeutic intervention.

fluoroscopy (*xray*) A technique which uses an image intensifier to give a real time x-ray image on video, cine-film or small format cut film (*see* Coltman, image intensifier).

flux (*phys*) Radiation fluence per unit time (*see* photon flux, photon flux (energy)).

flux gain (*phys*) Gain in light intensity between input and output phosphors (electronic gain of image intensifier).

flying focal spot (*ct*) A process where the number of measurement channels is doubled by rapid deflection of the x-ray tube focal spot for each projection increasing the image resolution. Achieved by electromagnetically deflecting the electron beam within the x-ray tube. For each focus position, two measured interlaced projections result, since the detector continues to move continuously. The sampling frequency is doubled enhancing the spatial resolution.

FM (*phys*) *See* modulation (frequency).

fMRI (*mri*) Functional magnetic resonance imaging. Measures changes in cerebral blood flow and cerebral blood oxygenation related to neuronal activity; also demonstrates function of the heart and other organs.

focal length (*us*) Distance from a focused transducer to the centre of a focal region or to the location of the spatial peak intensity.

focal region (*us*) Region of minimum beam diameter and area.

focal spot (*xray*) The target area on the anode which forms the real focal spot of the electron beam. The anode angle determines the projected or effective focal spot size of the x-ray beam (sometimes called the apparent focal spot). Focal spot size influences the sharpness of the image and the tube rating (loadability). Due to the rotation of the anode, the electronic focus traces out a ring-shaped focal track on the surface of the anode disk. The size of the effective focal spot is determined by the line focus principle (*see* dual focal spots, focal spot (effective), focal spot (real)).

focal spot (effective) (*xray*) The projected dimensions from the angled anode target as calculated from the line-focus principle. The effective focal spot for general radiography is 0.6–1.2 mm and for mammography 0.4 mm. The dimensions of the effective focal spot differs over the image plane.

focal spot (real) (*xray*) The rectangular area on the anode, bombarded by the electron beam. The area and angle of the real focal spot determines the effective focal spot. Single filaments are used in x-ray tubes having a single anode target; dual-sized focal spots can be obtained by altering the electron beam size. Dual filaments, operated in parallel on a single focal spot, are used in mammography tubes to overcome the space charge limitations; these are operated as the single filament to obtain dual focal spot sizes. Separate dual focal spots are also used (fluoroscopy), but are operated independently and focused on separate differently angled targets to give dual focal spots. Focal spots can be moved to slightly different positions on the target surface by control coils which surround the x-ray tube; used in some CT machines as flying focal spots to increase image resolution (*see* focal spot (effective), filament).

sometimes present. Multifocal tracks are each supplied by a separate filament.

focal zone (*us*) Length of the focal region. This is the narrowest region of the ultrasound profile. Two focal zones are present in a multi-element ultrasound array. The focal zone across the width of the transducer decides slice width and is controlled by a shaped lens with a fixed radius. The focal zone parallel with the transducer face depends on aperture size and signal delay. This decides the lateral resolution.

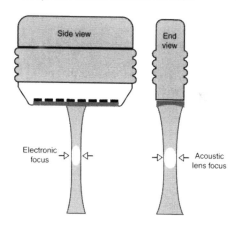

Real FS 11° Anode
Real FS 20°
Effective focal spots

(*see* focus (ultrasound)).

focus (*xray, us*) Determines the slice thickness by shaping the crystal or matching layer, or an electronic focus can influence lateral resolution. Concentration of a sound beam into a smaller beam area than would exist otherwise (*see* focal spot).

focal spot size (*ct*) While the electronic focal spot has a nonquadratic shape on the anode surface, the tube is installed on the fan beam assembly so that the optical focal spot approximates a quadratic shape at the centre of the detector array; for CT, the focal spot size does not need to be small, since a finite beam width due to an increased focal spot size is suitable for the suppression of aliasing artefacts.

focal surface (*us*) The surface which contains the smallest of all beam cross-sectional areas of a focusing transducer assembly. Unit: centimetre squared (cm^2).

focal track (*xray*) The target area on the circumference of a rotating anode x-ray tube. Dual tracks giving two focal spot sizes (two different angles) or multiple focal tracks carrying different target material (mammography) are

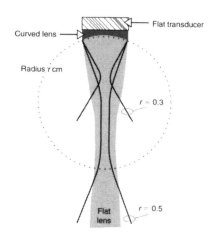

Flat transducer
Curved lens
Radius *r* cm
r = 0.3
Flat lens
r = 0.5

focus (dynamic) (*us*) When a transducer array is receiving echoes, the receiving focus depth may be continuously increased by altering receiver delay as the transmitted pulse travels forward. The contiguously changing echo receiver window is dynamic focusing which increases image resolution with depth.

focus–image–distance (FID) (*image*) A measure from the focal spot to the imaging surface (film, image plate or digital image surface).

focusing coils (*xray*) These control the electron beam geometry magnetically, using coils which control and focus the beam. Cathode ray and camera tubes both used x and y-axis coils to give focused scanning geometry. Some x-ray tubes for computed tomography (CT) can have beam steering which shifts the x-ray spot between two focused points on the target.

focusing cup (*xray*) *See* cathode assembly.

focusing electrodes (*xray*) High voltage electrodes accelerating electrons (*see* image intensifier).

foetus (exposure risk) (*dose*) The mean foetal dose limit (ICRP60) is 5 mSv over a period of 1 year. The added risk to the foetus *in utero* for a 5 mSv exposure is 0.05%. The normal incidence of no abnormality being 95.93% or an approximate abnormality incidence of 1 in 24 live births. Deterministic threshold of between 200 and 400 mGy for severe mental retardation resulting from foetal exposure. Lower doses of 10 mSv have been a suggested risk. (*mri*) At present, there is no known evidence linking MRI exposures to disorders in embryogenesis, but high gradient slew rates should be reconsidered ($20\,\mathrm{T\,s^{-1}}$ rise time >10 ms National Radiological Protection Board (NRPB) in the UK and $>6\,\mathrm{T\,s^{-1}}$ in the United States). Field strengths are limited to 2.0–2.5 T.

■ Reference: Doll and Wakeford, 1997.

fog level (*film*) *See* characteristic curve.

foot (ft) (*phys*) Non-SI, imperial measure of length where:

1 ft	0.3048 m (30.48 cm)
1 m	3.28 ft (39.37 in)
1 ft²	0.093 m²
1 m²	10.76387 ft²

footprint (*us*) Area of transducer in contact with the patient. Also applied to certain computer hardware.

forbidden band (*phys*) *See* energy bands.

force (F) (*phys*) A vector quantity where $F = ma$, the quantity m is the mass of a body and a its acceleration. Since $a = F/m$, then the acceleration of the body is directly proportional to the resultant force acting on it and that the acceleration is inversely proportional to the mass of the body. This is a point considered with x-ray anode design; lighter anodes accelerate faster to their working speed and, if greater surface area is required, graphite is used as it is a very light material which adds very little mass.

Mammography compression paddle
Stated maximum range (*F*) is 150–200 newtons. Since mass $m = F/a$ and acceleration due to gravity $a = 9.8\,\mathrm{m\,s^{-2}}$, the actual pressure felt by the patient under maximum compression is equivalent to 15–20 kg.

(*see* weight).

forced convection (*xray*) *See* convection.

form filter (*ct*) Device for x-ray beam filtration; the thickness of the form filter increases with the distance from the central ray, so that the difference in intensity measured at the detector between rays through the centre of the object and peripheral rays, which experience low or no attenuation, is decreased. Applying form filters reduces the intensity of scattered radiation from peripheral parts and therefore patient dose is decreased. A common name is the 'bow-tie' filter due to its shape.

forward bias (*phys*) *See* junction diode.

Fourier Jean (1768–1830) French mathematician and scientific adviser to Napoleon in Egypt. Developed analysis of complex waveforms into simple sine waves.

Fourier analysis (*math*) A method of waveform analysis. Any periodic function (sine-wave, square wave, etc.) is a summation of sinusoidal components consisting of fundamental and harmonic frequencies of the system (ultrasound pulse, FID, etc.). The simplest example is the sine wave where:

$$X_{(t)} = A = \sin(\omega_o t + \theta).$$

A is a constant for the peak amplitude and ω_o is the angular frequency ($2\pi f$ where f is in Hz); θ is the phase angle in radians. A Fourier series where each harmonic component repeats itself can be represented as:

$$X_{(t)} = A_o + A_1 \sin(\omega_o t + \theta_o) + A_2 \sin(2\omega_o t + \theta_o) + A_n \sin(n\omega_o t + \theta_n)$$

or

$$X_{(t)} = \sum_{n=1}^{n=\infty} A_n \sin(n \times \omega_o t + \theta_n) \quad (n = 1,2,3,...)$$

The summation is the Fourier series and the analysis of the composite periodic function into simple harmonic components is its Fourier analysis. A complimentary process, the inverse Fourier transformation allows regeneration of the original signal (*see* discrete Fourier transform, fast Fourier transform (FFT)).

Fourier space (*mri*) Raw data matrix axes, k_x and k_y dividing the matrix into four squares. The plane spanned by the two axes is the Fourier space or k space.

Fourier's theorem (*math*) This states that it is possible to synthesize or construct any signal (one-dimensional function $f(x)$) as a summation of a series of sine and cosine terms of increasing frequency (*see* Fourier transform).

Fourier transform (FT) (*math*) A measure of the relative amplitude of the frequency components of a signal x takes the exponential notation developed in Euler's formula to give the Fourier transform $F(u)$.

$$F(u) = \int_{-\infty}^{\infty} f(x) \cdot e^{-j\omega x} \cdot dx$$

where $\omega = 2\pi f$. The variable x represents time, so functions in the time domain. The transform F represents frequency so exists in the frequency domain. Given F, it is possible to recover the original time domain function as the inverse:

$$f(x) = \int_{-\infty}^{\infty} F(u) \cdot e^{j\omega x} \cdot du.$$

This can also be used as a 2D transform for image analysis and reconstruction (*see* discrete Fourier transform, Fourier's theorem).

Fourier transform imaging (*mri*) MR imaging techniques in which at least one dimension is phase-encoded by applying variable gradient pulses along that dimension before reading the MR signal with a magnetic field gradient perpendicular to the variable gradient. The Fourier transform is then used to reconstruct an image from the set of encoded MR signals An imaging technique of this type is spin warp imaging.

FOV (*nmed*) Field of view. Central field-of-view (CFOV) of a gamma camera detector, corresponding to 75% of the detector diameter. Useful field of view (UFOV) of a gamma camera detector corresponding to 95% of the detector diameter. Typical values for intrinsic flood field uniformity:

Field	UFOV (%)	CFOV (%)
Integral	±2.5	±2.2
Differential	±2.0	±1.5

Fowler JF British medical physicist and radiobiologist. Pioneer of the investigation of radiation biology and dose response for plant and mammalian tissue.

fraction (*math*) Consists of a numerator n and denominator d (or divisor): n/d, a vulgar fraction is written as $\frac{2}{4}$, a decimal fraction as 0.5. A proper fraction is a vulgar fraction that has a numerator smaller than the denominator $(\frac{1}{2})$; an improper fraction is a vulgar fraction having the numerator bigger than the denominator $(\frac{6}{2})$.

fractional bandwidth (*image*) Bandwidth divided by operating frequency.

fractional error (*math*) The inaccuracy associated with measurement. If original value is V_o and measured or nominal value V_n, then fractional error f is: $(V_n - V_o)/V_o$ (*see* accuracy, precision).

fractionated dose (*dose*) A total dose delivered in successive fractions with periods of days or weeks between each fraction. Contrast with protracted doses given by irradiation continuously over a long period.

frame (*image*) A single image from a series either analogue (cine-angiography) or digital (nuclear medicine, digital subtration angiography (DSA)) (*see* interlacing).

frame averaging (*image*) If image frames (F) are summed, the composite image signal to noise is improved as $\sqrt{F}$, so improving image contrast at the expense of image resolution.

frame rate (*us*) Number of complete scanned images per second. (*image*) The number of complete matrices completed per second.

frame relay (*comp*) A high-speed, low-latency packet switching technology, based on a switched virtual network topology; popular for LAN-to-LAN connections (*see* FDDI).

Fraunhofer zone (*us*) That region of the field in which the acoustic energy flow proceeds essentially as though coming from a point source located in the vicinity of the transducer assembly. (For an unfocused transducer assembly, the far field is commonly at a distance greater than $S/\pi\lambda$, where S is the radiating cross-sectional area and λ is the acoustic wavelength in the medium.) The far field divergence related to wavelength and transducer diameter as:

$$\sin\theta = 0.612 \times \left(\frac{\lambda}{r}\right)$$

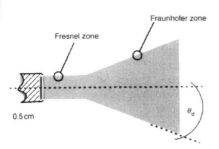

Fresnel zone

Fraunhofer zone

0.5 cm

θ_d

(*see* Fresnel zone).

FRE (*mri*) Field reversal echo (*see* GRE).

free electron (*phys*) *See* electron (free).

free induction decay (FID) (*mri*) The signal induced by an RF excitation of the nuclear spins; decreases exponentially without external influence at a characteristic time constant T2*. When transverse magnetization, M_{xy}, is produced (e.g. 90° RF pulse), a transient MR signal will be produced decaying toward equilibrium M_o with a characteristic time constant T2 or T2*. In practice, the first part of the FID is not observable due to residual effects of the exciting

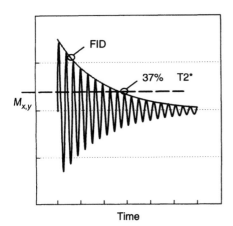

FID

37%   T2*

$M_{x,y}$

Time

RF pulse on the receiver. Signal is induced by the RF excitation of the nuclear spins and that decreases exponentially without external influence at a characteristic time constant T2*.

free radicals (*phys*) An atom or group of atoms that have unpaired valency electrons. They are extremely reactive and are responsible for most cellular damage (DNA, cell membranes) caused by radiation exposure. Ionization is defined as the formation of free radicals and does not apply to simple dissociation of molecules into ions seen in other non-radiation events (e.g. NaCl → Na^+ and Cl^-). Water molecules, the most common constituent of tissue, enter a state of excitation, forming free radicals (H^o and OH^o). These are highly reactive and are responsible for indirect protein damage. Ionization of the water can occur ($H_2O \rightarrow H^+ + OH^-$). Both indirect and direct reactions can lead to self-perpetuating chain reactions. A chain reaction may occur causing further damage in adjacent molecules. Radiation damage to living systems occurs almost exclusively by free-radical production and not by the direct ionizing event.

Direct and indirect damage

Direct damage where R = protein molecule

1 $RH^* \rightarrow R^o + H^o$
2 $R^o + O_2 \rightarrow RO^o_2$ (peroxy radical)
3 $RO^o_2 + RH \rightarrow RO_2H + R^o$ (return to start of 2)

Indirect damage: (the radiolysis of water)

4 $H_2O^* \rightarrow H_2O^+ + e^-$
5 $H_2O + e^- \rightarrow H_2O^-$
6 $H_2O^+ \rightarrow H^+ + OH^o$
7 $H_2O^- \rightarrow H^o + OH^-$

The ions OH^- and H^+ are removed since they recombine to form water:

$H^+ + OH^-$ H_2O.

H^o and OH^o have unpaired electrons so are free radicals and extract hydrogen from organic molecules:

8 $RH + OH^o \rightarrow R^o + H_2O$
9 $RH + H^o \rightarrow R^o + H_2$

which joins the chain reaction in (1) above.

FREEZE (*mri*) Respiratory selection of phase-encoding steps, Elscint. Respiratory ordered phase encoding (*see* RESCOMP, RSPE, PEAR).

freeze frame (*image*) An ability to hold in storage and display a single image frame from a series of frames.

frequency (Hz) (*phys*) For electromagnetic wave-forms, the relationship between frequency f, wavelength λ and velocity c, is:

$$f = c/\lambda$$

$$c = f\lambda$$

$$\lambda = c/f.$$

(*us*) Measured in cycles per second. Typical ultrasound values 2–10 MHz.

Frequency (MHz)	Wavelength (mm)
2.0	0.74
3.5	0.42
5.0	0.30
7.5	0.20
10.0	0.15

frequency domain (*math*) When a periodic sig-nal is broken down into its frequency compo-nents (e.g. MR spectroscopy), the signal exists in the frequency domain (*see* Fourier transform).

frequency encoding (*mri*) Encoding MR signals using a steady magnetic field gradient. Without other position encoding (phase), the Fourier transform is a projection profile of the object. During data acquisition, a gradient is applied in one spatial direction, giving nuclear spins with linearly increasing precession frequencies. The MR signal is then a mix of frequencies which must be filtered individually. In the row direction, the location of the nuclear spin can be reconstructed from the frequency; this is the frequency encod-ing axis. The perpendicular axis is the phase-encoding axis.

frequency offset (*mri*) Difference between the given signal frequency and a reference frequency.

frequency response (*image*) The output signal spectrum is the product of the input frequency spectrum and the system's gain together with its phase shift. The impulse response characterizes a system in the time domain; the frequency response characterizes a system in the frequency domain.

frequency response function (*math*) Describing a circuit in the frequency domain by applying an arbitrary frequency input and measuring the Fourier transform of its output. The output signal spectrum is the product of the input fre-quency spectrum and the system's gain, together with its phase shift. The impulse response characterizes a system in time domain; the fre-quency response characterizes a system in the frequency domain. The identified frequency

component or frequency response function uniquely defines the system (amplifier, filter) in the frequency domain (*see* impulse response function).

frequency selective RF pulse (*mri*) An RF pulse having energy only within a specified fre-quency range. Commonly used for slice excita-tion or for selective saturation pulses.

frequency tuning (*mri*) The RF system fre-quency is set to the resonant frequency of tissue in the main magnetic field (Larmor frequency).

Fresnel zone (*us*) or 'near zone'. This dimension is dependent on transducer diameter d and aperture as:

$$\frac{d2}{4\lambda}.$$

The length of the Fresnel zone is proportional to the square of the transducer diameter and inversely proportional to wavelength; increas-ing transducer frequency extends the Fresnel zone. Also the Fresnel zone length depends on

$$\frac{\alpha^2}{\lambda}$$

where α is half width (or radius) of the trans-ducer. Diversion angle (*Fraunhofer zone*) depends on $\sin^{-1}(0.61\lambda/\alpha)$.

freeze frame (*di*) An ability to hold in storage and display a single image frame from a series of frames.

frequency (Hz) (*us*) Cycles per second. Typical ultrasound values 2–10 MHz.

frequency spectrum (*us*) The range of frequen-cies present. In a Doppler instrument, the range of Doppler shift frequencies present in the returning echoes.

friction (*phys*) Energy loss commonly seen as an increase in system heat. Since friction always opposes motion, a moving body experiences a frictional force. This is not confined to solids; it is also experienced by fluids and gases caused by viscous drag between layers of molecules.

FRF (*mri*) Field reversal echo.

fringe field (magnetic) (*mri*) Region surrounding a magnet. The earth's magnetic fringe field is typically 0.05–0.1 mT. Due to the physical properties of magnetic fields, they form closed field lines. Depending on the magnet construc-tion, the returning flux will penetrate large open spaces (unshielded magnets) or will be confined largely to iron yokes or through secondary coils (shielded magnets).

Frost, Edwin Brant American professor of astronomy asked by his brother (a clinician) to carry out the first radiograph on a patient on February 3rd 1896 (*see* Campbell-Swinton).

FS (*mri*) Fast scan.

FSE (*mri*) *See* Fast spin echo.

F-SHORT (*mri*) Steady-state gradient echo with spin echo sampling. Short-repetition technique based on free induction decay (Elscint). Rewinding of phase-encoding and no intentional spoiling (*see* GRASS, FGR, FISP, FAST, GFEC, SSFP).

FSPGR (*mri*) Fast spoiled gradient recalled. Gradient-echo imaging techniques T1-weighted contrast (GE) (*see* FLASH, SPGR, HFGR, RE spoiled, 3D-ME-RAGE, T1-FEE, STAGE-T1W).

FTP (*comp*) File transfer protocol. A means of transferring files from one computer to another across the Internet, and one of the principal tools that is available on the Internet (the three other key functions are e-mail, news groups and the web).

full-scan interpolation (*ct*) Synonymous with 360° interpolation.

full-wave rectifier (*elec*) The preferable method for rectifying an a.c. waveform since both halves of the cycle contribute to the d.c. output. Full wave rectification applies to single phase (×4 rectifiers) and three-phase (×12 rectifiers) supplies.

full-width-at-half-maximum (FWHM) (*phys*) A commonly used measure for resolution of peak events such as point spread function in visual image separation, energy resolution measured on the photopeak of a scintillation detector, NMR spectral lines and slice profiles in tomography. (*ct*) Distance on the abscissa of a 1D or 2D distribution between the points where the function reaches one half of its maximum value.

full-width-at-tenth-maximum (FWTM) (*phys*) Sometimes used as an additional measurement with the FWHM to measure the degree of scattered radiation entering the photopeak or, in the case of spatial resolution, the collimator penetration or light diffusion within the scintillation detector.

function (*math*) A variable that can take a set of values, each of which is associated with the value of an independent variable or variables. The notation $f(x) = y$ reads that y is a function of x.

functional groups (*nmed*) Small group of linked atoms with chemically active bonds. These are important in nuclear medicine labelling reactions.

functional imaging (*mri*) *See* fMRI.

fuse (*elec*) A short length of wire acting as a circuit weak-link which breaks if excessive current is present that could damage electrical equipment. Wire fuses have a relatively long dead time and are not suitable for protection against fast pulsatile current surges.

fusion (nuclear) (*phys*) *See* nuclear fusion.

fuzzy logic (*comp*) A method of analyzing a data set which considers the probability of set membership. A measurement that cannot be defined precisely but is judged relatively, e.g. hot/cold, loud/quiet. The term was coined in 1965 by Lofti Zadeh (USA). In radiology, it finds a use for controlling x-ray tube loadability and dose measurement in CT or fluoroscopy.

FWHM (*nmed*) *See* full-width-half-maximum.

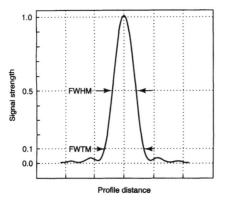

G

Gx, Gy, Gz (*mri*) Conventional symbols for magnetic field gradient. Used with subscripts to denote spatial direction component of gradient, i.e. direction along which the field changes.

gadobuterol (*cm*) Generic name for Gd–DO3A-buterol and paramagnetic magnetic resonance imaging (MRI) contrast agent (*see* Gadovist®).

gadolinium (Gd) (*elem*) Lanthanum element

Atomic number (Z)	64
Relative atomic mass (A$_r$)	157.25
Density (ρ) kg/m³	7900
Melting point (K)	1585
K-edge (keV)	50.2

Relevance to radiology: As rare-earth scintillators for intensifying screens. Gd2O2S:Tb. MR contrast agents in a chelated form, such as DTPA, because of its effect of strongly decreasing the TI relaxation times.

^{153}Gadolinium

Nuclear data	Emission
Half-life	242 d
Decay mode	β–
Decay constant	0.0028 day^{-1}
Photon (abundance)	97 (0.40)
	103 (0.59)

As a dual energy source for bone mineral estimation and for attenuation correction fitted to gamma cameras.

gadolinium contrast medium (*mri*) Lanthanide element used in its trivalent state. Used as the active component of some paramagnetic contrast agents; strongly decreases the TI relaxation times of the tissues to which it has access. It is given in a chelated form, such as DTPA (*see* contrast agent (MRI)).

gadolinium oxy-orthosilicate (GSO) (*phys*) Cerium-activated gadolinium oxyorthosilicate (Gd$_2$OSiO$_4$:Ce or GSO). This scintillator gives a better energy resolution and higher light output than LSO. It also has better attenuation for 511 keV photons; its light decay time is slightly higher.

gadolinium phosphor (*xray*) Gadolinium compounds used in the manufacture of rare earth intensifying screens in the form of Gd$_2$O$_2$S:Tb; these emit light in the green spectrum (*see* intensifying screen).

gadoteridol (*clin*) Generic name for magnetic resonance image (MRI) contrast agent Prohance®.

Gadovist $^\times$ (*cm*) Commercial (Schering) preparation of gadobutrol Gd-BT-DO3A, a paramagnetic contrast agent.

Compound	Concentration (mg mL^{-1})	Osmolality (mosm/kg)
Gadobutrol (Gd-BT-DO3A)	0.5 and 1.0 mol/L	557 and 1603

gain (*elec*) Increasing amplification by either potentiometric adjustment or by altering feedback. Certain charge amplifiers have unity gain, merely acting as impedance matching devices; ratio of amplifier output to input electric power. (*us*) Ratio of amplifier output to input electric power.

gain control (*us*) The signal amplitude changed by either altering the amplitude of the transmitted pulse or the gain of the receiving circuits. The first method increases transmitted power and image depth, the second method increases displayed noise levels.

gallium (Ga) (*elem*)

Atomic number (Z)	31
Relative atomic mass (A$_r$)	69.72
Density (ρ) kg/m³	5950
Melting point (K)	302.9
K-edge (keV)	10.36

Relevance to radiology: As a low melting point alloy lubricating x-ray tube bearings.

^{67}Gallium (tumour imaging)

Production	$^{68}_{30}$Zn (p,2n)$^{67}_{31}$Ga
Decay scheme (e.c.) ^{67}Ga	^{67}Ga (γ 93 185 300 keV) → ^{67}Zn stable
Photons (abundance)	91 (0.032)
	93 (0.376)
	185 (0.212)
	209 (0.024)
	300 (0.168)
	394 (0.047)
Half-life	78 hours
Decay constant	0.00885 h^{-1}
Gamma ray constant	2.2 × 10^{-2} mSv hr^{-1} GBq^{-1} at 1 m
Half value layer	0.7 mm Pb, 47 mm water

Radiation attenuation factors for lad (^{67}Ga).

Pb (mm)	Attenuation factor
0.66	0.5
4.10	10^{-1}
12.0	10^{-2}
25.0	10^{-3}
	10^{-4}

Hours	Fraction remaining
0	1.00
6	0.95
12	0.90
24	0.81
36	0.73
48	0.65
60	0.59
72	0.53
84	0.48
96	0.43
120	0.35
144	0.28
168	0.23

⁶⁷Gallium citrate (*nmed*) Binds to the intracellular lactoferrin of leukocytes and is transported to infection sites where it is deposited when the leukocytes excrete some of their lactoferrin. Gallium is believed to localize in inflammatory lesions by diffusing across 'leaky' capillaries into the extracellular space and binding to iron-binding proteins. An iron analogue that reacts with iron-binding proteins including:

- transferrin: a primary transport protein for ⁶⁷Ga within the circulatory system;
- lactoferrin: stored within specific leukocyte granules and is released by the leukocytes at sites of inflammation;
- ferritin: an intracellular protein, which mediates uptake of iron/gallium within bacteria;
- siderophores: low molecular weight compounds produced by bacteria that also mediate uptake of iron/gallium within bacteria.

⁶⁸Gallium (*nmed*) Generator derived, it decays by positron emission and is used for positron emission tomography.

Production (generator)	⁶⁸Ge/⁶⁸Ga
Decay scheme (β+) ⁶⁸Ga	⁶⁸Ga (β+ 2.9 MeV, 2γ 511 keV) → ⁶⁸Zn stable
Eluent	0.005 M EDTA
Half-life	1.13 hours
Half value layer	4.1 mm Pb (511 keV)

gamma (-γ) (*math*) A symbol used to indicate: chemical shift, electrical conductivity, gyromagnetic ratio, gamma photon, slope of film characteristic curve (film gamma), mathematical function, Γ, and specific gamma ray constant (dose constant), Γ.

gamma camera (*nmed*) A position-sensitive imaging device invented by Anger Hal O, that displays the distribution of radioactivity within a source or body. Uses a bank of photomultipliers behind a large thin NaI:Tl scintillation detector to given positional information with the aid of collimation. It records the quantity and distribution of photons emitted by the radioactive material in the area of interest. The principal imaging device used in nuclear medicine.

gamma decay (*phys*) A nuclear decay process involving the emission of gamma radiation either as a single or multiple event.

gamma fit (*math*) A method used for approximating the shape of a dilution (time–activity) curve, so that mixed curves can be separated for quantitation.

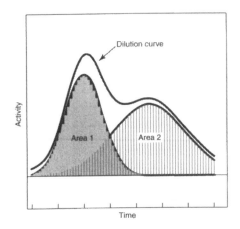

gamma radiation (*phys*) Electromagnetic radiation emitted during gamma decay. The range extends to several MeV. The diagnostic imaging energy range is roughly 80–200 keV.

gamma-ray dose rate constant (*nmed*) This constant, which has the symbol F, represents the radiation dose rate (mR/hr) present when an unshielded 1 mCi source is positioned 1 cm from a detector. Each radionuclide has a characteristic F value (*see* specific gamma ray constant).

gamma spectrum (*nm*) For gamma energies <100 keV, the absorption in NaI(Tl) is predominantly photoelectric. Iodine escape peak due to absorption of photoelectron from iodine x-rays mainly from front surface of the crystal. The photopeak corresponds to absorption of photoelectrons from the gamma photoelectric event; depends on scintillator crystal dimensions. At <200 keV, most scintillation pulses occur in the photopeak. Between 200 keV and 1 MeV Compton events are more appreciable and the

Compton edge, *C*, is visible. The maximum energy when the photon is scattered through 180° is then:

Compton peak = $E2/(E + 256)$.

For a gamma energy of 662 keV (^{137}Cs), the peak of the Compton continuum would be 447 keV. The backscatter peak is due to incomplete absorption; no iodine escape peak is visible. At energies greater than 1.02 MeV, pair production becomes a prominent feature.

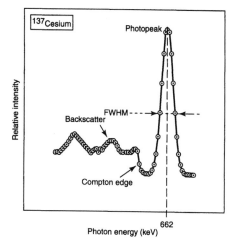

(*see* detector spatial resolution).

gantry (*ct*) Scanner structure containing the x-ray tube, collimators and the detector array.

gantry aperture (*ct*) Diameter of the physical opening of the gantry through which the patient is moved for the examination.

gantry rotation time (*ct*) The time for a full 360° rotation of the gantry around the patient table. Single-section helical CT scanners typically have a 360° gantry rotation speed of about one second. With multislice CT, gantry rotation speeds of 0.4 or 0.5 s; twice as fast as that of single-section helical CT (*see* g-force).

gantry tilt (*ct*) The angle between the vertical plane, and the fan beam assembly containing the x-ray tube and the detector array. The tilt of the CT gantry with respect to the patient can be altered typically up to 30°; the scan plane is rotated around the x-axis such that the axis of rotation and the direction of table feed are not orthogonal.

GARP (*mri*) Globally optimized alternating phase rectangular pulse.

gas ionization detector (*ct*) A detector design for CT scanners, employing vessels filled with noble gas under high pressure (xenon). For multislice CT machines, gas detectors are not suitable, especially in terms of overall spatial resolution. Their major limitation is the low quantum detection efficiency of <50%, caused primarily by low x-ray absorption in the xenon gas and by the absorption of x-rays in the thick container housing the pressurized gas (*see* Geiger counter, proportional counter, ionization chamber).

gas laws (*phys*) The variation of pressure, volume and temperature on a gas, Boyle's law (Robert Boyle 1627–91, Irish physicist) together with Charles' law (JA Charles, 1746–1823; French physicist) form basic relationships in physics and also feature in the propagation of sound through air. Boyle's law states that pressure is inversely proportional to volume at constant temperature and Charles' law states that volume and temperature are proportional at constant pressure. Summarizing these two statements gives:

$$PV/T = \text{constant.}$$

The gas laws play an important academic role in the derivation of the SI scale for temperature (*see* equations of state).

gas multiplication (amplification) (*phys*) A property of the Geiger counter where at reduced gas pressure, electrons released from the ionizing event, can gain sufficient velocity under the influence of a high electrical field, to cause secondary ionization by colliding with other gas atoms. This enables a large electrical signal to be generated without electronic amplification.

Gastrografin® (*cm*) Commercial (Bracco) preparation of 66% meglumine diatrizoate and 10% sodium diatrizoate for the examination of the gastrointestinal tract. Oral or rectal administration.

Compound	Viscosity (cP)	Osmolality (mOsm/kg)	Iodine (mg I mL^{-1})
Meglumine diatrizoate	18.5 at 20°, 8.9 at 37°	1940	370

Gastromiro® (*cm*) Preparation containing 612.4 mg mL^{-1} of iopamidol (Bracco) for investigating the gastrointestinal tract.

Gastroview® (*cm*) Commercial preparation of meglumine diatrizoate 66% and 10% sodium diatrrozoate; gastrointestinal tract, osmolality 2000 mOsm/kg iodine content 367 mg I mL^{-1} (Mallinckodt/Tyco Healthcare Inc).

---

gated acquisition (*xray*) Image data acquisition under the control of a gating signal either electrocardiogram (ECG) or respiration. Linking physiological timing (cardiac, respiration) to data acquisition in order to either freeze motion or collect a series of temporal images (cardiac cycle: end diastole to end systole). Synchronization of imaging with a phase of the cardiac or respiratory cycles. A variety of means for detecting these cycles can be used, such as the ECG, peripheral pulse, chest motion, etc. The synchronization can be prospective or retrospective.

gateway (*comp*) A network station used to interconnect two or more dissimilar networks or devices: may perform protocol conversion.

GATOR CIST (*mri*) Respiratory gated imaging.

gauss (*phys*) G unit of magnetic flux in the c.g.s. system (1 Tesl = 10 000 G) and $1\,G\,cm^{-1} = 0.01\,T\,m^{-1}$ ($10\,mT\,m^{-1}$).

gaussian curve (*math*) *See* Gaussian distribution.

gaussian distribution (*stats*) This describes the distribution of random events and is represented by:

$$y = e^{-x^{2/d}}$$

where *d* is the width of the distribution measured as the full width of the curve at half its maximum (FWHM). The gaussian distribution describes both energy and spatial resolution of a detector system, and approximates the spread of frequencies (bandwidth) of an RF or ultrasound pulse. Other gaussian distributions occur in dosimetry (*see* normal curve).

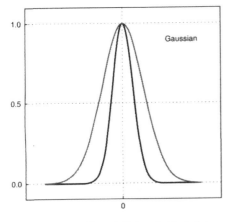

gaussian noise (*image*) Noise distributed in a normal (Gaussian) pattern. In such a distribution, approximately 65% of all points fall within one standard deviation(s) of the mean.

GBP (*mri*) Global bolus plot.

GDI (*image*) Graphical device interface, the native graphical language of Windows. A GDI-compliant printer will print exactly what is displayed on the Windows screen without having to transpose it into a printer language.

GE/GFE (*mri*) Gradient echo or gradient field echo, general sequence, Hitachi (*see* FFE, GRE, MPGR, GRECO, FE, PFI, Turbo-FLASH, TFF, SMASH, SHORT, STAGE).

Geiger, Hans W (1882–1945) German physicist who developed a form of gas detector for counting alpha particles. Geiger and Marsden performed the original experiment with alpha particles and gold foil that led Rutherford to propose his model of the atom. He also demonstrated that two alpha particles are emitted from uranium during decay. With Nuttall, he demonstrated the relationship between alpha particle range an decay constant known as the Geiger–Nuttall rule. He became professor at Kiel University where he developed his particle counter with Walther Müller to give the Geiger–Müller counter.

Geiger counter (*phys, nmed*) More correctly, Geiger–Müller counter used as an inexpensive contamination radiation monitor. A higher voltage supply encourages the ionization events (ions and electrons) to multiply and give a large signal output; this multiplying effect prevents it being photon energy sensitive. A damped Geiger counter is often calibrated in terms of events per second or dose rate ($\mu Sv\,hr^{-1}$) (*see* gas multiplication, ion chamber).

gelatin (*film*) The suspending medium for silver halides in the emulsion.

gene (*clin*) A locality on the chromosome carrying specific genetic information in the form of DNA.

generator (*xray*) The electrical system which provides the high voltage (typically up to 150 kV) and low voltage (typically 8–12 V) which drives the x-ray tube. Present day generators are all high frequency designs with multiple feedback circuits controlling voltage, output and timing (*see* high frequency generator).

generator (radionuclide) (*nmed*) A device for generating clinically useful daughter products from a long-lived parent, i.e. ^{99}Mo/^{99m}Tc and ^{81}Rb/^{81m}Kr. Two types of generator exist commercially. Those showing:

- transient equilibrium, where the parent has a very much longer half-life than the daughter product;

- secular equilibrium where the parent has only a somewhat longer half-life than the daughter product (*see* individual generator types ^{99}Mo/^{99}mTc, Rb/Kr, etc.).

generator (shielding) (*nmed*) Radiation levels from a medium-size technetium generator would be an unshielded core of 18.5 GBq (500 mCi) generator $6 \, \text{mSv} \, \text{h}^{-1}$ at 0.5 m. For $7.5 \, \mu\text{Sv} \, \text{h}^{-1}$, this would require 6.8 cm Pb (HVL for ^{99}Mo, 740 keV γ 7 mm Pb). A typical shielded core with 5.0 cm Pb, additional lead shielding 4.5 cm Pb, total lead shielding 9.5 cm Pb. The total shielding supplied by the manufacturer typically exceeds the minimum levels.

genetically significant dose (GSD) (*dose*) The dose that, if given to every member of a population, should produce the same hereditary damage as the actual doses received by the gonads of an individual receiving radiation. It is calculated as:

$$\frac{\Sigma[N_{xy}P_{xy}D_{xy}]_m + [N_{xy}P_{xy}D_{xy}]_f}{\Sigma N_x P_x}$$

where N_{xy} is the number of patients in age groups x undergoing patient examination y; P_{xy} is child expectancy for persons in age group x undergoing examination y; D_{xy} is the average gonad dose for patients in age group x undergoing examination y; N_x is the number of people of age group x in the population; P_x is the child expectancy for age group x. The subscripts m and f denote male and female subsets. The GSD value has steadily declined over the years, some values are:

Sweden	0.46 mSv
Germany	0.41 mSv
USA	0.20 mSv
Japan	0.17 mSv
UK	0.12 mSv

Natural radiation delivers a GSD of about 1 mSv. Medical values are primarily an indicator of the care with which the reproductive organs are protected in medical procedures and the amount of radiography of pregnant women and children that is done in the country.

genetic effects (*nmed*) Radiation effects induced in the offspring of irradiated persons (or animals), if conception occurs after exposure (*see* somatic effects).

genome (*clin*) Basic haploid set of chromosomes.

genotype (*clin*) Genetic constitution of an organism.

geometric dose efficiency (*ct*) The quantity of radiation striking the detector as a fraction of the total radiation dose leaving the patient. In practice, the geometrical efficiency is less than 100% mainly due to post-patient collimation and due to inactive areas (dead space) between adjacent detector channels (the septa); especially with multi-row detectors, the geometrical efficiency is an important parameter of the system (*see* **dose efficiency**).

geometric efficiency (G_{eff}) (*ct*) A measure of the best dose utilization in the z-axis, as the ratio of the imaged slice section profile (SSP) relative to the z-axis slice dose profile (SDP). High geometric efficiency is a requirement for multi-slice detectors. Dead spaces are as small as possible Antiscatter collimators should be as thin as possible. Geometric efficiency should be 100%, but it is often less, especially for narrow beam collimations where post-patient collimation may be necessary to bring the imaged slice thickness closer to the chosen value. Values of 80–90% are typical. In arrays with a finer separation of detector elements in the z direction, a reduction in geometric efficiency is seen. The geometric efficiency (G_{eff}) of the detector array can be calculated by comparing the FWHM of the SDP with the SSP:

$$G_{eff} = \frac{\text{FWHM (SSP)}}{\text{FWHM (SDP)}} \times 100\%.$$

If the SSP and SDP dimensions are identical, as in the case of sequential CT, the geometric efficiency is 100%. For single slice and multislice spiral CT, the geometric efficiency can fall as low as 60%. As the number of slices increases, the excess dose not contributing to the image ('wasted dose') becomes less. The value for a quad slice scanner having 1.25 mm slice thickness is about 64%, whereas an eight-slice scanner with the same slice width gives a figure closer to 76%.

geometric mean (*stats*) The average value of a set of n numbers expressed as the nth root of their product. Thus the geometric mean of n numbers $x_1, x_2, \ldots x_n$ is:

$$\sqrt[n]{x_1 \cdot x_2 \cdots x_n}.$$

(*see* mean, average).

Geometric mean

If the annual percentage change in patient workload for a particular examination for 5 years is: 15.8, 8.3, 13.4, 18.0, 11.9%, then the overall scaled effect is:

$1.158 \times 1.083 \times 1.134 \times 1.180 \times 1.119 = 1.878$.

So the average patient workload increases by

$\sqrt[5]{1.878} = 1.134$ or 13.4%. = 1.134 or 13.4%.

geometrical resolution (*ct*) The ability to display small structures of high contrast (line pair grating). The geometrical resolution can be quantitatively described by means of the limiting spatial frequency (as line pairs), the point spread function, the edge spread function, the line spread function and the modulation transfer function.

geometrical resolution limit (*ct*) Resolution limit for high contrast, expressed as the minimum size of an object detail that can be resolved (*see* line pairs).

geometric unsharpness (*xray*) *See* unsharpness (geometric).

geometry (detector) (*math*) Relating to detector surfaces 2π describes a flat surface, e.g. a gamma camera which has a 180° acceptance angle; a 4π detector describes a volume device with a 360° or spherical acceptance, e.g. dose calibrator.

germ cell (*clin*) Pertaining to the gametes: sperm, ovum or a cell from which they originate.

germanium **(Ge)** (*elem*) Non metallic semiconductor.

Atomic number (Z)	32
Relative atomic mass (A_r)	72.59
Density (ρ) kg/m³	5400
Melting point (K)	1210.5
K-edge (keV)	11.1
Relevance to radiology: high resolution volume semiconductor detectors as hyper-pure germanium (HpGe).	

^{68}Germanium (*nmed*) As a long-lived calibration source for PET scanners:

Production (cyclotron)	$^{66}_{30}Zn(\alpha, 2n)^{68}_{32}Ge$
	or $^{69}_{31}Ga(p, 2n)^{68}_{32}Ge$
Decay scheme (β+) ^{68}Ge	^{68}Ge (electron capture) → ^{68}Ga (*see* ^{68}Ga decay scheme)
Half-life	270 days
Half value layer	4.1 mm Pb (511 keV γ)

germinal tissue (*dose*) Tissue associated with the gonads in which sperm or ova are developing.

GFE (*mri*) Gradient field echo, Hitachi. Term for any GRE sequence.

GFEC (*mri*) Gradient field echo with contrast, Hitachi. Enhanced intensity; rewinding of phase-encoding and no intentional spoiling (*see* GRASS, FGR, FISP, FAST, F-SHORT, SSFP).

g-force (*units*) Both centripetal and centrifugal force use this value, $F = mv^2/r$, where m is mass, v velocity and r the radius of rotation.

G-force

The forces on an x-ray tube and HF generator of 150 kg having a rotation radius of 0.6 m and rotation time of 0.5 s. The velocity is therefore $2\pi \times 0.6 \times 2 = 7.54 \, m \, s^{-1}$ and the force (F) is

$$\frac{150 \times 7.54^2}{0.6} = 14213 \, N.$$

ghosting (*mri*) During periodic movement (respiration), some phase-encoding steps are acquired during inspiration, and others during expiration. This misregistration gives a displaced false image of the body region. The distance between ghosting images determined by movement period and relaxation time, TR.

Gibbs' artefact (*image*) Truncation artefact due to Gibbs' phenomenon.

Gibbs' phenomenon (*image*) Ripples in the calculated value that occur near a discontinuity when reconstructing a mathematical function from a limited portion of its Fourier transform. In MR imaging, it is visible as linear artefacts parallel to sharp edges in the object, particularly with the use of zero filling. CT images show poor delineation and black spaces between bone and soft tissue (i.e. the skull) (*see* truncation artefact).

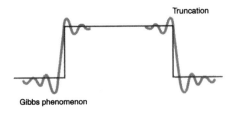

Gibbs phenomenon

GIF (*comp*) Graphics interchange format. A raster graphics format developed to handle 8-bit (256) colour with high compression ratios. Combines palette-based indexing and LZW compression. Contains a maximum of 256 colours taking full advantage of the ability to store images with fewer colours at lower bit-depths. Since GIF restricts the number of colours, the typical flat-coloured GIF image is more suitable for LZW compression. Apart from its minimized file size, GIF offers a number of other advantages. Interlacing means all even scan lines are stored first and then odd rows are split into three sets; the image appears in four passes with a 'Venetian blind' effect, so a viewer can grasp the essence of the image after only 50% of the data has downloaded. The 256-colour limit and LZW compression result in both poor image quality and large files. JPEG was developed by the Joint Photographic Experts Group to solve this problem.

gigabyte (GB) (*comp*) 1024 megabytes.

gigabit Ethernet (*comp*) an extension of the 10 and 100 Mbps (megabits per second) ethernet standards that describes 1000 Mbps transmission speeds. Originally required fibreoptics, but the specification now supports these speeds over copper cable.

GINSEST (*mri*) Generalized interferography using spin echoes and stimulated echoes.

glare (*x-ray*) *See* veiling glare.

glass crown (*mat*)

Density (ρ) kg m⁻³	2600
Melting point (K)	1400 K

glass flint (*mat*)

Density (ρ) kg m⁻³	4200
Melting point (K)	1500 K

glass (lead) (*xray*) Density $4800 \, kg \, m^{-3}$ Pb content 48%; Ba content 15%.

Approximate thickness (mm)	Pb equivalent (mm Pb)	Weight (kg m⁻²)
6.5	1.5	35
8.5	2.1	45
10	2.5	50
13	3.3	65

Global bolus plot (*mri*) Global time–density curve (GBP).

global maximum (*us*) The greatest value of a quantity evaluated over all times, over all locations, and over all operating conditions for any given operating mode.

global shim (*mri*) Fat saturation, EPI, or spectroscopy require high magnetic field homogeneity where shim coils are used to optimize homogeneity.

Glofil-125 (*nmed*) Commercial preparation of sodium ¹²⁵I Iothalamate (QOL Medical Inc).

glow curve (*dose*) The important properties of a practical thermoluminescent detector are the photon energy response and allowing light emission at about 200°C forming a glow-curve in or near the blue region of the spectrum. The light output is proportional to radiation exposure.

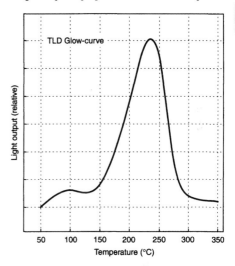

TLD Glow-curve

gluceptate/gluconate (*nmed*) As labelled ⁹⁹ᵐTc-gluceptate (⁹⁹ᵐTc-D-glycero-D-glucoheptonate as the calcium salt (calcium glucoheptonate/gluconate) used for scintigraphy of kidney function and cerebral perfusion. ⁹⁹ᵐTc-gluconate also tends to accumulate in intracranial lesions. Renal retention is greater in the cortex than the medulla.

Generic name	⁹⁹ᵐTc-gluceptate
Gluceptate	Draximage®
	(Mallinckrodt)
Glucoheptonate	TechneScan®
Gluconate	Amerscan®
Imaging category	Renal function and
	brain perfusion

gluconate (*nmed*) *See* gluceptate.

GMC (*mri*) Gradient moment compensation. Instrumentarium FC, flow compensation, GE Philips. Reduction of motion-induced phase shifts during TE (*see* GMR, GMN, FLOW-COMP, CFAST, MAST, FLAG, FC, STILL, SMART, GR).

GMN (*mri*) Gradient moment nulling GE. Reduction of motion-induced phase shifts during TE (*see* GMR, FLOW-COMP, CFAST, MAST, FLAG, GMC, FC, STILL, SMART, GR).

GMR (*mri*) Gradient motion rephasing, Siemens. Reduction of motion–induced phase shifts during TE (*see* GMN, FLOW-COMP, CFAST, MAST, FLAG, GMC, FC, STILL, SMART, GR).

Golay coil (*mri*) Term commonly used for a particular kind of gradient coil. Commonly used to create magnetic field gradients perpendicular to the main magnetic field.

gold (Au) (*elem*)

Atomic number (Z)	79
Relative atomic mass (A_r)	196.97
Density (ρ) kg/m^3	19 300
Melting point (K)	1336.1
Specific heat capacity, $J\,kg^{-1}K^{-1}$	128
Thermal conductivity, $W\,m^{-1}K^{-1}$	317
K-edge (keV)	80.7

^{195m}Au (*nmed*) Daughter product of ^{195m}Hg/ generator. Used for vascular imaging giving a steady-state picture of circulation.

Production (cyclotron)	$^{197}_{79}$Au(p,3n)$^{195m}_{80}$Hg
Decay scheme (i.t.) ^{195m}Au	^{195m}Hg $T\frac{1}{2}$ 41.6 h
	(γ keV) $\rightarrow$ ^{195m}Au
Eluent	Sodium thiosulphate/ sodium nitrate
Half-life	30.5 s
Half value layer	mm Pb

^{198}Au (*nmed*) Used for intracavity therapy.

Decay scheme ($\beta-$) ^{198}Au	^{198}Au ($\beta - 1.37$ MeV) $\rightarrow$ ^{198}Pt
Half-life	2.7 days
Decay mode	$\beta- 0.961$ MeV
Decay constant	0.256 year^{-1}
Photons (abundance)	412 keV

goodness of fit (*stats*) How well a particular set of data fits a given relationship or distribution. The goodness of fit may be measured by using a chi-squared test.

GPF (*comp*) General protection fault. A Windows warning that a protected part of RAM is being accessed. Caused by a program trying to access an area of memory being used either by another program or the operating system.

GPRS (*comp*) General packet radio services. Provides packet-switched data radio technology for GSM networks. Being always on, GPRS connections offer mobile users network availability comparable to that of a corporate network.

GPU (*comp*) Graphics processing unit. Graphics cards with GPUs handle a great deal of the resource-intensive functions that are traditionally handled by the main processor. Image processing is an example.

GR or GRE (*mri*) Gradient rephasing, Hitachi. Reduction of motion–induced phase shifts during TE (*see* GMR, GMN, FLOW-COMP, CFAST, MAST, FLAG, GMC, FC, STILL, SMART).

gradient (*mri*) The magnitude and rate of change in space of a magnetic field strength seen in magnetic gradients of an MRI machine.

gradient coils (*mri*) These supply magnetic gradients which define the strength and direction of the magnetic field in the field of view. Gives a linear change in the magnetic field in a specific direction and determines the spatial orientation and resolution of the image. Magnetic gradients are defined by rise time, duty cycle, gradient linearity, gradient strength and slew rate. Gradient coils operate in pairs in the *x*-, *y*- and *z*-axis, having identical properties, but opposite polarities. Each coil increases the magnetic field by a specific fraction; the opposing coil reduces the field by the same amount. This provides the linear gradient.

gradient echo (GRE) (or gradient recalled echo or field echo) (*mri*) The formation of an echo by the application of a single excitation pulse followed by switching of the gradient polarity; echo signal generated by a magnetic gradient field reversal instead of the 180° pulse in spin echo). The method chosen for fast imaging, but does not refocus field inhomogeneity. The gradient echo is generally adjusted to be coincident with the RF spin echo. When the RF and gradient echoes are not coincident, the time of the gradient echo is denoted TE and the difference in time between the echoes is TD, while T_{ER} refers to the time of the RF spin echo. The method is chosen for fast imaging but does not refocus field inhomogeneity. Gradient echo images are sensitive to static field perturbations.

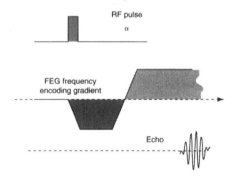

gradient field reversal (*mri*) Switching gradient polarity.

gradient magnetic field (*mri*) *See* magnetic field gradient.

gradient moment nulling (*mri*) Adjustment to zero at the time TE of the net moments of the amplitude of the waveform of the magnetic field gradients with time. The aim is to minimize the phase shifts acquired by the transverse magnetization of excited nuclei moving along the gradients, including the effect of refocusing RF pulses, and reduces image artefacts due to motion.

gradient motion (*mri*) *See* flow compensation, rephasing.

gradient pulse (*mri*) The magnetic field gradient briefly switched. This is used in gradient echo pulse sequences.

gradient recalled echo (*mri*) *See* gradient echo.

gradient strength (*mri*) Magnitude and rate of change in space of magnetic field strength seen in magnetic gradients of an MRI system. Unit is $mT\,m^{-1}$ (milliT per metre). Typically, $20–35\,mT\,m^{-1}$ for a 1.5 tesla machine and $45\,mT\,m^{-1}$ for a 3 T machine (*see* slew rate).

gradient swap (*mri*) Exchange of phase-encoding and readout directions in the image. Flow and motion artefacts are rotated 90°. Prevents artefacts.

grain (*film*) The film emulsion is composed of a random distribution of silver halide crystals in gelatine. Light or x-ray photons expose this random distribution. Although the photons are randomly distributed (even in a structured image), they encounter a much greater grain randomicity leading to quantum error. On development, the silver halide is transformed into silver specks or grains which give the structural property. Low photon images yield 'grainy' images with a high quantum error or mottle. Fine-grain emulsion is typically slower and has a larger latitude or dynamic range than coarser grained emulsion. Film grain size limits the enlargement or magnification of a film image. High developer temperatures increase film graininess.

gram (*phys*) Fundamental unit of mass in the c.g.s. system. In SI units, the kilogram (1000 g) is the base unit.

graph (*math*) A data plot depicting the relationship between certain sets of numbers or quantities by means of a series of dots, lines, etc. When empirical data are plotted, the points are not necessarily joined; a best fit may be drawn through them. A Cartesian graph has two uniform scales on perpendicular axes *x* and *y*. The *x*-axis is usually for the independent variable, the *y*-axis for the dependent variable. Linear and logarithmic scales can be used. Polar graphs are centred on a particular point; the size of the variable depends on its direction; they are used for sound or RF intensity over distance. Normal distributions of statistical data can be plotted on probability graph paper.

graphics adapter/card (*comp*) An expansion board that converts images created by the central processing unit (CPU) into video signals required by the monitor. It determines the maximum resolution, refresh rate and colour depth. The VGA card is the basic graphics adapter. The on-board graphics memory must be capable of handling specified resolution, etc. For a resolution of 1024×768 and a colour depth of 32 bits this requires a minimum of:

$$\frac{1024 \times 768 \times 32}{8 \times 1024} = 3072 \text{ kBytes}$$

or 4 MByte installed. Typical RAM installed is 16–32 MByte, which will cater for 2000×1500 resolution 32-bit colour, a refresh rate of between 75 and 100 Hz and bandwidths of 250 MHz. Often incorporates a graphics accelerator (AGP) (*see* AGP, VGA, SVGA, XVGA).

graphite (*chem*) An allotrope of carbon used as an alternative to tungsten as a backing material for x-ray tube anodes. It increases their rating (loadability) without increasing the anode weight; offers a large increase in surface area and mass.

	Graphite	Tungsten
Melting point	3500°C	3650
Density	$2300\,kg\,m^{-3}$	19 320
Thermal conductivity	$5.0\,W\,m^{-1}K^{-1}$	1.78
Specific heat capacity	$710\,J\,kg^{-1}K^{-1}$	

GRASE (*mri*) Gradient and spin echo hybrid. Fast imaging technique using multiple gradient and spin echoes. Both gradient-echo and spin-echo techniques are combined to acquire multiple lines in k-space during measurement following a single spin-echo excitation.

GRASS (*mri*) Gradient recalled acquisition in the steady state (GE Medical Systems). Enhanced intensity, rewinding of phase-encoding and no

G

intentional spoiling (*see* FGR, FISP, FAST, GFEC, F-SHORT, SSFP, FLASH).

grating lobes (*us*) Side lobes produced by a multi-element transducer. Grating lobes. Additional weaker beams of sound travelling out in directions different from the primary beam as a result of the multi-element structure of transducer arrays.

gravity (*g*) (*units*) The standard value $9.8062 \, \mathrm{m\,s^{-2}}$. This is $9.78 \, \mathrm{m\,s^{-2}}$ at the equator and $9.832 \, \mathrm{m\,s^{-2}}$ at the north pole (*see* **g-force**).

Gray LH (1905–65) British physicist who developed and rationalized radiation protection. The SI unit for absorbed dose is the gray (Gy).

gray (Gy) (*dose*) An SI unit of radiation absorbed dose equal to 1 joule of absorbed energy per kg of absorber. Measure of absorbed dose $1 \, \mathrm{J\,kg^{-1}}$. It replaces the rad; $100 \, \mathrm{rad} = 1 \, \mathrm{Gy}$; $1 \, \mathrm{rad} = 10 \, \mathrm{mGy}$ or $1 \, \mathrm{cGy}$ (*see* **sievert**).

grey level (*image*) The value associated with a pixel in a digital image, representing the brightness in the original scene at the point represented by that pixel. It is inversely proportional to the degree of blackening at the corresponding point (a low degree of film optical density corresponds to a high value of grey level).

grey scale (*image*) The number of steps between extremes of white and black used in image formation. A typical computer display is represented by a pixel depth of 8 bits representing 2^8 or 256 different grey levels. A good quality photographic print can reproduce 20–30 grey levels, the human eye can discern about 35 and a photographic negative transparency about 40–50. A computer video display unit (VDU) typically registers 10–15 levels (*see* **colour scale, transfer function**).

GRE (*mri*) Gradient-recalled echo or gradient echo, general sequence, GE, Siemens. Allows faster imaging than spin-echo. Gives T2* information (*see* FFE, MPGR, GRECO, FE, PFI, GE, Turbo-FLASH, TFF, SMASH, SHORT, STAGE).

GREAT (*mri*) Ghost reduction by equalized acquisition triplets.

GREC (*mri*) Gradient field echo with contrast.

GRECO (*mri*) Gradient-recalled echo, general sequence, Resonex (*see* FFE, GRE, MPGR, FE, PFI, GE, Turbo-FLASH, TFF, SMASH, SHORT, STAGE).

grid (*xray*) A device which is positioned close to the entrance surface of an image receptor to reduce the quantity of scattered radiation reaching the receptor (*see* **anti-scatter grid**).

grid control (*xray*) An x-ray tube whose cathode assembly receives a separate negative voltage which when applied switches off the beam. This is a method of achieving very fast (<1 ms) beam switching with very little inertia. Can also dynamically alter the focal size or, if the negative charge is large enough, switch off the electron beam entirely. The grid controlled x-ray tube is used in cine-fluorography, digital subtraction angiography (DSA) units and computed tomography (CT) where rapid pulses of x-rays are required.

grid factor (*xray*) Also known as the grid exposure factor or Bucky factor. It is calculated as:

$$\frac{\text{Exposure with grid}}{\text{Exposure without grid}}.$$

Using the same kV_p, if the two exposures giving the same film density are 30 mAs (with) and 10 mAs (without), then the grid factor would be 3. The grid factor changes with kV_p, thickness of lead septa and the type of interspace material. Mammography grids have the lowest factors (2–3), while high kV (chest radiography) have the highest factors (4–6).

grid line density (*xray*) In an anti-scatter grid, this is measured as the number of lead strips per cm. This is calculated as $10/(d + D)$, where d and D are thickness in mm, of the lead septa and interspace material, respectively. A superfine grid used for chest radiography ($d = 0.025 \, \mathrm{mm}$ and $D = 0.05 \, \mathrm{mm}$) would have 133 lines per cm. A standard grid ($d = 0.05 \, \mathrm{mm}$, $D = 0.1 \, \mathrm{mm}$) would have a density of 66 lines per cm.

grid ratio (*xray*) Ratio of grid height h to interspace distance D as h/D. For three grid types Pb6/28, Pb12/44 and Pb12/100, complete specifications are:

L/mm	Ratio	Factor	Selectivity
28	6	4.1	4.5
44	12	5.2	6.6
100	12	6.2	8.4

grid selectivity (Σ) (*xray*) This parameter is influenced by both grid ratio and lead septa thickness, so considers all three measurements of spacer thickness, lead septa height and thickness. It measures transmitted scatter T_s as a percentage of the primary beam T_p reaching the imaging surface: $\Sigma = T_p/T_s$. A perfect anti-scatter grid would stop all scatter and pass all the primary beam so $\Sigma = \infty$. If 20% of x-ray scatter is transmitted ($\Sigma = 5$), this would seriously degrade image quality. Improved grids would therefore have higher values than this ($\Sigma = 6$ to 8).

grid tagging (*mri*) *See* tagging.

GROPE (*mri*) Generalized compensation for resonance offset and pulse length errors.

ground state (*phys*) The lowest energy state of a system (molecule, atom, nucleus).

group classification (*nmed*) A radionuclide toxicity classification ranging from group 1 (most toxic) to group 4 (least toxic). Group classification determines limits for safe disposal.

GSD (*dose*) *See* genetically significant dose.

GSM (*comp*) Global support for mobiles. Currently, GSM systems operate at 800, 900, 1800 or 1900 MHz. GSM standards bodies have been defining data networking technologies, such as GPRS, to build on GSM. Three non-compatible mobile wireless protocols are being developed for the wireless mobile market. They are GSM, TDMA and CDMA.

GSO (*rad*) *See* gadolinium oxy-orthosilicate.

GUI (*comp*) Graphical user interface. A system that simplifies selecting computer commands by enabling the user to point to symbols or illustrations (called icons) on the computer screen with a mouse. The basic Windows and Linux screen format.

gyromagnetic ratio (*mri*) The precessional frequency *f* of the nucleus can be calculated as:

$$f = \frac{\mu B_o}{2\pi L}$$

where μ is the proton magnetic moment, L the proton spin angular momentum and B_o the magnetic field strength in Tesla. It can be simplified where μ and $2\pi L$ are treated as constants being fixed for any particular nucleus (in this case a hydrogen proton). Together they describe the gyromagnetic ratio γ as:

$$\gamma = \frac{\mu}{2\pi L}.$$

The gyromagnetic ratio for the hydrogen proton is calculated in the example below. Simplifying the above equation by substituting γ yields $\omega L = \gamma B_o$ relating the precession frequency to magnetic field strength (B_o) and is the Larmor equation. ωL is the Larmor frequency, where ω represents the angular frequency of precession.

The gyromagnetic ratio γ for hydrogen
Proton magnetic moment: 1.41031×10^{-26} J T^{-1}
The proton spin angular momentum is:

0.527×10^{-34} J s^{-1} so

$$\gamma = \frac{\mu}{2\pi L} = \frac{1.41 \times 10^{-26}}{2\pi \times 0.527 \times 10^{-34}} = 42582252 \text{ Hz}$$

or 42.58 MHz T^{-1}.

A 200 Hz variation due to magnet inhomogeneity, would give a variation of: 0.0002/42.582252 or 4.7 ppm.

Clinical magnet strengths
The precession frequency of a ^{1}H (proton) for a

High 3 T	$f = 42.58 \times 3.0$	
Medium 1.5 T	$f = 42.58 \times 1.5$	
Low 0.3 T	$f = 42.58 \times 0.3$	12.77 MHz

Ho (*mri*) *See* magnetic field intensity.

H1 (*mri*) *See* magnetic field intensity.

H and D curve (*film*) F Hurter (H) and VC Driffield (D) pioneers in the evaluation of film emulsion performance and speed. Their work led to the production of the modern characteristic curve. The ASA/DIN/BS/ISO are now the internationally quoted speed ratings for film.

haematocrit (Ht) (*clin*) Separating the blood cells from the plasma, by centrifugation, so that the volume percentage of cells (erythrocytes) can be estimated. The normal value varies with age, being 56.6% at birth, 35.2% at 1 year, 39.6% at 12 years and about 43% for an adult (male 46%; female 40%). Also called the packed cell volume (PCV).

haemodynamics (*clin*) The study of blood circulation. Achieved by either following x-ray contrast bolus transit (digital subtration angiography (DSA) or computed tomography (CT)), nuclear medicine ^{99m}Tc bolus transit (*in vivo* red blood cell (RBC) labelling, diethylene triamine pentaacetic acid (DTPA)), ultrasound (Doppler) or magnetic resonance imaging (MRI).

haemopoiesis (*clin*) The formation of red blood cells. There is a clinically significant depression for acute radiation exposure at 500 and 400 mGy y^{-1} over many years.

hafnium (Hf) (*elem*)

Atomic number (Z)	72
Relative atomic mass (A$_r$)	178.49
Density (ρ) kg/m^3	133 00
Melting point (K)	2423
K-edge (keV)	65.3

Hagen–Poiseuille law (*us*) This describes the relationship between volume flow of a liquid of known viscosity to diameter and length of a blood vessel The vascular resistance (R) is:

$$R = 1 \Big/ \frac{\pi \times r^4}{8 \times \eta \times l}$$

where η is fluid viscosity, r and l are vessel radius and viscosity, respectively. The volume flow (Q) per unit time is given as:

$$Q = \frac{\pi \cdot \Delta p \cdot r^4}{8\eta}$$

where Δp is the pressure difference between the ends of the blood vessel (perfusion pressure). Simplified to:

$$Q = \frac{P}{R}$$

where P is the perfusion pressure gradient (*see* blood flow).

Hahn echo (*mri*) The formation of a spin-echo after applying two or more RF pulses.

Hahn, Otto (1879–1968) German physicist, who trained under William Ramsay and Ernest Rutherford in London and Montreal. At the Kaiser Wilhelm Institute, he worked with Lise Meitner on the irradiation of uranium and thorium with neutrons, which (with Fritz Strassmann) led to the discovery of nuclear fission. Hahn was involved with the discovery of several radioelements. He received the Nobel prize for chemistry in 1944.

Hahn (von Hahn) filter (*di*) *See* Hanning filter.

halation (*film*) Commonly applied to intensifying screens where the incident radiation is fully absorbed, but the light is emitted at all angles causing radiographic unsharpness or penumbra formation and loss of resolution.

Half-Fourier matrix (*mri*) The MRI raw data matrix has a specific symmetry, which suggests sampling of only half the matrix is sufficient. The other half can be symmetrically reconstructed; mathematically, the matrices are conjugated complexes. Unavoidable phase errors due to minor magnetic field inhomogeneity require a phase correction, therefore a little more than half of the phase-encoding steps are acquired. Measurement time is reduced by 50%.

half (partial) Fourier (*mri*) Method for acquiring image data using approximately half the usual number of phase-encoding steps.

half-life (*nmed*) *See* half-life (physical).

half-life (biological) (*nmed*) Time required for clearing one half the amount of a substance from a biological system. The time required for the mass of a drug substance to be reduced to exactly 50% of its original value due solely to biological elimination. For each drug there is a single organ biological half-life and a whole body biological half-life. They are almost never identical.

half-life (effective) (*nmed*) The time required for the radioactivity level of a living thing to be reduced to exactly 50% of its initial value as a result of both biological elimination and radioactive decay. The sum of the biological and physical half-lives (see **effective half-life**).

half-life (physical) (*nmed*) The time required for the radioactivity level of a source to decay to exactly 50% of its original value. The half-life of a radionuclide, the energy type and energy of emission are all identifying characteristics. The common formula used for half-life determination uses the exponential function *e* is:

$$A_t = A_o \times e^{-\lambda t}$$

where A_o is the original activity and A_t is the value representing new activity at time *t*, influenced by λ, the decay constant, which is the quotient:

$$\lambda = 0.693/t_{\frac{1}{2}} \quad \text{since } e - \lambda t_{\frac{1}{2}} = 0.5 \text{ and}$$
$$\ln 2 = \lambda t_{\frac{1}{2}}.$$

Isotope decay
The half-life for ^{99m}Tc is 6 h. If the original activity A_o was 800 MBq. Then the activity after 1 day where $A_t = A_o \times e^{-\lambda t}$ and after time *t* (24 h) with λ, (decay constant) for ^{99m}Tc as 0.693/6.0 = 0.1155 h, then:

$$A_t = 800 \times e^{-0.1155 \times 24}$$
$$= 800 \times 0.06253$$
$$= 50 \text{ MBq}$$

(*see* **decay constant**).

half-scan interpolation (*ct*) *See* **180° interpolation**.

halftone (*image*) Since inkjet printers only have the four process colours, they produce other shades by laying down patterns of primary colour dots, varying the pattern and ratio of each colour; this is half-toning.

half-value layer (HVL) (*phys*) The thickness of an absorber that reduces the intensity of a photon beam to 50% of its initial value; the fraction of photons (x- or gamma radiation) removed from a beam per unit thickness of absorber (m^{-1}). The **linear attenuation coefficient** μ for a particular tissue at a particular energy is a measure of the ability of the tissue to remove photons from a photon beam. From the general exponential relationship:

$$I_x = I_o \times e^{-\mu x}.$$

If the thickness *x* absorbs half the radiation, the half-value-layer (HVL) is defined as:

$$\frac{I_x}{I_o} = 0.5 = e^{-\mu^* HVL}$$

Since $e^{-0.693} = 0.5$, then $\mu^* HVL = 0.693$ and so

$$\mu = \frac{0.693}{HVL}$$

The influence on the incident beam of a certain number of half-value layers can be calculated from 1/2n, where *n* is the number of half-value layers; plotted below for intensity versus absorber HVL.

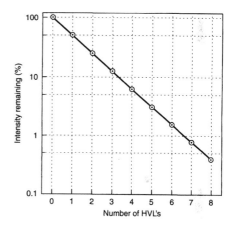

Accurate determination of HVL can be calculated from the formula:

$$HVL = \frac{x_1 \times \ln\left[\frac{2 \times y_2}{y_0}\right] - x_2 \times \ln\left[\frac{2 \times y_1}{y_0}\right]}{\ln\left[\frac{y_2}{y_1}\right]}$$

where y_0 is the incident radiation intensity measured without absorber, y_1 the intensity measured after x_1 mm filtration added, and y_2 the intensity measured after the x_2 mm filtration is added. The radiation intensity can be given in mR or mGy. The HVL defines the x-ray beam quality being the thickness of aluminium which reduces the x-ray beam intensity by half. This should be at least 2.5 mm aluminium at 80 kVp.

Half value layer, mammography
A mammography unit gives the following readings for aluminium:
Measurement with no absorber = 718 (y_o)
Measurement with 0.1 mm aluminium = 583 (y_1)
Measurement with 0.5 mm aluminium = 275 (y_2)

$$HVL = \frac{0.1 \times \ln\left[\frac{2 \times 275}{718}\right] - 0.5 \times \ln\left[\frac{2 \times 583}{718}\right]}{\ln\left[\frac{275}{583}\right]}$$

$$HVL = \frac{-0.02665 - 0.2424}{-0.7514} = 0.358 \text{ mm.}$$

---

half-wave rectification (*elec*) A rectifier circuit where only alternate half-waves of either a single or three-phase a.c. supply are effective in forming the d.c. supply.

Hall effect (*elec*) An effect occurring when a conductor is placed in a magnetic field and orientated so that the field is at right angles to the current direction. There is a small potential difference (the Hall voltage) set up across the conductor. Semiconductor Hall effect generators are used for calibrating magnetic field strengths.

Hamming filter (*image*) A filter formed by altering the relative proportions of the d.c. and cosine component in the Hanning filter, so improving the sidelobe levels (*see* filters (signal), Bartlett filter).

handshake (*comp*) The exchange or recognition of a coded signal between electronic (computer) devices or peripherals. Modems use this prior to linking and transmitting data.

Hanning filter (*image*) A signal filter with a cosine shape having a main spectral lobe similar to a triangular window but with a d.c. level that makes all the sampled values positive. Used in magnetic resonance imaging (MRI) to reduce truncation artefacts. (*nmed*) Also a common filter used in nuclear medicine which reduces higher spatial frequencies, so losing fine detail. The graph compares Hanning (Hn), Hamming (Hm), Butterfield (B) and simple ramp (R) (*see* filters (signal), Bartlett filter, Hamming filter).

haploid (*clin*) Relates to single-stranded DNA cells: bacteria and gametes.

hard copy (*di*) Recording the image on film or paper (*see* film formatter).

hard disk drive (HDD) (*comp*) The major bulk magnetic storage device for small and large computers. Non-volatile data storage using multiple stacked platters/disks made from light aluminium alloy or glass and coated with a thin layer of magnetic cobalt-ferrous alloy. Large-scale, reliable storage led to the introduction of configurations such as the redundant array of independent disks (RAID), network attached storage (NAS) systems and storage area network (SAN) systems that provide efficient and reliable access to large volumes of data. Common storage capacity ranges from 100 Gb to 1 TB (1000 GB) and above; these have data transfer rates of 1 Gbit s^{-1} or higher.

hard radiation (*xray*) *See* beam hardening.

harmonic imaging (*us*) As the transmitted ultrasound signal propagates within tissues or is scattered by contrast medium microbubbles, the echo signals will show non-linear effects and have more than just fundamental frequencies. They will also exhibit multiples of the transmit frequency (second, third, etc., harmonic frequencies). These are utilized in harmonic imaging, where fundamental and harmonic echo signals are separated either by:

- Second-harmonic or narrow band harmonic imaging separates the strongest second harmonic from the fundamental components using a high-pass filter. There is some degree of frequency overlap.
- Wide-band harmonic imaging applies phase inversion to the transmit pulse and uses the transducer's full bandwidth. There is a smaller degree of frequency overlap allowing a wider transmit frequency spectrum. Narrow-band harmonic imaging (1) requires a long transmit pulse and the suppression of the echo fundamental frequency by using a high pass filter.

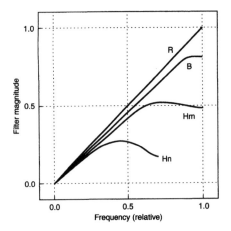

Wide-band harmonic imaging (2) uses two short phase-inverted transmit pulses and the suppression of uneven echo frequencies by signal addition. The side lobes seen in conventional imaging are reduced. The narrower width of the second harmonic main lobe gives better lateral resolution, but degrades axial resolution. Wide-band harmonic imaging preserves axial resolution. The images appear sharper and exhibit higher contrast resolution and less noise (*see* contrast medium (ultrasound)).

HASTE (*mri*) Half-Fourier acquisition single shot turbo spin-echo (Siemens). A turbo spin-echo technique with one very long echo train that uses k-space reordering and half-Fourier reconstruction to control the contrast and maximize resolution in the T2-weighted image. All of the echoes are recorded in one TR; the effective TE is <100 msec. Half of k-space is filled on each acquisition in an interleaving lines fashion. Equivalent pulse sequences are SS-FSE (GE Medical Systems, Philips), FSE-ADA (Hitachi) and FASE (Toshiba).

havar foil (*nmed*) Commonly used target window for medical cyclotrons designed for pressurized water target for ^{18}F production. An alloy of Co, Cr, Fe, Ni, Mn, W and Mo. Since this is exposed to a high flux of protons and secondary neutrons, when replaced the foil must be treated as radioactive waste and treated accordingly.

Hayes command set (*comp*) A standard set of coded instructions for controlling basic modem functions, such as dialling and hanging up, devised by the modem manufacturer Hayes.

HDP (*nmed*) See oxidronate.

HD-TV (*di*) High definition television. Video scan line density greater than 512/625 domestic standard. European standards are now 2459 lines giving an image matrix of 2590 × 2048, non-interlaced (progressive scan) with a 54 cm diagonal and a refresh frequency of 72 Hz (horizontal frequency 150.2 kHz). Special closed circuit video exceeds 3000 lines (*see* video).

heat (*phys*) This is now strictly defined as the transfer of energy from a body at high temperature to one at a lower temperature due to the temperature difference. This process can be by conduction, convection and radiation; all radiation wavelengths emitted are considered as heat (ultraviolet, visible, infrared, etc.), since they all inject energy into the system. The SI unit of heat is the joule (J) (*see* energy, work, heat units (HU)).

heat capacity (*phys*) The heat required (in joules) to raise a body's temperature by 1 K or 1°C measured as JK^{-1} (or $J°C^{-1}$). It is the characteristic of the material independent of its size or unit mass (unlike specific heat capacity). Heat capacities of common materials used for anode materials, with mass 2 kg are:

Anode material (2 kg)	Heat capacity (JK^{-1})
Tungsten	272
Titanium	1046
Zirconium	560
Molybdenum	492
TZM	692

Heat capacity is simply specific heat capacity × mass; So for 2 kg tungsten, the heat capacity is 136×2 or $272 JK^{-1}$.

heat loading (*xray*) The amount of heat energy deposited in the anode during an x-ray exposure. The loading depends on peak kV, waveform, tube current, exposure time and rate of exposures per unit time. Heat loading is assessed by reference to a rating chart (*see* heat storage, rating).

heat loss (*xray*) The removal of heat from the focal spot of an x-ray tube involves conduction, convection and radiation. All three maintain an acceptable anode cooling rate which affects the loadability of the x-ray tube.

heat storage (*xray*) Heat storage of an x-ray tube is the product of anode mass, specific heat and temperature rise. If the maximum heat capacity of the anode is 150 kHU in the diagram then this may be exceeded if the rate of heat production is high (A in $HU s^{-1}$) and must be reduced to B (*see* rating).

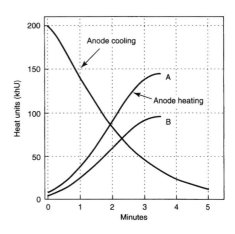

heat units (HU) (*xray*) A measure of heat storage for an x-ray tube. The heat capacity of an anode is sometimes expressed in heat units HU for three-phase and single-phase supply, calculated as the product of kV, mA and seconds $HU = V \times mAs$. For a three-phase supply: $HU = 1.35 \times kV \times mA \times sec$. The 35% increase is due to the increased efficiency of the waveform; for constant current generators (high frequency generators) this is 1.4. Heat units were common when single phase and three-phase electrical generators supplied x-ray sets, since the high voltage electrical supply had a ripple component which produced a cyclic variation in x-ray (and hence heat) production. Contemporary x-ray equipment now use high frequency generators and are virtually constant current so the ripple component is negligible. The heat unit has been superseded by measuring heat capacity in joules (J) and heat loss in joules per second or watts (W).Conversion: $HU \times 0.71 = $ joules (J); $J \times 1.41 = HU$ (*see* x-ray tube rating).

heating (ultrasonic) (*us*) The heating of tissue (including bone) due to ultrasound absorption (*see* ultrasound (safety)).

heel effect (*xray*) The diminishing intensity across the x-ray beam toward the anode; the non-uniform distribution of air kerma rate in an x-ray beam in a direction parallel to the cathode-anode axis. The x-rays produced by bremsstrahlung in the target pass through the tungsten target material and are attenuated. The thickness of tungsten and therefore x-ray attenuation, is greater on the anode side of the beam, so the intensity is reduced asymmetrically. As the target surface wears, the heel effect becomes more pronounced. Beam uniformity changes with anode angle. Collimating the useful field of view reduces the heel effect, but does not eliminate it. The heel-effect decreases with increase in anode angle: 7°, 12° and 20°, but increasing the angle adversely affects image resolution and thermal rating (loadability) (*see* field size).

helical/spiral CT (*ct*) A particular technique of scanning in which there is continuous rotation of the x-ray tube coupled with continuous linear translation of the patient through the gantry aperture in order to achieve volumetric data acquisition. Also known as spiral or volume CT.

helical scan (acquisition) (*ct*) Continuous rotation of a fan beam assembly while the scan bed moves incrementally; also known as spiral scan.

helium (He) (*chem*) An inert/noble gas belonging to group 18 of the periodic table. The element has the lowest boiling point of all substances and can be solidified only under pressure.

Atomic number	2
Relative atomic mass (atomic weight)	4.0026
Density	$0.166\,kg\,m^{-3}$
Melting point	0.95 K at 26 atm
Boiling point	4.21 K
^{4}He	≈100%
^{3}He	0.00013%

Relevance to radiology: As a cryogen for MRI and cyclotron superconductor magnets. Negative helium ions ^{3}helium and ^{4}helium are used for cyclotron beam production.

^{3}Helium ($^3_2$He) (*nmed*) Stable isotope of helium with fractional abundance of 0.00013%. Used as a negative ion beam 3He$^-$ carrying three electrons, stripped to yield a 2p,1n cyclotron beam for radionuclide production (*see* hydrogen, deuterium).

^{4}Helium ($^4_2$He) (*nmed*) The most stable isotope of helium with approximately 100% abundance. It is the decay product of the alpha particle. Used as a negative ion beam 4He$^-$ carrying three electrons, stripped to yield a 2p,2n (alpha) cyclotron beam for radionuclide production (*see* hydrogen, deuterium).

Helmholz coil (*mri*) A pair of identical current-carrying coils used to create a uniform magnetic field.

henry (H) (unit) A measure of inductance. The inductance has a value of one henry, if a current changing at the rate of one ampere per second induces an electromotive force of one volt.

$$H = V\,(A\,s^{-1})^{-1} = V\,s\,A^{-1} = Wb\,A^{-1}.$$

Magnetic permeability is measured as $H\,m^{-1}$. The inductance of a closed loop that gives a magnetic flux of 1 weber for each ampere.

hepatic angiography (*clin*) Imaging the vascularity of liver, spleen and pancreas: intra-arterial DSA is being effectively replaced by contrast enhanced magnetic resonance angiography (MRA).

hepatic arteriography (*clin*) Opacification and visualization of the hepatic artery using an iodinated contrast medium (*see* TIPS, transarterial chemo-embolization (TACE)).

Hepatolite® (*nmed*) A CIS commercial product of $^{99\,m}$Tc disofenin (DISIDA).

hereditary (*dose*) Affecting future generations (*see* genetically significant dose).

Hertz, Heinrich R (1857–94) German physicist. Confirmed Maxwell's predictions of electromagnetic transfer by experimental discovery of 'Hertzian waves' or radio waves; further developed by Marconi.

hertz (Hz) (*phys*) The SI unit for frequency as cycles per second.

Very low frequency (VLF)	<1–10 Hz	Atmospheric
Low frequency	50–100 Hz	A.C. power
Medium frequency	20 kHz	Sound
High frequency	1 MHz	AM radio
Very high frequency (VHF)	100 MHz	FM radio
Ultra high frequency (UHF)	1 GHz	Mobile (cell) phones
Infra-red, x-rays	1014 Hz	
Gamma rays	>1023 Hz	

HESPA filter (*nmed*) High efficiency sub-micron particulate air filter. Recommended for clean air installations and conforming with Hosch Class 100 and the US Federal Standard 209B (0.003%).

Hevesy von, George Charles (1885–1966) Hungarian physicist. Studied in Freiburg, Zurich and Manchester where he worked with Rutherford. His work with radioactive tracers to study chemical processes in biology started the idea of nuclear medicine. Awarded the Nobel prize for chemistry in 1943.

Hexabrix (*cm*) Preparation of ionic dimer of ioxaglic acid, introduced by (Mallinckrodt Inc.). Consists of meglumine ioxaglate 39.3% and sodium ioxaglate 19.6%.

Compound	Viscosity (cP)	Osmolality (mOsm/kg)	Iodine (mg I mL^{-1})
Meglumine ioxaglate, sodium ioxaglate	15.7 at 20°, 7.5 at 37°	600	320

hf (*hv*) (*phys*) Depicting the energy E of a single photon: $E = hf$, where h is Planck's constant and f frequency. Substituting c/λ for f then $E = hc/\lambda$. The product hc is 12.4, so the relationship between energy and wavelength is $E = 12.4/\lambda$.

HFGR (*mri*) Inversion-recovery fast GRASS rapid gradient-echo imaging techniquesT1-weighted contrast GE (*see* FLASH, SPGR, FSPGR, RE Spoiled, 3D-ME-RAGE, T1-FEE, STAGE-T1W).

hibernating myocardium (*clin*) *See* myocardium.

HIDA (*nmed*) A dimethyl-substituted analogue of imino-diacetic acid (IDA); complexed with ^{99m}Tc, it is used for hepatobiliary imaging. Chemical form: N-[N′-(2,6-dimethylphenyl-carbamoyl-methyl] imidodiacetic acid. Hepatic iminodiacetic acid. Used for functional hepatobilliary imaging when labelled with ^{99m}Tc as ^{99m}Tc-lidofenin (HIDA) or ^{99m}Tc-EHIDA. This family also includes EHIDA, DISIDA (Hepatolite®, Technescan®).

HFI (*mri*) Half Fourier imaging. Sampling only part of *k*-space and using phase conjugate symmetry to fill in the rest of the image plane.

high contrast resolution (*image*) *See* spatial resolution.

high frequency generator (*xray*) The most recent design for all x-ray tube supplies which translate (invert) the 50/60 Hz a.c. single or three-phase supply into a 5–20 kHz supply which then feeds the a.c. circuitry. There is a significant decrease in transformer size with increasing frequency of supply. The cross-section, A, of the transformer and its number of turns, n, are related to output voltage, V, and frequency, f: $A = V/(n\times f)$. The high frequency circuit is controlled by microprocessor to stabilize kV and exposure.

high-osmolarity (*cm*) A solution having a higher osmolar concentration when compared to blood plasma or intracellular fluid; cells shrink as a consequence. A solution that has a higher osmolality than blood and body fluids, i.e. higher than 300 mOsm/kg water, is hypertonic. Commonly describes contrast media with a significantly higher ion concentration than body fluids (between five and seven times, termed high-osmolar contrast media (HOCM)). These contrast media may show adverse patient reactions than contrast media having low osmolarity (LOCM) (*see* isotonic saline).

high pass filter (*di*) A filter designed to reject low frequencies, while retaining high frequencies. Seen in edge enhancement filters or kernels (*see* filters (spatial)).

High performance liquid chromatography (HPLC) (*nmed*) Formerly known as high pressure liquid chromatography. Used for the ultimate purification of radiopharmaceuticals and for their analysis. HPLC can separate all impurities in one analysis and can give chemical, as well as radiochemical, purity information.

hippuran (*nmed*) *See* iodohippurate.

histogram (*math*) A chart which displays grouped data in which the area of each bar is proportional to the occurrence or frequency that it represents.

histamine release (*cm*) The release of histamine from mast cells; a major cause of allergic reactions (*see* chemotoxicity).

HL7 (*comp*) Health Level Seven, Inc., a 'not-for-profit' volunteer organization centred at Ann Arbor, MI, USA. The term describes a seven-layer International Organization of Standards (ISO) communication model. HL7 allows the interchange of non-imaging data between electronic patient administration systems, practice management systems, laboratory information systems, dietary, pharmacy and billing systems, as well as electronic medical record (EMR) and electronic health record (EHR) systems. Each layer has a function. Layers 1–4 deal with communication; comprising physical, data link, network and transport communication layers. Layers 5–7 deal with functions like session, presentation and application. Level 7 is regarded as the application level dealing with the data definition to be exchanged and supports various functions, such as security checks, operator identification, availability checks, exchange mechanism negotiations and data exchange structuring.

HMDP (*nmed*) Hydroxy-methylene-diphosphate. A radiopharmaceutical which when reconstituted with ^{99m}Tc forms a bone imaging agent. Rapid uptake enables earlier imaging than with MDP.

HMPAO (*nmed*) Hexa-methyl-propylene amine oxime (exametazine): a ^{99m}Tc radio-pharmaceutical used for brain perfusion imaging and white cell labelling (Ceretec®, Amersham/GE Healthcare). The labelled compound readily passes the intact blood–brain barrier and is retained in brain tissue. The uptake closely matches regional cerebral blood flow (rCBF).

holmium (Ho) (*elem*) A metallic element sometimes used as a K-edge filter.

Atomic number (Z)	67
Relative atomic mass (A$_r$)	164.9
Density (ρ) kg/m^3	8800
Melting point (K)	1734
K-edge (keV)	55.6

home page (*comp*) The main page of a website and the first screen that a visitor sees displayed when connecting to that site; usually has links to other pages, both within that site and to other sites (*see* URL).

homogeneity (image) (*ct*) Image quality parameter that describes the degree with which a test object made from a homogeneous material (water phantom) is displayed with uniform mean value of the CT number at varying positions within the image (central and peripheral).

homogeneity (magnet) (*mri*) This refers to the uniformity of a magnetic field with no object present. A magnetic field is considered homogeneous when it has the same field strength across the entire field; measured in parts per million (ppm) of main field. Homogeneity of the main magnetic field defines the quality of the main magnet over a large field of view; a relative measure independent of field strength that uses as reference the Larmor frequency for water 42.5759 MHz T^{-1}. A 200 Hz variation would give an inhomogeneity of:

$$\frac{200}{42.5759 \times 10^6} = 4.7 \times 10^{-6} = 4.7 \text{ ppm.}$$

Superconducting magnets have typically <0.03 ppm for a 10-cm spherical volume and <0.5 ppm for 40 cm. Permanent and resistive magnets have typical inhomogeneities of 40 ppm. Homogeneity is important for spectral fat saturation, a large measurement field, echo planar imaging and MR spectroscopy.

homomorphic filter (*image*) Usually applied to an image to increase edge detection and reduce overall brightness. It achieves the separation of illumination and reflectance components, which roughly corresponds to slow or abrupt image variations, respectively.

homospoil (*mri*) Of a magnetic field gradient to effectively eliminate residual transverse magnetization by producing a strong position dependence of phase within a resolution element. Also called 'spoiler pulse'.

homospoil pulse (*mri*) *See* spoiler gradient pulse.

hormesis (*dose*) Hormesis has been defined as 'the stimulating effect of small doses of substances which in larger doses are inhibitory.' The meaning has been modified referring not only to a stimulatory effect, but also to a beneficial effect. Hormesis now contains a value judgement whereby a low dose of radiation is considered beneficial to an organism.

- Reference: BEIR VII, 2006.

Hotelling observer (*stats*) Demonstrates maximum discrimination ability, in terms of the SNR figure of merit, among all observers that are limited to performing only linear operations on the data. When the data are normally distributed, including the unequal variance case, this observer also demonstrates maximum discrimination as specified by the area under the ROC curve. When the data are not normally distributed, the SNR figure of merit may no longer be predictive of the area under the ROC curve. It will then be necessary to obtain that area to test for optimality of observers.

hot-pluggable (*comp*) The ability to remove or change circuit boards or connectors from a working computer without interruption of power supply or computer service (*see* USB).

hot spot imaging (*nmed*) Small regions of a radioactive source observed in scintigraphy where the activity of the source is significantly greater than its surroundings. If the region of the source is smaller than the resolution of the gamma camera system, the image of the hot spot will appear in size equal to the gamma camera resolution element.

Hounsfield, Sir Godfrey Newbold (1919–2004) British engineer. Inventor of computed axial tomography using x-rays which led to the computed axial tomography (CAT) scanner. Awarded a Nobel prize in 1981 (*see* Cormack).

Hounsfield unit (HU) (*ct*) The comparative attenuation value that represents the mean x-ray attenuation associated with each elemental area (voxel) of the CT image; the Hounsfield unit expresses the relative deviation of the measured linear attenuation coefficient from that of pure water, multiplied by 1000; the unit of x-ray absorption used in computed tomography relating linear attenuation coefficient $\mu_{unknown}$ to μ_{water} at a fixed kV as:

$$HU = 1000 \times \frac{\mu_{unknown} - \mu_{water}}{\mu_{water}}$$

Water is taken as reference zero; air has the lowest negative value at about -1000 and bone has the highest value at about $+3000$. Since values are scaled to water, the Housfield unit is independent of beam energy (voltage).

CT number calculation

	80 kV	100 kV	150 kV
μ_{muscle}	0.1892	0.1760	0.1550
μ_{water}	0.1835	0.1707	0.1504

At 80 keV: $1000 \times \dfrac{0.1892 - 0.1835}{0.1835} = 31$

At 100 keV: $1000 \times \dfrac{0.1760 - 0.1707}{0.1707} = 31$

At 150 keV: $1000 \times \dfrac{0.1550 - 0.1504}{0.1504} = 31$

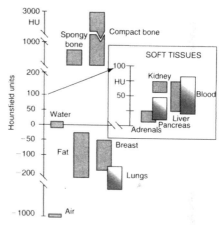

hour (h) (*phys*) Not an SI unit, but can form compound units with SI units, e.g. kWh.

housing (*xray*) The x-ray tube is enclosed in a sealed housing. **Heat loss**: circulating air is sufficient to cool mobile and mammography units (fan-assisted cooling can halve tube cooling time), but circulating oil is necessary within the enclosure for cooling conventional and DSA equipment. The total **heat capacity** of the tube enclosure is largely dependent on the volume of oil it contains.

HSA (*nmed*) Soluble human serum albumin used for blood pool imaging. Largely replaced by ^{99m}Tc labelled red **blood cells**.

H$_T$ (*dose*) *See* equivalent dose.

HTML (*comp*) Hypertext markup language, the authoring language of the Internet, used to create web pages. Browsers interpret the codes to give the text structure and formatting (such as bold, blue, or italic) (*see* hypertext).

HTTP (*comp*) Hypertext transfer protocol. A common system used to request and send HTML documents on the world wide web, defining how information is formatted and transmitted. It is the first portion of all URL addresses on the world wide web (e.g. http://www.hospital.com).

HTTPS (*comp*) Hypertext transfer protocol secure. Often used in within-company Internet sites. Passwords are required to gain access.

HU (*xray, ct*) *See* CT number (Hounsfield units), heat unit.

hub (*comp*) The central device in a star-configured network; useful for centralized management, the ability to isolate nodes from disruption, and extending the distance of LAN coverage. A device used on a star network to connect all workstations together.

hue (*image*) The colour's position along the colour spectrum (*see* saturation).

Huygen's principle (*us*) Every point or element of a multi-element transducer acts as a source of spherical wavelets producing a combined wavefront. The wavelets advance with speed and frequency of the primary wave.

hv (*phys*) *See* hf .

hybrid magnet (*mri*) Magnet system employing both current carrying coils and permanently magnetized material to generate the magnetic field.

hybrid spectroscopy (*mri*) Combing single volume spectroscopy (SVS) with chemical shift imaging (CSI). The CSI measurement is performed over a selectively excited volume of interest. Through volume selection, areas with strong distorting signals (e.g. fat) are not stimulated and therefore do not contribute signal to the spectra.

hybrid subtraction (*xray*) This combines the advantages of both dual energy subtraction and temporal filtering to remove interfering tissue (bone) and vessel movement.

HyCoSy (*clin*) Hysterosalpingographic contrast sonography. Ultrasound technique using appropriate ultrasound contrast medium for demonstrating uterus and ovaries, and tubal patency.

hydrogen (*elem*) Consists of three isotopes: ^{1}Hydrogen (proton and electron); ^{2}hydrogen or deuterium (proton, neutron and electron); ^{3}hHydrogen or tritium (proton 2 neutrons and electron).

Atomic number (Z)	1
Relative atomic mass (Ar)	1.00
Density (ρ) kg/m³	0.089
Melting point (K)	14.01

^{2}**Hydrogen** (*nmed*) *See* deuterium.

^{3}**Hydrogen** (*nmed*) *See* tritium.

Nuclide	^{3}H
Production (cyclotron)	^{6}Li(n,α) ^{3}H
Half-life	12.3 years
Decay mode	β−

hydrogen bond (*chem*) An electrostatic bonding that occurs in molecules that have hydrogen atoms linked to electronegative atoms (F, N, O). Hydrogen bonds impart significant effects on a compound's physical property causing liquid water to be liquid at room temperature with higher than expected boiling point. In water molecules (H–O–H), the oxygen atom attracts the electrons in the O–H bonds, and since the hydrogen atom has no inner shell of electrons which shield the nucleus, there is an electrostatic interaction between the hydrogen proton and a lone pair of electrons on the electronegative atom (oxygen). It is of great importance in biological compounds, occurring between bases in DNA and between the C=O and N–H groups in proteins. Strengths of hydrogen bonds are about one tenth of a normal covalent bond (*see* contrast media).

hydrophilic/hydrophilicity (*clin*) Having an affinity for or associating with water; the preference (solubility) of a contrast medium for aqueous solvents; a property of polar radicals or ions. Non-ionic contrast media do not dissociate and their water-solubility is generally achieved by several hydrophilic hydroxyl groups. Several non-ionic monomeric contrast media are available that have hydrophilic hydroxyl groups attached to all three side chains; a feature contributing to their reduced toxicity. The multiple hydrophilic side groups of second-generation non-ionic monomers protect the inner hydrophobic benzene ring from interaction, thereby reducing their chemotoxicity. Relative hydrophobic/hydrophilic properties of the molecule is its partition coefficient; a low partition coefficient is advantageous since high hydrophilicity contributes to low protein binding. Non-ionic contrast media are sufficiently hydrophilic to only make small differences in the partition coefficient (*see* lipophilicity).

hydrophobic (*clin*) Lacking an affinity for water molecules; a property of apolar radicals.

hydrophone (*us*) An instrument for detecting sounds under water. Used for measuring the power output from an ultrasound transducer.

Hypaque" (*cm*) A commercial preparation (Amersham/GE Healthcare Inc) of ionic diatrizoate-meglumine and diatrizoate sodium salt. Supplied in 50, 60 and 76% solution concentrations.

Compound	Viscosity (cP)	Osmolality (mOsm/kg)	Iodine (mg I/mL)
Diatrizoate-meglumine 50%	3.43 at 20°, 2.43 at 37°	1550	300
Diatrizoate-meglumine 60%	6.16 at 20°, 4.10 at 37°	1415	282
Diatrizoate-meglumine 76%	9 at 37°	2016	370

Hypaque-Cysto" (*cm*) A commercial preparation (Amersham/GE Healthcare Inc) of diatrizoate-meglumine consisting of 30% solution (w/v) of meglumine salt of diatrizoic acid. Formulation for retrograde cysto-urethrography.

Compound	Viscosity (cP)	Osmolality (mOsm/kg)	Iodine (mg I/mL)
Diatrizoate-meglumine salt	1.94 at 25°, 1.42 at 37°	633	141

hyperechoic (*us*) Having relatively strong echoes.

hyperlinks (*comp*) Embedded text in web pages that allow users to jump from one document to another related document, regardless of where it is stored on the Internet. By selecting the text or image with a mouse, the computer jumps to and displays the linked site (*see* HTML, hypertext).

hyperosmolar/hyperosmolality/hyperosmolarity (*clin*) An increase in the osmotic concentration of a solution measured as osmoles of solute per kilogram (osmolarity (Osmol)/osmolality (Osm)) or litre of solution (osmolarity). Ionic contrast media dissociate in solution into anionic and cationic components and are markedly hyperosmolar. Non-ionic contrast media do not dissociate in solution and are less hyperosmolar or isosmolar with blood. The ionic contrast media for intravascular use are hyperosmolar, having an osmolality seven to eight times that of blood plasma. This hyperosmolality is partly responsible for several subjective and objective adverse effects, i.e. pain, endothelial damage, thrombosis and thrombophlebitis, disturbance of the blood–brain barrier, bradycardia in cardioangiography and increased pressure in the pulmonary circulation (*see* contrast medium (radiographic)).

hypertext (*comp*) A method of presenting information that allows the user to jump between places in a document by clicking on a highlighted word or an icon, rather than being forced to navigate it in a linear fashion. Both the Help files and web pages make extensive use of this technique (*see* HTML).

hyperthyroidism (*clin*) A condition in which an overactive thyroid gland produces excessive thyroid hormone, leading to a characteristic clinical picture. Since the thyroid uses iodine to make its hormone (thyroxine or T-4), radioactive iodine in small dosages can be used to image the thyroid and in large dosages to treat it (reduce its function).

hypertonic (*cm*) *See* high osmolarity.

hyper-threading technology (*comp*) In order to improve performance in early computers, threading was enabled in the software by splitting instructions into multiple streams so that multiple processors could act upon them. Hyper-threading technology (HT technology) is now hardware built into the CPU and provides the ability to run multiple parallel threads on each processor, resulting in more efficient use of processor resources, higher processing throughput, and improved performance on multithreaded software. Hyper-threading technology improves the performance of existing software in multitasking server environments. Many applications are already multithreaded and will automatically benefit from this technology, but performance will vary depending on the specific hardware and software (*see* duo core processors).

hypo (*film*) Sodium thiosulphite.

hypoechoic (*us*) Having relatively weak echoes.

hypo-osmolar (*cm*) *See* low osmolarity.

hysteresis (*phys*) Phenomenon seen in electromagnetic behaviour of materials in which a lag occurs between application or removal of a magnetic force (examples can be found in MRI and magnetic recording).

hysteresis loss (*mri*) Dissipation of energy that occurs when a magnetic material is subjected to magnetic field change. Important factor with gradient field switching.

hysterosalpingography (*clin*) Injection of contrast material into the uterus and uterine tubes and imaging the uterus and fallopian tubes thereafter. Also known as salpingography.

H

I

i (*math*) The complex variable representing $\sqrt{-1}$. Sometimes represented by *j* or *q* (*see* complex numbers).

I (*units*) Induction. (*phys*) *See* spin quantum number.

IAEA (*dose*) International Atomic Energy Authority. Established by the United Nations in 1957 to advise member countries on the application of nuclear power and on security matters. Headquarters in Vienna.

ibitumomab (*nmed*) ^{90}Y-labelled antibody for non-Hodgkin's lymphoma therapy.

ICRP (*dose*) International Commission on Radiological Protection. Established in 1928, associated with the International Commission on Radiation Units and Measurements, The World Health Organization and the International Atomic Energy Agency. The ICRP only concerns itself with ionizing radiation and with the protection of man. The ICRP recommendations have helped to provide a consistent basis for national and regional regulatory standards; the recommendations carry no regulatory powers, but form the basis of most national legislation. The most recent (September 2008) ICRP reports of interest to medical applications are:

ICRP publication No.

106 Radiation dose to patients from radiopharmaceuticals. ISBN-13: 978-0-7020-3450-3, ISBN-10: 0-7020-3450-9, 2009

105 Radiological protection in medicine, ISBN-13: 978-0-7020-3102-1, ISBN-10: 0-7020-3102-X, 2008

103 Recommendations of the ICRP: user's edition. ISBN-13: 978-0-7020-3063-5, ISBN-10: 0-7020-3063-5, 2007

102 Managing patient dose in multi-detector computed tomography (MDCT). ISBN-13: 978-0-7020-3047-5, ISBN-10: 0-7020-3047-3, 2007

95 Doses to infants from ingestion of radionuclides in mother's milk. ISBN-13: 978-0-08-044627-1, ISBN-10: 0-08-044627-2, 2004

93 Managing patient dose in digital radiology. ISBN-13: 978-0-08-044469-7, ISBN-10: 0-08-044469-5, 2004

92 Relative biological effectiveness (RBE), quality factor (Q), and radiation weighting factor (wR). ISBN-13: 978-0-08-044311-9, ISBN-10: 0-08-044311-7, 2004

90 Biological effects after prenatal irradiation (embryo and foetus. ISBN-13: 978-0-08-044265-5, ISBN-10: 0-08-044265-X, 2004

88 ICRP Supporting Guidance 2: Radiation and your patient: a guide for medical practitioners.

ISBN-13: 978-0-08-044211-2, ISBN-10: 0-08-044211-0, 2003

87 Managing patient dose in computed tomography. ISBN-13: 978-0-08-044083-5, ISBN-10: 0-08-044083-5, 2002

84 Pregnancy and medical radiation. ISBN-13: 978-0-08-043901-3, ISBN-10: 0-08-043901-2, 2001

73 Radiological protection and safety in medicine. ISBN-13: 978-0-08-042738-6, ISBN-10: 0-08-042738-3, 1997

60 1990 Recommendations of the International Commission on Radiological Protection, ISBN-13: 978-0-08-041144-6, ISBN-10: 0-08-041144-4, 1991.

ICRU (International Commission on Radiation Units and Measurement) (*dose*) Formed in 1925 for developing internationally acceptable recommendations regarding quantities and units of radiation and radioactivity and makes recommendations for radiation protection. Cooperates with the **ICRP**. Selected ICRU reports:

- Receiver operating characteristic (ROC) analysis in medical imaging (report 79) 2008
- Prescribing, recording and reporting proton-beam therapy (report 78) 2007
- Measurement quality assurance for ionizing radiation dosimetry (report 76) 2006
- Patient dosimetry for x rays used in medical Imaging (report 74) 2005
- Image quality in chest radiography (report 70) 2003
- Tissues substitutes, phantoms and computation modelling in medical ultrasound (report 61) 1999
- Fundamental quantities and units for ionizing radiation (report 60) 1998
- Medical imaging – the assessment of image quality (report 54) 1996
- Quantities and units in radiation protection dosimetry (report 51) 1993
- Tissue substitutes in radiation dosimetry and measurement (report 44) 1989
- Modulation transfer function of screen-film systems (report 41) 1986.

IDA (*nmed*) *See* HIDA.

IDE (*comp*) Integrated drive electronics. A control system which allows a computer and a device to communicate. Now replaced by **EIDE** (enhanced IDE) which offers improved performance.

ideal filter (*image*) An ideal low-pass filter has a rectangular transfer function. Commonly used filters are radially symmetrical about the origin

(3D plot), so they can be specified by a cross-section extending from the origin in a 2D graph. On the graph D_o is the cut-off frequency; all frequencies inside a circle of radius D_o are passed with zero attenuation, whereas all frequencies outside D_o are stopped. The ideal high-pass filter has a transfer function that attenuates low frequencies without disturbing high frequencies (*see* Butterworth, Hanning, Hamming, Shepp-Logan).

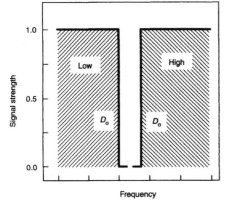

ideal observer (*stats*) The ideal observer is the Bayesian decision-maker who minimizes the 'cost' or 'risk' when determining a decision strategy for a given task.

IEEE (*comp*) The Institute of Electrical and Electronics Engineers, a body that defines standards and specifications: IEEE 802 Standards govern networking.

IEEE 1394 (*comp*) An external bus that transfers data from one computer to another at up to 400 Mbps. Thanks to its high speed, IEEE 1394 is the standard for multimedia and will clash head on with USB 2.0 should it establish a foothold in the market. At present IEEE 1394 is in a dominant position, mainly thanks to manufacturers including it in their computer devices, complementing their digital cameras and camcorders. IEEE 1394 is known as FireWire at Apple and i-link at Sony, where it has been adopted as the standard across its popular Valo notebook range. Although SCSI (small computer systems interface) has provided an invaluable medium-term solution for users who need extra speed; these ports also have serious disadvantages. Having installed a SCSI card, the user has to attach a thick,

unwieldy parallel cable linking the PC to the peripheral. In addition, unlike the smaller and more robust USB 2.0, SCSi cable ports are easily damaged.

IHE (*comp*) Integrating the healthcare enterprise. Developed by the Radiological Society of North America (RSNA) and Healthcare Information Management Systems Society (HIMSS). There are ambiguities and conflicting interpretations between standards like DICOM and HL7. IHE coordinates the use of these established standards and answers issues that remain unresolved in DICOM/HL7 operations.

iliocavography (*clin*) *See* pelvic venography.

illuminance (*phys*) The total luminous flux received by a unit area of surface expressed in lux (lumen m^{-2}). Non-SI units are illuminance (lumen ft^{-2}) or phot (lumen cm^{-2}). One lux $= 10^4$ phots. Illuminance is analogous to irradiance, but illuminance refers only to visible light weighted to the non-linear luminous efficiency of the human eye (*see* radiance).

image (*image*) A 2D representation of a volume distribution either as a landscape or object. A volume object in diagnostic imaging can be interrogated by x-rays, gamma rays, ultrasound or radio frequencies to give an image distribution in x and y dimensions (height and width). Signal strength is represented as a change in image density either as a grey or colour scale. This can be analogue (film) or digital (computer matrix). A computer matrix has a third dimension given by the pixel depth which determines the dynamic range (latitude) of the image (*see* tomography).

image (latent) (*image*) Light reacting with a photographic emulsion causes some silver ions to be converted into silver atoms. Developing this emulsion causes further silver atoms to form in the vicinity of these original atoms, giving a latent or hidden image which can be revealed by fixing with a chemical that removes the remaining unaffected emulsion silver salts.

image acquisition time (*image*) Time required to carry out an imaging procedure. The number of encoding signals required for reconstruction. Applicable to ultrasound and nuclear medicine. (*mri*) Time required to carry out a magnetic resonance (MR) imaging procedure comprising only the data acquisition time. The total image acquisition time will be equal to the product of the repetition time. The time required

T is: $T = TR \times Lines \times Nex$, where TR is the repetition time, $Lines$ the number of image lines (phase encoding steps) and Nex the data averaging. For a TR of 0.5 s, an image matrix of 512 and $\times 2$ averaging the image acquisition would be 512 seconds or 8.5 minutes. The additional image reconstruction time will also be important to determine how quickly the image can be viewed. In comparing sequential plane imaging and volume imaging techniques, the equivalent image acquisition time per slice must be considered, as well as the actual image acquisition time.

image archiving (*image*) Recording a raw image matrix on to bulk storage by compressing the information and so achieving the maximum utilization of the data medium capacity; there are loss-less compression and lossy compression methods for image archiving.

image contrast (*xray*) *See* contrast. (*mri*) The strength of the image intensity in adjacent regions of the image is compared, or object contrast, where the relative values of a parameter affecting the image (such as spin density or relax-at ion time) in corresponding adjacent regions of the object are compared. There are more object parameters affecting the image in magnetic resonance imaging (MRI) and their relative contributions are dependent on the imaging technique used.

image depth (*us*) Maximum penetration that will yield image information. Decreases with increasing frequency and with decreasing transducer size or aperture (Fresnel or near zone shortened). The useful image depth is also dependent on pulse repetition frequency. Proportional to 75/PRF (pulse repetition frequency). The displayed distance from transducer face determined by the pulse repetition period (PRP) and transducer frequency. Calculated from the speed of sound in soft tissue ($1500\,\mathrm{m\,s^{-1}}$) and allowing for a return path (so halving this distance), then $D_{max} = 150\,000 \times 0.5 \times PRP$ or $75\,000 \times PRP$ cm. For a PRP of 200 μs this would give an imaging depth of 15 cm. Alternatively, D_{max} can be calculated as $75\,000/PRF$. Similarly, for soft tissue imaging: $PRF = 1500/2 \times D_{max}$. Higher frequency transducers have higher PRP values so give shallower image depths. Since sound attenuation increases with frequency, this is the major determining factor for image depth. The graph

plots the relationship between PRP and imaging depth for a speed of sound of $1500\,\mathrm{m\,s^{-1}}$; transducer frequencies used at various PRP values are superimposed on the graph; higher frequency transducers give improved image resolution and owing to faster PRP are more able to give real-time displays and follow pulsatile (cardiac) movement.

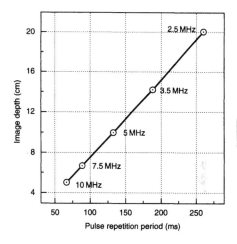

(*see* dispersion, axial resolution, lateral resolution).

image fusion (*image*) Combination of two or more registered images, with the objective of producing a single image of additional diagnostic information.

image intensifier (*xray*) An electronic method for increasing the light intensity from a fluorescent screen. The input fluorescent phosphor is typically CsI:Na which has several advantages:

- good absorption for x-ray energies above the K-edges of Cs (33 keV) and iodine (36 keV);
- spectral matching with $SbCs_3$ photocathode material;
- vapour deposition of CsI:Na produces monoclinic crystalline structure (150 μm thick) which channels light quanta and prevents light diffusion.

The photocathode is in optical contact with the input phosphor transforming light quanta into an electron flux density distribution. The electrons are accelerated on to an output phosphor screen which is generally ZnCdS:Ag, a few micrometres thick on a glass base. A thin aluminium skin on the phosphor acts as the anode and also prevents transmission of light back to the photocathode. Large field image intensifiers are typically metal sheathed with a titanium input window up to 40 cm diameter and 2.5 cm output window coupled to either a video camera tube or CCD. X-rays are converted to light by a caesium iodide scintillator; the light is then converted to electrons by a photocathode. The electrons are accelerated by a high voltage (typically 30 kV) on to a phosphor applied to the output window. Minification and electronic gain intensify the original x-ray photon flux to give a visible image (*see* Coltman, fluoroscopy, conversion efficiency).

image intensifier (contrast ratio) (*xray*) The degree of contrast loss measured using a lead disc covering the central area of the image intensifier face. The lead disc should be at least 2 mm thick. Contrast ratio is then:

$$\frac{\text{Conversion factor without lead disc}}{\text{Conversion factor with lead disc}}$$

The contrast loss is then defined as:

$$\frac{100\%}{\text{Contrast ratio}}.$$

Typical values are 20 to 25:1.

image intensifier (conversion efficiency) (*xray*) A measure of efficiency for image intensifiers, as the ratio of output phosphor luminance (cd m^{-2}) to input dose (μGy^{-1}s^{-1}). Other methods use microCoulombs (cd m$^{-2}\mu$C kg^{-1}s^{-1} or use millirads (cd m^{-2}mR^{-1}s^{-1}). Conversion factor multipliers:

Given	Required (multiplier)		
	μGy^{-1}	μC kg^{-1}	mR^{-1}
μGy^{-1}	1.0	34.0	8.7
μC kg^{-1}	0.03	1.0	0.256
mR^{-1}	0.115	3.9	1.0

For a 40 cm (16 in) diameter image intensifier typical values are: 1280 cd m^{-2} μC kg^{-1}s^{-1}; 327 cd m^{-2}mR^{-1}s^{-1}; and 38 cd m$^{-2}\mu$Gy^{-1}s^{-2}

image intensifier (low frequency drop, LFD) (*image*) The modulation transfer function (MTF) for an image intensifier shows a rapid drop from 1.0 to about 0.8. The percentage drop is the LFD and represents a fall of 8 to 13% in resolution, responsible for the degradation of all spatial frequencies. Two main factors are responsible: (1) x-ray scatter in the input window and phosphor; (2) light diffusion at the output window. The first factor can be reduced

by using titanium input windows and CsI phosphor; the second can be reduced by using a fibreoptic plate between output window and video/CCD device.

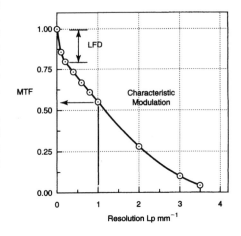

image intensifier (resolution) (*xray*) Spatial resolution is often conveniently measured in terms of line pairs per millimetre (Lp mm^{-1}) by using a line pair test pattern consisting of an etched tungsten or tantalum grating, measuring high contrast fine object detail in the output image. Overall resolution of the image intensifier improves with increased dose rate at the image intensifier face, but low contrast visibility is the limiting factor. Dose rate at the face is restricted to within 0.15–0.2 μGy s^{-1} and 3.5–4.0 Lp mm^{-1} is currently the best performance value. Typical performance figures for an image intensifier have three zoom values 29, 22 and 16 cm, respectively; resolution is measured in Lp mm^{-1}:

Operating mode	Normal	Zoom 1	Zoom 2
Entrance field size	29 cm	22 cm	16 cm
Limiting resolution			
Centre	4.4	5.0	5.6
93% radius	3.8	4.6	5.2
Contrast ratio			
Large area	22:1	25:1	30:1
Small detail	13:1	15:1	17:1

image intensifier (speed) (*image*) This is the reciprocal of the mean kerma in air at the input face of the image intensifier (μGy21). For optimum performance under automatic control, values should not exceed 1.0 μGy s21. For single film and serial fluorography, it should be within the range 0.43–1.74 µGy per frame and within 0.087–0.348 µGy per frame for cinefluorography.

image lag (*image*) Temporal response time, affecting dynamic events when viewed as a series of images (cine). A common artefact in fluoroscopy when the video camera has a poor response time compared to the speed of the physiological event.

image matrix (*image, ct*) The 2D arrangement of values (i.e. CT numbers) at discrete positions; the single elements stored are voxels. The display image matrix are called pixels (*see* matrix).

image noise (*ct*) Noise contributions to the final image. Caused by many factors, notably sampling error, electronic noise, mechanical misplacement (*see* noise).

image orientation (*mri*) A recommended standard orientation for the presentation of nuclear magnetic resonance (NMR) images is: (1) transverse: patient's right on the left side of the image, anterior or ventral on top; (2) coronal: patient's right to left side of image, superior or head to the top; (3) sagittal: patient's head to the top, anterior to the left side of image. R (right), L (left), P (posterior), A (anterior), and if necessary S (superior) should be shown on the screen and the hardcopies, as appropriate.

image plate (*image*) Filmless recording using either phosphor material or selenium. The thermoluminescent material used for the phosphor image plate is commonly a complex barium fluorohalide BaFX:Eu2+ where X is the halide atom Cl, Br or I. Under x-ray exposure, the europium ion changes from divalent to trivalent state. On stimulation with laser light of a particular wavelength, this valency state is reversed releasing a UV (ultraviolet) luminescence (photostimulated luminescence (PSL)) whose intensity is proportional to the original x-ray intensity. This is captured by a photomultiplier whose signal forms a digital image.

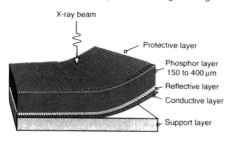

X-ray beam

Protective layer

Phosphor layer 150 to 400 µm

Reflective layer

Conductive layer

Support layer

image processing (*image*) A method applied to digital image matrices using precise filters or selecting thresholds within the image data to accentuate certain information or accentuate certain details (edge enhancement) or reduce noise (smoothing, unsharp masking, histogram equalization).

image quality (*image*) Described by the maximum/minimum range of contrast and resolution registered by the image and its noise content (*see* signal to noise, DQE, NEQ, contrast detail diagram, MTF, Wiener spectrum).

image reconstruction (*ct*) Calculation of the CT image from the projection data. Attenuation coefficients that have been collected as single-dimensional values must now be displayed as a 2D image. The data matrix of these coefficients is obtained from the scanning pattern of the fan beam and is commonly represented in a 512 × 512 format. The total absorption figure is known: this is the ray sum. The separate matrix values are found by mathematical reconstruction. The individual values in the matrix can be calculated by using either: iterative reconstruction technique or backprojection (or its derivatives). The calculations are performed in a dedicated array processor in order to provide almost instantaneous image display.

image reconstruction algorithm (*ct*) A method used to reconstruct images from the measured attenuation profiles (as CT numbers) using algebraic (iterative) reconstruction or filtered backprojection reconstruction.

image reconstruction (back projection) (*ct*) A tightly collimated x-ray beam is used and its total absorption provides the ray-sum signal for each matrix row, which is stored in the array processor image memory. This is shown in the diagram (a) for 0° 45° and 90° rotated scan positions (a). Other projections (b) provide the complete data set. The central high uptake from the original is now distinguishable, but it has a star-burst interference pattern. Early attempts at this form of reconstruction used photographic methods and the final images contained star artefacts (there is only one star artefact shown here matching the single high data point in the original image). The artefacts can be removed by just accepting the high values, but this is not a satisfactory solution.

image reconstruction (filtered backprojection) (*ct*) The star interference may be removed. A mask signal with negative going edges acts as a high-pass filter removing the remaining backprojected low frequency interference pattern.

I

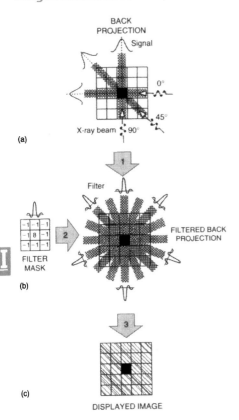

(a) BACK PROJECTION

(b) FILTER MASK / FILTERED BACK PROJECTION

(c) DISPLAYED IMAGE

image reconstruction (iterative) (*ct*) This uses an exact mathematical solution for reconstructing the image slice from the attenuation data. This was the original method for image reconstruction used by Godfrey Hounsfield (British engineer, 1919–2004) in the first CT machine. Its disadvantages are that it takes a considerable amount of computer time and is slow. It also suffers from rounding errors (0.95 = 1.0, etc.) which give imprecise CT values and all the data must be collected before reconstruction can begin.

image reconstruction algorithm (*ct*) Method used to reconstruct images from the measured attenuation profiles (as CT numbers) using algebraic (iterative) reconstruction or filtered backprojection reconstruction.

image reconstruction time (*ct*) The additional time taken to display the image after acquisition and axial reconstruction protocol. Important in CT and MRI, since reconstruction of the images can occupy a significant proportion of the delay. (*image*) Additional time after

completion of image data acquisition before the display of the first image. Dedicated array processor, CPU speed and available memory influence this.

image resolution (*image*) *See* resolution element.

image segmentation (*image*) Partition of an image into disjoint regions, each of which is uniform with respect to a certain characteristic (such as brightness or texture), but such that no union of adjacent regions is uniform.

image set reconstruction time (*image*) Total additional time after completion of data acquisition until all images of a set (e.g. multiple plane or volume imaging) are available for display.

image transform (*image*) Mapping of image data into image data. An image transform generates one or several resultant images out of one or several given images. It is generally considered to be a process of analysis, breaking the image down into its elemental components (basic images) and providing further information that is not readily available in the raw image data.

imaginary signal (*math*) Out-of-phase component of the signal from a quadrature detector.

imaging depth (*image*) Maximum penetration that will yield image information. Proportional to 75/PRF.

imaging volume (*image*) *See* volume of investigation.

Imagopaque® (*cm*) Commercial form of iopentol introduced by Nycomed in 1991.

Compound	Viscosity (cP)	Osmolality (mOsm/kg)	Iodine (mg I/mL)
Iopentol	12.0 at 25°	680	350

imciromab (*nmed*) *See* Myoscint®.

Imeron® (*cm*) Commercial form of iomeprol, introduced by Bracco in 1994.

Compound	Viscosity (cP)	Osmolality (mOsm/kg)	Iodine (mg I/mL)
Iomeprol	1.4–12.6	300–726	150–400

impedance Z (*phys*) A varying a.c. power source connected to an electrical network sees an impedance: $Z = A + iB$, where A is the 'real' part of the impedance representing the resistive component which is energy dissipating. B is the 'imaginary' part of the impedance, made up mainly of capacitance or inductance. Both are loss-less energy storage elements and can retrieve energy stored at some previous time without loss, so they produce phase shift. An RF signal is affected by both the capacitance and inductance of a circuit, as well as its resistance; this total opposition to the signal is the impedance. The matching of the impedances between circuits is essential to prevent signal loss. (*us*) Defined as material density × sound propagation speed. Typical range 1.3×106 to 1.7×106 rayls (*see* input impedance).

impedance matching (*phys*) Adjusting the electrical impedance of two circuits that are being connected so that they are equal, so preventing signal loss or ringing.

impulse (*phys*) A very short duration electrical signal which can be represented by a Dirac function. An important property of ultrasound and MRI-transmitted pulses. (*elec*) A brief excursion of electric voltage from its normal value, usually zero.

impulse response function (*di*) The response, in the time domain, of a circuit (amplifier) or filter to a precisely known input and measuring the resulting output function. The total response expressed as a weighting function is the impulse response function, uniquely defining the system. Usually seen as a decaying waveform in ultrasound or MRI pulses (*see* frequency response function).

incandescence (*xray*) The emission of visible radiation from a material at high temperature. It is applied to illumination (e.g. viewboxes), x-ray anodes when bombarded by an electron beam.

incidence (angle of) (*us*) The angle between the incident ray and the reflected ray. Angle between incident sound direction and a line perpendicular to the boundary of the medium.

incidence (incidence rate) (*dose*) The rate of occurrence of a disease within a specified period of time, often expressed as a number of cases with a disease per 100 000 individuals per year (or per 10 000 person-years).

incident (radiation) (*phys*) The primary radiation striking a surface. Either electromagnetic or sound.

incidence (screening) (*clin*) The number of newly diagnosed cases (cancer) in a defined population within a defined period. Usually expressed as an incident rate of x per 1000 for small populations or x per 100 000 per year for large populations. An incidence of 8 per 1000 means eight new cases of disease per year per 1000 of the defined population (*see* incident screen, interval disease).

incident (radiation) (*phys*) The primary radiation striking a surface. Either electromagnetic or sound.

incident screen (screening) (*clin*) The screening investigation carried out after the first screen, which detects the incident disease.

incoherent spins (*phys*) A state of a set of spins in which the ensemble of spins in a voxel are uniformly distributed with phases between 0 and 2p reducing the transverse magnetization in a voxel to essentially zero.

independent event (*stats*) Events which have no influence on each other. Independent variable is a random variable.

independent variable (*stats*) (or explanatory variable) The independent variable appears on the right hand side of the equation.

indirect splenoportography (*clin*) *See* splenoportography.

Indichlor^{x} (*nmed*) ^{111}Indium chloride preparation from Amersham/GE Healthcare.

indium (In) (*elem*)

Atomic number (Z)	49
Relative atomic mass (A$_r$)	114.8
Density (ρ) kg/m^3	7310
Melting point (K)	429.8
K-edge (keV)	27.9

Relevance to radiology: As a low melting point alloy for lubricating anode bearing in x-ray tubes.

^{111}Indium (*nmed*) $T\frac{1}{2}$ as a scintigraphic label for radiopharmaceuticals (listed below)

Production (cyclotron)	$^{111}_{48}Cd(p,n)^{111}_{49}In$
	or $^{109}_{47}Ag(^{4}He,2n)^{111}_{49}In$
Decay scheme (e.c.) ^{111}In	^{111}In (γ 171, 245 keV) $\rightarrow$ ^{111}Cd stable
Gamma ray constant	$8.4 \times 10^{-2} mSv h^{-1}$ GBq^{-1} at 1 m
Half-life	2.8 days
Decay constant	0.2475 day^{-1}
Annual limit on intake	150 MBq (4.0 mCi)
Half value layer	0.23 mm Pb, 51 mm water

Uses for labelling biological agents (somatostatin, antibodies and white cells). ^{111}In-DTPA used for imaging the cerebrospinal fluid (CSF) pathway. ^{113m}In generator also used for general imaging (now uncommon).

Radiation attenuation for lead

Thickness (mm Pb)	Coefficient of attenuation
0.23	0.5
2.03	10^{-1}
5.13	10^{-2}
8.34	10^{-3}
11.20	10^{-4}

Physical decay: ¹¹¹Indium

Hours	Fraction remaining
0	1.000
3	0.970
6	0.940
12	0.885
24	0.781
36	0.690
48	0.610

¹¹¹Indium DTPA (*nmed*) *See* ¹¹¹Indium pentetate.

¹¹¹Indium chloride (*nmed*) Used as a label for a variety of radiopharmaceuticals including monoclonal antibodies and peptides (*see* OncoScint® and Octreoscan®).

¹¹¹In-oxyquinoline (*nmed*) ¹¹¹In-oxine, a diagnostic radiopharmaceutical (Amersham/GE Healthcare) for radiolabelling autologous leucocytes (white blood cells). The presence of red blood cells or plasma will lead to reduced leucocyte labelling efficiency. The transferrin in plasma competes for ¹¹¹indium-oxyquinoline.

¹¹¹Indium pentetate (*nmed*) As ¹¹¹In DTPA, a radiopharmaceutical for cyeternography CSF.

¹¹¹Indium satumomab pendetide (*nmed*) *See* OncoScint®.

¹¹¹Indium tropolone (*nmed*) A neutral, lipid-soluble metal complex of ¹¹¹In and tropolone used as a tracer for white blood cell and platelet labelling. Unlike oxine, which is soluble in ethyl alcohol, tropolone is soluble in isotonic saline.

¹¹³ᵐIndium (*nmed*) Generator-derived nuclide for brain, liver and blood pool imaging.

Production	$^{112}_{50}$Sn (n, γ)$^{113}_{50}$Sn → ^{113m}In
Decay scheme (i.t.) ^{113m}In	^{113}SnT $\frac{1}{2}$118 days → ^{113m}In (γ 393 keV) → ^{113}In stable
Eluent	0.05 M HCl
Gamma ray constant	4.6×10^{-2} mSv hr^{-1}GBq^{-1} at 1 m
Half-life	1.7 hours
Half value layer	(mm Pb)

individual dose (*dose*) (ICRP60) A distinction between the collective dose of a selected population and the dose to an individual in that population.

inductance (*phys*) Measure of the magnetic coupling between two current-carrying loops of an RF circuit. A property of a conductor resulting from the magnetic field induced when a current flows. The SI unit of self and mutual inductance is the henry (H) which is the inductance of a closed loop that gives a magnetic flux of 1 Wb A^{-1}.

induced genomic instability (*dose*) The induction of an altered cellular state characterized by a persistent increase over many generations in the spontaneous rate of mutation or other genome-related changes.

induction B (*phys*) *See* magnetic induction.

inductor (*phys*) A device (e.g. a coil) possessing inductance.

in-elastic scattering (*phys*) *See* Compton scattering.

inert gases (noble gases/rare gases) (*chem*) A group of gaseous elements forming group 18 (previously group 0) in the periodic table. The relative abundance of these gases in air together with the major constituents is as follows:

Gas	Symbol	Z	Abundance (%)	Density (kg m^{-3})
Air	–	7.78 (eff)	100	1.293
Nitrogen	N_2	7	78	1.25
Oxygen	O_2	8	28	1.429
Carbon dioxide	CO_2	–	0.04	1.97
Helium	He	2	–	0.166
Neon	Ne	10	0.0018	0.839
Argon	Ar	18	0.93	1.66
Krypton	Kr	36	0.0001	3.5
Xenon	Xe	54	0.0009	5.5
Radon	Rn	86	–	9.73

inertia (*phys*) Any mass when in motion tends to resist being retarded. In the case of a rotating anode, it can be shown that its tendency to preserve its state of motion (its inertia) is determined by its mass and its radius. The inertia I of a disc of uniform density having mass M and radius R is given by $I = \frac{1}{2}MR^2$ from which it is seen that the inertia can be increased by increasing either the mass or the diameter of the disc.

inferior mesenteric arteriography (*clin*) Arteriography of the inferior mesenteric artery usually demonstrating gastrointestinal bleeding or mesenteric ischaemia, and sometimes tumours of the large bowel (*see* superior mesenteric arteriography).

inferior venocavography (*clin*) Angiography of the inferior vena cava (IVC), using a common femoral vein approach.

inflow technique (*mri*) *See* time of flight angiography (TOF).

inflow amplification (*mri*) Slowly moving blood perpendicular to the slice returns a stronger signal than the surrounding tissue. If a bolus within a selected slice is excited using a 90° pulse, the spins fully recover within a short repetition time (TR). They retain their saturation, but the signal is weaker than that from a long TR in relationship to T1. Conversely, spins outside the slice are fully magnetized and spins flowing out of the slice are replaced by fresh inflowing spins. The overall effect is that vascular magnetization within the slice decreases.

information density (*nmed*) The count density in units of counts/cm^2 of gamma camera images.

information technology (IT) (*comp*) A wide range of techniques used to handle and distribute information. Incorporating computing and all forms of electronic communication.

infrared radiation (*phys*) A section of the electromagnetic spectrum capable of producing heat. Situated between wavelengths $0.7\,\mu m$ to 1 mm. It has subregions IRB and IRC.

inherent filtration (*xray*) *See* filtration.

inhomogeneity (*mri*) Degree of lack of homogeneity; for example, the fractional deviation of the local magnetic field from the average value of the field.

input impedance (*elec*) The impedance presented by an electronic circuit at its input. Charge amplifiers connected to the output of a photomultiplier have a very high input impedance, RF-coil amplifiers (MRI) have a low input impedance (*see* impedance).

instantaneous dose rate (*dose*) The dose rate averaged over 1 minute at a particular location.

insufflation (peri-renal) (*clin*) Obsolete procedure which injects air or CO_2 around the kidneys in order to visualize the adrenal glands.

insulator (*phys*) A material having a wide forbidden zone between electron orbits and conduction zone, thus preventing orbital electrons acting as electrical carriers. The permeability indicates the degree to which the medium can resist the flow of electric current compared to free space. The value εr varies from unity (for a vacuum) to over 4000 for some composite materials. Gases including water vapour have relative permittivity values marginally greater than 1. Plastics have values between 2 and 3.5, glass between 5 and 10 and pure water is 80.4.

intake (i) (*dose*) Activity that enters the body through the respiratory tract or gastrointestinal tract from the environment.

integer (*math*) A whole number.

integral (*math*) The area underneath a curve describing a function.

integral dose (*dose*) The total dose received by a cell culture, tissue or population over a period of time.

integral uniformity (*nmed*) *See* uniformity (integral).

integrated panorama array (IPA) (*mri*) An integrated panorama array (Siemens) accelerates set-up time and increases patient throughput by employing up to 4, 8 or 16 independent array coil systems linked simultaneously.

integrated imaging (diagnostic) (*stats*) Combining two or more diagnostic tests, which utilize different imaging functions, improves the overall sensitivity and specificity for detecting disease. For tests x and y reporting two sensitivities Sen_x and Sen_y and two specificities $Spec_x$ and $Spec_y$, then for these two test conditions:

1 If x and/or y are positive or x and y are negative, integrated sensitivity is:

$Sen_x + ((100 - Sen_x) \times Sen_y)/100\%$

Integrated selectivity is: $(Spec_x \times Spec_y)/100\%$.

2 If x and y are positive or x and/or y are negative, the integrated sensitivity is:

$(Sen_x \times Sen_y)/100\%$

Integrated selectivity: $Spec_x + ((100 - Spec_x) \times Spec_y)/100\%$.

If the following percentage diagnostic accuracies have been reported:

	Sensitivity (%)	Selectivity (%)
Nuclear medicine	80	60
Computed tomography	90	90

For condition (1), sensitivity becomes 98% and specificity 54%; for condition (2), sensitivity becomes 72% and specificity 96%. High sensitivity excludes disease and is most valuable when screening. High selectivity confirms that disease is present and prevents unnecessary treatment.

integration/differentiation (*math*) Integration is the inverse of differentiation; it is the area under a curve. The integral of a function $f(x)$ with respect to x is written as $\int f(x).dx$. The symbol $\int$ being the old English for S, representing sum.

The definite integral f(x) defined by an interval a to b is:

$$\int_b^a f(x).dx$$

The infinite integral applies if one or both of the limits tends to infinity. The integral dose or exposure over an organ or surface can be represented as a gaussian distribution which serves to demonstrate the integration process. Differentiation is concerned with studying the rate of change of a function with respect to its variable (e.g. time); integration is the converse.

- Reference: Gonzalez and Wintz, 1987.

intensification factor (*xray*) Product of minification gain and electronic gain.

intensifying screen (*image*) Thin sheets of plastic impregnated with phosphor which converts x-radiation into UV/visible light. Early phosphors used calcium tungstate; current phosphors are complexes of lanthanum and gadolinium (rare earth phosphors); other phosphors which emit exclusively in the UV spectrum are complexes of yttrium, tungsten and tantalum. Either a single or double screen is used in the film cassette applied directly to the film emulsion (single- or dual-sided film). A large increase in quantum efficiency enables the film to be exposed with a significantly lower patient radiation dose. Intensifying screens are graded according to speed (sensitivity). Conventional or 'par' speed is 100. Detail screens with a thinner phosphor layer have speeds below par. Fast screens which offer very low dose investigations (e.g. paediatrics, lumbar spine) have speeds up to 400.

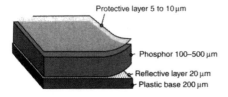

Protective layer 5 to 10μm

Phosphor 100–500 μm

Reflective layer 20 μm

Plastic base 200 μm

intensity (*phys*) The power carried by a wave or oscillation divided by the area (W m⁻²) (*see* photon fluence). (*us*) *See* ultrasound (intensity).

intensity, instantaneous (*i*) (*us*) The instantaneous ultrasound intensity transmitted in the direction of acoustic wave propagation, per unit area normal to this direction, at the point considered. It is given by: $i = P^2/2\rho c$, where P is the instantaneous **acoustic pressure**; ρ is the density of the medium; and c is the speed of sound in the medium. The unit is Watt per square-centimetre, $W\,cm^{-2}$.

intensity (maximum) I_m (*us*) The intensity averaged over the time of the half cycle (half period). The unit is $W\,cm^{-2}$.

intensity modulation (*image*) The variation of signal intensity (video signal) in a light image on a video screen (CRT (cathode ray tube) or flat field: LCD (liquid crystal display) or TFT (thin film transistor)) (*see* video display, **video signal**).

intensity profile (*us*) Acoustic intensity across the ultrasound transducer has an approximately gaussian distribution having a spatial peak intensity (SP) and spatial average intensity (SA) (*see* intensity).

intensity reflection coefficient (IRC) (*us*) Defined as reflected intensity/incident intensity. Both units measured in $W\,cm^{-2}$.

intensity transmission coefficient (ITC) (*us*) Defined as transmitted intensity/incident intensity. Approximately equal to $1 - IRC$ (**intensity reflection coefficient**), both units measured in $W\,cm^{-2}$.

intensity reflection coefficient. Reflected intensity divided by incident.

intensity, temporal average (I_{TA}) (*us*) The time average for the intensity at a point in space from the transducer. For **non-autoscan** systems, the average is taken over one or more pulse repetition periods. For **autoscan systems**, the intensity is averaged over one or more scan repetition periods for a specified operating mode. For autoscan modes, the average includes contributions from adjacent lines that overlap the point of measurement. For combined modes, the average includes overlapping lines, from all constituent discrete operating mode signals. Measured in $mW\,cm^{-2}$.

intensity, temporal peak I_{TP} (*us*) The peak value of the intensity at the point considered. The unit is Watt per square-centimetre, $W\,cm^{-2}$.

intensity transmission coefficient Transmitted intensity divided by incident intensity; the fraction of incident intensity transmitted into the second medium.

interactive real time (*mri*) Changing the measurement parameters in real time by operator control.

interactive shim (*mri*) Manual tuning of the shim coils to improve magnetic field homogeneity. Shim currents are set individually for a selected pulse sequence.

interface (*comp*) The interconnection (either hardware or software) that allows a device, a program or a person to interact. Hardware interfaces are the cables that connect the device to its power source and to other devices. Software interfaces allow the program to communicate with other programs (such as the operating system), and user interfaces allow the user to communicate with the program (e.g. via mouse, menu commands, icons, voice commands, etc.).

interference (*phys*) The interaction of an unwanted structured signal (not noise) with the wanted signal. Examples would be interfering signals from adjacent slices in MRI which degrade the information contained within the targeted slice. When waveforms having the same frequency but slightly different phase combine, they interfere with each other as shown in the figure. Waveforms in-phase (coherent) show constructive interference and produce a resultant of greater amplitude (*Cn*). Waveforms out of phase (incoherent) show destructive interference (*Ds*). Increasing phase differences give greater degrees of destructive interference until a 180° phase difference cause the signal to disappear giving a zero resultant.

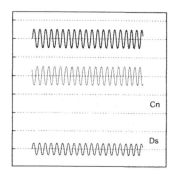

(*see* beat frequency).

interlacing (*image*) A method for reducing the bandwidth necessary to give a video display. Fields are interlaced to give each frame. Non-interlaced (progressive scan) displays require higher bandwidth, but have better resolution.

interleaved image acquisition (*mri*) Combined collection of data for two or more separate images; a subset of k-space samples for the second image is acquired immediately after the first image. This avoids misregistration between the two images and allows for accurate subtraction of the two images.

interleaved k-space coverage (*mri*) The sequential collection of raw data from multiple excitations such that each excitation samples multiple lines or curvilinear paths in k-space.

interleaved slices (*mri*) *See* slice sequence.

internal conversion (*nmed*) A nucleus in an excited state may interact with K or L shell electrons and transfer excess energy to these electrons. This internal conversion compliments electron capture. Internal conversion is a competing process with gamma ray emission and an internal conversion coefficient. The number of particles emitted per transition, or the fractional abundance, takes part in MIRD calculations. Since internal conversion creates a vacancy in an electron orbit of the atom characteristic x-rays and Auger electrons will be emitted which contribute to the total tissue radiation dose.

internal conversion coefficient (*nmed*) Describes the proportion of internal conversion events in a gamma decay process which blocks gamma emission as:

$$\frac{\text{Internal conversion process}}{\text{Gamma emission}}$$

This ratio can range from zero (all transitions result in gamma emission) to infinity (all transitions are internally converted: no gamma emission). It is estimated that 10.4% of all ^{99m}Tc nuclear transformations involve internal conversions by the K, L and to a lesser extent M shell electrons. About 40% of nuclear transformations involve internal conversion in the decay of ^{81m}Kr.

internal focus (*us*). A focus produced by a curved transducer element.

internal reflection (*phys*) This occurs when the reflection angle for the light source is >90° (*see* fibreoptics).

International Commission on Radiation Units and Measurement (*dose*) *See* ICRU.

International Commission on Radiological Protection (*dose*) *See* ICRP.

Internet (*comp*) A global network able to link up a large number of computers (millions). A computer joins the Internet via a modem or broadband router and adopts the standards and software set-up that allows it to take advantage of the services (e-mail, web, FTP file transfers) (*see* FTP, TCP/IP, e-mail, worldwide web).

interpolation (*math*) Estimation of a value of a variable between two known values. A mathematical method of averaging or smoothing images that are being displayed on a larger number of pixels than that for which they were originally reconstructed.

interpolation (nearest neighbour) (*image*) The simplest interpolation method basically making the pixels bigger. The greyscale or colour of an introduced pixel in the new image is the colour of the nearest pixel of the original image. Most image viewing and editing software use this type of interpolation for enlarging a digital image for closer examination; this does not change the greyscale/colour information of the image and does not introduce aliasing. It will increase the visibility of jaggies or pixelation.

interpolation (bicubic) (*image*) Produces smoother edges than bilinear interpolation. A new pixel is a bicubic function using 16 pixels in the nearest 4×4 neighbourhood of the pixel in the original image. This is the method most commonly used by image editing software, printer drivers and many digital cameras for resampling images.

interpolation (bilinear) (*image*) This determines the value of a new pixel based on a weighted average of the four pixels in the nearest 2×2 neighbourhood of the pixel in the original image. The averaging has an anti-aliasing effect and therefore produces relatively smooth edges with hardly any jaggies/pixelation.

interpolation (fractal) (*image*) Mainly useful for extreme enlargements; it retains the shape of features more accurately with cleaner, sharper edges and fewer halos and less blurring around the edges than would bicubic interpolation. An example is Genuine Fractals Pro from The Altamira Group.

interpolation algorithms (*ct*) To reconstruct an axial image from a helical data set, single-slice scanners have commonly used 180° linear interpolation algorithms. The z-sensitivity profile (imaged slice width) for the helical scan, with a $pitch_x = 1$, is similar to that of an axial image. On multi-slice scanners, the use of a 180° linear interpolator, in conjunction with $pitch_x = 1$, results in wider z-sensitivity profiles, and increased artefacts, in comparison to single-slice systems. Helical interpolation algorithms for multi-slice CT are different than those for single-section CT, but in general do not cause any increase in image artefacts compared with the algorithms for single-section helical CT and are generally much less noticeable in multi-slice CT because most scanning is performed at lower pitch values than was practical with single-section systems.

interpulse times (*mri*) Times between successive RF pulses used in pulse sequences. Particularly important are the inversion time (TI) in inversion recovery and the time between 90° pulse and the subsequent 180° pulse to produce a spin echo, which will be approximately one half the spin echo time (TE). The time between repetitions of pulse sequences is the repetition time (TR).

interscan delay time (ISD) (*ct*) Limitations to collecting data as sequential axial slices particularly when small lesions are being imaged since these can be missed if they are located between adjacent slices. The sequential slice protocol, although giving complete disc-like sections, includes delays between slices since the sequential process consists of:

- fan beam assembly accelerated to scan speed;
- x-ray tube pulsed and data collected;
- fan beam assembly halts and returns to its home position;
- table indexed to next longitudinal position while x-ray tube cools.

This series of events constitutes the interscan delay time and adds a significant time to the clinical study causing problems if the patient must hold their breath or patient movement is present.

inter-slice distance (*ct*) The distance between the adjacent nominal margins of consecutive slices in serial CT scanning. It is dependent upon the couch increment between slices.

intervention (*dose*) (ICRP60) Those activities which subtract from a person's overall radiation exposure. Controls applied to the source are usually the most effective interventional methods, e.g. improved quantum efficiency of detection (imaging) and heavier shielding (*see* practices (ICRP)).

intra-arterial (*clin*) Relating to substances (contrast media) injected or deposited into an artery.

intracellular (*clin*) Within the cell.

intrathecal (*clin*) Within either subarachnoid or subdural space.

intrathecal contrast media (*cm*) Water-soluble contrast media can enter the brain by diffusion. Penetration of brain tissue by contrast media after intrathecal injection has been observed by both ionic and non-ionic contrast material, causing a variety of changes and reactions due to chemotoxic effects. Unlike the blood–brain barrier, there appears to be nothing similar between the cerebral spinal fluid and extracellular fluid of the brain.

■ Reference: Dawson and Clauss, 1999.

intravenous (*clin*) Relating to substances (contrast media) injected or deposited into a vein.

intravenous cholangiography (*clin*) Where intravenously injected, contrast medium is excreted into the bile by hepatocytes. The contrast medium concentrates in the gall bladder and is excreted in the faeces and urine unchanged. There is strong binding to plasma proteins.

intravenous cholecystography (*clin*) Slow injection of contrast medium over a period of 1 hour. Replaced in some instances by endoscopic retrograde cholangiography (ERC) or percutaneous transhepatic cholangiography (PTC).

intravoxel incoherent motion (*mri*) Diffusion and perfusion both act to reduce the signal observed *in vivo*; the two effects are difficult to separate and the term 'intravoxel incoherent motion' is used to describe their combined effect.

intravoxel phase dispersion (*mri*) Signal loss due to spread of spin phases within a voxel (usually because of motion or susceptibility effects).

intrinsic efficiency (*image*) The quantum efficiency of a system (imaging detector) when all external devices (collimation) have been removed.

intrinsic resolution (*image*) The primary resolution of the gamma camera crystal without its collimator. This is usually measured by using a slit source placed directly on the crystal face and a line spread function obtained.

interval cancer (screening) (*clin*) The incidence of disease between screening intervals and after a negative test result. Results are false negative if a cancer becomes known within 1 year of a screening result. After that time it becomes an interval cancer (*see* incidence (screening)).

interventional level (*dose*) (ICRP60) A value of equivalent or effective dose at which intervention measures should be considered.

intranet (*comp*) An internal network of computers (RIS or HIS) controlled by a network administrator who decides access privileges and controls the software. A network maintained by a company that is only available to its staff or other authorized users and looks like a private Internet.

intra-osseus venography (*clin*) Intra-osseus venography visualizes the pelvic veins or lower limb veins where the contrast medium is introduced via a cannula directly inserted into the medullary space of the greater femoral trochanter or lateral malleolus.

intravascular space (*clin*) Within the vessel (blood or lymphatic).

intravenous angiocardiography (*clin*) Usually performed on children or young adults when catheter procedures are unsuitable.

intravenous cholangiography (*clin*) Radiography of the bile ducts opacified by hepatic secretion of intravenously injected contrast medium.

intravenous cholecystangiography (*clin*) Demonstrates the extrahepatic biliary tree and gall-bladder (*see* Biligrafin).

intravenous pyelography (IVP) (*clin*) *See* intravenous urography (IVU).

intravenous urography (IVU) (*clin*) Radiography of kidneys, ureters and bladder following injection of contrast medium into a perpheral vein (also called excretory urography) (*see* nephrotomography, zonography).

intravoxel incoherent motion (*mri*) Diffusion and perfusion both act to reduce the signal observed *in vivo*; the two effects are difficult to separate and the term 'intravoxel incoherent motion' is used to describe their combined effect.

intravoxel phase dispersion (*mri*) Signal loss due to spread of spin phases within a voxel (usually because of motion or susceptibility effects).

intrinsic filtration (*ct*) Filtration of an x-ray beam by the component parts of the x-ray housing (x-ray tube envelope glass or exit window); the intrinsic beam filtration is also caused by the anode itself, the oil used for cooling (*see* added filtration).

intrinsic quantum efficiency (*ct*) Absorption of an x-ray photon by the scintillator host lattice generates numerous free electrons and holes in the conduction and valence bands, respectively. Once the electron-hole pairs are captured and bound to a selected site, the recombination energy of these pairs is transferred to that site where radiative (luminescence) energy is emitted. Ideally, there is a fast recombination of electron-hole pairs at the activator sites (luminescent centres). In this way, a useful scintillator will produce several thousand visible photons from the absorption of one x-ray photon.

intrinsic resolution (*nmed*) The primary resolution of the gamma camera crystal without its collimator. This is usually measured by using a slit source placed directly on the crystal face and a line spread function obtained.

intrinsic semiconductor (*elec*) A pure semiconductor where hole and electron densities are practically equal. Used for the manufacture of detectors; the so-called hyperpure germanium (HpGe).

invalid page fault (*comp*) Caused when a page of data or program code in the swap file cannot, for various reasons, be loaded into the main memory.

invariant (*image*) The response of a system is the same at every position of the x axis (*see* convolution).

invasive probe (*us*) An ultrasound probe that is intended to contact tissue other than intact skin or the surface of the eye. These include transvaginal, transoesophageal, transrectal, transurethral, intravascular and intraoperative probes.

inverse Fourier transform (*math*) Form of the Fourier transform that reverses the process, e.g. if the Fourier transform is used to analyze a function of time into its equivalent frequency components, the inverse Fourier transform will synthesize that function of time from these frequency components.

inverse image transform (*di*) Process of synthesis, reassembling the original image from its components via summation.

inverse square law (*phys, dose*) The reduction of radiation intensity from an isotropic point source (I_d) at a distance d will vary as I_d/d^2. Variations on this basic formula can be used for calculating intensities or doses at different distances.

Inverse square law

1 The radiation dose rate at 30 cm from a point source is $7.5\,\mu Sv\,hr^{-1}$. If the known dose $7.5\,\mu Sv$ is I_d at distance d, then dose rate I_{dn} at 80 cm (d_n) is:

$$I_{dn} = \frac{I_d \times d^2}{d_n^2} = \sim 1\mu Sv\,h^{-1}.$$

2 The distance that reduces $7.5\,\mu Sv\,h^{-1}$ at 10 cm to $2.5\,\mu Sv\,h^{-1}$ is:

$$d_n^2 = \frac{I_d \times d^2}{I_{dn}} = 55\,cm.$$

---

inversely proportional (*math*) Describes two numbers, one of which is in a constant ratio to

the reciprocal of the other, $x \propto 1/y$, so x is inversely proportional to y. Examples would be resolution and sensitivity in nuclear imaging and distance and dose from a point source: the inverse square law.

inversion (*mri*) The magnetization vector orientated opposite to the magnetic field produced by 180° pulse or gradient switching. A nonequilibrium state where the macroscopic magnetization vector is oriented opposed to the magnetic field; produced by adiabatic fast passage or 180° RF pulses.

inversion recovery (*mri*) A pulse sequence where the nuclear magnetization is inverted prior to a spin-echo pulse sequence by an initial 180° pulse. The time between the 180° pulse and the SE sequence is the inversion time TI. The signal is dependent primarily on T1 (the image is T1 weighted). Imaging time is relatively long due to long TR.

inversion recovery sequence (*mri*) A pulse sequence where the nuclear magnetization is inverted prior to a spin-echo pulse sequence. The time between the 180° pulse and the SE sequence is the inversion time TI; an initial 180° pulse to invert the magnetization followed by a spin-echo or gradient-echo sequence. Representation of data from image acquisition as a two-dimensional matrix of points. The coordinates of each point represent a unique combination of frequency and phase corresponding to the time-integral of the frequency- and phase-encoding gradients, respectively.

inversion-recovery-spin-echo (IRSE) (*mri*) Form of inversion-recovery imaging in which the signal is detected as a spin echo. For YE short compared to the 72 relaxation time, there will be only a small effect of T2 differences on image intensities; for longer TEs, the effect of T2 may be significant.

inversion time (TI) (*mri*) *See* inversion recovery.

inversion transfer (*mri*) *See* saturation transfer.

inverter (*phys*) Any circuit that converts d.c. to a.c. A common component in high frequency x-ray generators.

in vitro (*xray*) Literally 'in glass', referring to a preparation outside the body, e.g. *in vitro* labelling of red blood cells; the radionuclide labelling is carried out under sterile conditions in the laboratory and then the preparation reinjected.

in vivo (*xray*) Literally 'in life', referring to a procedure that occurs within the body, e.g. *in vivo* labelling of red cells when the radionuclide is

---

post-injected after a previous injection prepares the cells for labelling (pyrophosphate).

I/O port (comp) A connector on the back of a computer for accepting input or output data from an
external device.

iobenguane (nmed) m-Iodobenzylguanidine, a
Bristol-Myers-Squibb preparation for MIBG.

iobitridol (cm) For angiography, venography,
urography, arthrography, angiocardiography
and hysterosalpingography (Guerbet).

Compound	Viscosity (cP)	Osmolality (mOsm/kg)	Iodine (mg I/mL)
Iobitridol	4–10	585–915	250–350

iocetamic acid (clin) An x-ray contrast medium;
generic name for Cholebrine.

iodamide compounds (clin) Ionic monomer x-ray
contrast material. A water-soluble, monomeric,
ionic x-ray contrast medium based on tri-
iodinated benzoic acid (see Uromiro).

iodecol (cm) Non-ionic dimer with low toxicity,
but insufficiently water soluble for clinical
applications.

iodine (I) (elem)

Atomic number (Z)	53
Relative atomic mass (A$_r$)	126.9
Density (ρ) kg/m^3	4940
Melting point (K)	386.6
K-edge (keV)	33.1

Relevance to radiology: Complex compounds of iodine
are used as x-ray contrast for vascular studies.

^{123}Iodine (nmed) Used for Na^{123}I in capsules for
thyroid function and morphology (scintigraphy).
An important radionuclide for imaging; ideal for
imaging using labelled compounds (hippuran,
MIBG), thyroid tests and labelling fatty acids,
monoclonal antibodies and proteins.

Production (cyclotron)	$^{122}_{52}$Te(d,n)$^{123}_{53}$I
	or $^{124}_{54}$Xe(p,2n)$^{123}_{55}$Cs
	$\rightarrow ^{123}$Xe $\rightarrow ^{123}$I(preferred)
	(European: ^{127}I(p,5n)^{123}Xe)
Decay scheme (e.c.)^{123}I	^{123}I $T_{\frac{1}{2}}$ 13 h(159keV)
	$\rightarrow ^{123}$Te 1.2 × 1013 years
Gamma ray constant	4.4 × 10^{-2} mSv h^{-1}GBq^{-1}
	at 1 m
Photons (abundance)	27 keV (0.86)
	159 keV (0.834)
	529 keV (0.014)
Half value layer	0.4 mm Pb, 46 mm water

^{125}Iodine (nmed) As a label for in vitro radioimmunoassay tests and sometimes as a thyroid
therapy agent.

Production (reactor)	$^{124}_{54}$Xe (n,γ) $^{125}_{54}$Xe $\rightarrow ^{125}$Xe $\rightarrow ^{125}$I
Decay scheme (e.c.) ^{125}I	^{125}I (27 keV x-ray) :^{125}Te stable
Gamma ray constant	3.4 × 10^{-2} mSv h^{-1}GBq^{-1} at 1 m
Annual limit on intake	1.5 MBq (0.04 mCi)
Photons (abundance) x-rays	35 (0.07)
	27–32 (1.40)
Half value layer	0.02 mm Pb

Physical decay for ^{125}iodine

Days	Fraction remaining
1	0.989
2	0.977
5	0.944
10	0.891
15	0.841
20	0.794
25	0.750
30	0.708
40	0.631
50	0.562
60	0.501

Shielding for ^{125}iodine

Lead thickness (mm)	Attenuation factor
0.017	0.5
0.058	10^{-1}
0.12	10^{-2}
0.2	10^{-3}
0.28	10^{-4}

^{125}Iodine (iothalamate) (nmed) Sodium iothalamate having been iodinated with ^{125}iodine; for
the determination of the glomerular filtration
rate (GFR) (see Glofil®).

^{125}Iodine (albumin) (nmed) Radioactive iodinated serum albumin (RISA) (see Isojex®).

^{129}Iodine (nmed) As a substitute calibration
source for ^{125}iodine.

Production	^n_nX(x,x) ^n_nY
Decay scheme (first stage) ^{129}I	^{129}I $T_{\frac{1}{2}}$ 1.57 × 107 years (38 KeV)
	$\rightarrow ^{129}$Xe stable
Photons (abundance)	30–35 keV (0.69)
	40 keV (0.075)
Half-life	1.57 × 10^{7}y
Decay constant	4.414E-8 y^{-1}
Gamma ray constant	1.7 × 10^{-2} mSv h^{-1}GBq^{-1} at 1 m
Half value layer	0.02 mm Pb

^{131}Iodine–iodixanol

^{131}Iodine (*nmed*) Thyroid function tests. Therapy for thyrotoxicosis and thyroid cancer

Production (reactor)	$^{235}_{92}$U $(n,f)\,^{131}_{52}$Te $\rightarrow ^{131}$I
Decay scheme (first stage) ^{131}I	^{131}I $T\frac{1}{2}$ 8.0 days $(\beta-,\,\gamma$ 364 keV) $\rightarrow ^{131}$Xe stable
Photons (abundance)	80 (0.026)
	284 (0.061)
	364 (0.812)
	637 (0.073)
	723 (0.018)
Decay constant	0.086194 day^{-1}
Gamma ray constant	5.7×10^{-2} m Svh^{-1} GBq^{-1} at 1 m
Half value layer	2.4 mm Pb, 63 mm water

Physical decay for ^{131}iodine

Days	Fraction remaining
0	1.000
1	0.917
2	0.842
3	0.772
4	0.708
5	0.650
6	0.596
7	0.547
8	0.502
9	0.460
10	0.422
11	0.387
12	0.355
13	0.326
14	0.299

Shielding for ^{131}iodine

Lead thickness (mm)	Attenuation factor
2.40	0.5
8.90	10^{-1}
16.0	10^{-2}
25.5	10^{-3}
37.0	10^{-4}

iodine content (contrast medium) (*cm*) Viscosity and osmolality of a contrast medium are related to the iodine content or concentration of the contrast medium solution, referred to as its strength in milligrams of iodine per millilitre (mg I mL^{-1}). The opacifying power of the contrast medium solution increases with its strength along with osmolality and viscosity; the physiological tolerance declines. This makes it necessary to have several different strengths (in mg I mL^{-1}) for each contrast medium preparation.

Contrast agent	Iodine content (mg mL^{-1})		Viscosity (mPa.s)
	20°C	37°C	
Iotrolan	300	17.8	9.5
Diatrizoate	306	–	5.0
Ioxaglate	320	14.6	9.5
Iodixanol	320	24.6	12.2
Iopentol	350	21.9	11.2
Iohexol	350	21.9	11.2
Iopromide	350	20.1	9.5
Iopamidol	370	18.7	9.8

iodine ratio (contrast medium) (*cm*) Iodine content is a measure of radiopacity; this is measured as a ratio of iodine atoms to particles or ions. The ionic-monomer contrast material dissociates into two ions: anion and cation. The anion carries three atoms of iodine between the two ions, so the ratio of iodine atoms to ions is 3:2 or 1.5:1 (ratio 1.5). The ionic dimer carries six iodine atoms for the two ions, so has an iodine ratio of 6:2 or 3:1 (ratio 3). The nonionic-monomer does not dissociate so has an iodine ratio of 3:1 (ratio 3). Their osmolalities are about half that of ionic monomer, or 2.5–3 times the osmolality of blood at the highest available concentrations. The non-ionic dimer has a ratio of 6:1 (ratio 6). Non-ionic dimeric contrast media have two linked iodinated benzene rings. These molecules have six iodine atoms per particle ('ratio 6').

iodine release (contrast medium) (*cm*) Elemental iodine is normally not a degradation product of contrast media. The release of colourless iodide ion occurs in both non-ionic and ionic CM. This is catalyzed by heavy metal ions, pH value, light exposure and increased temperature.

■ Reference: Dawson and Clauss, 1999.

iodipamide (*clin*) The group of ionic x-ray contrast media that contain the meglumine salt of iodipamide. A large molecule contrast medium appearing commercially as Biligrafin and Endografin.

iodixanol (*cm*) Non-ionic dimer for cerebral angiography, cardiac and peripheral arteriography, urography, venography, ERCP, hysterosalpingography and gastrointestinal studies.

Iodine (mg/mL)	Osmolality	Viscosity
150–320	290	12.2

(*see* Visipaque®).

iodohippurate (*nmed*) A compound which is completely excreted by the renal tubules and completely extracted on its first pass through the renal capillary system. ^{123}I-ortho-iodohippurate is used in scintigraphy/renography for the accurate estimation of renal function.

Iodotope˟ (*nmed*) ^{131}Iodine-labelled sodium iodide (Bracco) for thyroid uptake and therapy.

iodoxamic acid (*clin*) Generic name for Endomirabil.

iofetamine/iofetaminal (*nmed*) An amphetamine analogue, rapidly taken up by the lungs and from there redistributed primarily to the brain and liver. Labelled with ^{123}I, it is used as a brain imaging agent in the localization and evaluation of certain kinds of stroke.

ioflupane (*nmed*) Radio-iodinated cocaine analogue (^{123}I-FP-CIT or ^{123}I-β-CIT-FP). Chemical form: N-w-fluoropropyl-2β-carbomethoxy-3β-(4-iodophenyl)-nortropane. As ^{123}I-ioflupane used for detecting loss of functional dopaminergic neuron terminals in the striatum of patients with clinically uncertain Parkinsonian syndromes helping to differentiate essential tremor from Parkinsonian syndromes related to idiopathic Parkinson's disease (PD), multiple system atrophy (MSA), progressive supranuclear palsy (PSP). It is claimed that the binding of ioflupane reflects the number of dopaminergic neurons in the substantia nigra (*see* DaTSCAN®).

ioglycamide compounds (*cm*) Aliphatic acid salts as meglumine salt of ioglycamic acid for cholecystographic contrast media. Has pharmacokinetic action similar to iodipamide group of compounds. Preferentially excreted into the bile and a small proportion enters enterohepatic reabsorbtion (*see* Biligram®, ipodate group).

iohexol (*cm*) Low osmolar 880, non-ionic monomer contrast media and tri-iodinated substituted ring compound do not dissociate in solution, so that hypertonicity is avoided. Side chains have been altered to make molecules highly hydrophilic to increase solubility without dissociation. Increased ratio of iodine per osmotic particle (3:2 for ionic) versus (3:1 for non-ionic) osmolality halved (non-ionic).

Agent	Viscosity (cP)	Osmolality (mOsm/kg)	Iodine (mg I mL^{-1})
Iohexol	11.2	862	350

(*see* Omnipaque®).

iomeprol (*cm*) Non-ionic monomer for angiography and CT introduced by Bracco in 1995; containing up to 400 mg I mL^{-1}

Agent	Viscosity (cP)	Osmolality (mOsm/kg)	Iodine (mg I mL^{-1})
Iomeprol	1.4–12.6	300–726	150–400

(*see* Imeron®, Iomeron®).

Iomeron˟ (*cm*) Commercial form of iomeprol (Bracco) produced in iodine concentrations of 150, 200, 250, 300, 350 and 400 mg I mL^{-1} (30.62–81.65%)

Compound	Viscosity (cP)	Osmolality (mOsm/kg)	Iodine (mg I mL^{-1})
Iiomeprol	2.0–27.5 at 20°C, 1.4–12.6 at 37°C	300–726	150–400

ion (*phys*) An electrically charged particle formed when one or more electrons is lost by an atom either by ionizing radiation *hf*:

$$H_2O + hf \rightarrow H^+ + OH^-$$

or when an ionic compound is dissolved in water:

$$(NaCl \rightarrow Na^+ + Cl^-).$$

ion beam (**cyclotron**) (*nmed*) Most hospital cyclotrons accelerate negative hydrogen ions (H$^-$) since negative ions have a higher extraction efficiency. A filament in the ion source assembly puts a negative charge on the hydrogen ion by the addition of two electrons. These are stripped to protons by a carbon stripper foil prior to bombarding the target. H$^- \rightarrow$ p + e$^-$. Larger cyclotron accelerate both negative and positive ions.

Ion source	Name
H$^-$ (p)	Negative hydrogen ion, as proton source
^{2}H$^-$ (D)	Deuteron
^{3}H$^-$ (t)	Triton
^{3}He$^+$	Helium ion
^{4}He$^+$	Alpha (α)

At the extraction port, carbon stripper foils remove electrons from the negative ions leaving positively charged ions (a H$^+$ proton or a D$^+$ deuteron). A single or dual beam can be obtained.

---

ion dose (I) (*dose*) The dose delivered by ionizing radiation. It is the quotient of dQ and dm, where dQ is the electrical charge of the ions of one sign produced by radiation in air having a volume of dV; d$m_a = \rho_a \times$ dV is the mass of air with density ρ_a so that $I =$ dQ/dm_a. Ion dose is measured in Coulombs per kilogram (C kg^{-1}), replacing the roentgen (*see* dosimetry, cavity ion dose, standard ion dose).

ion pair (*phys*) A pair of negative and positive charged ions caused by ionizing radiation. Ion pairs are formed in gas detectors which give the signal.

ion source (cyclotron) (*phys*) A source of charged particles in a particle accelerator. Hydrogen or helium gas is ionized by means of an electron beam or electric discharge, yielding positive and negative ions The latter are either simple electrons or added electrons to a neutral atom. Conversion of negative ions to the positive state (protons) is achieved in a gas or thin metal foil strippers. In radio frequency (20 MHz) ion sources, a plasma is produced in a gas contained in a glass vessel. Some common ions used in particle accelerators are: ^{1}H$\pm$, ^{2}H, ^{3}H, D+, ^{3}He++, ^{4}He++) (*see* cyclotron).

ion toxicity (*cm*) A surplus or deficit of various ions in the solution.

ionic (*clin*) Ionic compounds will dissociate into anions and cations when dissolved in water. Contrast media which are chemically salts of organic compounds containing iodine. Ionic contrast media will dissociate into two particles, one anion and one cation when dissolved in water. The anions are iodinated benzoic acid. They might occur as single benzoic rings (monomeric contrast media) like diatrizoate, metrizoate or iothalamate, or as two connected rings (dimeric contrast media) like iocarmate or ioxaglate. The cations are either metals: Na+, Ca++, Mg++ or organic cations like meglumine (methylglucosamine). Ionic monomeric contrast media will have a high osmolarity of greater than seven times the osmolarity of blood at the highest clinical concentrations. Ionic dimeric contrast media have a lower osmolarity, but most often higher chemotoxicity.

ionic contrast medium (*cm*) These are salts of weak organic acids containing iodine, water soluble that will split into an anion and cation (ions or particles) when dissolved. These agents are based on the six-carbon benzoic acid ring rather than the earlier five-carbon pyridine ring. This structure is able to carry three atoms of iodine and is therefore more radiopaque. Two substituted benzoic acids came into common usage: diatrizoate and its predecessor, iothalamate. These fully substituted benzoic acids include three iodine molecules per unit and are completely dissociated in solution. The anion component is the iodinated benzene ring, where one of the side chains is a weak organic acid (benzoic acid). They are either single rings; monomeric contrast media, such as diatrizoate, metrizoic acid/metrizoate compounds or iothalamate, or double-linked rings as dimeric contrast media, such as ioxaglate or iocarmate. In summary:

- ionic monomer: one tri-iodobenzene ring (metrizoate, Isopaque, diatrizoate, Hypaque);
- ionic dimer with two tri-iodobenzene rings (ioxaglate, Hexabrix).

Cations (not radiopaque) are either inorganic such as sodium, calcium or magnesium, or organic such as meglumine. Current formulations have meglumine, sodium, or a mixture of both depending on the formulation of the manufacturer. Ionic contrast media have high osmolality five to ten times that of normal serum, which is associated with unwanted side effects.

ionic dimer (*clin*) These have intermediate viscosity, intermediate i.v. tolerance.

Ionic dimer

Examples: ioxaglate, iodine atoms to particles ratio: 6:2 or 3:1, osmolar concentration to blood at 300 mg: ×2.

Generic name	Trade name	Iodine ratio	Viscosity (cP)	Osmolality (mOsm/ kg H$_2$O)
Ioxaglate	Hexabrix	3:1	12 at 20°C, 6 at 37°C	600

ionic monomer (*clin*) These x-ray contrast materials have the lowest viscosity, the highest osmotoxicity and the lowest i.v. tolerance. (*cm*) Hypertonic contrast medium between 1500 and

2000 mOsm/kg water (blood, 300 mOsm/kg). The general structure being:

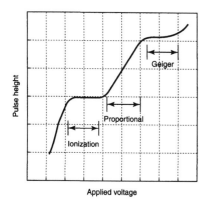

Ionic monomer

Generic name	Trade name	Iodine ratio	Viscosity (cP)	Osmolality (mOsm/ kg H₂O)
Iothalamate	Conray	1.5:1	5–9 at 20°C, 3–5 at 37°C	1500–1600
Diatrizoate	Vasoray			
Metrizoate	Isopaque			
Amidotrizoate	Urografin			
Ioxithalamate	Angiografin			
	Gastrografin			
	Telebrix			

ionization (*phys*) Loss of an orbital electron from an atom forming a charged ion. The production of negative or positive ions. A neutral atom or molecule acquires or loses an electric charge. Certain compounds (electrolytes) ionize in solution: $NaCl \rightarrow Na^+ + Cl_2$ forming cations and anions, respectively.

ionization chamber (*phys*) An enclosed volume of gas (air, nitrogen, argon, xenon), the enclosure forming one electrode and the other electrode centrally placed. A high voltage is applied (typically 200–400 volts) and the small ionization currents collected by a charge amplifier. These detectors are integration devices and if air filled are tissue equivalent. The thickness of

the enclosure can be increased to encourage secondary electron formation (*see* **gas** ionization chamber (CT), Geiger counter, proportional counter).

ionization potential (*phys*) The minimum energy necessary to remove an orbital electron from an atom causing ionization.

ionizing radiation (*phys*) Electromagnetic radiation (x- or gamma rays) or particulate radiation (alpha particles, beta particles, electrons, positrons, protons, neutrons and heavy particles) capable of producing ions by direct or secondary processes in passage through matter (*see* radiation (ionizing)).

Ionising Radiations Regulations (1985) IRR85 (*dose*) (UK) ICRP 26 recommendations were published as directives 80/836, then 84/467 EURATOM Basic Safety Standards adopted by the UK as the Ionising Radiation Regulations 1985 (IRR85). ICRP60 and subsequent directive 96/29/EURATOM revised the basic safety standards and were adopted by the UK as Ionising Radiations Regulations (1999) IRR99 which replaced this IRR85 legislation (*see* Ionising Radiation (Protection of Persons undergoing Medical Examination or Treatment) 1988).

Ionising Radiations Regulations (1999) IRR99 (*dose*) (UK) ICRP60 and subsequent directive 96/29/EURATOM revised the basic safety standards and were adopted by the UK as IRR99, replacing Ionising Radiations Regulations (1985) IRR85. They relate principally to the protection of workers and the public, but also address the equipment aspects of patient protection. The essential legal requirements arising out of this legislation are: authorization, notification, prior risk assessment, restriction of exposure, maintenance and examination of controls, contingency plans, radiation protection adviser, information, dose limits, instruction, training, designated areas, local rules, classified persons, duties of manufacturers, QA programmes.

Ionising Radiation (Medical Exposure) Regulations (2000) IR(ME)R2000 (*dose*) (UK) These relate to patient protection as set out in European Council Directive 97/43/Euratom of June 30, 1997 'The Medical Exposures Directive', derived from ICRP60, replacing Ionising Radiation (Protection of Patients Undergoing Medical Examination or Treatment (POPUMET) Regulations 1988. The essential legal requirements dealt with in these regulations are: duties

Applied voltage

of employers, duties of the practitioner, operator and referrer, justification of medical exposures, optimization, clinical audit, expert advice, equipment and training.

Ionising Radiation (Protection of Persons Undergoing Medical Examination or Treatment) Regulations (POPUMET) (1988) (*dose*) (UK) ICRP 26 recommendations were published as 84/466/EURATOM (Patient Protection) and adopted by the UK as these regulations. Directive 97/43/EURATOM 'The Medical Exposures Directive', derived from ICRP60 replaced this 1988 Act with Ionising Radiation (Medical Exposure) Regulations (2000) IR(ME)R2000.

Ionising Radiations Incident Database (IRID) (*dose*) (UK) In 1996, the National Radiological Protection Board (NRPB), the Health and Safety Executive (HSE) and the Environment Agency (EA) jointly established the Ionising Radiations Incident Database (IRID) extending back to 1974 in the UK. The objectives of the database are to act as a reference for radiation incidents, primarily in the non-nuclear sector and provide analyses of data that help in assessing priorities in resource allocation.

ion toxicity (*cm*) A surplus or deficit of various ions in the solution.

Iopamidol* (*cm*) Introduced in 1981 by Bracco, available as monomeric, low osmolar, water-soluble, non-ionic contrast medium, tri-iodinated substituted ring compound. Does not dissociate in solution so that hypertonicity is avoided. Side chains have been altered to make molecules highly hydrophilic to increase solubility without dissociation. An aqueous solution (Gastromiro®) for oral administration is used for gastrointestinal diagnosis.

Compound	Viscosity	Osmolality	Iodine (mg/mL)
Iopamidol	2.0–9.4	413–796	200–370

(*see* Iopamiron®, Iopamiro®, Solutrast®, Niopam®, Isovue®).

Iopamiro* (*cm*) Preparation of the non-ionic monomer iopamidol introduced by Bracco in 1981.

Compound	Viscosity (cP)	Osmolality mOsm/kg	Iodine (mg I mL^{-1})
Iopamidol (306.2–755.3 mg)	2.0–9.4 @ 37°C	413–796	150–370

(*see* Iopamiron®).

Iopamiron® (*cm*) A preparation of the non-ionic monomer iopamidol introduced by Bracco as Iopamiro® in 1981 having 370 mg I mL^{-1} and an osmolarity of 796 (*see* solutrast, Niopam, Isovue).

iopanoic acid (*clin*) Generic name for Telepaque.

iopentol (*clin*) A non-ionic monomer for vascular use produced by Nycomed/Amersham (GE Healthcare)

Compound	Viscosity (cP)	Osmolality mOsm/kg	Iodine (mg I mL^{-1})
Iopentol	12.0	680	350

(*see* Imagopaque®).

iopodate compounds (*clin*) Ionic x-ray contrast media comprising sodium and calcium ipodate manufactured by Schering AG for oral administration as Biloptin.

iopromide (*cm*) Non-ionic monomeric x-ray contrast material for angiography, digital subtraction angiography (DSA), intravenous urogram (IVU), venography, hysterosalpingography, fistulography and general CT applications.

Compound	Viscosity (cP)	Osmolality mOsm/kg	Iodine (mg I mL^{-1})
Iopromide 62.3%	9.5 at 20°C; 4.6 at 37°C	610	370

(*see* Ultravist).

iothalamic acid/iothalamate compounds (*cm*) Conventional high osmolar monomeric ionic contrast medium developed in the 1960s; salts of tri-iodinated benzoic acid (sodium) as the anion iothalamate is the radiopaque portion, but both the anion and cation are osmotically active so will be hypertonic to plasma.

Compound	Viscosity (cP)	Osmolality mOsm/kg	Iodine (mg I mL^{-1})
Na-iothalamate	2.7 at 37°C	1843	325

(*see* Conray®, osmolality).

Iothalamate [^{125}I] (*nmed*) Sodium iothalamate having been iodinated with ^{125}iodine; for the determination of the glomerular filtration rate (GFR).

Generic name	Iothalamate
Commercial names	Glofil®
Non-imaging category	Glomerular filtration (GFR)

iotrolan/iotrol (*cm*) Hydrophilic non-ionic dimeric aqueous preparation isotonic with CSF.

Compound	Viscosity (cP)	Osmolality mOsm/kg	Iodine (mg I mL^{-1})
Iotrolan	9.1 at 37°C	360	300

(*see* Isovist®).

iotroxate (meglumine) (*cm*) For intravenous cholegraphy and cholecystography (*see* Biliscopin®).

ioversol (*cm*) A non-ionic x-ray agent for cerebral angiography produced by Mallinckrodt as Optiray.

Compound	Viscosity (cP)	Osmolality mOsm/kg	Iodine (mg I mL^{-1})
Ioversol	5.0 at 37°C	780	339–741

ioxaglate/ioxaglic acid (*cm*) Ionic dimer produced as Hexabrix®

Compound	Viscosity (cP)	Osmolality mOsm/kg	Iodine (mg I mL^{-1})
Ioxaglate	6.2 at 37°C	560	300

ioxilan (*cm*) Intra-arterial (cerebral, cardiac and aortography), intravenous (CT head and body, excretory urography)

Compound	Viscosity (cP)	Osmolality mOsm/kg	Iodine (mg I mL^{-1})
Ioxilan	5.1–8.1	585–695	300–350

(*see* Oxilan®).

ioxithalamate compounds (*clin*) Ionic monomer x-ray contrast material (*see* Telebrix®).

IP (*comp*) Internet protocol, an addressing system of TCP/IP that governs packet forwarding.

IP (Internet protocol) address (*comp*) An Internet protocol address is a unique set of numbers used to locate another computer on a network. The format of an IP address is a 32-bit string of four numbers separated by periods. Each number can be from 0 to 255. Within a closed network IP addresses may be assigned at random, but IP addresses of web servers must be registered to avoid duplicates.

IPA (*mri*) See integrated panorama array.

iPAT (*mri*) Integrated parallel acquisition techniques. Siemens' procedure for reducing acquisition time.

IPP (*mri*) Integrated panoramic positioning.

ipodate group (*cm*) Sodium and calcium ipodate absorbed after oral administration and excreted in the bile. These compounds undergo entero-hepatic re-absorption (*see* cholegraphic contrast agents, ioglycamide group, Biligrafin®, Biloptin®).

IPX (*comp*) Internet packet exchange, a NetWare protocol that provides connectionless communications between devices on a network. (*mri*) See inversion recovery.

IRC (*comp*) Inter relay chat; using the Internet like a CB (citizens' band) radio.

IR-EPI (*mri*) Inversion recovery echo planar imaging.

IRFGR (*mri*) Inversion recovery fast gradient recalled acquisition in the steady state.

iridium (Ir) (*elem*)

Atomic number (Z)	77
Relative atomic mass (A$_r$)	192.2
Density (ρ) kg/m^3	22 420
Melting point (K)	2716
K-edge (keV)	76.1

Relevance to radiology: ^{192}Ir used as a short half-life (74 days) therapy nuclide. $^{191\,m}$Ir has been used as a generator-derived nuclide for cardiology.

iris (*xray*) A circular diaphragm placed behind a lens system for adjusting its aperture and improving the image depth.

iron (Fe) (*elem*)

Atomic number (Z)	26
Relative atomic mass (A$_r$)	55.84
Density (ρ) kg/m^3	7870
Melting point (K)	1808
Specific heat capacity, J kg^{-1}K^{-1}	449
Thermal conductivity, W m^{-1}K^{-1}	80.2
K-edge (keV)	7.1

Relevance to radiology: As a general x-ray shielding material or as shielding for low background laboratories (old stock).

^{55}Iron

Nuclear data ^{55}Fe	
Half-life	2.7 years
Decay mode	e.c. 100% x-rays
Decay constant	0.2566 years^{-1}
Photons (abundance)	5.9–6.5 keV

^{59}Iron

Production	
Half life	44 days
Decay mode	β − 1.562 MeV
Decay constant	0.01575 years^{-1}
Photons (abundance)	1.0 MeV (0.56)
	1.2 MeV (0.43)

Uses in radiology: Both nuclides are used for tracer studies in iron metabolism.

iron-binding (*nmed*) Forming protein complexes, particularly concerned with trapping ^{67}Gallium. Gallium is believed to localize in inflammatory lesions by diffusing across 'leaky' capillaries into the extracellular space and binding to proteins that are in relatively high concentrations in inflammatory lesions. Other iron binding proteins are:

- Transferrin: a primary transport protein for ^{67}Ga within the circulatory system;
- Lactoferrin: stored within specific leucocyte granules and is released by the leucocytes at sites of inflammation;
- Ferritin: an intracellular protein, which mediates uptake of iron/gallium within bacteria;
- Siderophores: low molecular weight compounds produced by bacteria that also mediate uptake of iron/gallium within bacteria.

IRQ (*comp*) Interrupt request signals are used by devices to interrupt the processor in order to gain priority. For example, a keyboard generates an interrupt signal indicating that an event has occurred when a key is pressed that requires an action. Each device must have its own IRQ or conflicts will occur.

IRR99 (*rad*) See **Ionising Radiations Regulations (1999) IRR99.**

IR(ME)R2000 (*rad*) See **Ionising Radiation (Medical Exposure) Regulations (2000) IR(ME)R2000.**

IRSE (*mri*) See **inversion-recovery-spin-echo.**

irradiance (*phys*) The flux per unit area received by a surface element or radiant flux falling on an area of surface divided by the area. The unit is $W\,m^{-2}$. It describes the irradiance level on a surface and is used in hazard and safety analysis (*see* flux).

irradiation (*phys*) Exposure of a material (or tissue) to radiation, either non-ionizing (UV) or ionizing (x-rays, gamma rays, alpha/beta particles, neutrons etc.).

ISA (*comp*) Industry standard architecture. The original PC set up which allows extras to be added to a system by connecting plug-in adapter cards into slots on the computer motherboard.

ischaemia (*clin*) Insufficient blood supply. Myocardial ischaemia being insufficient blood supply to the myocardium, usually caused by reduced diameter of the coronary arteries, ultimately causing myocardial infarction (myocardium (stunned), hibernating myocardium).

ISDN (*comp*) Integrated services digital network. A telecommunications standard for sending digitized voice, video and data signals over the existing public switched telephone network. It increases the amount of information that can be transmitted over regular phone lines, supporting speeds of up to 64 Kbps. Routers and other communication devices connect to ISDN through standardized interfaces. Two channels combine to give 128 kbits per second data transfer or one channel giving a 64 kbps Internet access, while using the other channel for voice analogue (*see* ADSL, modem).

ISIS (*mri*) Image selected *in vivo* spectroscopy. Single voxel localization achieved without forming an echo like STEAM and PRESS. A localization scheme consisting of eight scans with different combinations of three inversion pulses and receiver phase for each scan. Summation in the correct manner causes all the signals outside of the desired volume to cancel. Widely used for phosphorus ^{31}P spectroscopy.

ISO (International Organization for Standardization) A large, worldwide developer and publisher of international standards. A network of the national standards institutes of 157 countries, one member per country, with a central secretariat in Geneva, Switzerland, that coordinates the system. ISO is a non-governmental organization that forms a bridge between the public and private sectors. Many of its member institutes are part of the governmental structure of their countries, or are mandated by their government. Other members are in the private sector, having been set up by national partnerships of industry associations. ISO enables a consensus to be reached on solutions that meet both the requirements of business and the broader needs of society. ISO 9000, 14000, 22000 and 27000 are international management standards. ISO 9000:2005 describes fundamentals of quality management systems, which form the subject of the ISO 9000 family, and defines related terms.

isobars (*nmed*) Nuclides having a constant mass, but varying proton and neutron number. An example series would be:

$$^{201}_{80}\mathrm{Hg}_{121} : ^{201}_{81}\mathrm{Tl}_{120} : ^{201}_{82}\mathrm{Pb}_{119}$$

isobaric transition (*phys*) A nuclear decay process where the atomic mass is unchanged, where neutron: proton or proton : neutron. Beta decay is an example:

$$^{131}_{53}I \rightarrow \, ^{131}_{54}Xe + \beta - (+gammas)$$
$$^{22}_{11}Na \rightarrow \, ^{22}_{10}Ne + \beta + (paired\ 511\ keV\ gammas)$$

isocentre (*ct*) Centre of gantry. (*ct*) Intersection of the axis of rotation with the scan plane.

isodiapheres (*phys*) Series of radionuclides where the difference between the number of neutrons and protons is the same. For example, losing an α–particle, the uranium series are isodiapheres where each stage emits an alpha particle $_2\alpha_2$:

$$.... \, ^{230}_{90}Th_{140} \rightarrow \, ^{226}_{88}Ra_{138} \rightarrow \, ^{222}_{86}Rn_{136}$$
$$\rightarrow \, ^{218}_{84}Ra_{134} \rightarrow \, ^{214}_{82}Ra_{132} ....$$

(*see* isotopes, isotones, isodiapheres, isobars).

isodose (*dose*) A series of contours drawn over a target area depicting areas expected to receive the same dose rate. Used to plot radiation treatment plans.

isomeric states (*phys*) States of a nucleus having different energies and observable half-lives.

isomeric transition (*nmed*) The decay of a metastable state yielding a single gamma photon only (pure gamma emitter). Isomers would be ^{99m}Tc and ^{99}Tc. These excited states usually last for extremely short times (picoseconds), but others can last for relatively long periods (many seconds or even hours) and are called metastable states. These can be considered as transition processes (*see* internal conversion, generator, internal conversion).

isomers (*nmed*) An atomic nucleus having the same atomic number and mass as another or others, but a different energy state. Two atoms of the same element in which the numbers of protons and neutrons are the same, and the atomic mass is the same, but the nuclear energy levels are different (e.g. ^{99m}Tc and ^{99}Tc).

Isojex ˣ (*nmed*) ^{125}I-RISA (human serum albumin, HSA) for plasma volume determination (Mallinckrodt Inc.).

isolated array coils (*mri*) Array coils, the signals whose elements are kept separate until after processing.

isolating transformer (*xray*) A transformer with equal primary and secondary windings used for isolating equipment from the a.c. mains supply. The electrical safety of the equipment is improved since there is no leakage path to earth.

isomeric states (*phys*) States of a nucleus having different energies and observable half-lives.

isometric venography (intra-osseous spinal venography) (*clin*) Visualizing the long saphenous vein for evaluating its suitability as a graft in arterial reconstruction surgery; achieved by contrast medium injection into a foot vein in the supine patient during isometric tension of the limb muscles.

Isopaque ˣ (*cm*) An ionic monomer used as a radiographic contrast agent; generic name metrizoic acid/metrizoate compoundsate.

Compound	Viscosity (cP)	Osmolality mOsm/kg	Iodine (mg I mL^{-1})
Na-metrizoate	–	2100	370

(*see* Triosil®).

isotonic saline (*clin*) Also called physiological saline. A solution of sodium chloride (9.448 g) in 1000 g of water, giving approximately 0.9% sodium chloride which possesses the same osmotic pressure as intracellular fluid: 290 mOsm/L. Plasma has an osmolality of 285 mOsm/kg water.

isotones (*nmed*) Nuclides having different proton numbers and different atomic mass, but the same number of neutrons. Two examples are the series:

$$^{30}_{14}Si_{16} : \, ^{31}_{15}P_{16} : \, ^{32}_{16}S_{16} \text{ and } \, ^{88}_{38}Sr_{16} : \, ^{89}_{39}Y_{50} : \, ^{90}_{40}Zr_{50}$$

isotonic (isotonicity) (*clin*) A fluid having the same osmolality or osmolarity as another fluid or surrounding tissue. Used synonymously with iso-osmolar. All ionic and non-ionic monomeric contrast media are hypertonic compared to blood, ionic contrast media having osmolarities up to ×7 of blood, non-ionic monomers up to ×3 times. Non-ionic dimers are much less hypertonic and are supplied as isotonic with blood in lower iodine concentrations. One of the non-ionic dimers, iodixanol, is actually isotonic with blood in all concentrations. This gives a very low osmotoxicity.

isotope (*phys*) Nuclides with the same proton number, but different neutron numbers. The three stable isotopes of oxygen are

$$^{16}_{8}O_{8} : \, ^{17}_{8}O_{9} : \, ^{18}_{8}O_{10}.$$

The corresponding radioactive isotopes would be $^{14}_{8}O_{6}$ (*T* ½ 1.2 m) and $^{15}_{8}O_{7}$ (*T* ½ 1/2 2 m). The three isotopes of hydrogen are known as hydrogen $\left(^{1}_{1}H_{0}\right)$, deuterium $\left(^{2}_{1}H_{1}\right)$ and tritium $\left(^{3}_{1}H_{2}\right)$. Various isotopes have different nuclear magnetic moments and hence, have quite different resonant frequencies (*see* isotones, isodiapheres, isobars).

isotopic abundance (*phys*) The number of atoms of a particular isotope in a mixture of the isotopes of an element expressed as a fraction of all the atoms of the element.

isotropic (*phys*) Independent of direction, having properties which are uniform and do not vary with direction. A point source of activity is isotropic, emitting in all directions over a spherical volume.

isotropic motion (*mri*) Motion which is uniform in all 3D dimensions. This is generally used in reference to molecular diffusion or rotation which gives rise to relaxation of the spin system through dipole–dipole interactions (*see* diffusion imaging).

isotropic sampling (*ct*) A coordination system giving equal dimensions in the x-, y- and z-axes. Images can be created in any plane with the same spatial resolution as the original sections. The x,y axis represents the normal transversal CT view of the body with the x-axis in a lateral direction and the y-axis in an anterior–posterior direction. The perpendicular to the x,y axis oriented z-axis is parallel to the longitudinal axis of the body and the system axis. An isotropic data set is achieved by using the small focal spot with thin section collimation (0.5 mm), giving a longitudinal resolution (z-axis) nearly identical to the in-plane (x-, y-axes) resolution. Images (coronal, sagittal and axial) can be reconstructed from one multi-slice acquisition and will have the same spatial resolution as sections from the original acquisition.

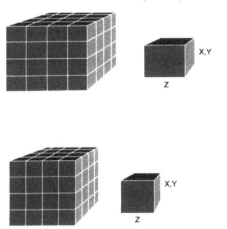

Isovist® (*cm*) Commercial (Schering) form of iotrolan, a non-ionic dimer

Compound	Viscosity (cP)	Osmolality mOsm/kg	Iodine (mg I mL⁻¹)
Iotrolan 512.59 mg mL⁻¹	6.8 at 20°C, 3.9 at 37°C	270	240

Isovue® (*cm*) Commercial (Bracco) preparation of iopamidol.

Compound	Viscosity (cP)	Osmolality mOsm/kg	Iodine (mg I mL⁻¹)
Isovue M200 41%	3.3 at 20°C, 2.0 at 37°C	413	200
Isovue M300 61%	8.8 at 20°C, 4.7 at 37°C	616	300
Isovue M370 76%	20.9 at 20°C, 9.4 at 37°C	796	370

isowatt (*xray*) Describes the characteristic curve for tube voltage and current in fluoroscopy where at a certain threshold current the tube kilovoltage is steadily reduced maintaining the same power in watts (isowatt). Automatic control based on this curve is not suitable for imaging so an 'anti-isowatt' control is available where tube voltage and current are increased over a restricted range giving optimum image contrast and brightness for all object sizes. The graph plots kilovoltage against tube current control and shows the maximum permitted level (450 W in this case) which forms the 'isowatt' limit for the particular x-ray tube.

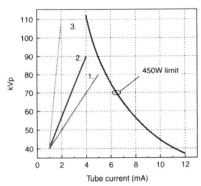

The linear functions plotted in the graph differ according to the emphasis placed on mA or kV; slope (1) predominantly alters mA, while

(2) alters mA and kV with equal measure; slope (3) rapidly alters kVp to a maximum of 110 kVp. During isowatt/anti-isowatt operation, the value of tube voltage and tube current relate directly to the transparency of the examined object since dose rate at the input screen of the image intensifier is kept at an optimum fixed value (typically 0.175 µGy/s).

ISP (*comp*) Internet service provider. A commercial concern controlling connection to the Internet.

iteration (*math*) A repeated procedure which allows better and better approximation to the true answer. Iterative reconstruction is sometimes used in tomographic imaging.

iterative reconstruction (*ct*) This uses an exact mathematical solution for reconstructing ray sums. This was the original method for image reconstruction. Its disadvantages are that it takes a long time and suffers from rounding errors. All data must be collected before reconstruction can begin.

IUP (*clin*) Intravenous urography.

IVIM (*mri*) Intravoxel incoherent motion.

IVP (*xray*) Intravenous pylorogram.

J

j (*math*) One of the symbols used for representing the complex variable (*see i*, complex numbers).

J-coupling (*mri*) *See* spin–spin coupling.

J-modulation (*mri*) Changes in the relative phase of the component lines of a multiplet (see spin–spin coupling) caused by differential phase accumulations, dependent on the particular acquisition parameters employed. For example, in multiple spin echo sequences the resulting modulation of the net intensity of the multiplet can affect the apparent $72\,s$ in a manner dependent on the choice of interpulse delays employed to observe the echo (*see* spin–spin coupling).

jaggies (*image*) *See* pixilation.

Java (*comp*) An object-orientated program language that enables interactive elements to work across operating systems making it an ideal language for web page design. Java allows programmers to create small programs or applications (applets) to enhance web sites.

Javascript/ECMA script (*comp*) A scripting language, similar to Java, which allows web programmers to create dynamic content, such as interactive games, or search engines on their web sites.

jaz drive (*comp*) Transportable disks capable of storing 1-Gbytes with access times of $17.5\,ms$ and transfer rates of $5.4\,M$-bytes s^{-1} (*see* zip disk).

JCAHO (*USA*) Joint Commission on the Accreditation of Healthcare Organizations. Establishes dosimetry standards.

jet effect (*mri*) Signal loss where spin dephasing occurs with complex flow patterns like turbulence. The degree of signal loss depends on the flow patterns and pulse sequence used; important when quantifying vascular stenosis.

Joliot-Curie Irène (1897–1956) and **Frédéric** (1900–58) continued the work of Marie and Pierre Curie observing the penetrating radiation ejected from paraffin wax (later identified as neutrons by Chadwick). They produced the first artificial radioisotope by bombarding aluminium with alpha particles to produce phosphorus. They were jointly awarded the Nobel Prize for chemistry in 1935.

Joule, James Prescott (1818–89) British physicist. Investigated the heating effect of electrical current on conductors. The mechanical equivalent of heat. His ideas were recast in terms of the principle of the conversion of energy. Gave his name to the SI unit.

joule (*phys*) A measure of the quantity of energy, work or heat. The SI unit of work $1\,J = 1\,N\,m^{-2}$; $1\,eV = 1.602 \times 10^{-19}\,J$ and $1\,Gy = 1\,J\,kg^{-1}$. The derived units are:

Measure	Joule equivalent
Energy density	$J\,m^{-3}$
Specific energy	$J\,kg^{-1}$
Absorbed dose (Gy)	$J\,kg^{-1}$
Equivalent dose (Sv)	$J\,kg^{-1}$
Watt (W)	$J\,s^{-1}$
Heat capacity	$J\,K^{-1}$
Coulomb (C)	$J\,V^{-1}$
Volt (V)	$J\,C^{-1}$
Specific heat capacity	$J\,kg^{-1}\,K^{-1}$

Measure	Joule equivalent
$10^{7}\,ergs$	$1\,J$
$1\,W\,s$	$1\,J$
$1\,kW\,h$	$3.6\,MJ$
$6.24 \times 10^{18}\,eV$	$1\,J$
$6.24 \times 10^{15}\,keV$	
$6.24 \times 10^{12}\,MeV$	
$1\,eV$	$1.602 \times 10^{-19}\,J$
$1\,keV$	$1.602 \times 10^{-16}\,J$
$1\,MeV$	$1.602 \times 10^{-13}\,J$

JPEG (*di*) Joint Photographic Experts Group. Compression algorithm and also popular graphics format (JPG). Usually referring to a graphic image format defined by this group that has become an alternative to GIF for compact images. All JPEG images can use 16.7 million colours at a higher compression rate that GIF.

jumper (*comp*) A method for altering a hardwired connection on the motherboard by plugging a small wire connector across two pegs.

junction diode (*phys*) The n-type and p-type semiconductors are combined to form the p–n junction diode. The junction diode exhibits different properties when connected to different polarity (+, −). Before current supply (battery) is connected, a small depletion layer exists between the p- and n-boundary. Electrons migrate from the n-type a small way into the p-type layer. Holes from the p-type also migrate into the n-type material. If the positive pole of the battery is connected to the p-type and the negative pole to the n-type then a current flows; the diode is then forward biased. Reversing the polarity causes a wide depletion layer to be formed and no current is able to flow; the diode is reverse biased.

justification (ICRP) (*dose*) A control measure to restrict exposure from practices. It implies that the detriment from exposure should be justified by the benefit resulting from the practice and thus preventing frivolous applications involving radiation (*see* practices (ICRP)).

J

K

K56Flex (*comp*) A proprietary protocol developed by Lucent Technologies and Rockwell specifying a 56 Kbits/sec download speed and 33.6 Kbits/sec upload. Employs pulse code modulation technology similar to ISDN and requires the line on the host side to be digitally terminated. K56Flex is incompatible with X2.

K6, K6-2, K6-III (*comp*) Central processing units manufactured by AMD Corporation.

k bits/s (kbps) (*comp*) Abbreviation for kilobits per second. Used for measuring serial data transfer in modems or other serial devices. $1\,\mathrm{kb\,s^{-1}}$ is exactly 1024 bytes per second. A megabyte (Mb) is 1024 kb or 1 048 576 bytes (*see* baud rate).

K-edge (filters) (*xray*) The abrupt increase in photon absorption when the incident photon energy equals the K-orbit binding energy. Metals with higher K-edge values (20–30 keV) are useful filters in radiology since they preferentially remove higher energy photons, unlike aluminium and copper filters that remove low energy photons. K-edge filters are commonly found in mammography where they reduce patient radiation dose by removing energies above 28 keV which only play a minor role in image formation for this examination. Common K-edge metals used for x-ray beam filtration are shown in the table from Z = 42 onwards. The K-edge for tin is useful since this allows this metal to be used as lightweight shielding in protective aprons.

Element	Z	K-shell energy (keV)
Carbon	6	0.28
Nitrogen	7	0.4
Oxygen	8	0.5
Phosphorus	15	2.1
Sulphur	16	2.5
Calcium	20	4.0
Molybdenum	42	20.0
Rhodium	45	23.2
Palladium	46	24.3
Tin	50	29.2
Barium	56	37.4
Iodine	53	33.2
Samarium	62	46.8
Erbium	68	57.5
Tungsten	74	69.5
Lead	82	88.0
Uranium	92	115.6

(*see* filters (radiation)).

k-space (*mri*) A convenient way for describing data sampling process in MRI. The data acquired for MR image reconstruction generally correspond to samples of *k*-space; they represent values of the Fourier transform of the image at a particular set of locations in *k*-space; a two dimensional map with most of the signal concentrated at the centre (low frequencies) and high frequency component on the periphery. The low frequency components of central *k*-space contain most signal intensity (contrast); the high frequency components in the periphery contain edge information (resolution). The Fourier transformation of *k*-space yields the spin density function. *k*-space and image space are inversely related through the Fourier transform (*see* spatial frequency, truncation error).

k-space filling (*mri*) The matrix position and order of data in two-dimensional spatial frequency space (*k*-space); the Fourier transform of this matrix gives the MR image. Conventional MR pulse sequences (spin-echo and gradient-echo imaging) fill a single line of k-space with each data measurement. A different phase encoding step fills out another parallel line of *k*-space. The full set of measurements completes a Cartesian grid of points in *k*-space. Other options for *k*-space filling include radial filling (back-projection imaging) or spiral filling (spiral imaging).

k-space trajectory (*mri*) The path traced in the spatial-frequency domain during data collection as determined by the applied field gradients.

Kaiser window (*di*) The filter windows such as Hanning and Hamming have fixed shapes giving a trade-off between width of main spectral lobe and side-lobe levels. The Kaiser window

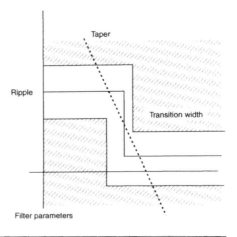

Filter parameters

allows this trade-off to be adjusted based on the allowable ripple, controlling taper and side-lobes, and transition width (see filters (spatial)).

kappa statistics (coefficient) (*stats*) Corrected index of agreement between two quantities. The value takes unity where there is perfect agreement. Commonly used to judge diagnostic accuracy. The assessment of a series of images for the presence of a subtle abnormality improves if more than one imaging procedure is used (e.g. mixing plane film radiograph, MRI and nuclear medicine) or more than one clinician views the images. In the latter case it is essential to establish that the clinicians concerned are looking for the same features. The kappa measure of agreement (κ) is used for this purpose; its value ranges from 0 (no agreement) to 1.0 (perfect agreement). The ROC analysis would answer the question 'is there an improvement between imaging techniques?'; the kappa statistic would answer the question 'is there an agreement between investigators?'

	Pos (A).	Neg (A).	Totals
Pos (B).	150 (*a*)	10 (*b*)	160 (*a* + *b*)
Neg (B).	20 (*c*)	20 (*d*)	40 (*c* + *d*)
Totals	170	30	200
	(*a* + *c*)	(*b* + *d*)	*n*

Kappa statistics

A special selection of 200 mammograms containing known lesions of varying significance are given to two radiologists (A and B) for assessment (positive + or negative −). The results are:
The observed measure of agreement (l_o) and the expected measure (l_e) are now computed as:

$$l_o = \frac{(a + d)}{n}$$

$$l_e = \frac{(a + c) \times (a + b) + (b + d) \times (c + d)}{n^2}$$

For the data given above, $l_o = 0.85$ and $l_e = 0.71$. The kappa statistic (κ) is computed as:

$$\kappa = \frac{l_o - l_e}{1 - l_e} = 0.48$$

This signifies a fair consistency of assessment between the two radiologists, but would require improvement if breast cancer screening were contemplated (see diagnostic accuracy).

■ Reference: Armitage and Berry, 1996.

kBytes s⁻¹ (kBps) (*comp*) Kilobytes per second. A measure of data transfer. 1 kBps is exactly 1024 bytes per second. One megabyte (MB) per second is 1024 kB or 1 048 576 bytes per second (see byte).

kelvin (K) (*phys*) The SI unit of temperature. kelvin K (*phys*) the SI unit of temperature starting at absolute zero where $T = 0$ K. Degrees Celsius (°C) have identical intervals to degrees kelvin.

	K	°C	°F
Absolute zero	0	−273.15	−459.67
Freezing point of water	273.15	0	32
Boiling point of water	373.15	100	212

Kelvin, William, Thomson (1824–1907) British scientist, proposed the absolute (Kelvin) scale of thermodynamic temperature adopted as an SI unit.

kerma (K) (*dose*) This term has replaced exposure in radiation dosimetry and is an acronym for Kinetic Energy Released per unit Mass. It is a measure of the removal of energy from the photon beam by ionization creating secondary electrons in the absorber. At diagnostic energies (20–200 keV) the photon energy is lost as a two-stage process:

1 Photon radiation transfers energy to electrons through photoelectric and Compton scattering.
2 The electron energy transfered to the absorber via atomic excitations and ionization.

The absorber material must be specified (air, water, tissue, etc.). When the absorbing medium is air, the term air kerma or kerma in air is used (K_{air}). For x- and gamma radiation, kerma can be calculated from the mass energy absorption coefficient of the material (μ_{en}/ρ) and the photon energy fluence as: $K = \Psi(\mu_{en}/\rho)$. The SI units for photon energy fluence are J m⁻², and for the mass energy absorption coefficient are m² kg⁻¹. Therefore the product, kerma, has units of joule per kilogram (J kg⁻¹) and is given the special name gray (Gy). For diagnostic energies (20–200 keV), kerma in air (K_{air}) and absorbed dose in air (D_{air}) can be treated as equal. The energy to form one ion pair in air is 34 J C⁻¹ (34 eV per ion pair) for diagnostic radiation energies and over a wide range of biological materials. Since 1 Gy = 1 J kg⁻¹ then Dose$_{(air)}$ (Gy) = 34 E (C kg⁻¹). Converting a dose in air to dose in an absorber (patient) for the same incident photon flux, the energy absorbed per unit mass of absorber depends only on the mass energy absorption coefficient of the medium. At diagnostic energies the mass energy transfer coefficient and mass energy absorption coefficient are inter-changeable (*see* f-factor).

kernel (*ct, image*) A discrete filter for image reconstruction. The mask used for producing a Laplace filter in a two-dimensional image convolution. The kernel contains weighting factors that will alter the image system in the frequency domain. Each pixel of the filtered image is calculated as the sum of the pixel of the original image at the same position and the surrounding points encompassed by the kernel (3×3) in this example:

Smoothing kernel

0.1	0.1	0.1
0.1	0.1	0.1
0.1	0.1	0.1

Edge enhancement kernel

−1	−1	−1
−1	+8	−1
−1	−1	−1

Thus the kernel is shifted uniformly over each pixel in the original image matrix. Kernel size and values decide filter behaviour (*see* filter (spatial)).

Kety–Schmidt principle (*clin*) A technique for reliable measurement of cerebral blood flow in man. The subject breathes an inert gas and the rate at which the gas comes to an equilibrium between blood and tissue is determined by serial measurements of gas concentration in arterial and venous samples. From curves of arterial and venous concentration over the period of equilibrium the blood flow per unit mass of tissue can be calculated from:

$$Q = \frac{C_t}{\int_0^t (C_a - C_v)dt}$$

$(C_t = S \times C_v)$ where C_a is the arterial, C_v the venous and C_t the tissue concentration of gas at time t. The partition coefficient between blood and tissue is S. Radioactive gases ^{133}Xe and ^{85}Kr are used with external detection.

▪ Reference: Veall and Vetter, 1958

keV (*xray*) Thousands of electron volts. Used as a precise measure of x-ray photon energy.

Kevlar™ (*chem*) A stiff chain polymer plastic, which is both strong and lightweight. It is used as an alternative to carbon fibre in the manufacture of x-ray couches and as a spacer material in anti-scatter grids.

kilobytes (kB) (*unit*) The terms kilo- and mega- do not strictly work out to 1000 and 1 million respectively:

- $2^{10} = 1024$ bytes $= 1$ kilobyte (kB)
- $2^{20} = 1048$ kB $= 1$ megabyte (MB)
- $2^{30} = 1073$ megabytes $= 1$ gigabyte (GB)

The term kilobyte has become confusing as a unit for computer storage since it can be either 1024 bytes or 1000 bytes (10^3), depending on context. This name has been discontinued as an SI standard. It has been recommended that the quantity of 1024 bytes is now called a kibibyte (KiB), the term kilobyte reserved for 1000 (10^3) bytes. Similarly the term megabyte (MB) describes strictly 1000^2 bytes and mebibyte (MiB) to describe 1024^2 bytes. The International Electrotechnical Commission (IEC) approved the names and symbols for prefixes for binary multiples for use in the fields of data processing and data transmission. The prefixes are as follows:

Factor	Name	Symbol	Origin	Derivation
2^{10}	kibi	Ki	kilobinary: $(2^{10})^1$	kilo: $(10^3)^1$
2^{20}	mebi	Mi	megabinary: [2] (2^{10})	mega: $(10^3)^2$
2^{30}	gibi	Gi	gigabinary: $(2^{10})^3$	giga: $(10^3)^3$
2^{40}	tebi	Ti	terabinary: $(2^{10})^4$	tera: $(10^3)^4$
2^{50}	pebi	Pi	petabinary: $(2^{10})^5$	peta: $(10^3)^5$
2^{60}	exbi	Ei	exabinary: $(2^{10})^6$	exa: $(10^3)^6$

Examples of the revised nomenclature and comparisons are:

One kibibit	1 Kibit = 2^{10}bit = 1024 bit
One kilobit	1 kbit = 10^3bit = 1000 bit
One mebibyte	1 MiB = 2^{20}B = 1 048 576 B
One megabyte	1 MB = 10^6B = 1 000 000 B
One gibibyte	1 GiB = 2^{30}B = 1 073 741 824 B
One gigabyte	1 GB = 10^9B = 1 000 000 000 B

kilo-electron volt keV (*phys*) Thousands of electron volts. Used as a precise measure of x-ray photon energy.

kilogram kg (*phys*) The mass of a body is the quantity of matter it contains. The basic SI unit is the kilogram 1000 grams for all m.k.s. systems including SI. 1 gram is 10^{-3} kg and 1 milligram is 10^{-6} kg. Some derived units are:

- kg $\times$ m^{-3} for density
- kg $\times$ m^{-1} $\times$ s^{-2} or pascal for pressure
- kg $\times$ m $\times$ s^{-2} or Newton for force (*see* weight).

kilowatt hour (*phys*) Used to describe electrical work 1 kWh = 1 kW $\times$ 3600 s = 3.6×10^6 J.

kinematic viscosity (*phys*) The ratio of viscosity to density. measured as m^2 $\times$ s^{-1}.

kinetic energy (E_k) (*phys*) Energy associated with movement so that: $E = \frac{1}{2}mv^2$. Increases with mass m and velocity v. If an object is brought to rest in time t the final velocity is zero as:

$$F = ma \text{ or } momentum\ change\ s^{-1} = mv/t.$$

Work done (kinetic energy) is:

$$E_k = F \times s = (mv/t) \times (vt/2)$$

cancelling t to give: $E_k = \frac{1}{2}mv^2$. If the velocity moved by the object diminishes uniformly over distance d, in time t, from v to zero, then:

$$d = average\ velocity \times time = vt/2.$$

The forms of kinetic energy include:

- *Translational* where the entire object moves.
- *Vibrational* where small masses move back and forth. Simple gas molecules, having one atom (hydrogen, helium, oxygen, etc.) only have translational kinetic energy. More complex gas molecules (H_2O, NH_4) may have rotational and vibrational kinetic energy.
- *Rotational* given by object spin.

Electron kinetic energy

Computer display screen:
Velocity of electron beam with kinetic energy of 30 kV (typical applied display tube voltage).

1 eV = 1.602×10^{-19} J so 30 keV = 4.906×10^{-15} J

Electron rest mass: 9.109×10^{-31} kg
Since $E = \frac{1}{2}mv^2$ then $v = \sqrt{2E/m}$ = 1.02×10^8 m s^{-1}.
The electron is travelling at 1/3 the speed of light.

X-ray tube:
Applied voltage 100 keV
Electron beam velocity: 1.87×10^8 ms^{-1} or almost two-thirds the speed of light.

---

krypton (Kr) (*elem*)

Atomic number (Z)	36
Relative atomic mass (A$_r$)	83.8
Density (ρ) kg/m^3	3.49
Melting point (K)	116.5
K-edge (keV)	14.3

^{81m}Krypton (*nmed*) A lung ventilation agent capable of steady state scintigraphy. The generator demonstrates secular equilibrium.

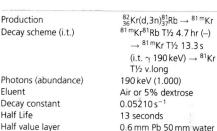

Production	$^{82}_{36}$Kr(d,3n)$^{81}_{37}$Rb → ^{81m}Kr
Decay scheme (i.t.)	^{81m}Kr^{81}Rb T½ 4.7 hr (–)
	→ ^{81m}Kr T½ 13.3 s
	(i.t. γ 190 keV) → ^{81}Kr
	T½ v.long
Photons (abundance)	190 keV (1.000)
Eluent	Air or 5% dextrose
Decay constant	0.05210 s^{-1}
Half Life	13 seconds
Half value layer	0.6 mm Pb 50 mm water

kV$_{eff}$ (*xray*) See effective energy.

kV$_{eqv}$ (*xray*) See equivalent energy.

kVp (*xray*) The peak photon energy of an x-ray beam.

L

labelled compound (*nmed*) A compound in which one or more of the molecules is replaced by a radioactive isotope (^{75}Se-seleno-methionine) or a radiopharmaceutical to which a radionuclide is attached (^{99m}Tc-DTPA). The radiolabel must not change the chemical nature or geometry of the original compound and so alter its original physiological property.

labelling (blood cells) (*nmed*) *See* blood cells (labelling).

lambert (L) (*phys*) A non-SI unit of luminance where 1 lambert = $(10^4/\pi)$ candela m^{-2} or $1/\pi$ candela cm^{-2}.

Lambert–Beer law (*ct*) See x-ray attenuation.

Lambert's Law (*phys*) This states that equal paths in the same absorbing medium absorb equal fractions of radiation that enters them. Originally conceived for light absorption but applies to all radiation (x and gamma) as well as ultrasound. Expressed as:

$$I = I_0 \cdot e^{-kx}$$

where k is the absorption coefficient and x the path length (*see* Beer's Law, attenuation).

laminar flow (*phys*) A non-turbulent flow pattern in which the gas or liquid moves in layers (*see* Reynold's number).

laminar flow cabinet (*nmed*) An enclosed or contained workstation for preparing and dispensing radiopharmaceuticals. The cabinet should conform to a recognized standard of air purity and flow pattern (e.g. Class I and II British Standard BS5295, German TUV DIN 12950). The air is required to be cleaner than the room environment and maintained at positive pressure. Negative pressure cabinets are also used (*see* HESPA filter).

LAN (*comp*) See local area network (*see* WAN).

Langmuir, Irving D (1881–1957) American physical chemist. Studied electron emission and temperature relationships of a heated tungsten filament in a vacuum, recognizing that electron emission depends only on the temperature of the filament. From this work Coolidge developed his version of the x-ray tube. In 1937 he proposed a design for an electronic image intensifier. A practical version was made by Coltman in 1948.

lanthanum (La) (*elem*)

Atomic number (Z)	57
Relative atomic mass (A$_r$)	138.9
Density (ρ) kg/m^3	6150
Melting point (K)	1190
K-edge (keV)	38.9

Relevance to radiology: Its complex compounds are used for intensifying screens, emitting blue light.

Laplace transform (*math*) A method for solving differential equations by transforming them into an algebraic equation so considerably simplifying their solution (*see* integration/differentiation).

Laplace equation (sound) (*math*) Relates to the speed of sound c in a gas to the density ρ pressure P and heat capacities h of a gas as $c = \sqrt{(hP/\rho)}$.

LAPM (*comp*) Link access protocol for modems. One of the two protocols specified by V.42 used for detection and correction of errors on a communications link between two modems.

large area (macro) transfer factor (*image*) The factor describing the scaling of information between the input and output of an imaging system. It is concerned with changes in the signal over a large area, c.f., spatial detail transfer characteristic.

Larmor, Sir Joseph (1857–1942) Irish physicist, demonstrated the precessive motion of the nuclear orbit in a magnetic field.

Larmor equation (*mri*) This describes the frequency of precession of the nuclear magnetic moment being proportional to the magnetic field as:

$$f = \frac{\mu B_0}{2\pi L} \text{ hertz.}$$

where μ is the proton magnetic moment, L the proton spin angular momentum and B_0 the magnetic field strength (tesla). Since μ and $2\pi L$ are fixed for any particular nucleus, they can describe a gyromagnetic ratio where $\gamma = \mu/2\pi L$. Simplifying the first equation by substituing γ gives the precessional frequency:

$$\omega_L = \gamma B_0$$

which is the Lamor equation relating precessional frequency ω_L to magnetic field strength.

Gyromagnetic ratio for hydrogen

Proton magnetic moment: $1.41031 \times 10{-}26$ J T^{-1}
Proton spin angular momentum: $0.527 \times 10{-}34$ J s^{-1}
Hence $\gamma = \mu/2\pi L = 42\,582\,252$ Hz

Larmor frequency (*mri*) The frequency at which magnetic resonance can be excited (f_0 or w_0);

given by the Larmor equation. For H^+ the Larmor frequency is 42.58 MHz T^{-1}; the frequency at which the nuclear spins precess about the main field. Depends on the nucleus type and strength of the magnetic field applied. By varying the magnetic field across the body, a magnetic field gradient can be used to encode position due to variation in Larmor frequency.

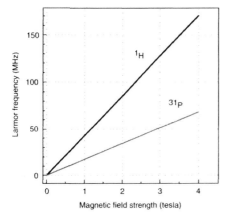

Magnetic field strength (tesla)

(*see* gyromagnetic ratio, precession).

laryngography (*clin*) Radiography of the larynx after coating mucosal surfaces with contrast medium.

laser (*phys*) Light Amplification by stimulated emission of radiation. A strong monochromatic coherent light source can be produced by causing many atoms to make transitions from one excited state to another so that all the light waves are in phase (coherent). Lasers produce:

- An intense coherent beam
- Monochromatic
- Virtually noise free
- Highly directional beam
- Can be tightly focussed

Many materials can be made to lase ruby, carbon dioxide, helium/neon. These are high power devices commonly found in laser film formatters. A material such as a ruby or gas mixture (helium–neon) is optically pumped continuously or in bursts to excite atoms from their ground state to a metastable state from where electrons fall back to their ground state emitting coherent monochromatic light. Semiconductor laser diodes are low power devices producing red/infrared light used

for optical transmission and reading laser-disks and CD-ROMs (*see* fibre optics, CD-ROM, DVD).

laser diode (*elec*) This is a semiconductor light emitting diode (LED) operating at high current. The *p–n* regions are manufactured from gallium arsenide and gallium aluminium arsenide. Stimulated emission produced by making the semiconductor faces optically flat. Spectral spread is much less than an LED, typically 1–2 nm, giving low dispersion in fibre optics.

laser imager (*image*) *See* film formatter.

laser printer (*image*) A tightly focussed laser beam can be used for imaging by:

- Exposing a charged selenium plate (paper printer)
- Reading an image phosphor plate
- Exposing a photographic film as in wet laser film formatters.
- Selectively removing a carbon or silver film from a plastic surface to produce an image (the dry laser process).

The resolution of a laser printer is measured in dot pitch; typical values are 300, 600 and 1200 dpi (*see* image plate, laser imager).

last image hold (LIH) (*xray*) Storing and displaying the most recent image from (commonly) a fluoroscopy study. The image can be held digitally (computer image matrix) or on video disc. The patient is not exposed to further radiation during this procedure so is a significant dose reduction facility.

late somatic effects (*dose*) Radiation effects occurring a considerable time (years) after exposure to radiation; these effects include mutagenesis, teratogenesis and carcinogenesis.

latency/latent period (*dose*) The period between exposure to ionizing radiation and the appearance of radiation effects (i.e. cancer). The median period is 8 years for leukaemia and two to three times longer for solid tumours (e.g. breast, lung). There is a minimum latency period of approximately 2 years for myeloid leukaemia.

latent heat (*phys*) The amount of heat per unit mass that is added to or removed from a substance undergoing a change of state, i.e. from solid to liquid or liquid to gas. The heat required to change the ice to water is the hidden or latent heat. The latent heat of fusion; a change of state from solid to liquid. The latent heat of vapourization; a change of state from liquid to vapour. Latent heat is the energy necessary to overcome the forces of attraction between the molecules of a substance. The latent heat of vapourization (liquid to gas) is therefore greater than the latent heat of fusion (solid to liquid). The latent heat of vapourization for helium is $21 \, kJ \, kg^{-1}$, this is a cooling process so requires energy when changing from gas to a liquid. Units are $(J \, kg^{-1})$. The table gives latent heat of fusion and vaporization for some common substances in $MJ \, kg^{-1}$.

Substance	Lf (fusion)	Lv (vapourization)
Alcohol	–	1.1
Water	0.335	2.260
Aluminium	0.400	12.3
Copper	0.205	4.80
Iron	0.275	6.29
Tungsten	0.192	4.35
Lead	0.023	0.87
Helium	–	0.021

(*see* specific heat, specific heat capacity).

lateral (*us*) Perpendicular to the direction of sound travel.

lateral resolution (*us*) Minimum reflector separation perpendicular to the sound path that is required to produce separate echoes; equal to the beam width in the scan plane. Also called azimuthal, angular or transverse resolution (*see* axial resolution, ultrasound (resolution)).

latitude (film) (*film*) This refers to the dynamic range of exposures (LogE values) which can be given to a film over which density continues to increase at a useful rate – that is, the maximum luminance range that can be differentially reproduced. The film latitude should be broad enough to register all tissue types of interest (bone and soft tissue in the chest radiograph) but should give high contrast between similar tissue types (mammogram).

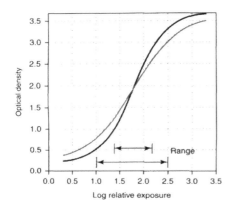

Contrast and latitude are therefore balanced; the greater the film gamma the smaller the latitude (*see* dynamic range, film speed, film contrast, film gamma).

lattice (*mri*) A property seen by nuclear magnetic resonance in solids. The magnetic and thermal environment with which nuclei exchange energy in longitudinal relaxation.

Lauterbur, Paul C. (1929–2007) American chemist who developed nuclear magnetic resonance in 1973 as an imaging technique using gradient fields. Awarded a Nobel Prize for this work in 2003.

Lawrence, Ernest Orlando (1901–1958) American physicist/engineer, who was the first director of Berkeley Radiation Laboratory in 1936 (now Lawrence Berkeley Radiation laboratory). Constructed the first cyclotron particle accelerator from ideas developed in 1929 with M. Stanley Livingston Edlefsen and others, extending the linear accelerator techniques of Cockcroft and Walton. Awarded the Nobel Prize for physics in 1939.

LD₅₀ (radiation) (*dose*) The lethal dose where 50% of the population die within a standard time, usually 30 days. Large mammals (including man) have an LD_{50} between 2.5 and $3 \, Gy$, whereas smaller mammals have LD_{50}s of approximately double this value. Intermediate symptoms are apparent 1 hour after partial exposure of about $0.5 \, Gy$ ($500 \, mGy$). These are prodromal reactions and include nausea, vomiting and diarrhoea if the gut wall has been exposed. The prodromal reactions are followed by a latent period before the main phase of the damage becomes apparent (*see* dose–mortality curve).

LD₅₀ (contrast media) (*cm*) The amount of contrast medium (usually expressed in g iodine per kg) that will kill 50% of a group of treated animals (mice). The LD_{50} value is inversely related to toxicity. Iodine contrast media are normally well tolerated and the LD_{50} value is correspondingly high.

	CM	LD₅₀
Ionic	Meglumine iothalamate	6
	Ioxaglate	10
Non-ionic	Metrizamide	15
	Iopamidol	20
	Iohexol	25
MRI		

Non-ionic contrast agents have higher LD_{50} due to low chemotoxicity. LD_{50} data published for various non-ionic contrast media relate to concentrations greater than 21 g iodine/kg (mice), exceeding the maximal anticipated clinical dose in humans by an order of magnitude (×10).

lead (Pb) (*elem*)

Atomic number (Z)	82
Relative atomic mass (A$_r$)	207.1
Density (ρ) kg/m^3	11340
Melting point (K)	600.4
Specific heat capacity J kg^{-1} K^{-1}	129
Thermal conductivity W m^{-1} K^{-1}	35.3
K-edge (keV)	88.0

Relevance to radiology: used as a radiation shielding material although its K-edge is awkwardly placed in the diagnostic range (see lead (shielding)).

^{210}Lead (^{210}Pb)

Half life	22y
Decay mode	β−3.7 MeV
Decay constant	0.0315y^{-1}
Photons (abundance)	17 keV (0.21)
	46 keV (0.04)

Freshly mined lead contains sufficient ^{210}Pb as contaminant to cause problems when used for shielding in low background equipment or laboratories.

lead equivalent (*dose*) A standard method for estimating the effectiveness of shielding materials (e.g. concrete, glass, brick, etc.) and protective clothing (e.g. aprons, gloves). Lead equivalent is normally quoted in mm Pb-equivalent.

lead glass (*xray*) The density of lead-glass varies between 4360 and 6200 kg m^{-3}. For this highest density the following measurements are:

Thickness (mm)	Weight (kg m^{-2})	Pb-equivalent (mm Pb)
4	18	1.0
6	28	1.5
8	37	2.0

(*see* Clear-Pb®, glass (lead)).

lead (shielding) (*xray*) For a density of 11 350 kg m^{-3} the following weights are given for lead sheet:

Thickness (mm)	Code	Weight (kg m^{-2})
0.5	–	5.4
1.0	–	10.76
1.32	3	14.6
1.5	–	17.20
1.80	4	19.5
2.0	–	21.50
2.24	5	24.4
2.65	6	29.3
3.15	7	34.2
3.55	8	39.1

The lead sheet must be firmly fixed to a rigid structure (e.g. wood or concrete) or sandwiched between wood laminate (plywood). The half value layer is affected by its K-edge at 88 keV.

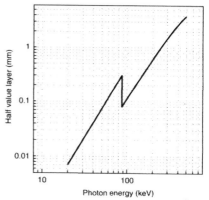

lead time (screening) (*stats*) The period between the time of detection by screening and the date it would have been diagnosed if not screened (*see* length time bias, screening (population)).

lead time bias (screening) (*stats*) Since survival is measured from the time of diagnosis then screening brings this time forward. Survival time is therefore lengthened even if the point of eventual death is not altered. This is the lead time bias (*see* length time bias, screening (population)).

lead zirconate titanate (LZT) (*us*) A ceramic piezoelectric material.

leakage radiation (*xray*) Measured from an x-ray tube housing with collimators (diaphragms) closed. Leakage measured at a distance of 50 mm over an area not exceeding 100 cm^2. It should be expressed as mGy hr^{-1} at 1 m and should not exceed 1 mGy. USA maximum leakage is 100 mR (1 mGy); the acceptable level being 50 mR (0.5 mGy).

least significant figure/bit (*math*) The rightmost figure in a number (decimal or binary) (*see* significant figure).

least squares, method of (*stats*) A way of estimating the best fit straight line for a plotted set of values and as a criterion for best fit.

LED (*elec*) Light emitting diode. A forward biased gallium arsenide semiconductor light source. Recombination of electron hole pairs causes light to be emitted (*see* laser diode).

Lenard von, Philipp Anton (1862–1947) Czech/German physicist. Demonstrated the magnetic deflection of cathode rays and electrostatic properties and on this work suggested that atoms contain both positive and negative units. Nobel Prize for physics, 1905.

length biased sampling (*stats*) The bias in a screening or sampling protocol where some members are more likely to be selected than others (*see* length time bias, screening (population)).

length time bias (screening) (*stats*) There is a tendency for screening to detect preferentially cancers that have a long asymptomatic phase. The extended duration of this phase implies slower growth and therefore good prognosis. More invasive cancers become symptomatic earlier and may be detected as interval cancers (*see* lead time bias, screening (population)).

Lenoscint [x] (*nmed*) Preparation of ^{99m}Tc-MDP (Bristol–Myers–Squibb).

lens (*us*) Curved material that focuses the sound beam in an ultrasound transducer.

LET (*dose*) *See* linear energy transfer.

leukaemia (*dose*) Forms of cancer due to the multiplication of malignant bone marrow cells. Leukaemias are differentiated depending on their marrow cell origin. The four main types identified include acute and chronic versions of myeloid and lymphatic forms. Acute lymphoid occurs most commonly in young children. Leukaemia is the first manifestation of radiation damage to a population and shows a linear dose response characteristic. *In-utero* exposure to radiation can increase the risk of childhood leukaemia by 40%.

 ▪ Hall and Brenner, 2008

Levovist [x] (*cm*) Commercial (Schering) preparation for ultrasound imaging consisting of galactose/palmitic acid granules containing microbubbles of gas.

Lexidronam [x] (*nmed*) Generic name for ^{153}Samarium used as a palliative treatment for bone pain (see Quadramet® samarium).

lidofenin (*nmed*) *See* HIDA.

life span study (*dose*) Refers to the long-term cohort study of health effects on the Japanese atomic bomb survivors in Hiroshima and Nagasaki.

lifetime risk estimates (*dose*) Several estimates are used for calculating the risk over a lifetime that an individual will develop or die from a specific disease caused by an exposure:

• Excess lifetime risk (ELR), the difference between the proportion of people who develop or die from the disease in an exposed population and the corresponding proportion in a similar control population without exposure;

• Risk of exposure-induced death (REID) defined as the difference in a cause-specific death rate for exposed and unexposed control populations of a given gender and age at exposure, as an additional cause of death introduced into a population,

• Loss of life expectancy (LLE) which describes the decrease in life expectancy due to the exposure.

• Lifetime attributable risk (LAR) an approximation of the REID and describes excess deaths (or disease) over a follow-up period with population background rates determined from control unexposed individuals.

ligand (*chem*) An ion or molecule that donates a pair of electrons to a metal at or ion in forming a complex compound. A double bond is formed between the metal and the ligand. Certain ligands are seen in chelating agents.

light (*phys*) Normally concerning the visible wavelengths of the electromagnetic spectrum from 390 to 740 nm, appreciated by the visual system as a series of colours. The absorption of light by various materials (air, water, glass, etc.) depends on the wavelength.

light exposure (*phys*) A measure of the total amount of light energy incident on a surface per unit area, measured in lux (*see* luminance, illuminance).

light guide (*phys*) A transparent material which conducts light onto a detecting system. A fibre optic cable as a transmission system is a light guide. Transparent plastic is used as a light guide for scintillation detectors; between the fluorescing substance and the light detector (photomultiplier or photodiode). Light guides area also found in the gamma camera.

likelihood ratio (L) (*stats*) Ratio of the probability that the data set (image data, **g**) would occur from a specified hypothesis H1 to the probability that it would occur from the alternative hypothesis, H2.

limiting diameter (*image*) the diameter of the smallest holes in a hole pattern test object which still appear separated in an image with given scan and reconstruction parameters (*see* geometrical resolution limit, low contrast resolution limit).

limiting spatial frequency (*ct*) The spatial frequency at which the modulation transfer function falls off to a certain minimum contrast level which can be distinguished. The minimum contrast is not commonly defined, but is often taken as 2% of the modulation transfer function (*see* limiting diameter, geometrical resolution limit).

limiting value (*qc*) A value of a parameter which, if exceeded, indicates that corrective action is required, although the equipment may continue to be used clinically (used in CEC 1993). Limiting values for dose or air kerma are derived differently from reference values, i.e. reference ESD is based on third quartile values derived during surveys whereas limiting values are derived from results which can be achieved in practice.

limulus test (*nmed*) Derived from the horseshoe crab; *Limulus polyphemus*. Hemolymph (amoebocyte), the circulating blood cell of the horseshoe crab, is extremely sensitive to bacterial endotoxins and endotoxin-like substances which induce coagulation of the haemolymph lystae. This established a Limulus test for detection of endotoxin in radiopharmaceutical products.

linac (*phys*) A linear accelerator for charged particles (electrons) using an RF signal aligned co-axially with the chamber. The electron beam bombards a transmission target to give high-voltage (4 MV) x-rays with high efficiency. Energy gain in current linacs are 7 MeV m^{-1} for electrons and 1.5 MeV m^{-1} for protons. Linacs can also produce narrow spectrum x-rays which have been used for phase contrast mammographic imaging.

line density (*xray*) *See* grid line density.

line focus principle (*xray*) The formation of a symmetrical (square) effective focal spot from an angled real focal spot on the anode surface achieved by choosing an angle that projects the same length as the real focal spot width. The example uses the geometry in the diagram.

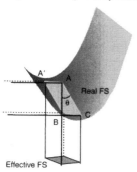

The line focus principle
From the diagram the electron beam of width *A-A'* strikes the anode target area. Distance BC is determined by *sin* θ × AC. If the real focal spot (*AC*) is 2 mm, the effective or apparent focal spot is then 0.2588 × 2 or 0.5 mm square. Doubling the real focal spot size (4 mm) will give a 1 mm effective focal spot.

line imaging (*image*) *See* sequential line imaging.

line of response (LOR) (*nmed*) Identified in PET when an event is detected in coincidence, the line passing through the site of annihilation.

line pairs (*image*) Resolution measurement using a millimetre grating of paired light and dark lines. Line pair spacings are available up to 20 Lp mm-1 for testing radiographic imaging systems. The resolution limit is reached when two lines are just resolvable spaced $1/x$ mm apart, representing x Lpmm^{-1}. A 1 mm line separation would represent 1 Lp mm^{-1} and 0.1 mm separation 10 Lpmm^{-1}. The eye can resolve about 30 to 35 Lp mm^{-1}. Nuclear medicine measures resolution as Lp per centimetre.

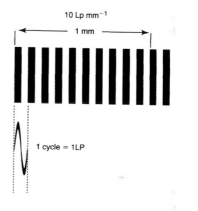

10 Lp mm^{-1}

1 mm

1 cycle = 1LP

line response function (LRF) (*ct*) *See* line spread function.

line scanning (*image*) *See* sequential line imaging.

line shape (*mri*) Distribution of the relative strength of resonance as a function of frequency which establishes a particular spectral tine. Common line shapes are Lorenizian and Gaussian.

line spectral (*mri*) *See* spectral line.

line spread function (LSF) (*image*) Obtained by imaging a slit source rather than a point, as used in the point spread function. If the imaging system is shift invariant, the shape of the line spread function perpendicular to the slit must have practical dimensions similar to the point source. The radiant exposure distribution in the image of an infinitely narrow and infinitely long slit (line source) of unit radiant energy per unit length (ICRU report, 1986) (*see* point spread function).

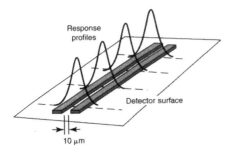

Response profiles

Detector surface

10 μm

line standard (*di*) The standard number of video lines in a display, i.e. 525, 625, 1024, 1249, etc. (*see* HD-TV).

line width (*mri*) Spread in frequency of a resonance line in an MR spectrum. A common measure of the line width is full-width at half-maximum (F WHM).

linear absorption coefficient (μ_{en}) (*phys*) Part of the linear attenuation coefficient attributable to absorption (photoelectric effect) sometimes given the symbol μ_τ. The unit is the reciprocal meter m^{-1}. The total attenuation of the photon beam (μ_{tot}) is the sum of linear absorption coefficient μ_{en} (photoelectric) and linear scatter coefficient μ_{scat} (Compton scatter) events, so: μ_{tot} = μ_{en} + μ_{scat}.

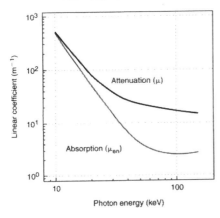

Attenuation (μ)

Absorption (μ_{en})

Linear coefficient (m^{-1})

Photon energy (keV)

linear acceleration (*phys*) When the velocity of a moving mass is changing the mass is accelerating. The rate at which the velocity of a mass is increasing is its acceleration, measured as the change of velocity (*x/t*) per unit time *t* expressed as 'per second, per second':

$$acceleration = \frac{x}{t} \, m \, s^{-1} \, s^{-1}$$

When the rate of change of velocity is increasing, the acceleration is +*a*, although the + sign is not usually shown. If the rate of change of velocity is decreasing, the body is retarding (or decelerating), and this is negative acceleration −*a*.

linear accelerator (*phys*) *See* linac.

linear array (*ct*) A solid state symmetrical x-ray detector where all the detectors have identical sizes. Unlike the adaptive array design, the linear array configuration is easily developed to provide more than four slices per rotation. The dimension of the z-axis is enlarged by increasing the width of the detector, increasing the z-dimension to give 4, 16 and 64 slice machines which allows a much wider coverage of the anatomy for each rotation. A four slice linear array is shown. Currently 16, 64, 128 and 256 slice linear arrays are available.

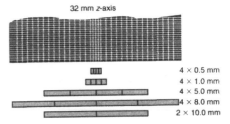

32 mm z-axis

4 × 0.5 mm
4 × 1.0 mm
4 × 5.0 mm
4 × 8.0 mm
2 × 10.0 mm

(*us*) Array made of rectangular elements arranged in a line whose elements are pulsed in a sequence to give a rectilinear shaped image or curvilinear for a curved face.

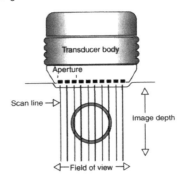

Transducer body

Aperture

Scan line

Image depth

Field of view

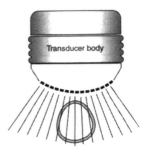

Transducer body

linear attenuation coefficient (μ) (*phys*) The fractional reduction in intensity per unit thickness of material as an x-ray beam passes through an absorber. For a polychromatic beam, the effective linear attenuation coefficient depends on the effective energy of the beam, and the density and atomic number (composition) of the material. For narrow beam geometry and a monoenergetic photon beam incident on the detector (I_o) with no absorber in the beam, the rate at which photon energy crosses a unit cross section perpendicular to the beam direction is measured as the photon fluence $\Phi = N/A$ m^{-2}, or photon flux is $\varphi = \Phi/t$ m^{-2} s^{-1}. As absorbers are introduced, the intensity now incident on the detector (I_x) will decrease according to an exponential law

$$I_x = I_o \cdot e^{-\mu x}$$

where absorber thickness is x and the symbol μ is the linear attenuation coefficient, a function of the photon energy and the atomic number of the absorber. Rearranging the above equation:

- $\dfrac{I_x}{I_o} - e^{-\mu x}; \dfrac{I_o}{I_x} = e^{\mu x}; \dfrac{I_x}{I_o} = e^{-\mu x}; \dfrac{I_o}{I_x} = e^{\mu x};$

- $\ln(I_x) = \ln(I_o - \mu x)$ and $\ln\dfrac{I_o}{I_x} = \mu x$

The logarithmic difference between the transmitted photons is directly proportional to the difference in thickness x. The fractional decrease in intensity is constant, relating to attenuation of wave or beam of particles along the medium's path attributable to all processes (absorption and scattering). The unit is the reciprocal meter m^{-1}. The value of μ decreases with increasing photon energy. Since μ has greater differences at high keV they are used preferentially for computing Hounsfield units. The total attenuation of the photon beam (μ_{tot}) at diagnostic x-ray energies, is the sum of photoelectric absorption (the absorption coefficient μ_{en}) and Compton scatter events (the scatter coefficient μ_{scat}) so: $\mu_{tot} = \mu_{en} + \mu_{scat}$.

Attenuation coefficient for aluminium
The value obtained for I_o is 718 and for I_x is 516 for 1 cm thickness at 200 keV. The attenuation coefficient for 1 cm aluminium is then $\ln\left(\dfrac{I_o}{I_x}\right) = 0.33$ cm^{-1} or 33.0 m^{-1}.

Linear attenuation keV	Coefficient for aluminium μ (m^{-1})
50	99.3
100	45.9
200	33.0

(*see* linear absorption coefficient, mass attenuation coefficient).

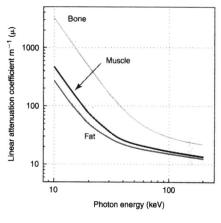

linear dose response (*dose*) A dose response model that expresses the risk of an effect (cancer) being proportional to dose.

linear energy transfer LET (*dose*) Energy transferred to material absorber by charged particle or photon throughout its path. A measure of the density of ionising events along a radiation path as keV μm^{-1}. Used for estimating radiation weighting factor (w_R).

- Gamma and x-rays = 1,
- α radiation = 20
- Beta radiation between 1 and 1.5.

(*see* weighting factor (radiation)).

linear momentum (I) (*phys*) Mass × velocity the SI unit of measurement is therefore the kilogram multiplied by the meter per second: kg m^{-1} s^{-1}. The product of the mass (m) and the velocity (v) of the body so: $I = mv$. Since force is momentum change per second (mass × velocity change) and velocity change per second is acceleration a then momentum change (ΔI) is also described by $F = ma$. The conservation of momentum is fundamental when considering elastic and inelastic collisions between objects (radiation and orbital electrons).

Radiation dosimetry: Nuclear recoil

^{238}U nuclear recoil due to alpha particle emission. The nuclear mass m_n due to 92 protons and 146 neutrons is 3.97×10^{-25} kg. Alpha particle mass m_α (2 protons: 2 neutrons) is 6.68×10^{-27}, the alpha particle velocity (v_α) is measured as 6.25×10^7 ms^{-1}. The original nucleus, before α emission, is at rest so linear momentum is zero (v_n and $v_\alpha = 0$). Conservation of momentum requires $m_n \times v_n + m_\alpha \times v_\alpha = 0$.

The nuclear recoil velocity (v_n) therefore is:

$-(m_a/m_n) \times v_a$
$= -1.05 \times 10^6$ ms^{-1} (recoil has minimum velocity)

When a force has set a body in motion, the body is stopped only by the application of other forces (such as friction, braking, magnetic force, etc.).

Linear parameters

Distance	ℓ (m)
Velocity	v (ms^{-1})
Acceleration	a (ms^{-2})
Mass	m
Force	$F = ma$
Momentum	$p = mv$
Work	$W = Fs$
Power	$P = Fv$
Kinetic energy	$\frac{1}{2} mv^2$

linear-non-threshold hypothesis (*dose*) A dose response model suggesting that, in the low dose range, radiation doses above zero will increase the risk of excess cancer and/or heritable disease proportionately.

linear phased array (*us*) Linear array operated by applying voltage pulses to all elements, but with small time differences (phasing) to direct ultrasound pulses out in various directions.

linear-quadratic dose-response (*dose*) A dose response model that suggests the risk of an effect (e.g. disease, death or abnormality) is the sum of a two component effect, one proportional to dose (linear term) and the other proportional to the square of dose (quadratic term).

linear relationship (*stats*) A relationship between two variables (e.g. dose and effect) which gives rise to a straight line on a Cartesian graph, conforming to the formula $y = mx + c$; m being the gradient and c the intercept with the y-axis.

linear scatter coefficient (σ) (*phys*) The Compton scattering process results in beam attenuation and in energy loss. The linear scattering coefficient σ decreases steadily with increasing energy: high energy radiation is less scattered than lower energy radiation: $Total = \sigma_s + \sigma_a$. Not only the amount of energy transferred to the recoil electron increases with increasing incident photon energy, but an increasing proportion of the total beam energy is taken by the recoil electron. Consequently, at higher energies the energy of the scattered photon is a smaller fraction of the total. A 30 keV photon scattered at a 90° angle retains 97% of its energy; a 100 keV retains 91%; a 1 MeV retains 67% and a 10 MeV retains only 9%.

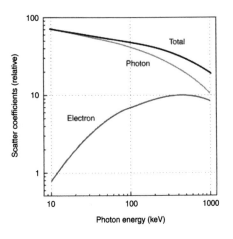

linear sequenced array (*us*) An ultrasound transducer array operated by applying voltage

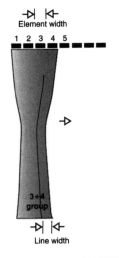

pulses to groups of elements sequentially. The linear array is formed from a large number of individual transducer elements arranged in groups. During each transmission/receive cycle a transducer group from 16 to 32 elements is active.

linear shift-invariant system (*image*) An imaging system which is both linear, i.e. the magnitude of the output signal is a linear function of that of the input signal, and shift invariant, i.e. shifting the position of the input signal results only in a displacement of the output by the same amount (or a simple scaling if magnification is allowed).

linear tomography (*xray*) Longitudinal sectional information obtained by moving the x-ray tube and film in synchrony about a fulcrum or axis. The fulcrum defines the sectional plane. The sectional images are degraded by blurring caused by interfering absorption on either side of the plane of interest (*see* tomography, computed tomography). Linear tomography has suffered a sharp demise with the widespread availability of computed tomography but is being reintroduced using digital imaging (*see* direct radiography).

linear velocity (*v*) (*phys*) The velocity of a moving point, or of a body is the rate of its displacement or the rate at which it changes its position, in a given direction. The rate of displacement of the body is the distance it moves during each unit of time. If it moves through s m in t seconds then $v = s/t \, \text{m s}^{-1}$. Velocity is a vector quantity having both magnitude and direction, but when the direction is constant (a straight line) and the body covers equal distances in equal times, the velocity is uniform and is measured by the displacement per unit time.

Units of linear velocity

SI m s^{-1}	
CGS cm s^{-1}	$1 \, \text{cm s}^{-1} = 1 \times 10^{-2} \, \text{m s}^{-1}$
Other miles hr^{-1}	1 m.p.h. = 0.44 m s^{-1}

Photon time of flight

The distance travelled by a 0.511 MeV gamma photon after 1 nanosecond (10^{-9} s). All electromagnetic radiation has a velocity of approximately $3.0 \times 10^{8} \, \text{m s}^{-1}$.

Distance travelled = $(3.0 \times 10^{8}) \times 10^{-9} = 0.3 \, \text{m}$.

---

linearity (*ct*) In CT, the extent to which the CT number of a given material is exactly proportional to its density (in HU unit).

linearly polarized coil (LP coil) (*mri*) Designed to excite or detect spins using one RF transmit and/or receive channel. The magnetic field has predominately a single direction.

Linux (*comp*) A UNIX® based, open-source (freely available) operating system originally developed by Linus Torvalds. Linux is suitable for many platforms, both PCs and Macintoshes.

lipiodol (*clin*) The first practical x-ray contrast medium introduced for mylography by Sicard in 1921. Because of induced pulmonary and peripheral fat micro-emboli oily x-ray contrast media have been discontinued.

lipophilic agents (*cm*) *See* lipophilicity.

lipophilicity (*clin*) Refers to its preference for fat-like (lipid) organic solvents such as n-butanol. Found to correlate approximately with toxicity of ionic contrast media; readily cross the blood–brain barrier (BBB) during their first pass through the cerebral vasculature. On the other hand, water-soluble contrast media such as non-ionic iodinated contrast used in CT, and water-soluble paramagnetic media used for MRI, are not lipophilic, have a high affinity for plasma water, and do not pass the normal BBB. Certain radiopharmaceuticals (HMPAO, IMP, HIPDM) are lipophilic compounds crossing the blood–brain barrier; conversion occurs within the brain tissue into a hydrophilic agent which traps the compound. Properties other than lipophilicity (e.g. hydrogen bonding) can also be responsible for interactions with biological molecules and membranes.

liquifier (*mri*) System for reliquification of cryogenic gases: if closely matched with a superconducting magnet, zero net cryogen boil-off can be achieved.

LIS (*mri*) Lanthanide-induced shift. A technique involving the substitution of a paramagnetic lanthanide ion for the calcium ion in a selected protein which results in lanthanide-induced shifts and broadening in the ^{1}H NMR spectrum of the protein. These shifts are sensitive monitors of the precise geometrical orientation of each proton nucleus relative to the lanthanide ion.

lithium (Li) (*elem*)

Atomic number (Z)	3
Relative atomic mass (A$_r$)	6.94
Density (ρ) kg/m^3	534
Melting point (K)	452

lithotripsy (*xray*) A non-invasive procedure which uses high power ultrasound to fracture kidney stones in situ (*see* extracorporal shock lithotripsy).

litre (L) (*phys*) The SI unit of volume. Up to 1964 the definition was the volume occupied by a mass of 1 kg of pure water at maximum density ($\approx 4°C$) under normal atmospheric pressure (101 325 Pa). 1 litre then equalled 1.000028 dm^3. This was changed in 1964; the SI unit of m^3 is used for deriving the litre as equal to 1 dm$^3 = 10^{-3}$ m^3. For practical purposes the millilitre (L^{-3}; ml) and cm^3 are equivalent.

liver (biliary contrast media) *See* cholegraphic contrast agents.

LMR (*mri*) *See* localized magnetic resonance.

LNT (*dose*) *See* linear no threshold.

loadability (*phys*) The thermal loadability of an x-ray tube for short, medium and long exposures is determined by the anode's heat capacity and heat loss (cooling rate). A high loadability/high-output tube has two distinguishing characteristics:

- An anode disc with a large diameter, providing greater heat radiation and greater heat storage
- A high conduction through larger surface area sleeve bearings

Short term loadability is a measure for very short exposure time of 0.1 s or less, and is determined by the size of the region which is directly bombarded by the electrons. The focal track of a rotating-anode tube is exposed to direct bombardment by electrons, and therefore represents the region with the highest thermal load. *Long term loadability*; determined by the anode cooling rate; achieved by rapidly restoring the heat capacity of the anode by providing suitable cooling (heat loss) for the anode.

Loadix" (*xray*) A device attached to the rear envelope of an x-ray tube used by Siemens to monitor the temperature of the anode and protect it from excessive heat damage.

loading (*mri*) *See* coil loading.

local (*comp*) Typically refers to devices attached to the user's workstation, as opposed to remote devices that are accessed through a server.

local area network (LAN) (*comp*) A small network that is generally confined to a single office or building. Workstations and computers that are tied together in a specific work area in the same general location. Peer-to-peer networks are a type of LAN architecture. Each workstation doubles as a server in this network, providing the ability to share peripherals and resources with any other workstation. Peer-to-peer resource sharing can be effective on small networks, but security and reliability issues are important.

local bus (*comp*) Also known as the system bus. An internal bus line between CPU, memory and other peripheral devices.

local coil (*mri*) Anatomically specific coils used for each region of the body to be examined (surface coils). The signal-to-noise ratio is significantly improved but over a smaller measurement field (*see* integrated panorama array).

local rules (*dose*) A list of recommendations and regulations drawn up by a hospital to serve all localities (radiology, surgery, laboratory, etc.) that use radiation sources. The local rules supplement, emphasize and clarify the national legislation, identifying the various categories of controlled, supervised and high radiation areas, together with procedures for decontamination. Estimations of risk to the foetus from radiation exposure *in-utero* should be included for reference as well as recommended radiographic protocols for low dose examinations.

localization techniques (*mri*) Means of selecting a restricted region from which the signal is received. These can include the use of surface coils, with or without magnetic field gradients. Generally used to produce a spectrum from the desired region.

localized magnetic resonance (LMR) (*mri*) A particular technique for obtaining NMR spectra, for example of phosphorus, from a limited region by creating a sensitive volume with inhomogeneous applied gradient magnetic fields, which may be enhanced with the use of surface coils.

localized MIP (*mri*) Localized maximum intensity projection. This improves image quality and significantly reduces reconstruction time. A partial data volume is collected containing the vessel of interest.

LocalTalk (*comp*) Apple Computer's proprietary LAN, based on the AppleTalk architecture.

location encoding (*mri*) Defining position and orientation of a slice using the frequency and phase-encoding gradients. The signal origin is encrypted in the MR signal and reconstructed with the image.

lock (*mri*) *See* field lock.

logarithm (*math*) The power to which a fixed number, the base, must be raised to obtain a given number. Abbreviated to *log* for base$_{10}$ and *ln* for base$_e$ (*see* exponential).

---

logarithmic subtraction (*xr*) *See* digital subtraction angiography (DSA).

logic circuit (*elec*) The component part of a digital circuit which acts as a gate, steering data according to a logical sequence. The gates operate according to Boolean logic giving AND, NAND, OR, NOR operations.

logical gradients (*mri*) Each of the three physical gradients has one task: slice selection, frequency encoding and phase encoding. For oblique slices, the logical gradients are a mix of the physical gradients.

longitudinal magnetization (M_z) (*mri*) The macroscopic magnetization aligned along the Z-axis. After the RF pulse, M_z returns to equilibrium M_0 with a characteristic time constant T1.

$$M_{z(t)} = M_0(1 - e^{-t/T1})$$

(*see* transverse magnetization).

longitudinal relaxation (*mri*) Return of M_z to M_0 after excitation. Requires an exchange of energy between the proton spin and the molecular lattice. Measured by time constant T1 (*see* magnetic vector).

longitudinal relaxation time (*mri*) T1 constant.

longitudinal spatial resolution (*ct*) *See* spatial resolution.

longitudinal wave (*us*) Compression wave in parallel to wave direction; the same direction as the direction of travel. The most common example is a sound wave where compressions and rarefactions move along with the speed of the wave-form each particle vibrating about a mean position transferring energy to the next particle (*see* transverse wave).

look-up table (LUT) (*di*) A series of stored values in memory which is used for mathematical transformations (log or non-linear image processing) on incoming signals. LUTs also control displayed grey scale.

Lorentzian line (*mri*) Typical line shape in an NMR spectrum, with a central peak (central resonance frequency) having long tails; proportional to:

$$\frac{1}{[(\frac{1}{T2})^2 + (f - f_0)^2]}$$

where f is frequency and f_0 is the frequency of the peak. The Lorentzian function is the Fourier transform of a decaying exponential.

LOTA technique (*mri*) Long term averaging. Data averaging for reducing motion artefacts.

LP (*mri*) Linear prediction.

LP (*mri*) Linear polarization.

low contrast resolution (*image*) A measure of the ability to discriminate between structures with slightly differing attenuation properties (CT number). It depends on the stochastic noise and is usually expressed as the minimum detectable size of detail discernable in the image, for a fixed percentage difference in contrast relative to the adjacent background. (*ct*) The geometrical resolution for low-contrast details within the object; a measure of the ability to discriminate between structures with slightly differing attenuation properties (CT number). In addition to the modulation transfer function of the CT system, quantum noise and other sources of noise inherent to the scanner determine the limit for separation of small low-contrast details within the image (see image noise, contrast detail diagram, contrast noise ratio).

low frequency drop (LFD) (*xray*) *See* image intensifier (low frequency drop).

low osmolarity (*cm*) A solution of salts, sugars, proteins, acids, etc. with a moderate osmolality or concentration. Describes a contrast medium with a slightly higher concentration than body fluids (two to three times). Such contrast media cause less pain and heat when injected compared to high-osmolar contrast media (*see* high osmolarity).

low-pass filter (*di*) A filter designed to reject frequencies above a certain value while retaining the lower frequencies. They are used in smoothing filters or kernels which reduce the influence of noise in the signal (*see* ideal filter).

LS (*mri*) Line scanning.

LSR (*mri*) Lanthanide shift reagent

LSO (*rad*) *See* Lutetium oxy-orthosilicate.

Lucite"/Perspex" (*phys*) *See* PMMA

lumen (lm) (*phys*) The SI unit of luminous flux, which is the amount of light passing through a unit area at a unit distance per second. One lumen is also defined as the light falling on a unit area at unit distance with a luminous intensity of 1 candela. One lumen of visible light at 555 nm wavelength dissipates an energy of 1.47×10^{-3} watts. Lamp output is measured in 10^3 lumens and efficiency as lumens W^{-1}. For a theoretical 100% efficiency, a white lamp would give 220 lm W^{-1}. In practice, a tungsten lamp gives 15 lm W^{-1} and fluorescent tubes approximately 50 lm W^{-1} (*see* luminance).

luminance (*phys*) A measure of the light coming from a surface. It is the photometric brightness measured in candela per unit area (SI-unit cd m^{-2}; also known as a nit). The non-SI unit is the lambert.

Quantity	SI unit	Abbr.
Luminous flux	lumen (cd × sr)	lm
Luminous energy	lumen second	lm × s
Illuminance	lux (lm m^{-2})	lx
Luminous intensity	candela (lm sr^{-1})	cd
Luminance	candela per square metre	cd m^{-2}

Source	Luminance
Film viewing box	2000 cd m^{-2} or 0.2 cd cm^{-2}
Video (TV) screen	
Display monitor	300 cd m^{-2} to 600 cd m^{-2}
Computer colour display	100 cd m^2
HD-TV	1.0 cd m^{-2} (L_{min}) and a maximum of 263 cd m^{-2} (L_{max}) giving a contrast of L_{max}/L_{min} or 263

- Reference: Assessment of Display Performance. Task Group 18 AAPM 2002.

(see radiance).

luminescence (*phys*) A general property of some inorganic crystals and plastics involving electron transition between valency and **conduction bands**. Gamma, x-radiation or particulate radiation (alpha, beta, electrons) interacts with the phosphor or scintillator producing a light event whose intensity is proportional to the photon energy deposited. Light production can be instantaneous or delayed and the duration of the light signal can be measured in nano-seconds (10^{-9}s) or tenths of seconds (10^{-1}s). Properties of a good luminescent scintillator are:

- transparency to emitted light
- large light output
- high photon absorption for γ-and x-rays
- available in large sizes.

The term luminescence covers three major phosphor types that are commonly found in radiology and used for both imaging and radiation dose measurement such as counters or storage devices. These are:

- phosphorescence
- fluorescence
- thermoluminescence.

Summary of luminescent detectors:

Scintillator	Application
Fluorescence	
NaI:Tl	Scintillator for NM
CsI:Tl	Scintillator for CT

Summary of luminescent detectors (*Contd.*):

Scintillator	Application
$CaWO_4$	Intensifying screen
Gd_2O_2S:Tb	Intensifying screen
Phosphorescence	
ZnS complex (P4)	Video monitor
ZnCdS:Ag (P20)	Image intensifier
Thermoluminescence	
LiF	Dosimeter
BaF(X) X = F, I or Br	Image plate

(*see* fluorescence, phosphorescence, thermoluminescence).

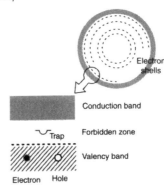

luminescent efficiency (*phys, ct*) The ratio of the total energy of visible emission to total x-ray energy. After irradiation the intensity of the visible emission quickly decreases with time. Once the luminescent intensity drops to a few percent of the luminescent light, further decay proceeds much slower (**afterglow**), caused by the trapping of electrons and/or holes in crystal imperfections. The intrinsic luminescent efficiency should be >5% (signifying efficient recombination of electron-hole pairs at the activator sites) so producing a good signal. Strongest **peak emission** should be at wavelengths between 500 and 900 nm where silicon **photodetectors** have highest sensitivity. Optical transparency at the peak emitting wave-length should be high to permit good optical light collection efficiency at the photodetector.

luminosity (*phys*) The arbitrary brightness of a colour on a scale from black to white (*see* hue, saturation).

luminous flux (*phys*) Luminous intensity integrated over a solid angle. The unit is the lumen.

luminous intensity (*phys*) The quantity of light emitted per second by a point source in unit solid angle. The unit is the candela (cd).

lutetium oxy-orthosilicate (LSO) (*rad*) Cerium activated lutetium oxyorthosilicate (Lu_2OSiO_4: Ce or LSO).LSO offers the best combination of properties for PET imaging. LSO has a higher effective Z (number of protons per atom) and density compared to BGO which results in a higher detection efficiency. It has a short decay constant for improved coincidence timing (decay constant 40 ns), and higher light output (compared to BGO). The crystal is rugged and non–hygroscopic and lends itself to precise machining.

lux (lx) (*phys*) A measure of illuminance as a lumen per square metre $lm\,m^{-2} = m^{-2}cd\,sr$.

lutetium (Lu) (*elem*)

Atomic number (Z)	71
Relative atomic mass (A_r)	174.9
Density (ρ) kg/m^3	9800
Melting point (K)	1925
K-edge (keV)	63.3
Relevance to radiology: lutetium yttrium aluminium perovskite Lu(Y)AP fast decay scintillator for PET.	

^{177}**Lutetium** (*nmed*) xxβ–497 keV, γ 208 keV T1/2 6.65 days. Short range beta 1–3 mm.

lymphocyte (*dose*) A white blood cell formed in the lymphatic tissue and in normal adults comprising approximately 22 to 28% of the circulating leukocytes (*see* **blood cells (labelled)**).

lymphangiography (*clin*) Imaging the lymphatic system (lymphatics and lymph nodes) by introducing CM into the lymph vessels.

lymphography (*clin*) Assessment of the regional lymphatics, lymph nodes and the thoracic duct, using an oily based contrast medium. Also gives contrast visualization of peripheral lymphatics in the extremities, the trunk, face and neck regions. Non-invasive methods using ultrasound, CT, MRI and radionuclides have largely replaced lymphography as a routine procedure. *Direct* (lymphangiography) is used in a few cases and involves direct puncture of lymph vessels and subsequent use of oily contrast media. *Indirect* uses a water based contrast medium infused into toes, fingers or backs of feet and hands. Depends on the CM rapidly diffusing through the lymphatic wall.

M

μ_o (*unit*) The symbol for permeability of free space having a value $4\pi \times 10^{-7}$ N/(ampere-turn)^2.

M_o (*mri*) Equilibrium value directed along the static magnetic field lines. Proportional to spin density.

M_{xy} (*mri*) *See* transverse magnetization.

M_z (*mri*) *See* longitudinal magnetization.

M mode (*us*) Mode of operation in which the display presents a spot brightening for each echo voltage delivered from the receiver, producing a two-dimensional recording of reflector position (motion) versus time.

MAA (*nmed*) Degradable macro-aggregates of human serum albumin. A radiopharmaceutical labelled with ^{99m}Tc and used for either lung scanning, venography or tracing the origins of artero-venous malformations.

Generic name	^{99m}Tc-MAA
Commercial names	Pulmonite®–CIS
Macrotec® (Bracco)	
Technescan® MAA	
Albumoscint®	
Draximage®	
Amersham® MAA	
Numbers of particles/vial	$8 \pm 4 \times 10^6$
Imaging category	lung perfusion

Aggregates of albumin ranging from approximately 10 to 60 μm (mean size 40 μm with 90% <90 μm); these lodge in the capillaries and precapillary arterioles.

Mackensie Davidson, James (1856–1919) pioneer British radiologist, president of the Roentgen Society, later to become British Institute of Radiology.

macro (*comp*) A script that operates a series of commands to perform a function. It is set up to automate repetitive tasks.

macroaggregates (*nmed*) *See* MAA.

macroscopic magnetization vector (*mri*) Net magnetic moment per unit volume of a sample, considered as the integrated effect of all the individual microscopic nuclear magnetic moments (*see* magnetic moment, magnetic vector).

MAG3 * (*nmed*) Benzoyl-mercapto-acetyl-triglycine, a kit for the preparation of ^{99m}Tc mertiatide, a renal diagnostic radiopharmaceutical manufactured by Mallinckrodt for labelling with ^{99m}Tc as Technescan – MAG3. High renal clearance primarily through proximal renal tubule, small amount of GFR and distal tubule secretion. It resembles the excretion pattern of ortho-iodohippurate.

magnesium (Mg) (*elem*)

Atomic number (Z)	12
Relative atomic mass (A$_r$)	24.3
Density (ρ) kg/m^3	1741
Melting point (K)	924
Specific heat capacity J kg^{-1} K^{-1}	1020
Thermal conductivity W m^{-1} K^{-1}	156
K-edge (keV)	1.3

magnet (*phys*) Ferrous material (commonly iron, cobalt or nickel) exhibiting permanent or electromagnetic behaviour.

magnet (homogeneity) (*mri*) Refers to the uniformity of a magnetic field with no object present. Homogeneity is quoted in parts per million (ppm) a relative measure independent of field strength that uses, as reference, the Larmor frequency for water 42.5759 MHz T^{-1}. A 200 Hz variation would give an inhomogeneity of:

$$200/(42.5759 \times 10^6) = 4.7 \times 10^{-6} = 4.7\,\text{ppm}$$

Permanent and resistive magnets have typical inhomogeneities of 40 ppm and superconducting magnets of 1–3 ppm.

magnet (permanent) (*mri*) Certain ferromagnetic alloys form a permanent magnetic field and need no power to maintain their field strength but will gradually lose their original magnetic strength over a period of several years. Permanent magnets have small fringe fields so can be operated in a small area. They are heavy (about 20 tonnes) and have field strength limitations of about 0.3 T but some are much smaller. Their open field aspect allows easy patient interventional studies; however, they cannot be switched off during emergencies and their magnet homogeneity is poor.

magnet (resistive) (*mri*) Operate using the basic electromagnetic principles. Consist of a collection of coils through which a large current is passed. They have a high electrical consumption and create considerable heat that must be removed by cooling. They have a practical upper limit of 0.3 T. They have larger fringe fields than the permanent magnet and their weight is between 5 and 10 tonnes. They can be switched off during an emergency so they are popular as interventional machines. Magnet homogeneity is fair.

magnet stability (*mri*) Temporal stability of the magnetic field. Factors that affect stability are: field decay of superconducting magnets in persistent mode, aging of permanent magnet material, temperature dependence of permanent magnet material, and temporal stability of magnet power supplies.

magnet (superconducting) (*mri*) These are a special type of electromagnet using windings made from alloys which become superconducting at liquid helium temperatures (4 K). An extremely high, stable magnetic field can be produced from 1 to 4 T although smaller magnets with field strengths of 9 T have been used for neonatal studies. The large field strengths allow spectroscopy and fast gradient switching pulse sequences (EPI) that are not available with other magnet designs. They have very high magnet homogeneity, which enables small volume acquisition and fat saturation routines.

magnetic dipole moment (μ) (*mri*) The ability of a current loop to produce a magnetic field at distances from the loop (signal coil). μ is the magnetic moment which is a vector quantity. The SI unit is the ampere-metre^2 (A m^2), weber metres or joules per tesla (J T^{-1}). An electric current loop or the effective current of a spinning nucleon can create a dipole equivalent to the north and south magnetic poles separated by a finite distance on a magnet (*see* magnetic moment).

magnetic disk (*comp*) *See* hard disk drive.

magnetic field (B) (*mri*) Other names are magfield, magnetic flux density, magnetic induction field and magnetic induction. A vector quantity describing the magnetic flux per unit area of a magnetic field at right angles to the magnetic force. The region surrounding a magnet (or current carrying conductor) where a small magnet in such a region experiences a torque that tends to align it in a given direction. The magnetic field produces a magnetizing force on a body within it. The net magnetic effect from an externally applied magnetic field and the resulting magnetization. B is proportional to H, the magnetic field intensity (B = μH) The fundamental quantity for describing a magnetic field. SI unit tesla or weber m^{-2} (Wb m^{-2}) or newton per ampere-meter (N $\times$ A $\times$ m^{-1}) (*see* magnetic field intensity, magnet homogeneity, safety limits (MRI)).

magnetic field gradient (*mri*) The rate of change of a component of the magnetic field with position. Gradients in each of three directions: $\partial Bz/\partial z$, $\partial Bz/\partial x$, $\partial Bz/\partial y$, a magnetic field which changes in strength in a certain given direction producing positional information. Such fields are used in NMR imaging with selective excitation to select a region for imaging and also to encode the location of NMR signals received from the object being imaged. The SI unit is tesla m^{-1}, (0.01 T m^{-1} = 1 gauss cm^{-1}). If the gradient coil imposes a change in the magnetic field of 0.01 T over 1 m then the magnetic field gradient is 10 mT m^{-1} (positive or negative). Typical values are 20 to 35 mT m^{-1} for a 1.5 T system and 45 mT m^{-1} for a 3.0 T system (*see* slew rate).

magnetic field intensity (H) (*mri*) or magnetic field strength. The alternative measurement to B where H = B/μ where μ is the permeability of the medium. The SI unit is ampere per metre (A m^{-1}) (*see* magnetic field).

magnetic field strength (H) (mri) *See* magnetic field intensity (H).

magnetic flux (Φ) (mri) A measure quantifying the magnetic field strength or magnetic field intensity (H); the magnetic flux density is another term for the magnetic field. The flux dΦ through a region of area dA perpendicular to B is given by dΦ = BdA. So the magnetic flux is the product of a magnetic field through a defined area, expressed as T m^2. The magnetic flux through a surface is proportional to the number of magnetic field lines that pass through the surface. The SI unit is the weber (Wb) or volt-second where: 1 Wb (V $\times$ s) = 1 T m^2.

magnetic flux density (B) (*mri*) *See* magnetic field.

magnetic forces (*mri*) Forces resulting from the interaction of magnetic fields. Pulsed magnetic field gradients can interact with the main magnetic field to produce acoustic noise. Induced magnetization reacts with the gradient of the magnetic field to produce an attraction toward the strongest area of the field. There is also a torque or twisting force on objects, for example, intracranial aneurysm clip tends to align along the magnet's field lines. The torque increases with field strength while the attraction increases with field gradient. The magnetic saturation of the object attraction is roughly proportional to object mass. Motion of conducting objects in magnetic fields can induce eddy currents that can have the effect of opposing the motion.

magnetic fringe field (*mri*) Region surrounding a magnet. The earth's magnetic fringe field is

M

typically 0.05–0.1 mT. Due to the physical properties of magnetic fields they form closed field lines. Depending on the magnet construction, the returning flux will penetrate large open spaces (unshielded magnets) or will be confined largely by a massive iron cage or through secondary coils (shielded magnets).

magnetic gradients (*mri*) *See* **gradient.**

magnetic induction (B) (*mri*) See **magnetic field.**

magnetic intensity (B) (*mri*) *See* **magnetic field.**

magnetic moment (m) (*mri*) The ratio between the maximum **torque** exerted on a magnet, current-carrying coil, or moving charge in a magnetic field and its strength. The maximum torque is given when the axis of the magnet is perpendicular to the field. The magnetic moment is a measure of the net magnetic properties of an object or particle. A nucleus with an intrinsic spin will have an associated **magnetic dipole moment**, so that it will interact with a **magnetic field** (resembling a tiny bar magnet). The SI unit is $Wb\,m^{-1}$.

magnetic permeability (μ) (*phys*) *See* **permeability.**

magnetic resonance (MR) (*mri*) Resonance phenomenon resulting in the absorption and/or emission of electromagnetic energy by nuclei or electrons in a static magnetic field. after excitation by a suitable RF magnetic field. The peak resonance frequency is proportional to the magnetic field, and is given by the Larmor equation. Only unpaired electrons or nuclei with a non-zero spin exhibit magnetic resonance.

magnetic resonance angiography (MRA) (*mri*) Allowing vascular structures to be seen without using contrast material. Produces images of blood vessels, for example with flow effects or relaxation time differences. Blood flow can be quantified and flow directions can be determined by using specific techniques and pulse sequences. Some common approaches use the washout of saturated spins from a region by blood flow to increase the relative intensity of blood vessels within images.

magnetic resonance cholangiopancreaticography (MRCP) (*mri*) Magnetic resonance imaging technique in which a two-dimensional (2D) multislice or three-dimensional (3D) RARE pulse sequence using partial Fourier techniques or a 3D gradient echo pulse sequence with heavy T2 weighting is used to acquire data from the liver and the pancreas. The T2 weighting gives essentially all signals from the liver; other solid parenchyma is suppressed and only fluid-filled structures, (gall bladder, bile and pancreatic ducts) contribute important signal intensity.

magnetic resonance signal (*mri*) The signal emitted by a sample in a strong magnetic field of a nuclear magnetic resonance system. A radio-frequency (1–100 MHz) signal is imposed at right angles to this main field and as the magnetic field or RF signal is altered there is a point where the RF signal is strongly absorbed. This resonance (detected by an inductor or antenna), produces a precise signal which is the magnetic resonance signal for the sample (typically hydrogen protons but also ^{31}Phosphorus) (*see* **free induction decay**).

magnetic resonance spectroscopy (MRS) (*mri*) Concerns itself with the free induction decay signal which carries information about the chemical nature of the material. The local magnetic field varies slightly within the compound molecule due to chemical bonds, size of atoms and position of the atom relative to others. The hydrogen atom in water will experience a different local magnetic field to a hydrogen atom in fat leading to a chemical shifts caused by slight variations in Larmor frequency (measured in **parts per million (ppm)** of the main magnetic field). The degree of chemical shift is characteristic of the chemical bonding. Spectroscopy is used for demonstrating the functional chemistry of compounds other than hydrogen. Phosphorus spectroscopy shows metabolic pathways and fluorine spectroscopy is used for following the fate of chemotherapeutic agents. All magnetic resonance spectroscopy requires field strengths higher than 1 T in order to provide resolvable peaks and also exceptional main magnetic field homogeneity (*see* **CHESS**).

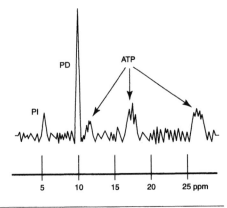

magnetic resonance venography (*clin*) Veins may be imaged and the flow rate determined directly, without the use of paramagnetic contrast media.

magnetic shielding (*mri*) Confining the region of strong magnetic field surrounding a magnet: most commonly the use of material with high permeability (passive shielding) or by employing secondary counteracting coils outside of the primary coils (active shielding). The high permeability material can be employed in the form of a cover or yoke, or an opposing coil immediately surrounding the magnet. Shielding is accomplished by forcing the magnetic return flux through more confined areas or structures, not by absorbing it. Soft iron (mu-metal) is a common material used for shielding against magnetic interference and can be placed around sensitive equipment (image intensifiers, photomultiplier tubes, etc.), since it can concentrate quite weak magnetic fields reducing the external magnetic flux and so protecting devices which are surrounded by the material.

magnetic shielding (mu-metal) (*phys*) Soft iron (mu-metal) is a common material used for shielding against magnetic interference and can be placed around sensitive equipment (image intensifiers, photomultiplier tubes, etc.), since it can concentrate quite weak magnetic fields reducing the external magnetic flux and so protecting devices which are surrounded by the material.

magnetic strength (*phys*) This is dependent on the pole strength m_1 and m_2 at a distance d. These attract or repel each other with a force F so that:

$$F = K \times \frac{m_1 \times m_2}{d^2}$$

where K is a constant, the force obeys the inverse square law. Intensity of the magnetic field is measured as:

$$F = \frac{m_1 \times m_2}{p \times d^2}$$

where p is the permeability of the medium (large for ferromagnetic materials; p for air $= 1$). The magnetic flux would be p times as great if the coils are wound over a magnetic core material (soft-iron); this is exploited in transformer design.

magnetic susceptibility (*mri*) An applied magnetic field induces magnetization of a material. The susceptibility measures the ability of a substance to become magnetized. A dimensionless unit whose value depends on the properties of the atoms and molecules of the material (*see* permeability).

magnetic tape (*comp*) *See* storage (bulk).

magnetic units (*units*) These are analogous to electrostatic units.

Quantity and symbol	SI unit
Magnetic dipole moment	A m^2 or J T^{-1}
Magnetic field strength (H)	
Magnetization	
Magnetic field intensity	H (A m^{-1})
Magnetic flux (Φ)	weber (Wb) T m^2
Magnetic field	
Magnetic flux density (B)	
Magnetic induction	tesla (T) Wb m^{-2}
Magnetic moment	henry (Wb m)
Magnetic constant (μ_0)	
Permeability of free space	henry m^{-1}
Inductance	Wb A^{-1}
Reluctance	ampere turn per weber (A Wb^{-1})

magnetic vector (*mri*) When a sample is exposed to an external magnetic field a net alignment of the individual magnetic moments (protons) will result in a preferred direction along the external field. The nuclei that make up this alignment contribute to a resultant magnetization vector (M). There is a longitudinal magnetization vector (M_L) and transverse magnetization vector (M_{xy}). A transverse component of the magnetization vector can be produced by applying a transverse magnetic field (90° RF pulse or other flip angle) which will move M away from the magnetic field; as the strength of the RF pulse increases the longitudinal component M_L of the magnetization vector decreases. M will assume a position between M zero and M_{xy}.

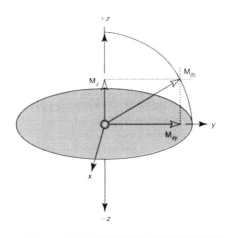

magnetization (*mri*) *See* magnetic field strength.

magnetization transfer (*mri*) The change in magnetization within a multi-component spin system when one of the component peaks is selectively perturbed. This is observed as a change in relative signal intensities. One of the most common forms of perturbation in imaging is selective saturation. For example, this phenomenon can be exploited as part of an imaging sequence to produce image contrast based on differential amounts of magnetization transfer, magnetization transfer contrast (MTC).

magnetization transfer contrast (MTC) (*mri*) Production of change in relative signal intensities by magnetization transfer. The signal from specific tissue regions such as the brain parenchyma is reduced and the signal from fluid components (blood and CSF) is retained, so enhancing these areas. More closely coupled states will show a greater resulting intensity change.

magneto-optical disk (*comp*) Removable optical disk which is re-writeable. Capacity 2.6 G-byte. Data transfer rates 3.4 M-bytes read, 1.7 M-bytes write. Average seek time 25 ms.

Magnevist (*cm*) Commercial (Schering/Berlex Labs. Inc) preparation of ionic gadopentetate dimeglumine for MR imaging.

Compound	Concentration mg mL^{-1}	Viscosity cP	Osmolality mOsm/kg
Gd-DTPA	469	4.9 @ 20°	
		2.9 @ 37°	1960

magnification (*xray*) Image enlargement re-displaying a section of the image to full display dimensions. No improvement in intrinsic resolution (*see* geometric unsharpness).

magnitude contrast angiography (MCA) (*mri*) Displaying a slow blood flow with good resolution across a large volume. Two data volumes are measured: the flow rephased image shows bright flow and the flow dephased image shows dark flow; tissue in unchanged in both data volumes. After subtraction the remaining image represents flowing blood.

magnitude image (*mri*) The normal image display, where the gray scale of a pixel corresponds to the magnitude of the MR signal at that location (*see* phase image).

main frame (*comp*) A large central computer having giga-bytes of memory and terabytes of disk storage.

Mallard JR (1927–) British medical physicist who pioneered developments in medical imaging, particularly nuclear medicine and magnetic resonance imaging.

mammography (*xray*) A low kV x-ray imaging technique for imaging breast tissue. Since photoelectric events predominate in the image formation, small soft tissue differences can be distinguished.

man-Sievert (*dose*) (ICRP60) Dosimetric quantities relating to exposed groups take into account the number of people exposed to the source. These quantities are the collective equivalent dose S_T which relates to a specified tissue or organ exposed (e.g. lungs in miners) and the collective effective dose S (e.g. equivalent whole body dose for miners). The unit of these collective quantities is the man-Sievert obtained from the product of the individual dose and population number. The patient population man-Sievert is used as the reference for reducing clinical dose rates (optimization).

manganese (Mn) (*elem*)

Atomic number (Z)	25
Relative atomic mass (A$_r$)	54.9
Density (ρ) kg/m^3	7440
Melting point (K)	1517
K-edge (keV)	6.5

Relevance to radiology: as a paramagnetic contrast agent in MRI as Mn-DTPA, also as manganese dipyridoxyl-diphosphate (Mn-DPDP) as a para-magnetic contrast agent for hepato-biliary imaging.

MAP shim (*mri*) Multi-angle projection. An early shim procedure that tunes the shim currents to a large region. The shim program can also be applied to the entire measurement field.

Marinelli formula (*nmed*) An early attempt at calculating internal dosimetry estimating organ and whole body radiation dose from beta, non-penetrating radiation $D\beta$ and gamma $D\gamma$ penetrating radiation. It uses a rough geometric factor g allowing for simple variations in organ shape (liver, lungs, kidney etc.) (*see* MIRD formula).

mAs product (*xray*) The product of tube current and exposure time. Since one milliampere is 1 mC s^{-1} then mC s^{-1} × seconds represents coulombs and 1 mAs = 1 mC (*see* exposure).

mask (*dsa*) An early image containing tissue detail which is subtracted from later images.

mask filter (*di*) *See* kernel.

mass (*phys*) The SI base unit is the kilogram (kg). The only base unit which is a multiple of a smaller unit, the gram.

- 1 kg = 1000 gm.
- 1 metric ton (tonne) = 10^3 kg.
- 1 pound = 0.453 kg (*see* kilogram).

mass absorption coefficient (*phys*) The equivalent of the linear absorption coefficient. It is the fraction of energy contained in the beam (gamma or x-radiation) which is absorbed per unit mass of the medium through which it passes when unit area is irradiated.

mass attenuation coefficient (μ/ρ) (*phys*) The quotient of linear attenuation coefficient and material density μ/ρ. The total mass attenuation coefficient is the fraction of radiation removed from the beam (gamma or x-radiation) of unit cross sectional area in a medium of unit mass. The linear attenuation coefficient μ has units of m^{-1}; the mass attenuation coefficient μ/ρ has units of m^2 kg^{-1}. The mass attenuation coefficient is independent of the state of the absorber (gas, liquid, solid). The table shows values for the same keV.

State	μ	ρ	μ/ρ
Ice	0.196	0.917	0.214
Water	0.214	1	0.214
Steam	1.2×10^{-4}	5.9×10^{-4}	0.214
Coefficient (at 150 keV)			
Muscle	0.0150	1.00	0.015
Fat	0.0135	0.91	0.015
Bone	0.0277	1.85	0.015

mass energy absorption coefficient (μ_{en}/ρ) (*xray*) charged particles (electrons) from photoelectric and scattering travel through the absorber and create bremsstrahlung. The mass transfer coefficient is related as:

$$\mu_{tr}/\rho \approx (1 - g)\mu_{tr}/\rho$$

where μen is the energy absorption coefficient, μtr is the energy transfer coefficient, g is the average fraction of kinetic energy of the secondary charged particles (electrons) produced in photoelectric and Compton interactions, subsequently lost in radiative processes (bremsstrahlung). In practice, since g is very nearly zero at diagnostic energies then the mass energy absorption coefficient is equal to the mass energy transfer coefficient ($\mu_{en}/\rho \approx \mu_{tr}/\rho$). The table shows values for water.

keV	μ(m^{-1})	μ_{en}	μ/ρ (m^2 kg^{-1})	μ_{en}/ρ (m^2 kg^{-1})
20	80.9600	55.03	8.096e-02	5.503e-02
40	26.8300	69.47	2.683e-02	6.947e-03
60	20.5900	31.90	2.059e-02	3.190e-03
100	17.0700	25.46	1.707e-02	2.546e-03
150	15.0500	27.64	1.505e-02	2.764e-03

mass energy transfer coefficient (μ_{tr}/ρ) (*xray*) This represents the energy transferred from the incident photons (X- or γ-radiation) to charged particles in the absorber. The mass energy transfer coefficient can be seen as the escape of secondary photon interactions at the initial photon/atom interaction site. For diagnostic x-ray energies (photon energies below 200 kV) the definition is: $\mu_{tr}/\rho = (f_{pe} + f_{scat})$, where μtr is the energy transfer coefficient, ρ the density, f_{pe} and f_{scat} represent the average fractions of the photon energy that is transferred to the kinetic energy of the charged particles (electrons) from the photoelectric (characteristic x-rays) and the Compton scattered photon. For diagnostic energies the contribution from pair and triplet production is ignored (*see* mass energy absorption coefficient).

mass number (*phys*) See atomic mass number.

MAST (*mri*) Motion artefact suppression technique. A pulse sequence for reducing motion induced phase shifts during TE (Picker Medical Inc.) (*see* GMR, GMN, FLOW-COMP, CFAST, FLAG, GMC, FC, STILL, SMART, GR).

matched sample (*stats*) A sample in which the same attribute, or variable, is measured twice under different circumstances or two samples in which the members are clearly paired.

matching (*elec*) See impedance matching.

matching layer (*us*) An additional material to the front of an ultrasound transducer for improving the inevitable mismatch between transducer face and the tissue. A layer ¼λ thick is chosen with an acoustic impedance as the geometric mean between transducer and tissue.

matching network (*mri*) An arrangement of reactive elements (inductors and capacitors) used to transform an input impedance of a given value to an output impedance of a second value. Such circuits are used in interfacing high impedance RF coils to low impedance (usually 50 or 75 ohms) transmission lines that feed RF energy to the coil or send the NMR signal to NMR preamplifier.

math co-processor (*comp*) Mostly incorporated into the CPU but a companion chip is sometimes included with the CPU that carries out arithmetic functions. Program speeds increase considerably when using image processing or graphics.

mathematical erosion (*image*) Mathematical morphology process that acts in a neighbourhood as a local minimum filter.

matrix (*image*) A two-dimensional *x, y* array, commonly stored in computer memory. Each location in the array can represent:

- a pixel containing a grey-level value for display;
- a voxel as an absorption coefficient or equivalent (CT number) representing a tissue volume (slice width dependent);
- ordered phase/frequency information for subsequent transfer into spatial domain for display.

An image matrix can be square or any rectangular pattern (DSA is typically 2048 × 2048, Image plate 1760 × 2140). (*ct*) 2D arrangement of CT numbers; used synonymously with **image matrix**.

matrix algebra (*math*) Many problems of numerical analysis can be reduced to the problem of solving linear systems of equations. Ordinary and partial differential equations by finite difference methods, eigen value problems, least squares fitting of data and polynomial approximation can conveniently use matrix notation and matrix algebraic procedures. Since any kind of matrix can be given a unique symbol it means that this symbol represents a whole array or matrix of numbers. These numbers may be manipulated as single entities are in ordinary algebra.

matrix element (*ct*) *See* voxel, picture element, pixel.

matrix of magnitudes of wavelet coefficients (*image*) Matrix of the magnitudes of the horizontal and vertical wavelet coefficient matrices. Magnitudes of wavelet coefficients represent local intensity variations, corresponding to edges.

matrix size (*mri*) The size of the raw data matrix which influences both the measurement time, resolution and image signal-to-noise ratio.

maximum intensity projection (MIP) (*image*) MIP allows the selection of bright pixels in 2D slices or in 3D volume, displaying maximum pixel value along a given path. Only high signal intensity pixels are projected into the final image and does not convey depth relationships. It is threshold independent. It is most useful when displaying rotating 3D anatomy. It lacks discrimination between tissue types (vascular/non-vascular) where blood is represented as white on black background. Generally, several 3D reconstructions are made at regular angular increments around a given axis. These can then be viewed in sequence to give more information, for example about vessel origins:

- displays maximum pixel value along given path;
- does not convey depth relationships;
- threshold-independent;
- gives attenuation information;
- depicts calcification;
- editing of bone necessary (*see* minimum intensity projection (mIP)).

Maxwell coil (*mri*) A particular gradient coil, commonly used to create gradient magnetic fields along the direction of the main magnetic field.

Mayneord, William Valentine (1902–1988) British physicist who was a pioneer developer of nuclear medicine imaging building a rectilinear scanner in 1958. Also produced early work on ultrasound in medicine and carcinogenetic effect of hydrocarbons.

MBS–MRA (*mri*) Minimum basis set magnetic resonance angiography.

mCi (*nmed*) milliCurie. The non-SI measure for radioactivity. $1\,mCi = 3.7 \times 10^7$ Bq or 37 MBq (*see* curie).

MD-76[*x*] (*cm*) Commercial preparation of meglumine and sodium diatrizoate (66%:10%).

Compound	Viscosity (cP)	Osmolality mOsm/kg	Iodine mg I/mL
Meglumine/Na diatrizoate	16.4 @ 25° 10.5 @ 37°	1551	370

MDI (medium dependent interface) (*comp*) The predefined physical layer interface for 10 Mbps Ethernet.

MDP (*nmed*) Disodium dihydrogen methylene diphosphonate used for bone scintigraphy, labelled with ^{99m}Tc. Taken up in three phases: vascular, enzymatic and bone surface (hydroxyappatite) accretion.

Generic name	^{99m}Tc- medronate (MDP)
Commercial names	Osteolite® – CIS TechneScan® MDP MDP Draximage®
Imaging category	bone

Approximately 50% of the injected dose is retained by the skeleton.

mean (*stats*) The average usually the arithmetic mean:

Arithmetic mean: $\dfrac{x_1 + x_2 + x_3 \cdots + x_n}{n}$

Geometric mean: $\sqrt[n]{x_1 \times x_2 \times x_3 \cdots \times x_n}$

Harmonic mean: $\dfrac{1}{\dfrac{1}{n}\left(\dfrac{1}{x_1} + \dfrac{1}{x_2} + \dfrac{1}{x_3} \cdots \dfrac{1}{x_n}\right)}$

Weighted mean:

$$\frac{w_1 x_1 + w_2 x_2 + w_3 x_3 \cdots + w_n x_n}{w_1 + w_2 + w_3 \cdots + w_n}$$

where $x_1 \ldots x_n$ are n separate numbers and w are the appropriate weightings (*see* **geometric mean**).

mean absorbed dose (*dose*) In a tissue T or organ D_T: the **absorbed dose** D_T, averaged over the tissue or organ T (ICRP 100 (2006a)) which is given by:

$$D_T = \frac{\varepsilon_T}{m_T}$$

where ε_T is the mean total energy imparted to a tissue or organ T and m_T is the mass of that tissue or organ.

mean down time (MDT) (*stats*) The average time that a machine is broken or out of service, including the repair time, corrective and preventive maintenance and any delays due to organization. MDT includes all delays involved and **mean time to recovery/repair (MTTR)** concerns only repair time.

mean error (*stats*) *See* **standard errors**.

mean glandular dose (*dose*) This is difficult to measure directly so is calculated from tabulated conversion constants appropriate for the machine HVL. Glandular tissues receive varying doses depending on:

- depth from the skin entrance site;
- beam quality (kv and filtration);
- breast thickness;
- breast consistency;
- optical density of the image.

In general, the MGD to the standard breast should not exceed 5 mGy. Current values are typically 3 mGy with more modern sets giving 1.5 mGy.

A standard 50:50 breast phantom with a 0.5 cm adipose layer is used for the measurements.

■ Reference: Dance, 1990.

An estimated measure of the radiation dose to the total organ (breast) at a stated beam quality, this is difficult to measure directly so is calculated from tabulated conversion constants appropriate for the machine HVL. Glandular tissues receive varying doses depending on:

- depth from the skin entrance site;
- beam quality (kv and filtration);
- breast thickness;
- breast consistency;
- optical density of the image.

In general, the MGD to the standard breast should not exceed 5 mGy. Current values are typically 3 mGy with more modern sets giving 1.5 mGy. A standard 50:50 breast phantom with a 0.5 cm adipose layer is used for the measurements.

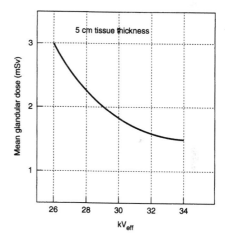

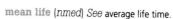

mean life (*nmed*) *See* **average life time**.

mean time between failures (MTBF) (*stats*) The mean or average time between failures of a system (computer or radiology imaging system), and is typically applied to the working life of a machine excluding the start and end of the bathtub curve. The average time between failing and being repaired is the mean down time (MDT) which includes the mean time to repair (MTTR). The MTBF is calculated as the sum of the recorded downtimes minus the uptimes divided by the number of failures:

$$\text{MTBF} = \frac{\Sigma(\text{downtime} - \text{uptime})}{\text{number of failures}}.$$

mean time to recovery/repair (MTTR) (*stats*) The average/mean time that a machine will take to recover from a non-fatal breakdown. This would include fuse replacement, circuit board replacement and mechanical part replacement/repair. The MTTR would be agreed as part of a maintenance contract. Computer systems (HIS/RIS/PACS) should have an MTTR of zero when back-to-back systems (built in redundancy) have secondary devices (computer systems) that can take over the instant the primary one fails. The MTTR can be measured from the repair efficiency (see **RAID**).

measurement field (*mri*) The spherical volume, or **field of view**, in the centre of the magnetic field where the field has a defined homogeneity and least distortion.

measurement geometry (*ct*) *See* **scanner geometry**.

measurement matrix (*mri*) Raw data matrix stored as voxels, not to be confused with the image matrix.

measurement time (*mri*) *See* **image acquisition time**.

mebrofenin (*nmed*) The generic name of iminodiacetic acid (HIDA) derivative as a hepatobiliary agent (*see* **Choletec®**, **CholeCis®**).

mechanical index (MI) (*us*) An indicator of non-thermal mechanism activity; equal to the peak rarefaction pressure divided by the square root of the centre frequency of the pulse bandwidth. The spatial-peak value of the **peak rarefaction pressure**, derated by 0.3 dB/cm-MHz at each point along the **beam axis**, divided by the square root of the **centre frequency**, that is:

$$MI = \frac{p_{-0.3}}{\sqrt{f_c}}$$

where $p_{-0.3}$ is the **peak rarefactional pressure** in megapascals (MPa) derated by 0.3 dB/cm-MHz to the point on the **beam axis** where the **pulse intensity integral** ($PII_{0.3}$) is maximum; and f_c is the **centre frequency** in megahertz. The mechanical index has no units.

MI exceeds 0.3	Minor damage to neonatal lung or intestine
MI exceeds 0.7	Risk of cavitation

■ Reference: AIUM/NEMA, 1998; AIUM, 2000.

mechanical transducer (*us*) A transducer that scans the beam by moving the element(s) or a beam reflector with a motor drive. Replaced by electronic switching.

median (*stats*) The middle value in a distribution. Thus if there are n values the median is that ranked $(n+1)/2$. For example 13, 11, 10, 9, 15, 12, 8 has a median value 11 (*see* **normal distribution**).

MEDIC (*mri*) Multi-echo data image. Multiple echoes are acquired and combined giving a higher SNR per time period and fewer artefacts.

medical exposure (*dose*) The intentional irradiation of a person (patient) either externally or internally, for the purpose of their own medical treatment or diagnosis or as the subject of medical research. It does not include the incidental exposure of others. ICRP 26 (1977) estimates that 1 man-Sievert can cause either 0.012 cases of cancer or 0.01 hereditary disorders. The population dose from medical x-rays is between 520 and 1300 µSv per person per year. The **genetically significant dose** (GSD) is 113 µSv. For 1 million people the population dose is estimated as 520–1300 man-Sv, which could cause between 6¼ and 15½ cancers in a population of this size (See **exposure**).

(The) Medicines (Administration of Radioactive Substances) Amendment Regulations 1995 (*dose*) In the UK these regulations amend the Medicines (Administration of Radioactive Substances) Regulations 1978, prohibiting the administration of radioactive medicinal products except by doctors or dentists. Prior authorization is required and certain controls implemented. Published by the UK Stationery Office Ltd. ISBN 01 10533607

■ Reference: Medicines (Administration of Radioactive Substances) Amendment Regulations, 1995.

medronate (*nmed*) A ^{99m}Tc-MDP preparation (Amersham/GE Healthcare).

mega-byte (M-byte) (*comp*) Approximately one million bytes or exactly 1024 kilo-bytes. A typical computer memory would be 16 to 128 M-bytes.

megahertz (*phys*) One million hertz, MHz.

meglumine (*cm*) A common non-radiopaque cation component associated with many ionic x-ray contrast material. the full chemical name is *N*-methyl-D-glucamine; the empirical formula is: $CH_3NHCH_2(CHOH)_4CH_2OH$ with a molecular weight of 195.22. Meglumine is an organic cation chosen because of its lower pharmacological activity than that of the sodium ion (and therefore better tolerance), but being a much larger ion, meglumine produces a medium of much higher viscosity. Meglumine is also diuretic. Meglumine sometimes shares the cation component of the contrast medium with sodium. Meglumine is used combined with radiopaque compounds such as diatrizoate meglumine and iodipamide meglumine. It also acts as an excipient which is an inert substance added to ensure the shelf-life of the product (contrast medium) that can be long enough to be active until internal use. Excipients also support the active ingredients *in vivo*.

meglumine diatrizoate (*clin*) Iodine containing x-ray contrast material simultaneously synthesized by Schering and Sterling Winthrop in 1954 (*see* Urografin®, Angiografin®, Gastrografin®, Angiovist®).

meglumine iodipamide (*cm*) *See* Biligrafin®, Endografin®.

meglumine iodoxamate (*cm*) *See* Endobil®.

meglumine ioglycamide (*cm*) *See* Biligram®.

meglumine ioxaglate (*cm*) *See* Hexabrix®.

meglumine iotroxate (*cm*) *See* Biliscopin®.

Meitner, Lise (1878–1968) Austrian physicist. Together with Otto Hahn in the Kaiser Wilhelm Institute, Berlin, set up a laboratory for nuclear physics. Co-discoverer of protactinium. Fled to Sweden in 1938. Made the original suggestion that Hahn's results with uranium were due to nuclear fission. Retired to England in 1960.

members of the public (*dose*) Individuals of the population, excluding exposed or designated workers or students during their working hours. Nurses and administrative staff in hospitals should be treated as members of the public along with patients' visitors (*see* public (exposure levels)).

memory (*comp*) The main temporary central storage for information, including applications and documents. Computer memory is measured in megabytes or gigabytes. More energy efficient DDR2 memory uses up to 30% less power than DDR1 and up to 58% less power than FBDIMM.

Mendelian disease (*dose*) An heritable disease attributed to a single gene mutation (*see* multifactorial disease).

mercury (Hg) (*elem*)

Atomic number (Z)	80
Relative atomic mass (A_r)	200.59
Density (ρ) kg/m^3	13590
Melting point (K)	234.3
K-edge (keV)	83.1

^{195m}**Mercury** (*nmed*) Parent of ^{195m}Hg/^{195m}Au generator

Production (cyclotron)	$^{197}_{79}$Au(p,3n)$^{195m}_{80}$Hg
Decay scheme (i.t.) ^{195m}Au	^{195m}Hg (γ keV) $\rightarrow$ ^{195m}Au
Half life	41.6 hours

^{197}**Mercury** (*nmed*) Early radionuclide for brain imaging, replacing ^{203}Hg. Now discontinued.

Decay scheme ^{197}Hg $\rightarrow$	^{197}Hg (ec 268 keV) $\rightarrow$ ^{197}Au
Half life	1.5 days

^{203}**Mercury** (*nmed*) Early radionuclide for brain imaging. Now discontinued.

Decay scheme ^{203}Hg	^{203}Hg (β–279 keV) $\rightarrow$ ^{203}Tl
Half life	46 days

Mertiatide (*nmed*) A carboxylated, diamido-, disulphur- compound as betiatide (N-[N-[N-[(benzoylthio) acetyl] glycyl]glycyl] glycine).; labelled with technetium ^{99m}Tc it forms ^{99m}Tc-mertiatide (disodium[N-[N-[N-(mercaptoacetyl) glycyl]glycyl] glycinato (2-) -N,N',N'',S']oxotechnetate (2-)) and is used in functional and anatomical renal imaging (*see* MAG3).

meson (*phys*) A nuclear family consisting of the pion, kaon and eta particles.

MESS (*mri*) Multiple echo single shot.

metabolic trapping (*nmed*) The uptake of certain compounds (e.g. ^{18}F-fluorodeoxyglucose) by tumours because of a higher metabolic rate for sugars than normal tissue. There is uptake, but little or no metabolism, causing trapping of the labelled sugar in the tumour.

metabolites (PET) (*nmed*) Compounds associated with energy transfer in cells (glucose, lipids). ^{18}FDG with a specific activity of 0.1–1.0 mCi per mole can image metabolic sites holding concentrations of 10^{-5} to 10^{-6} mole per gram or 0.2 to 1.0 mg per gram tissue (*see* receptor site (PET), neuro-transmitters (PET)).

metastable state (*phys, nmed*) An excited nuclear state existing after α or β decay lasting for seconds, minutes, hours or days. Sometimes called isomeric state. Indicated as ^{99}Tc^m or ^{99m}Tc. An excited state of an atom with a measurable half-life (e.g. ^{99m}Tc).

methionine (*nmed*) *See* selenomethionine.

metre (*unit*) The base SI unit of length. Fractions used in radiology are:

- 10^{-1} decimetres (dm); used for defining volume (litre);

- 10^{-2} centimetres (cm); a convenient distance measurement (radiation output);
- 10^{-3} millimetres (mm); image resolution as line pairs per mm;
- 10^{-6} micrometers (μm); image resolution (micro-calcifications);
- 10^{-9} manometers (nm); used for visible light wavelength.

A multiple is the kilometre 10^3. Converting between metres and non-SI units:

- Angstrom (Å) 10^{-10} m;
- 1 inch, 2.54×10^{-2} m;
- 1 yard, 0.914 m;
- 1 foot, 0.304 m;
- 1 mile, 1.6×10^3 m or 1.6 km (*see* area, volume).

metrizamide (*cm*) Developed by Torsten Almén. the first iodinated, water-soluble, non-ionic monomer contrast medium developed in the 1970s. Low osmolar. The molecule is highly hydrophilic, increasing solubility without dissociation and has an increased iodine ratio. Although this agent was inconvenient and expensive for routine intravascular applications, it was used extensively for lumbar myelography because of its favourable neurotoxic profile (*see* Amipaque®, diatrizoate, iothalamate).

metrizoic acid/metrizoate compounds (*cm*) Ionic contrast media monomeric salts of tri-iodinated benzoic acid with substituted side-chains at positions 3 and 5; iodine atoms at 2,4 and 6; cation at position 1. Both the anion and cation are osmotically active, therefore the solution will be hypertonic to plasma (*see* adverse reactions, contrast media (hypertonicity), contrast media (toxicity)).

MeV (*phys, nmed*) Million electron volts. Some gamma radiation used in radiology is measured in MeV (^{60}Cobalt has two gamma energies of 1.173 and 1.333 MeV). All alpha radiation is measured in MeV.

mFISP (*mri*) Mirrored FISP.

M$_{grad}$ (*image*) See film sensitometry.

MHz (*phys*) Abbreviation for megahertz.

MI (*us*) See mechanical index.

MIBG/mIBG (*nmed*) Meta-iodo-benzyl-guanidine. (Iobenguane® CIS/Shering). An analogue of nor-epinephrine with affinity for the sympathetic nervous system and related tumours; MIBG, labelled with ^{123}I is used for the diagnostic imaging of neuroendocrine tumours, disorders of the adrenal medulla and neuroendocrine tumours

such as phaechromocytoma. ^{131}I-iobenguane is used for local radiation therapy in the treatment of carcinoid syndrome, pheochromocytoma, and neuroblastoma. Scintigraphy as labelled compound ^{123}I-MIBG of sympathetic nervous system. Also used in therapy as ^{131}I-MIBG.

MIBI (*nmed*) Methoxy-isobutyl-isonitrile. Labelled with ^{99m}Tc and incorporated into mitochondria-rich sites (cardiac muscle, vertebral muscle, some tumours).

micro-dosimetry (*dose*) The absorbed dose levels at the cellular level (chromosomes, cell membrane, etc.). It is defined as the measurement or calculation of energy deposition by ionising radiation in volumes of the order of 1 μm or less.

- Reference: Kliauga *et al.*, 1996)

Micro-dosimetry parameters

Quantity	Definition	Unit
Energy imparted ϵ	Total energy deposited within micro-volume	keV
Lineal energy y	Quotient of energy imparted by single event and mean chord length of volume (equiv. LET)	keV μm^{-1}
Lineal energy distribution $f(y)$	The probability function of y	
Frequency mean lineal energy y_F	The expectation value of $f(y)$	keV μm^{-1}
Dose probability density $d(y)$	The fraction of absorbed dose delivered to the volume	
Dose mean lineal energy y_D	The expression value of $d(y)$	keV μm^{-1}

Microliteˣ (*nmed*) A kit for ^{99m}Tc labelled albumin colloid used for RES imaging.

Micopaqueˣ (*cm*) Barium sulphate suspension (Guerbet).

microprocessor (*comp*) A complete central processing unit (CPU) contained on a single silicon chip.

micro-spheres (*nmed*) A fixed size albumin or latex spheres labelled with radionuclide. Used for vascular flow studies or estimating the perfusion rate of selected tissues. The albumin is commonly labelled with ^{99m}Tc for imaging the vascular distribution, and after a short while becomes disassociated *in vivo*. The latex spheres are inert and insoluble and become permanently trapped in the selected organ.

micturating cystogram (*clin*) Voiding cystogram (*see* urethrography).

MII (*comp*) Medium independent interface. The predefined physical layer interface for **100BASE-T**.

millicurie (mCi) (*nmed*) The non-SI measure for radioactivity. Since $1 \, mCi = 3.7 \times 10^7$ Bq, then $1 \, mCi = 37 \, MBq$ (*see* curie).

MiniDisk[x] (*comp*) A magnetic-optical digital recording/playback disk produced by Sony. Used almost exclusively for audio recording, giving CD quality and 74 minute recording time. Track numbers can be marked for rapid location. Not used for computer bulk storage (*see* ZIP® drive).

minification gain (*xray*) Ratio of input to output screen area of an image intensifier.

minimum intensity projection (mIP) (*image*) Is employed where blood is represented as black on a white background (*see* maximum intensity projection).

MIP (*image*) Maximum intensity projections.

mips (*comp*) Millions of instructions per second.

Miraluma[x] (*nmed*) *See* Cardiolite®.

MIRD (*dose*) Medical Internal Radiation Dose Committee, Society of Nuclear Medicine which deals with internal radiation dosimetry. Publishes data on decay schemes for tracers used in nuclear medicine, tables for dose computation and reports on dosimetric analysis for specific radiopharmaceuticals.

MIRD formula (*dose*) An improved internal dose estimation with better organ geometry factor and the addition of contributing organ activity. An approach to internal dosimetry proposed by the Medical Internal Radiation Dose (MIRD) Committee in the USA. The MIRD technique:

- Groups both penetrating and non-penetrating radiations together.
- Considers biological and physical data regarding distribution and resident time
- The irradiation of adjacent organs by the target organ.

Dose calculations can be solved for:

- radio-tracers that accumulate mostly in one organ (liver colloid, lung perfusion);
- tracers that are distributed in a number of organs (vascular, hepatobiliary system);
- time varying distribution (bolus studies);
- dose variations to selected organs (the bladder depending on voiding frequency).

MIRD schema (*dose*) A series of MIRD equations used for estimating the absorbed dose to the tissue of interest, taking into consideration the many kind of radiations from the radionuclide as well as the distribution of the radionuclide which may be taken up in a number of different tissues adjacent or associated with the tissue of interest. The MIRD units used in the dose calculation are:

Physical quantity	MIRD symbol	Unit	Symbol
Activity	A	becquerel	Bq
Cumulated activity	Ā	becquerel second	Bq s
Absorbed dose	D	gray	
Mean dose per unit cumulated activity	S	$\dfrac{gray}{becquerel\text{-}sec.}$	$\dfrac{Gy}{Bq\ s}$
Mean energy emitted per nuclear transition	Δ	$\dfrac{gray\text{-}kilogram}{becquerel\text{-}sec.}$	$\dfrac{Gy\ kg}{Bq\ s}$
Residence time	τ	second	s
Energy per particle	E	joule	J
		electron volt	eV
Particle per transition	N	$\dfrac{1/becquerel}{second}$	$(Bq\ s)^{-1}$
Absorbed fraction	υ		
Specific absorbed fraction	Φ	1/kilogram	kg^{-1}
Mass of organ	M	kilogram	kg
Physical half-life	T		
Effective half-time	(Tj)eff	second	s
Physical decay constant	λ		
Biological decay	λj	1/second	s^{-1}

■ Reference: Loevinger, 1991.

mirror image (*us*) An artificial grey-scale, colour-flow or Doppler signal appearing on the opposite side (from the real structure or flow) of a strong reflector.

mission critical (*comp*) A term which emphasizes the importance of a continuous service, such as a hospital or radiology information system, which is expected to give 24 hour, 7 days a week reliability. Normally applied when specifying a control computer system (**file server**) whose reliability must approach 100% achieved by having dual processor design with hot-plugable capability (*see* down-time).

m.k.s. (*unit*) Metric measurement of metre, kilogram, second used in SI units.

M mode (*us*) Mode of operation in which the display presents a spot brightening for each echo voltage delivered from the receiver, producing a two-dimensional recording of reflector position (motion) versus time.

MNP (*comp*) Microcom networking protocol. A set of protocols designed to improve communications between modems but superseded by LAPM. MNP 4 error correction and MNP 5 compression are used as fallbacks if a remote modem does not support LAPM or V.42 bis.

M_0 (*mri*) Equilibrium value directed along the static magnetic field lines. Proportional to spin density.

mode (*stats*) The value of the variable which occurs most frequently; the value of a distribution peak (see normal distribution). (*us*) One of the following system operations: A-mode, M-mode, static B-mode, real-time B-mode, CW Doppler, pulse Doppler, static flow mapping, real-time flow mapping, or any other single display format for presenting clinical information. *Note* Under this definition, the Food and Drug Administration (FDA) considers amplitude Doppler to be a mode.

modem (*comp*) MOdulator/DEModulator. A device which allows a workstation or computer system to communicate and exchange information with other modem equipped computers using telephone lines. A device that connects two computers together over a telephone or cable line by converting the computer's data into an audio signal (*see* ISDN, ADSL).

moderator (*phys*) Neutron absorbing material (graphite or heavy water) lying between the fuel rods in the core of a nuclear reactor to slow down and reduce the energetic neutrons released during fission to thermal (slow) neutron energies. This increases the probability of further nuclear fission events. Typical moderators are graphite or heavy water (D_2O) (*see* hydrogen).

modulation (*elec*) Superimposition of an amplitude, frequency, phase or pulse train onto a carrier wave of high frequency. These various forms of modulation are seen in ultrasound, MRI and computer network communications (*see* PACS, LAN, WAN). (*ct*) A periodic variation of

a signal in the spatial or temporal domain; the modulation is assumed to be a sinusoidal (modulation transfer function) or rectangular (square wave modulation transfer function).

modulation (amplitude: AM) (*elec*) A high frequency carrier wave (sound or RF) whose amplitude varies at the signal frequency. The depth of modulation is measured by comparing the amplitude of the carrier to the signal. It is typically seen in a video signal where the very high frequency carrier is modulated in sympathy with the signal information.

modulation (frequency: FM) (*elec*) The frequency of the carrier wave is varied with the amplitude and polarity of the input signal. The amplitude of the carrier wave is unchanged. FM gives a higher signal to noise ratio than AM.

modulation (phase) (*elec*) Used in RF communications where the phase of the carrier frequency is varied by an amount proportional to the instantaneous amplitude of the input modulating signal.

modulation (pulse code: PCM) (*elec*) A train of pulses is used as the carrier wave, one or more of the signal parameters (amplitude) modifying the pulse train. A carrier wave can also be used which is modulated (FM) in a pulsatile pattern.

modulation transfer function (MTF) (*image*) A complete description of the display resolution. A varying frequency signal (supplied by a line pair grating or line spread function) is supplied to the imaging system. As the frequency of the input signal increases, the ability of the recording (imaging) device begins to fail. The ratio of the output signal amplitude to the input signal amplitude at each frequency is the MTF; a perfect system would register a straight line graph where the MTF = 1.0. It is measured in practice by taking individual readings across a line spread function. The formula used in the calculation involves a Fourier analysis of the response to reveal each frequency component:

$$\frac{\sum_{j=1}^{m} L(x_j, z) \times (\cos 2\pi v x_j - i \times \sin 2\pi v x_j)}{\sum_{j=1}^{m} L(x_j, z)}$$

where $L(x_j, z)$ is m individual line spread values at Δx sampling interval; v is the frequency in cycles cm^{-1} computed. The MTF graph compares two imaging surfaces on linear scales.

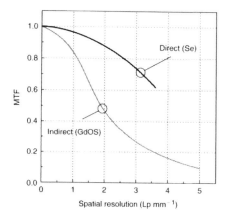

MTF plotted against Spatial resolution (Lp mm^{-1}), showing Direct (Se) and Indirect (GdOS) curves.

modulus (*image*) Magnitude.

modulus of elasticity E (*phys*) A measurement of material stiffness represented by *stress/strain*. The inverse is *compressibility* or 1/E.

mole (*phys*) The SI unit (mol) for the amount of a substance that contains as many elementary entities as there are atoms in 12 g (0.012 kg) of carbon as ^{12}C. The former name was the gram-atom. The elementary entities may be atoms, electrons, molecules, ions etc., but must be specified. Can also be defined as a millimole (mmol):

1 mol = molecular weight in grams

NaCl has a molecular weight of 58.45, so 58.45 g in 1 L of water is a molar solution. Isotonic (normal) saline is 300 mmol and contains 9.448 g NaCl per litre of water.

The number of elementary particles is a constant known as Avogadro's constant and is 6.022×10^{23} mol^{-1}; atoms per mole. The atoms per unit mass = N/A, where A is atomic mass. Since Z (atomic number) also represents the number of electrons, then electron density $e = N \times [Z/A]$. The lighter elements have a greater electron density (*see* osmolarity).

molecular imaging (*image*) Changes in size and structure are detected by anatomic imaging. Molecular imaging characterizes and monitors biological processes at the cellular and molecular levels. Molecular imaging techniques include positron emission tomography, planar nuclear medicine (NM) and single photon emission computed tomography (SPECT), optical fluorescence, optical bioluminescence, magnetic resonance spectroscopy, molecular MRI (mMRI), and functional MRI (fMRI). Molecular imaging positron

emission tomography provides functional information in patients following intravenous administration of tracers that are incorporated into various biochemical and cellular processes (*see* physiologic imaging).

molecular weight (*unit*) *See* relative molecular mass.

molybdenum (Mo) (*elem*)

Atomic number (Z)	42
Relative atomic mass (A$_r$)	95.94
Density (ρ) kg/m^3	10 200
Melting point (K)	2880
Specific heat capacity J kg^{-1} K^{-1}	250
Thermal conductivity W m^{-1} K^{-1}	138
K-edge (keV)	20.0

Relevance to radiology: as a support for the anode disk (axle) since it has relatively low thermal activity. As a K-edge filter material in mammography. Relevant nuclides.

^{99}Molybdenum (*nmed*) The parent radionuclide for the ^{99}Mo/^{99m}Tc generator.

Production	$^{235}_{92}$U(n,f)$^{99}_{42}$Mo(+ $^{135}_{50}$Sn)
Decay scheme (beta decay) ^{99}Mo	^{99}Mo (β–, γ 740 keV) : ^{99m}Tc T½ 6.02 h
Gamma ray constant	4.1×10^{-2} mSv hr^{-1} GBq^{-1} @ 1 m
Half life	2.76 days
Half value layer	mm Pb

^{99}Mo/^{m}Tc generator (*nmed*) The most commonly used radionuclide generator system found in all scintigraphic nuclear medicine departments. The production of the radionuclide Technetium-99 m is based on isomeric transition (i.t.) by the decay of its parent radionuclide:

^{99}Mo (T½ 2.76 d) (β–, γ 740 keV)
→ ^{99m}Tc (T½ 6.02 h) (i.t. 140 keV)
→ ^{99}Tc(β – 2.1 × × 10^5 y) → ^{99}Ru (stable)

The construction consists of glass or plastic column containing alumina (aluminium oxide, Al$_2$O$_3$) and the ^{99}Mo is loaded onto the column as ^{99}MoO$_4$$^{2-}$ (molybdate ion). The eluent is normal saline. Since ^{99}Mo is in the ^{99}MoO$_4$$^{2-}$ form with a 6+ oxidation state. ^{99}Mo decays into ^{99m}Tc as ^{99m}TcO$_4$– (the pertechnetate ion), having a 7+ oxidation state. The 6+ oxidation state of Mo probably provides a firm binding to the alumina, whereas the 7+ oxidation state of ^{99m}Tc provides a weaker binding and can be removed with 0.9% saline, the molybdate remaining bound to the column. The common QC tests include: breakthrough (Mo- and aluminium. The pH of the eluate should be in the range of 4.5–7.5. Radiochemical purity of the eluate can be analysed by chromatography. Sterility/apyrogenicity and freedom from particles should be checked (*see* quality control (nuclear medicine), limulus test).

momentum (*phys*) Mass × velocity. The SI unit of measurement is therefore the kilogram multiplied by the metre per second: kg m^{-1} s^{-1}.

momentum (angular) (*phys*) *See* angular momentum, angular displacement.

momentum (linear) *I* (*phys*) *See* linear momentum.

moment of inertia (*phys*) For a rigid body moving about a central fixed axis. Resembles linear motion with moment of inertia replacing mass, angular velocity replacing linear momentum. Moment of inertia is important to consider with x-ray anode design, keeping the surface area large but the mass (moment of inertia) low by using lightweight materials (graphite).

monitor (*dose*) To determine the level of ionizing radiation and radioactive contamination in a given region. Also a device used for this purpose.

Moniz, Egas (1874–1955) Portuguese radiologist first to use thorium dioxide suspension as contrast medium for carotid arteriography in 1929. Nobel Prize for Medicine and Biology 1949.

monochromatic beam (*nmed*) All the gamma-ray energy is the same (e.g. ^{99m}Tc is monochromatic because essentially all the photons have an energy of 140 keV).

monochromatic radiation (*phys*) Electromagnetic radiation having a single wavelength. Laser radiation is monochromatic; some phosphors also emit very nearly single wavelength light so can be termed monochromatic. (*ct*) x-ray beam with all its photons having one and the same energy or in practice a very narrow energy range (*see* polychromatic radiation).

monoclonal (*clin*) Describes a monoclonal antibody.

monomer (contrast medium) (*cm*) Contrast media consisting of one benzoic ring with three iodine atoms. Monomeric contrast media can be ionic (**Iodine ratio 1.5**) or non-ionic (**Iodine ratio 3**). All have osmolalities higher than blood/CSF, ionic CM 5–7 times as high, and non-ionic CM 2–3 times. Iodine-complex contrast media are built typically on a benzene ring structure where up to three iodine atoms can be chemically attached; this is the basis for monomeric contrast media like diatrizoate, metrizoate or iothalamate (*see* non-ionic monomer, dimer).

monomeric (contrast media) (*cm*) Contrast material consisting of one benzoic ring with three iodine atoms. Monomeric contrast media can be ionic ('Ratio 1.5 contrast media') or non-ionic ('Ratio 3 contrast media').

Monte Carlo analysis (*stats*) A technique for obtaining an approximate solution to certain mathematical and physical problems, characteristically involving the replacement of a probability distribution by sample values, usually performed using a computer. A method of finding the probability distribution of all the possible outcomes of a complex process by simulation where a theoretical analysis is not possible. The probabilities of various outcomes are estimated by repeated computer simulations to form a probability pattern.

morbidity (*clin*) The incidence of non-fatal illness. Disease of any type or the risk of such illness (e.g. number of illnesses per 1000 appendectomies).

mortality (*nmed*) Death or the risk of death, i.e. number of deaths per 1000 procedures. The number within a chosen population (e.g. women between the ages 50–84) who die within a defined period. Rates per 1000 or 100 000 are commonly quoted or a simple percentage.

mosaic images (*mri*) Where 16 to 64 EPI images are combined into one mosaic image. This increases the clarity of BOLD display. Motion artefact is reduced since random or involuntary movement (breathing, heartbeat, blood flow, eye movement, swallowing) and patient movement are obscured and appears as ghosting or smearing in the images in phase-encoding direction only.

motion artefact (*ct*) Artefact caused by movements of the object during data acquisition; the inconsistencies of the measured projections not only result in unsharpness, as in conventional radiography, but can also cause long-range artefacts in the CT image.

motion compensation (*mri*) Modifying the field gradients used in a pulse sequence such that flow and acceleration do not induce any additional phase effects.

motion (harmonic) (*phys*) When the force acting on a system is directly proportional to its displacement x from a fixed point, then the variation of x with time follows a sine relationship: $x = a \sin \omega t$, where a is the amplitude of the waveform or the greatest displacement from the equilibrium position. The constant ω equals

2π *f*, where *f* is the frequency of oscillation measured in cycles per second or Herz (Hz). The period *T* of the waveform which is a measure of the time to undergo one complete cycle is $1/f$ so $\omega = 2\pi/T$. When the waveform completes a cycle it moves forward a distance λ, the wavelength. In one second when *f* vibrations occur, the wave moves forward a distance *f*λ. Hence the velocity *c* of the waves, which is the distance a peak moves in one second is $c = f\lambda$.

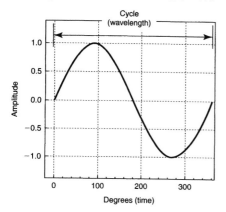

motion (rotational) (*phys*) A force is being applied to a disc or wheel so as to produce rotary motion, variation of the force will usually cause a proportional variation in the speed of rotation and therefore of the kinetic energy of the rotating part. Any mass when in motion tends to resist being retarded. In the case of a rotating anode it can be shown that its tendency to preserve its state of motion (its inertia) is determined by its mass and its radius. The inertia *I* of a disc of uniform density having mass *M* and radius *R* is given by:

$$I = \tfrac{1}{2}MR^2$$

Inertia can be increased by increasing either the mass or the diameter of the disc.

Rotational motion: CT assembly

Centripetal/centrifugal forces on a CT x-ray tube and support of mass 100 kg and 0.6 m radius revolving at 0.5 s or 2 rev per second.
Force $= ma = m(v^2/r)$
Velocity $= 2\pi r \times 2$ metres per second $= 7.54\,\mathrm{m\,s^{-1}}$
Centripetal or centrifugal force is $(100 \times (7.54)^2)/0.6 = 9466\,\mathrm{N}$

MOTSA (*mri*) Multiple overlapping thin slab acquisition.

moving average filter (*di*) A technique for reducing rapid temporal fluctuations (particularly image data in DSA). Each average or smoothed value is computed from the average of preceding raw data values. It is non-recursive since the output relies solely on input data.

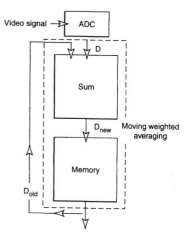

moving slit scan (*xray*) A technique for moving a line source of radiation over an object so that the whole of the object's surface is scanned by the radiation (*See* AMBER).

movement unsharpness (*image*) *See* unsharpness (movement).

MP3 (*comp*) MPEG audio layer 3. A standard for compressing and storing audio sequences in very small files while maintaining high-quality sound. MP3 encoders (or rippers) use a mathematical model of the human ear and removing frequencies that would not normally be detected.

MPEG (*comp*) Motion Picture Experts Group. A compression format for video enabling high quality picture sequences to be stored. A committee that defines the standards for digital video and audio compression techniques. MPEG-i compression allows video CDs to be played on PCs at 30 fps (frames per second) while MPEG-2 is used for digital TV broadcasts and OVO movies.

MPGR (*mri*) Multiplanar gradient recalled, general sequence, GE (*see* FFE, GRE, GRECO, FE, PFI, GE, Turbo FLASH, TFF, SMASH, SHORT, STAGE).

MPPS (*mri*) Modality performed procedure step.

MPR (*mri*) *See* multiplanar reconstruction.

MP-RAGE (*mri*) Magnetization prepared rapid gradient echo. A pulse sequence developed by Siemens for T1-weighted contrast. A rapid gradient-echo acquisition preceded by a magnetization preparation (MP) period that ensures proper image contrast.

MR signal (*mri*) Radiofrequency electromagnetic signal produced by the precession of the transverse magnetization of the nuclear spins.

MRA (*mri*) *See* magnetic resonance angiography.

mrad (*dose*) A fraction of a rad as 10^{-3} rad. The non-SI measurement of absorbed dose.

MRCP (*mri*) Magnetic resonance cholangiopancreatiography. This relies on the high contrast between the fluid-filled ductal structures, yielding high T2 signal intensities and the surrounding tissues, yielding lower T2 signal strengths. Usually implemented with a single shot RARE sequence.

mrem (millirem) (*dose*) The sum of the products of the absorbed dose in mrad and a quality factor: $mrem = (dose_1 \times QF) + (dose_2 \times QF)$.

MRS (*mri*) *See* magnetic resonance spectroscopy.

MSAD (*ct*) *See* multiple scan average dose.

MS-DOS (*comp*) An early operating system developed by Microsoft Corporation (Microsoft Disc Operating System).

MS-EPI (*mri*) Multi-shot echo planar imaging

MTBF (*stats*) *See* mean time between failures.

MTC (*mri*) *See* magnetization transfer contrast.

MTSA (*mri*) Multiple thin slab acquisition.

MUGA (*nmed*) Multi-gated-acquisition using the ECG for gating heart images according to their position in the cardiac cycle.

multi-core (*comp*) In April 2005, Intel announced a Pentium based duo-core processor, providing advantages for multitasking jobs and improve the throughput of multithreaded applications. A dual-core processor consists of two complete execution cores in one physical processor both running at the same frequency. Both cores share the same packaging and the same interface with the chipset/memory. Dual-core designs support hyper-threading technology and can process four software threads simultaneously. Currently, quad core processors have become available (Intel® Xenon® 5300 series). Processors with DDR2 memory are designed to offer a seamless upgrade path from dual-core to quad-core (*see* memory).

multidose (*nmed*) Refers to a vial, etc. that contains enough of a radiopharmaceutical whereby doses for more than one patient can be taken from it.

multi-echo sequences (*mri*) Differentiating the T1 and T2 contributions in an image can be achieved by using a 180° pulse train after the initial spin echo sequence. The successive 180° echoes have approximately the same T1 content but different T2 content. Multi-echo sequences can be run with multi-slice routines.

multifactorial disease (*dose*) Diseases that are attributable to multiple genetic and environmental factors.

Multihance™ (*cm*) Commercial (Bracco) preparation of gadobenic acid as the dimeglumine salt (Gd-BOPTA). MRI ionic paramagnetic contrast agent.

Compound	Concentration mg mL^{-1}	Viscosity (cP)	Osmolality mOsm/kg
Dimeglumine gadobenate (Gd-BOPTA)	529	9.2 @ 20° 5.3 @ 37°	1970

multimedia (*comp*) The use of sound and graphics. The PC to be supplied with sound card, speakers, multi-speed CD-ROM drive and equipped with memory and disk space for sound and image files.

multipath (*us*) Relating to paths to and from a reflector that are not the same.

multiphase study (*nmed*) A dynamic study using a mixture of frame timings.

multiplanar reconstruction (MPR) (*mri*) The ability to display not only axial images but also sagittal, coronal and selected oblique views from a data set. A new images or any orientation can be reconstructed as a post processing technique based on a 3D or continuous multi-slice measurement.

multiple echo imaging (*mri*) Spin echo imaging using spin echoes acquired as a train. Typically a separate image is produced from each echo of the train. Includes rapid acquisition with relaxation enhancement (RARE) techniques (fast-spin echo (FSE) or turbo-spin echo (TSE)) where more than one echo is acquired per excitation pulse. Carr–Purcell (CP) sequences and Carr–Purcell–Meiboom–Gill (CPMG) sequences are examples of multiple-echo imaging techniques where distinct images are constructed from signal echoes acquired at a different TE values, yielding different T2 weighting to each image set. Echo-train techniques speed image acquisition by applying a different phase-encoding to each echo but combining echoes with different T2 weightings into a single image set.

multiple line-scan imaging (MLSI) (*mri*) Variations of sequential line imaging techniques that can be used if selective excitation methods that do not affect adjacent lines are employed.

Adjacent lines are imaged while waiting for relaxation of the first line toward equilibrium, which may result in decreased image acquisition time. A different type of MLSI uses simultaneous excitation of two or more lines with different phase encoding followed by suitable decoding.

multiple quantum coherence (*mri*) Excitation by an RF pulse creates a transition or 'coherence' between different energy levels. Transitions are only allowable between states of the spin system differing in quantum number by one unit 'single-quantum coherence', but multiple RF pulses can act in cascade and produce multiple-quantum coherence. Only single quantum coherence produces a directly observable signal, however, requiring indirect observation of multiple-quantum frequencies.

multiple reflection (*us*) Several reflections produced by a pulse encountering a pair of reflectors; reverberation.

multiple scan average dose (MSAD) (*ct*) The MSAD is the average dose across the central slice from a series of N slices (each of thickness T) when there is a constant increment I between successive slices:

$$MSAD = \frac{1}{I} \int_{-0.5}^{+0.5} D_{N,I}(z)dz \text{ (mGy)}$$

where $D_{N,I}(z)$ is the multiple scan dose profile along a line parallel to the axis of rotation (z). For a sufficient number of slices such that the first and the last in the series do not contribute any significant dose over the width of the central slice:

$$MSAD = \frac{T}{I} * CTDI \text{ (mGy)}$$

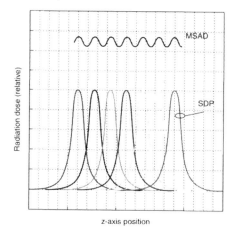

z-axis position

multiple sensitive point (*mri*) Sequential line imaging technique utilizing two orthogonal oscillating magnetic field gradients, an SFP pulse sequence. and signal averaging to isolate the NMR spectrometer sensitivity to a desired line in the body.

multiple slice imaging (*mri*) Sequential plane imaging used with selective excitation techniques that do not affect adjacent slices. Adjacent slices are imaged while waiting for relaxation of the first slice toward equilibrium. Reduces imaging time for a slice set.

multiple spin echo (*mri*) A pulse sequence leading to the production of multiple spin echoes after an initial excitation (*see* multiple echo imaging).

multislice (*ct*) *See* adaptive and linear array.

multiplet (*mri*) A pattern of multiple resonances (spectral lines) observed when the initially single Larmor frequency of a given nucleus is split by interactions with neighbouring spins through the scalar or spin–spin interaction. The magnitude of this interaction is independent of the applied magnetic field; referred to as J, the spin–spin coupling constant.

multiple tuned coil (*mri*) RF coil designed to operate at more than one resonance frequency. so that NMR of more than one kind of nucleus can be observed with the' same coil.

multiply tuned coil (*mri*) RF coil designed to operate at more than one resonance frequency, so that NMR of more than one kind of nucleus can be observed with the same coil.

multi-row detector (*ct*) Detector array with currently between 4 and 256 independent detector rows. The multi-slice machine has its focal spot-to-isocenter and focal spot-to-detector distances shortened in order to cover patient anatomy; the number of detector elements along the detector arc can then be increased. The multi-slice detector is divided into many elements along the z-axis (*see* multi-slice system).

multi-slice artefacts (*ct*) These include partial volume artefact, spiral artefacts, cone-beam artefacts, rod artefacts. Spiral interpolation artefacts, especially in structures that change rapidly in the z-axis, are an important issue for multi-slice scanners.

multi-slice imaging (*mri*) A variation of sequential imaging. The recovery period of the first excited slice is used to measure additional slices. The slices are interleaved.

multi-slice machine (*ct*) CT scanner capable of measuring more than one slice simultaneously, based on multi-row detectors. Multislice CT scanners (MSCT) which acquired two transaxial slices simultaneously, began in 1992 using two parallel banks of detectors. A variant is the electron-beam scanner also with a dual set of detectors. Multi-row detector CT scanning was made available in 1998 using solid detectors and simultaneously imaging four slices in each rotation of the x-ray source. Multi-slice CT helical scanners are all third-generation (fan beam variation) systems mostly with low voltage slip rings. Faster rotation sub-second times (0.5 s) reduce exam time while producing image quality similar to that of single slice scanners. Multi-slice helical CT performs differently from single-slice helical scanners, with respect to patient dose, pitch, image artefacts and its method for image reconstruction. Fundamental advantages of MSCT include:

- Shorter acquisition times with improved temporal resolution (less motion artefacts);
- retrospective creation of thinner or thicker sections from the same raw data;
- improved 3D rendering with diminished helical artefacts;
- increased volume coverage per unit time;
- high axial resolution; examination can be performed with thinner sections, leading to higher spatial resolution along the longitudinal axis;
- Intravenously administered iodinated contrast material can be delivered at a faster rate, increasing contrast enhancement in the images.

These factors improve the spatial, temporal and contrast resolution of the images, significantly increasing the diagnostic accuracy.

multistage tumorigenesis (*dose*) A progressive acquisition of cellular properties that can lead to the development of tumour from a single (target) cell.

multitasking (*comp*) Running more than one program or doing more than one job simultaneously on the same computer or connected group of computers; the ability to run two or more programs from one computer at the same time, controlled by the operating system. The number of programs that can be effectively multitasked in this way depends on several factors: the amount of main memory available, CPU speed, disk capacity as well as the efficiency of the multitasking program itself (*see* pre-emptive multitasking).

multithreading (*comp*) A feature which allows an appropriately designed operating system to run several tasks concurrently.

multi-venc sequence (velocity encoding) (*mri*) Phase contrast angiography. This sequence is not equally sensitive to various flow velocities and used for acquiring wide variations in flow velocity commonly in the peripheral arteries.

mu-metal (*phys*) A trade name for a nickel-based ferromagnetic alloy used for shielding magnetically susceptible devices (image intensifiers, photomultipliers). Also a ferromagnetic alloy used for magnetic shielding and transformer cores. Has a very high relative permeability. Consists of 78% Ni, 17% Fe, 5% Cu and some Cr and Mo (*see* magnetic permeability).

mutagenesis (*nmed*) Induction of a change in genetic material by radiation or any other agent; this could be either a somatic or a genetic effect, depending on whether body cells or germ cells are affected.

mutation (*dose*) A genetic change that can be transmitted to offspring as an inheritable divergence from the parent.

mutation component (MC) (*dose*) A measure of the relative change in disease frequency per unit relative change in mutation rate as a measure of responsiveness. MC values differ for different classes of heritable disease.

mutation rates (*dose*) The frequency, per gamete of mutations, in a given species per unit time.

M_{xy} (*mri*) *See* transverse magnetization.

myelography (*clin*) Radiological investigation of the central nervous system: spinal canal, subarachnoid space. Contrast medium is injected into the sub-arachnoid space, replacing and gradually mixing with the cerebral spinal fluid.

Mylar[x] (*chem*) A polyester film used in the manufacture of recording tapes.

myocardium (*clin*) The muscle composing the heart and some of the pulmonary vessels.

myocardium (hibernating) (*clin*) Hibernating myocardium occurs when coronary artery disease has chronically caused a significant reduction in myocardial perfusion. Contraction ceases through insufficient energy production but the tissue remains viable. Metabolism is maintained by a complete change from fatty acid to glycolytic metabolism. Removal of the stenotic lesion re-establishes normal myocardial function.

myocardium (stunned) (*clin*) Non-infarcted myocardium fails to regain contractility following removal of the stenotic lesion. The perfusion may be normal but the ischaemic damage has caused functional changes. Over a period of time the function may return to normal.

myelography (*clin*) Imaging the spinal chord and subarachnoid space by injecting CM via the cisteral or lumbar route. Either negative CM (gas/air) or oil based iodine compounds may be used. (*clin*) Radiography of the spinal cord and nerve roots using x-ray contrast medium into spinal subarachnoid space.

Myoscint⁺ (*nmed*) ^{111}Indium imciromab pentetate monoclonal for imaging myocardial necrosis.

Myoview⁺ (*nmed*) A version of tetrofosmin (GE Healthcare) for labelling with ^{99m}Tc. Myoview®.

M_z (*mri*) *See* longitudinal magnetization.

NanoCis (*nmed*) CIS/Schering preparation of colloidal rhenium sulphide (nanocolloid).

nanocolloid (*nmed*) Very small particle colloid with a particle size distribution 95% less than 80 nm; used for imaging reticulo-endothelial system. Typically a preparation of ^{99m}Tc-antimony trisulphide (*see* colloid).

narrow beam (*rad*) A collimated radiation beam (x-ray) preventing scatter events reaching any detector (*see* scatter coincidence events). The half value layer is less than broad beam measurements. (*us*) A beam focused laterally (*see* collimation).

National Council on Radiation Protection and Measurements (NCRP) A United States of America agency that seeks to formulate and widely disseminate information, guidance and recommendations on radiation protection and measurements which represent the consensus of leading scientific experts. The Council monitors areas in which the development and publication of NCRP materials can make an important contribution to the public interest. Recent reports are:

Report number	Title
157	Radiation Protection in Educational Institutions
149	A Guide to Mammography and Other Breast Imaging Procedures (2004)
148	Radiation Protection in Veterinary Medicine (2004)
147	Structural Shielding Design for Medical x-Ray Imaging Facilities (2004)
145	Radiation Protection in Dentistry (2003)
140	Exposure Criteria for Medical Diagnostic Ultrasound; II. Criteria Based on All Known Mechanisms (2002)

The information supersedes the recommendations that address such facilities in NCRP Report No. 49, Structural Shielding Design and Evaluation for Medical Use of X Rays and Gamma Rays of Energies Up to 10 MeV, which was issued in September 1976.

native image (*mri*) A contrast study without the use of contrast agent as in BOLD imaging.

navigator echo (*mri*) Additional spin or gradient echoes used for detecting changes in object position in a measurement volume, or other changes. Can be used for interventional procedures or respiratory gating.

NCRP *See* National Council on Radiation Protection and Measurements.

natural background radiation (*nmed*) Radiation originating from natural sources such as cosmic radiation, naturally radioactive minerals and gases in the earth and naturally radioactive elements in the body (14 C, 40 K), typically contributes a dose of 1–3 mGy per year in the United States and Europe.

near field/near zone (*us*) *See* Fresnel zone.

negative contrast medium (*cm*) *See* contrast medium (gaseous).

negative predictive accuracy (diagnostic) *See* predictive accuracy (negative).

negligible individual dose (NID) (*dose*) The NRCP Report 91 defines this as a risk level below which efforts to reduce exposure are not considered important. NCRP Report 116 further recommends that an annual effective dose of 0.01 mSv may be considered a negligible individual dose for a source or practice. ICRP has not defined this quantity.

neighbourhood (*image*) A set of pixels located near a given pixel.

neighbourhood operation (*image*) An image processing operation that assigns a grey level to each output pixel on the basis of the grey level of pixels located in the neighbourhood of the corresponding input pixel.

NEMA (National Electrical Manufacturer's Association) The trade association for the electrical manufacturing industry. Founded in 1926 and headquartered near Washington, DC, its approximately 450 member companies manufacture products used in the generation, transmission and distribution, control and end-use of electricity. These products are used in utility, medical imaging, industrial, commercial, institutional and residential applications.

neodymium (Nd) (*elem*)

Atomic number (Z)	60
Relative atomic mass (A$_r$)	144.24
Density (ρ) kg/m^3	6960
Melting point (K)	1297
K-edge (keV)	43.5
Relevance to radiology: used as a dopant in various phospors.	

neon (Ne) (*elem*)

Atomic number (Z)	10
Relative atomic mass (A$_r$)	20.18
Density (ρ) kg/m^3	0.839
Melting point (K)	24.5
Relevance to Radiology: used as a gas mixture in laser recording and printers.	

neoplastic transformation (*dose*) *See* cell modification.

Neoscan* (*nmed*) A 67 Ga-citrate preparation (Amersham/GE Healthcare).

Neospect* (*nmed*) A ^{99m}Tc imaging agent which binds to somatostatin receptors on malignant tumours; produced by (Amersham/GE Healthcare). The active substance is depreotide (as trifluoroacetate), a synthetic peptide. When reconstituted with pertechnetate, ^{99m}Tc-depreotide is formed which binds with high affinity to somatostatin receptors, which are expressed in both small cell and non-small cell lung carcinoma.

Neotect* (*nmed*) ^{99m}Tc-depreotide for somatostatin receptor bearing pulmonary neoplasms (GE Healthcare).

Nephroscint* (*nmed*) A preparation for ^{99m}Tc-DMSA (Bristol Myers Squibb).

nephrosography (*clin*) Radiography of the kidney by injecting contrast medium through nephrostomy tube and opacifying the renal pelvis.

nephrostomy (*clin*) Establishing a connection between pelvis of the kidney through its cortex to the exterior of the body. Opening between pelvis of the kidney through its cortex to the exterior of the abdomen under fluoroscopic control. *Percutaneous* drainage by collecting system via catheter inserted through skin of the flank, under fluoroscopic viewing.

nephrotoxicity (contrast medium) (*cm*) Disturbances of the kidney function. Iodinated contrast materials are nephrotoxic. The acute deterioration of renal function is sometimes seen following exposure to iodine contrast material, called contrast-induced nephropathy (CIN). Ionic contrast media can significantly reduce the glomerular filtration and affect the tubular function. Non-ionic and isosmolar contrast media have a very low risk of causing loss of kidney function. The effect on renal vascular supply is biphasic: first there is a mild vasodilatation, followed by a more prolonged vasoconstriction. Renal ischemia and breakdown of some renal basement membrane junctions is frequent. Studies have suggested that non-ionic agents have less nephrotoxicity.
- Reference: Dawson and Clauss, 1994.

NEQ (*image*) *See* Noise equivalent quanta.

net optical density (*film*) Optical density excluding base and fog.

network (*comp*) Several computers linked together with their output devices shared (printers, film-formatters etc.). The three most common wiring types for networks are twisted pair, fibre optic and coaxial. Local area (LAN) and wide area (WAN) network designs are available (*see* LAN, WAN, NOS).

network operating system (NOS) (*comp*) Software that manages the resources of a network, typically provides file sharing, e-mail, print services, security measures, etc.

Neurolite* (*nmed*) Produced by (Bristol–Myers Squibb) N N' -ethylenedi-L-cysteinato 3- oxo [^{99m}Tc V] diethyl ester dihydrochloride, Bicisate (ECD) a radio-pharmaceutical labelled with ^{99m}Tc demonstrates cerebral perfusion which crosses the blood–brain barrier by passive diffusion and exhibits uptake and retention in the normal brain.

neurotoxicity (contrast medium) (*cm*) The blood–brain barrier can be compromised (damaged) by hyper-osmolar contrast material. This is lessened with low osmolar agents. Where the blood–brain barrier is normally incomplete (choroid plexus, stalk of the pituitary etc), contact with iodine contrast materials can cause central nervous system reactions. Central nervous system neoplasms, infections and infarctions can also increase leakage across the blood–brain barrier. Neurotoxicity is related to both concentration and type of ions present in the contrast material. Charged ions can inhibit normal neuro-transmission. Consequently non-ionic agents have minimal electrical effects. Neurologic side effects include seizures, cortical blindness, paresis and encephalopathy. The carboxyl ion present in ionic contrast media is associated with high neurotoxicity in the subarachnoid space. Low neurotoxicity is particularly important with intravascular injections of contrast media if damage to the blood–brain-barrier is suspected. Neurotoxicity is most critical with myelography. Non-ionic contrast media tend to have a low neurotoxicity
- Reference: Dawson and Clauss, 1994.

neurotransmitters (PET) (*nmed*) Substances labelled with positron emitters resembling those produced by synaptic systems in parasympathetic and sympathetic nerve pathways (adrenaline, nor-adrenaline etc.). A specific activity of 10^2 to 10^3 mCi ($\approx$5–50 GBq) per mole, it has been estimated that tissue concentrations of 10^{-8} to 10^{-9} mole per gram (0.2–2.0 µg per gram) can be imaged (*see* receptor site (PET), metabolites (PET)).

neutrino (*phys*) A neutral elementary particle (fermion) that only takes part in weak interactions. The rest mass is zero and so moves at the speed of light. A neutrino transfers mass, energy and

N

momentum. It is produced during **beta decay** and its arbitrary mass energy transfer causes the beta particle to exhibit a range of energies in the form of a *continuous spectrum*. The particle responsible is now considered to be an anti-neutrino (*see* positron).

neutron (*phys*) A neutral particle within the nucleus. A member of the baryon family having zero charge with a rest mass and energy $(1.674 \times 10^{-27}\,\text{kg}$ and 939.550 MeV) slightly greater than the proton and a mean lifetime of 932 s (15 min).

neutron capture (*phys*) Slow and thermal neutron reaction of the form (n,γ) indicating gamma photon emission. A common method for preparing clinical nuclides, i.e. ^{60}Co, ^{125}I. Boron and cadmium have a very large cross section for neutron capture. Boron neutron capture is used as a technique for increasing tumour neutron dose by using boron-labelled, tumour-seeking agents. Cadmium, in the form of control rods, regulates the power output in nuclear reactors.

NeutroSpec" (*nmed*) A variety of fanolesomab, a murine IgM monoclonal antibody for labelling with $^{99\,m}$Tc. Manufactured by Mallinckrodt Inc.

newton (N) (*phys*) The SI unit of force: $F = ma$ provides a mass of 1 kg an acceleration of 1 m s^{-2} (*see* force, mass, weight).

NEX (*mri*) A term used to represent the number of signals averaged for each phase encoding step (*see* NSA).

NIC (*comp*) A network interface card. A PCI or ISA adapter card stalled in a PC in order to allow It to connect it to a network. Some motherboards have an integrated network chip (*see* adapter).

nickel (Ni) (*elem*)

Atomic number (Z)	28
Relative atomic mass (A$_r$)	58.71
Density (ρ) kg/m³	8900
Melting point (K)	1726
Specific heat capacity J kg^{-1} K^{-1}	444
Thermal conductivity W m^{-1} K^{-1}	90.7
K-edge (keV)	8.3
Relevance to radiology: in the manufacture of the cathode assembly in x-ray tubes.	

niobium (Nb) (*elem*)

Atomic number (Z)	41
Relative atomic mass (A$_r$)	92.90
Density (ρ) kg/m³	8570
Melting point (K)	2741
K-edge (keV)	18.9
Relevance to radiology: sometimes used as a K-edge filter.	

Niopam " (*cm*) Preparation of iopamidol, a nonionic monomer radiographic contrast agent introduced by Bracco in 1981.

nit (*phys*) Equivalent to candela per m² (cd m^{-2}).

nitrogen (N) (*elem*)

Atomic number (Z)	7
Relative atomic mass (A$_r$)	14.01
Density (ρ) kg/m³	1.165
Melting point (K)	63.3
Relevance to radiology: used as a refrigerant for cryogen protection surrounding the helium cryostat.	

^{13}**Nitrogen** (*nmed*) a positron emitter used in PET scintigraphy.

Production	$^{12}_{6}\text{C}(d,n)^{13}_{7}\text{N}$
Decay scheme	^{13}N T½ 10 m (β+, 2γ
(β+) ^{13}N	511 keV) → ^{13}C stable
Decay constant	0.0693 min^{-1}

Uses in radiology: cyclotron produced nuclide for PET imaging.

NMR signal (*mri*) Electromagnetic signal in the radiofrequency range produced by the **precession** of the **transverse magnetization** of the spins. The rotation of the transverse magnetization induces a voltage in a coil, which is amplified and demodulated by the receiver; the signal may refer only to this induced voltage.

noble gases (*elem*) *See* inert gases.

node (*comp*) Each of the individual computers or other devices on the network.

NOE (*mri*) *See* nuclear Overhauser effect.

nofetumomab merpentan (*nmed*) A fragment of a monoclonal antibody that when tagged with $^{99\,m}$Tc as $^{99\,m}$Tc-nofetumomab merpentan, can detect a protein found on the surface of most small cell lung cancers. determine the extent of disease in patients diagnosed with small cell lung cancer (SCLC). Distributed under the trade name Verluma® by the Dupont Merck Pharmaceutical Company, Billerica,

noise (*phys*) Any undesired signal whether electrical, RF or sound. Thermal noise in electrical circuits is due to the interchange between a material (resistive or semiconductor) and its surroundings. Thermal noise can be affected by ambient temperature and can be reduced by cooling. Impulse noise (switching transients) is an instantaneous disturbance. Both wideband and impulse noise can be reduced by signal filtering.

(image) Noise in an image is considered to be random events characterized by a probability density function (PDF), the most common noise PDFs being Gaussian noise, Rayleigh noise, uniform and impulse noise. *(ct)* The point-to-point variation in image density that does not contain useful information. The magnitude of noise is indicated by the percentage standard deviation of the CT numbers within a region of interest in the image of a uniform substance (generally water), relative to the difference in CT numbers between water and air. For a given CT system, noise is inversely proportional to resolution. Generally, image noise is proportional to $1/\sqrt{mAs}$ when mAs is doubled the noise decreases by $1/\sqrt{2}(\times 0.707)$. Factors affecting noise and low contrast detectability depend on:

- photon flux reaching the detector: influenced by kVp, filtration, mAs and patient size;
- system noise: mechanical or electrical noise within the CT system;
- detector efficiency;
- reconstruction algorithm;
- slice thickness;
- x-ray tube age.

Data acquisition using multi-slice systems covers more patient length per rotation, so for extended-length studies x-ray tube current can be increased compared to single-slice machines. The higher current reduces image noise and improves image quality, which is critical for thin-section extended-length studies, but at the expense of increased patient CT dose.

noise correlation *(ct)* The relationship between two quantities that carry statistical noise; for CT the reconstructed images show a noise correlation; the pixel noise at one position within the image is not independent from that at other positions, since each measured attenuation value contributes randomly with every pixel in the reconstructed image *(see* space invariant etc.).

noise equivalent power (NEP) *(image)* The RMS value of a modulated radiant power source incident on a detector surface that will give an RMS signal equal to the detector RMS noise voltage. The detectability $D = 1/NEP$. A detector generates a signal in the absence of any radiative flux; this is the dark current. If the dark current signal randomly fluctuates as σ_d then:

$$NEP = \sigma_d/R$$

where R is the responsivity of the detector defined as the ratio between incident flux and resulting signal. It is essentially the minimum radiative flux that can be measured with a particular detector for a specified frequency band (see Wiener spectrum).

noise equivalent quanta (NEQ) *(image)* A comprehensive measure of image quality involving the intensity transfer function (characteristic curve) (G), the modulation transfer function (MTF) and the noise power spectrum (W):

$$NEQ = \frac{G^2 \times MTF^2}{W}$$

It is a measure of the number of quanta which form the final image; the theoretical minimum photon density required for a visible image. With photon noise limited images, the effective number of input quanta (NEQ) per unit area will give the same signal to noise ratio (SNR) in an ideal imaging system, as the actual quanta required in a real imaging system. The relationship to the total number of photons at the detector face defines the DQE. The equivalent input exposure deduced from the measured noise and signal transfer characteristics for a photographic or radiographic system is:

$$NEQ(v) = \frac{\gamma^2 (\log_{10} e)^2 MTF(v)^2}{W_{\Delta D}(v)}$$

where γ is the slope of the curve of the density vs. log exposure, MTF the modulation transfer function and $W_{\Delta D}$ the noise power spectrum at the operating point of interest. Analogous quantities for other modalities are found throughout the image assessment literature with the large area factor K in the place of $\gamma(\log_{10} e)$. They are often loosely referred to as NEQ because they play the same role as NEQ in the ideal-observer signal-to-noise ratio.

- Reference: Dobbins JT 3rd, 1995.

noise figure *(mri)* A measure of the noise performance of an amplifier or chain of amplifiers such as an NMR receiver. In NMR systems the preamplifier should have a very low noise figure to prevent significant degradation of the signal-to-noise ratio of the NMR signal. Noise figure is a ratio in dBs, and is given by:

$$20 \log[V_o/V_i(G)]$$

where V_i is the input thermal noise voltage, V_o is the amplifier output noise level and G is the voltage gain of the amplifier, when the input and output impedances of the amplifier are equal.

noise power spectrum (*image*) An alternative name for the Wiener spectrum.

noise structure (*ct*) Non-regular patterns visible in a reconstructed CT image, caused by noise correlation.

nominal (tomographic) slice thickness (*ct*) The slice thickness selected and indicated at the control panel of the CT scanner.

nominal risk coefficient (*dose*) A gender and age (at exposure) averaged lifetime risk estimates for a representative population.

nominal slice thickness (*ct*) The slice thickness selected and indicated at the control panel of the CT scanner.

non-autoscan (non-autoscanning) (*us*) The emission of ultrasonic pulses in a single direction, where scanning in more than one direction would require moving the transducer manually.

non-cancer disease (*dose*) A disease other than cancer such as cardiovascular, cataract, fetal malformation.

non-circular orbits (*nmed*) Since humans in cross section are essentially ellipsoid, the distance between camera face and subject will vary with a circular camera orbit. Resolution deteriorates with distance and resulting tomographic images will show unsharpness. Non-circular orbits can be achieved by either moving the detector in an elliptical path or by moving the table towards and away from the camera face while the camera itself traces a circular orbit. With the moving table technique image reconstruction is simpler than with elliptical orbiting of the camera head.

non-ionic (*clin*) Compounds that will not dissociate or that dissociate minimally when solved in water. Non-ionic contrast media will not dissociate when dissolved in water. The number of ions in solution per iodine atom is therefore lower than for ionic contrast media. Non-ionic monomeric contrast media consist of one benzoic ring with three iodine atoms ('Ratio 3 contrast media'). These will have osmolalities of about half that of ionic monomeric contrast media, typically 2.5–3 times the osmolality of blood at the high estiodine concentrations. Non-ionic dimeric contrast media have two iodinated benzoic rings connected by a nondissociating bridge. Non-ionic dimeric contrast material have six iodine atoms per ion ('Ratio 6 contrast media').

non-ionic dimer (*cm*) Non-ionic dimers (e.g. iodixanol) combine dimerization with nonionicity to achieve isosmolality.

Nonionic dimer

Generic name	Trade name	Iodine ratio	Viscosity cP	Osmolality mOsm/kg H_2O
Iodixanol	Visipaque	6:1	25 @ 20°	300
Iotrolan	Isovist		10 @ 37°	

■ Reference: Dawson and Clauss, 1994.
(*see* anaphylactic/idiosyncratic reactions, blood–brain barrier, distribution coefficient, excretion/elimination half-life, osmolality/osmolarity, pH value, pharmacokinetics, protein binding, tissue-specific, toxicity, viscosity).

non-ionic monomer (*cm*) The elimination of charge and the masking of the hydrophobic iodinated core by multiple hydrophilic substituted groups gave monomeric nonionic agents which provided a marked reduction in osmolality and a reduction in chemotoxicity as compared with their ionic predecessors.

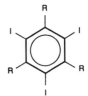

Non ionic monomer

Generic Name	Trade Name	Iodine Ratio	Viscosity cP	Osmolality mOsm/kg H_2O
Iohexol	Omnipaque	3:1	11 @ 20°	500–700
Iopamidol	Iopamiro		6 @ 37°	
Iopromide	Ultravist			
Ioversol	Optiray			
Iopentol				
Iobitridol	Xenetix			

non-ionizing radiation (*clin*) *See* radiation (non-ionizing).

non-parametric test (*stats*) Tests of significance making no assumptions about population distribution. Tests involve ranking. Examples would be: Kendall and Spearman's rank correlation, Mann-Whitney U-test. Anova may be carried out on ranks of data (*see* non-parametric test).

non-prewhitening matched filter (NPWMF) (*image*) The NPWMF is a sub-optimal observer in that, while using all known information regarding the signal parameters perfectly, is unable to undo any correlations in the data. The NPWMF observer uses a template matched to the expected difference image to form a test statistic, regardless of the sources of variability in the data.

nonquadratic shape (*xray*) Much larger in radial than in azimuthal direction (*see* focal spot size).

non-recursive filter (*di*) A signal processing technique where the output signal from the filter depends only on present and previous inputs. Inherently stable as a filter design. Since non-recursive filters have a finite impulse response they can be made symmetrical producing linear phase characteristics and no phase distortion. They are used for removing reconstruction artefacts in axial tomography (*see* side lobe, Hanning filter, Hamming filter, moving average).

non-selective pulse (*mri*) Transmitted pulses that affect all of the tissue within the coil. Used with other sequences to select and define slices (3D) or at a frequency removed from the resonant frequency (MTC).

non-specular reflection (sound) (*phys*) A rough surface will give non-specular sound reflection.

non-stochastic (*dose*) *See* deterministic.

non-uniformity (differential) (*nmed*) The percentage maximum difference between two adjacent pixels in an image matrix is the differential non-uniformity and is defined by NEMA as the high and low values obtained from image matrix pixel values measured over a range of five pixels in all rows and columns. percentage maximum difference between two adjacent pixels. Typical value $\leq \pm 1.5\%$. Companion measured to integral non-uniformity (*see* uniformity).

non-uniformity (integral) (*nmed*) Measured as the percentage difference between the maximum and minimum pixel counts in a sampling area (UFOV or CFOV). The formulas used in calculating integral and differential uniformities, where $U_i(+)$ and $U_i(-)$ are the measured extreme values for non-uniformity. C_{max} and C_{min} are the maximum and minimum pixel counts and C_x is the mean pixel count within the sampled area of an image matrix. Typical value $\leq \pm 2.0\%$. The NEMA (1980)

definition for integral non-uniformity is defined below. Both equations give the same result.

Integral non-uniformity	$U_i(+) = \dfrac{(C_{max} - C_x)}{C_x} \times 100\%$
	$U_i(-) = \dfrac{(C_{min} - C_x)}{C_x} \times 100\%$
Integral non-uniformity (NEMA)	$\dfrac{C_{max} - C_{min}}{C_{max} + C_{min}}$
Differential non-uniformity	$\dfrac{high - low\ pixel}{high + low\ pixel}$

(*see* uniformity).

normal distribution (*stats*) A continuous distribution of a random variable with its mean, median and mode equal. The shape of the normal curve is defined as:

$$y = \frac{N}{\sigma\sqrt{2\pi}} \cdot e^{-(x^2/2\sigma^2)}$$

where N is the number of observations, σ is the standard deviation and x is the magnitude of N the sample value. The normal curves, in the diagram above, show two standard deviations for the same sample size. In a normal distribution approximately two-thirds of the distribution lies less than 1 SD from the mean (34% each side) and 95% lies less than 2 SD.

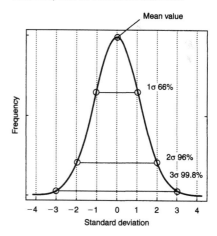

(*see* standard deviation, percentile, quartile).

normalization filter (*mri*) Signal intensity equalization by using surface coils. The greater signal intensity from locations close to the coil is reduced while signal intensity is increased in locations further from the coil.

NOS (*comp*) Network operating system. Software designed to run on a server that controls access from client PCs to services such as email or printer sharing. Windows NT Server and Novell NetWare are the two most common NOSs.

Noyce, Robert Norton (1927–1990) American physicist and engineer, was co-founder of Fairchild Semi-conductors where he developed the first integrated circuits. He also co-founded Intel.

NRC (USA) (*rad*) Nuclear Regulatory Commission.

NRPB (UK) (*rad*) National Radiological Protection Board.

NSA (*mri*) Number of signals averaged together, so reducing noise component before determining each position-encoded signal to be used in image reconstruction.

NTFS (*comp*) NTFile System. An advanced form of file coding used for hard disks. It allows file names of 255 characters. Replaces FAT file systems.

NTSC (*image*) National Television Systems Committee. Television transmission standard developed in the USA offering 525 lines at 60 fps.

nuclear fission (*phys*) Splitting of a transuranic element to give two or more lighter element fragments. A heavy nucleus splits into two approximately equal halves. Uranium and plutonium are the common fissionable elements in a nuclear reactor providing commercial quantities of numerous lighter element radionuclides: ^{131}I, ^{133}Xe, ^{125}I, ^{99}Mo:

$$^{237}U + n \begin{array}{c} > ^{99}Mo \\ > ^{131}I \\ > ^{133}Xe \end{array}$$

nuclear fusion (*phys*) If two light nuclei are combined to form a nucleus of Z, < 56 energy is released. The benefits over fission are that the light nuclei are plentiful and the end products are usually stable light nuclei. The reaction which has been chosen for power production is the *deuterium-tritium* or *D-T* reaction: $^2H + ^3H \rightarrow$ $^4H + n$ ($Q = 17.6\,MeV$). A disadvantage is that most of the energy is given to the neutron from which it is not easy to extract.

nuclear magnetic moment (*phys*) The magnetic moment of an atomic nucleus that arises from the spin of the protons and neutrons. It is mainly a magnetic dipole moment. The nuclear magnetic moment varies from isotope to isotope of an element. It can only be zero if the numbers of protons and of neutrons are both even. Odd numbered nucleons are detected in NMR.

Isotope	Natural abundance (%)	Γ (MHz)	Signal intensity
^{1}H (Proton)	99.98	42.58	1.0000
^{19}Fluorine	100	40.05	0.8300
^{23}Sodium	100	11.26	0.0930
^{31}Phosphorus	100	17.24	0.0660
^{17}Oxygen	0.037	5.77	0.0290
^{13}Carbon	1.11	10.71	0.0160
^{35}Chlorine	75.5	4.17	0.0084
^{15}Nitrogen	0.37	4.30	0.0010
^{39}Potassium	93.1	1.99	0.0005

nuclear magnetic resonance (NMR) (*mri*) A hydrogen proton can align its magnetic moment either parallel or antiparallel in a strong static magnetic field. A pulse of electromagnetic radio frequency of exactly the resonant frequency (equal to the difference between these levels) will excite them into a higher energy state. When the protons relax back to their ground state, they each emit energy of the same resonant frequency which can be detected. NMR spectroscopy depends on the phenomenon that the electrons in a molecule shield the protons to some extent from the main magnetic field, depending on the chemical construction. This effect changes the Larmor frequency very slightly so giving chemical shifts. Fourier analysis translates the frequency differences into peaks which can identify different compounds.

nuclear Overhauser effect (NOE) (*mri*) A change in the steady state magnetization of a particular nucleus due to irradiation of a neighbouring nucleus with which it is coupled by means of a spin–spin coupling interaction. This interaction must be the primary relaxation mechanism of these nuclei. Such an effect can occur during decoupling and must be taken into account for accurate intensity determinations during such procedures.

nuclear reactions (*elem*) A reaction where there is a change in the atomic nucleus, resulting in the formation of a different nuclide. The reaction may be a spontaneous natural one (uranium disintegration), obtained using a nuclear reactor (^{99}Mo fission product) or by a particle accelerator (cyclotron derived ^{18}F).

Nuclear reactor

An overall reaction in a nuclear reactor can be described as:

$$^{32}_{16}S + ^1_0n \rightarrow ^{32}_{15}P + ^1_1p + Q$$

where Q describes the overall energy requirements of the reaction. This is conveniently shortened to $^{32}S(n, p)\,^{32}P$.

Nuclear fission

$$^{235}_{92}U_{143} + {}^{1}_{0}n \rightarrow {}^{99}_{42}Mo_{57} + {}^{134}_{50}Sn_{84} + 2{}^{1}_{0}n$$

^{235}U (n,f) ^{99}Mo

$$^{235}_{92}U_{143} + {}^{1}_{0}n \rightarrow {}^{131}_{53}I_{78} + {}^{102}_{39}Y_{63} + 2{}^{1}_{0}n$$

^{235}U (n,f) ^{131}I

Cyclotron

Using accelerated charged particles in a cyclotron (protons, deuterium nuclei or alpha particles) give reactions of the form:

proton reactions $^{1}_{1}p_{0}$

$$^{11}_{5}B_{6} + {}^{1}_{1}p \rightarrow {}^{11}_{6}C_{5} + {}^{1}_{0}n \qquad {}^{11}B\ (p,n)\ {}^{11}C$$

deuteron reactions $({}^{2}_{1}d_{1})$

$$^{82}_{36}K_{46} + {}^{2}_{1}d_{1} \rightarrow {}^{81}_{37}Rb_{44} + 3{}^{1}_{0}n \qquad {}^{82}K\ (d,3n)\ {}^{81}Rb$$

alpha reactions $({}^{4}_{2}\alpha_{2})$

$$^{14}_{7}N_{7} + {}^{4}_{2}\alpha_{2} \rightarrow {}^{17}_{8}O_{9} + {}^{1}_{1}p \qquad {}^{14}N\ (\alpha,p)\ {}^{17}O$$

---

nuclear reactor (*phys*) A critical assembly of fissionable material (^{235}U, ^{238}U, ^{239}Pu) and moderator (carbon or heavy water). The nuclear reactor is used for thermal energy production and also as a source of neutrons for radionuclide production by either neutron irradiation of a prepared sample or from products of nuclear fission.

nuclear spin (*mri*) An intrinsic property of certain nuclei that gives them an associated characteristic angular momentum and magnetic moment. Shown by nuclei with an odd number of neutrons and protons. For imaging, mostly only hydrogen protons are used. For MR spectroscopy, other nuclei are used, such as phosphorous, fluorine and carbon (*see* sensitivity).

nuclear spin quantum number (*mri*) *See* spin quantum number.

nucleon (*phys*) General term to describe either the proton or neutron.

nucleus (*phys*) Central mass within an atom consisting in its simplest form, protons and neutrons (collectively called nucleons). The number of protons determines the atomic number Z. The variation in neutrons gives various isotopes of the same element. The total nucleons is the mass number A; the element is completely defined by the atomic and mass numbers:

$$^{238}_{92}U, \quad ^{99\,m}_{43}Tc, \quad ^{14}_{6}C, \quad ^{3}_{1}H$$

nuclide (*phys*) This defines a specific position in the periodic table of elements, described by proton and neutron number. A specific nuclear species identified by the form $^{A}_{Z}X_{N}$ where A is the atomic mass, Z the proton number and N the neutron number. Nuclides can be stable or unstable naturally occurring (^{40}K, ^{238}U) or man made ($^{99\,m}Tc$, ^{131}I).

null hypothesis (*stats*) Usually based upon the assumption that nothing special is different between two samples. A statistical test challenges this assumption. If the significance of the difference (probability) is sufficiently large then the null hypothesis is rejected.

number of measurements (*ct*) The total number of attenuation values measured during the acquisition of the raw data for a single slice.

nutation (*mri*) A displacement of the axis of a spinning body away from the simple cone-shaped figure which would be traced by the axis during precession. In the rotating frame of reference, the nutation caused by an RF pulse appears as a simple precession, although the motion is more complex in the stationary frame of reference.

nylon (*material*) Hard plastic used as a tissue substitute in dosimetry.

Density (ρ) kg/m^3	1150 kg/m^3
Melting point (K)	470 K

Nyquist frequency (*image*) An analogue signal containing components up to some maximum frequency f Hz may be completely represented by regular sampling provided the sampling rate is at least $2f$ samples per second where f is the Nyquist frequency. This corresponds to two samples per period of the highest frequency present. The sampling interval is then $1/2f$ (*see* aliasing, Shannon equations).

Nyquist limit (*image*) Frequency of a signal beyond which aliasing will occur in the sampling process. This frequency is equal to one half the sampling rate. (*us*) The Doppler shift frequency above which aliasing occurs; one half the pulse repetition frequency.

O

object (*image*) In pattern recognition, a pixel or connected set of pixels usually corresponding to a physical object in the scene represented by the image.

objective contrast (*film*) Optical density.

oblique incidence (*us*) Sound direction not perpendicular to transducer boundaries.

oblique slice (*imaging*) Obtained by rotating an orthogonal slice (sagittal, coronal or axial) about a coordinate axis in the slice plane (*see* orthogonal slice).

occupancy factor (*shld*) The occupancy factor is estimated from the fraction of an 8-hour day or 2000-hour year for which a particular area may be occupied by a single individual. It is estimated as a 'worst case' for the fraction of time spent by the single person who is in the area the longest. The critical groups for shielding purposes are not patients or patients' visitors, but radiology staff both clinical and non-clinical (secretaries, porters, etc). The constraint level of 3/10 of the maximum limit areas where exposure can be greater than 6 mSv per year should be controlled; design factors and assumptions on occupancy should reflect this limit. A lower limit of 0.5 mSv per annum or an occupancy factor of 0.05 (5%) is sometimes recommended. An assessment should use the 0.3 mSv per annum constraint value for public places, including the surrounding area/rooms. The table suggests some working values for occupancy and use factors. These values do not represent fixed rules but are suggestions.

T:	Occupancy
1.0	Control areas and offices
0.25	Corridors and wards
0.06	Toilets and outside areas

(*see* primary barrier).

occupational dose (*dose*) The dose received by an individual in a restricted area, or in the course of employment in which the individual's duties necessarily involve exposure to radiation (medical doses involving diagnosis or treatment of the exposed individual are excluded).

occupational dose limits (*dose*) There is mostly agreement between ICRP 60 (1991a) and NCRP report 116 (1993).

Based on stochastic effects	50 mSv annual effective dose limit and either 100 mSv over 5 years or 10 mSv × age cumulative effective dose limit
Annual limits on intake (ALI)	$\dfrac{20\,\text{mSv}}{E_{(50)}\text{Bq}^{-1}}$
Annual reference levels of intake (ARLI)	$\dfrac{20\,\text{mSv}}{E_{(50)}\text{Bq}^{-1}}$

occupationally exposed (*dose*) Exposed to radiation in connection with occupational duties, e.g. nuclear medicine technologists, nurses, physicians, etc.

OCR (*comp*) Optical character recognition. Software that analyses scanned images and translates the letters and numbers it recognizes into text for use in other applications such as word processors.

Octreoscan[*R*] (*nmed*) A kit for the preparation of [111]Indium-pentetreotide (Mallinckrodt). A diagnostic radiopharmaceutical. An agent for the scintigraphic localization of primary and metastatic neuroendocrine tumours bearing somatostatin receptors.

Octreotide[*R*] (*nmed*) Analogue of somatostatin produced for nuclear medicine imaging by Mallinckrodt Inc., which binds to receptor sites expressed by a range of neoplasms. Commonly labelled with [111]Indium for imaging.

oersted (Oe) (*unit*) The c.g.s. unit of magnetic field (H) where $1\,\text{Oe} = 79.6\,\text{A m}^{-1}$.

off-centre slice (*mri*) Moving the centre of a slice group from the centre of the magnetic field within the slice plane.

off resonance (*mri*) When the Larmor frequency of a spin isochromat is different from that of the exciting RF field.

ohm W (*phys*) The measure of electrical resistance when 1 A flows at a potential difference of 1 V.

oil (mineral) (*material*)

Density (ρ) kg/m^3	760–870
Melting point (K)	–
Boiling point (K)	533–603
Specific heat capacity J kg^{-1} K^{-1}	2130
Thermal conductivity W m^{-1} K^{-1}	0.150
Relevance to radiology: x-ray tube coolant	

Oldendorf technique (*clin*) An injection technique for obtaining a tight bolus when following organ flow (time activity curve). After positioning an antecubital butterfly needle, a sphygmomanometer cuff applied to the subject's arm is inflated slightly above arterial pressure. The cuff is quickly released and, at the same time, the small volume bolus injected. The action of reactive hyperaemia in the arm ensures a rapid transit of the intact bolus.

OLE (*comp*) Object linking and embedding. Allows files or data created by one application to be linked or embedded in another.

outlier (*stats*) Observation which is far removed from the others in a set.

Omnipaque* (*cm*) Commercial preparation of non-ionic iohexol introduced by Nycomed (Amersham/GE Healthcare) in 1982.

Compound	Viscosity (cP)	Osmolality mOsm/kg	Iodine mg I/mL
Iohexol 39%	2.81 @ 20° 2.05 @ 37°	411	180
Iohexol 52%	4.33 @ 20° 3.08 @ 37°	504	240
Iohexol 65%	10.35 @ 20° 6.77 @ 37°	709	300
Iohexol 76%	18.50 @ 20° 11.15 @ 37°	862	350

Omniscan* (cm) Generic name gadodiamide: gadolinium DTPA-bis methylamide (Gd-DTPA BMA). A non-ionic neutral analog of Gd-DTPA. Manufactured by GE- Healthcare for MRI.

Compound	Concentration mg mL^{-1}	Viscosity (cP)	Osmolality mOsm/kg
Gadodiamide (GdDTPA-BMA)	287	2.0 @ 20° 1.4 @ 37°	789

OncoScint* (*nmed*) [111]Indium-labelled pentetrotide used for imaging colorectal and ovarian metastatic disease. (Cytogen) (*see* satumomab).

open source (*comp*) Computer programs whose original source code was revealed to the general public so that they will be developed openly. Software licensed as open source can be freely changed or adapted to new uses. Programmers may redistribute and modify the code.

operating condition (*us*) Any one combination of the possible particular output control settings for a mode.

operating frequency (*us*) Preferred optimum frequency of operation of a transducer, i.e. maximum efficiency.

operating system (*comp*) A set of computer instructions automatically loaded into the machine at start up (boot-up) from hard disk, for operation when it is turned on, performing all the basic or housekeeping instructions, i.e. disk transfer of program material, erasing or relocating data, etc. It sets up a filing system to store files and sets the display information on the monitor display. Most operating systems are DOS. Well-known operating systems include UNIX®, Linux®, Macintosh® and Windows®.

operative cholangiography (*clin*) Demonstration of the biliary tree during surgery by direct injection of the CM into the gall bladder, cystic duct or common bile duct.

optical density (OD) (*film*) The logarithm of the ratio of the intensity of the incident light on a film to the light intensity transmitted by the film. The logarithm of the ratio of the reference intensity of perpendicularly incident light (I_o) on a film to the light intensity (I) transmitted by the film:

$$OD = \log_{10} I_o/I$$

Optical density differences are always measured in a line perpendicular to the tube axis to avoid influences by the heel-effect (*see* characteristic curve).

optical disk drive (*comp*) Larger version of the read/write CD having capacities of typically 2.6 G-bytes. Data write transfer 1.7 M-bytes s^{-1} and data read transfer of 3.4 M-bytes s^{-1} with an average seek time of 25 ms.

optical sensitisers (*film*) Dyes added to film emulsion to increase spectrum response.

optically stimulated luminescence (OSL) (*phys*) This technology was pioneered in 1992 in conjunction with Battelle Northwest National Laboratory and Oklahoma State University using crystalline aluminum oxide crystals (Al_2O_3), as the detector material, The first OSL dosimeter was first distributed in 1996. The radiation level experienced by this material is measured by stimulating the Al_2O_3 material with green light from either a laser or light emitting diode source. The resulting blue light emitted from the Al_2O_3 is proportional to the amount of radiation exposure. Optically stimulated luminescence is a significantly faster process than thermoluminescence readout which requires heating. The light exposure can be controlled with very high precision and, as a result, the accuracy of dosimetric measurements is greatly improved. Unlike TLDs, the green light OSL allows multiple readouts and can be used to reconfirm reported radiation doses. Measuring capabilities down to 10 µGy (1 mrad) up to exposures as high as 100 Gy (10 000 rad).

optical transfer function (OTF) (*image*) The two-dimensional Fourier transform of the point spread function. The values of the OTF on a line in a specified direction through the origin of the spatial frequency domain are given by the one-dimensional Fourier transform of the corresponding line spread function. The OTF is generally a complex function and can be separated into the MTF and the phase transfer function.

Optimark ^{x} (cm) Non-ionic MRI contrast agent (Mallinckrodt/Tyco Healthcare Inc) a preparation of gadoversetamide.

Compound	Viscosity (cP)	Osmolality mOsm/kg
Gadoversetamide	3.1 @ 20° 2.0 @ 37°	1110

optimization (dose) (ICRP60) Maintains the principle that radiation exposure should be as low as reasonably achievable (ALARA) taking social and economical considerations into account (see practices (ICRP)).

Optiray ^{x} (cm) Commercial (Mallinckrodt/Tyco Healthcare Inc) preparation of ioversol introduced in 1988, non-ionic monomer. Produced as Optiray 160, 300, 320 and 350 depending on concentration of iodine.

Compound	Viscosity (cP)	Osmolality mOsm/kg	Iodine mg I/mL
Ioversol 51%	4.6 @ 20° 3.0 @ 37°	502	240
Ioversol 63.6%	5.5 @ 37°	645	300
Ioversol 68%	9.9 @ 20° 5.8 @ 37°	720	320
Ioversol 74%	14.3 @ 20° 9.0 @ 37°	792	350

Optison ^{x} (cm) Echogenic ultrasound contrast agent produced by Amershassm/GE Healthcare. Consists of microspheres of human serum albumin entrapping the gas perflutren (empirical formula C_3F_8). Mean diameter 3.0–4.5 μm; a maximum diameter of 32.0 μm with more than 95% less than 10 μm (see Sonovue).

Oracle (comp) A large database and application software vendor. Oracle 8 is a database management system.

oral cholangiography (clin) Demonstrating extra-hepatic biliary tree and gall-bladder.

oral cholecystography (clin) Using water soluble choleographic contrast agent orally and images taken 10–12 hours after ingestion. Its role has been diminished by high quality ultrasound imaging, CT, endoscopic retrograde choledochography ERC and MR cholangiopancreaticography.

order of magnitude (math) An increase or decrease by a factor of 10.

ordinate (math) The y-axis of a graph.

orientation (mri) The three basic orthogonal slice orientations are: transverse (m), sagittal (S) and coronal (C). The basic anatomical directions are: right (CR) to left (L), posterior (P) to anterior (A), and feet (F) to head (H). Considered as positive directions. In the R/L and P/A, directions can be specified relative to the axis of the magnet; the F/H location can be specified relative to a convenient patient structure.

orthochromatic film (film) Film emulsion sensitive to blue/green light. Matched to gadolinium phosphors.

orthogonal slice (mri) Slices oriented perpendicular to each other. The basic orientations are: sagittal, coronal and transverse (axial).

Osborne, E.D. American physician who first observed and described x-ray opaque iodine compounds in 1923.

oscillation (phys) In the form of sound or radio-frequency, waveforms play a most important part in radiology. The interactions of sound waves and radiowaves show the same general behaviour:

- harmonic motion;
- signal decay;
- signal resonance;
- interference between signals having different frequency and phase. The waveform characteristics of oscillating signals can be analysed using a Fourier transform.

oscillator gate (us) The electronics of a pulsed Doppler system that converts the continuous voltage of the oscillator to a pulsed voltage.

OSI (comp) Open system inter-connection. A LAN communication model developed by ISO.

osmium Os (elem)

Atomic number (Z)	76
Relative atomic mass (A_r)	190.2
Density (ρ) kg/m³	22 480
Melting point (K)	3300
K-edge (keV)	73.8
Relevance to radiology: rarely used as a K-edge filter	

osmolarity (Osmol)/osmolality (Osm) (chem) The osmole (osm) is a unit used in biology and medicine and is a measure of the total number of particles (ions) dissolved in water.

- The osmolarity depends on the number of molecules dissolved in a litre of solution expressed in milliOsmol L^{-1} (mOsmol L^{-1}).

- The osmolality is the number of molecules per kilogram of water usually expressed in milliOsm kg^{-1} (mOsm kg^{-1}).

Except under very specific circumstances, these terms can be treated as the same. The osmole (osm) is a unit frequently used in biology and medicine. Ionic contrast media form anions and a cations in solution, whereas non-ionic contrast media have a solution of intact molecules; this effects the iodine ratio. Hyperosmolality is an important contributing factor to toxicity. Cations in solution account for 50% of the overall osmolality of ionic contrast materials. Osmotic pressure is one source of adverse reactions to radiographic contrast materials (osmotoxicity). Other clinically significant effects that can be attributed to the osmolality problem include damage to the blood–brain barrier, renal damage and disturbance of electrolyte balance.

Substance	Osmolality (mOsm)
Sea water	1000
Isotonic saline	290
Blood plasma	285–290
Ionic monomer	1530–1843
Ionic dimer	580
Non-ionic monomer	610–645
Non-ionic dimer	290–320

Osmalality of blood and cerebrospinal fluid is approximately 290 mOsm/kg H_2O. Almost all current ionic and non-ionic monomeric and ionic dimeric contrast material have osmolalities in excess of this figure, although some are very much higher than others (*see* hypertonic, isotonic saline).

osmole (osm) (cm) The amount of a solute that when dissolved in water gives a solution of the same osmotic pressure as that expected from one mole of an ideal non-ionized solute. The osmole (osm) is a unit frequently used in biology and medicine. It can be freely replaced by the mole, representing the mass of 6.023×10^{23} osmotically active particles (Avogadro's constant) in an aqueous solution and is therefore a mole related to the solution phase. It differs from the mole only when it relates to the undissociated solute. The total osmotic concentration or osmolarity of a solution is usually estimated by measuring the vapour pressure or the freezing point depression of the solution.

osmotic pressure/osmotic potential (clin) The pressure exerted by the flow of water through a semi-permeable membrane separating two solutions with different concentrations of solute. The osmotic pressure of physiological solutions and X-ray/MRI contrast material mostly control their toxicity. Using a version of the van't Hoff equation, the osmotic pressure p can be estimated for a given solution:

$$p = \phi iRTm$$

where i is the van't Hoff factor. The van't Hoff factor is normally 1 for each ion in solution so for a simple ionic solution (NaCl) $i = 2$, however random ion pairing reduces this; ϕ is the osmotic coefficient; a correction factor to adjust for random ion pairing; m is the molarity moles/litre (*see* mole); R is the gas constant which in the case of solutions is represented by solute molecules dispersed in solvent; this is 0.08206 L atm mol^{-1} K; T is the temperature in kelvin, commonly used values are 273.15 K (0°C), 293.15 K (20°C) and 310.15 K (37°C). Values for i and ϕ for solutes of physiological interest:

Solution	Mol. wt.	i	ϕ
NaCl	58.5	2	0.93
Glucose	180.0	1	1.01

The product ϕ im is called the osmolar concentration with units osmoles per litre.

Osmotic pressure

The osmotic pressure of 155 mM solution of sodium chloride (normal physiological saline) at 37°C; from the formula: $p = \phi iRTm$ and the table values above:

$$p = 0.93 \times 2 \times (0.08206 \times 310.15) \times 0.155 = 7.3 \text{ atm}$$

The osmolarity of this solution:

$$\phi im = 0.93 \times 2 \times 0.155 = 0.288 \text{ osmol L}^{-1}$$
$$= 288 \text{ mOsm.}$$

The osmolarity of blood plasma is between 285 and 300 mOsm L^{-1}.

Measurement of osmotic pressure of a solution (contrast medium) is more conveniently estimated from the depression of freezing point. The relation that describes this for water and a solute is:

$$\Delta T_f = 1.86 \phi ic$$

where ΔT_f is the freezing point depression in °C. The effective osmotic concentration (osmoles) is $\phi ic = \Delta T_f/1.86$. Red blood cells are commonly used to test osmolarity of contrast media. At a concentration NaCl of 155 mM (isotonic with 310 particles or ions) the volume of the cells is the same as that of plasma. At molar solutions greater than this the cells shrink (hypertonic) and conversely cells expand in hypotonic solutions and can burst, releasing haemoglobin at 1.4 times their original volume.

- Reference: Berne and Levy, 1999.

osmotoxicity (*cm*) Iodine contrast media have varying degrees of osmolality (*see* **osmolarity (Osmol)/osmolality (Osm)**), since the iodinated and negatively charged ions (diatrizote, iothalamate, metrizoate) are associated with non-iodinated positively charged ions (sodium ions, meglumine ions). A hyper-osmolar agent causes sudden shifts of fluid from the intracellular compartment to the extracellular compartment. This hypertonicity causes fluid loss from blood, endothelial cells and other tissues, causing consequent damage and patient reactions. A source of hyper-osmolality and therefore osmotoxicity, in ionic contrast media is that cations in solution account for 50% of the overall osmolality of iodine contrast material. Since they do not effectively attenuate x-ray photons they yield no diagnostic information.

osmotoxicity ratio (OTR) (*cm*) Osmotoxicity potential may be expressed with the osmotoxicity ratio (OTR). An isotonic solution having an OTR of 1.0. and typical low osmolar contrast media having an OTR of ≈2.0; ionic high osmolar contrast media will have an OTR of about 5–7. Osmotoxicity is directly responsible for a number of clinically important effects, including sensations of heat or even pain. Other clinically significant effects include damage to the blood–brain barrier, renal impairment and disturbance or electrolyte balance (*see* **chemotoxicity, toxicity, neurotoxicity**).

OsteoCis (*nmed*) Preparation by CIS/Schering of oxidronate as ^{99m}Tc-HDP.

OsteoScan " (*nmed*) (Mallinckrodt Tyco) Version of oxidronate.

Osterkamp formula (*xray*) Describes the x-ray tube loadability L, where:

$$L = \frac{2P}{A} \times \sqrt{\frac{t}{\pi \lambda \rho c}}$$

where P is the power input, A is the focal spot area, t is the load time, λ is the thermal conductivity, c is specific heat and ρ is the density (*see* **x-ray tube (loadability)**).

ounce (*phys*) An imperial measure of weight; there are 16 *avoirdupois* ounces to the pound. The common (avoirdupois) ounce is 2.834952×10^{-2} kg or approximately 28.35 g. There are 12 troy and apothecary ounces to the pound and both are approximately equivalent to 31.103 g.

outlier (*stats*) Observation which is far removed from the others in a set.

output control settings (*us*) The settings of the controls affecting the acoustic output of an ultrasound instrument. Such controls would include but are not limited to the **power** output control, the focal zone control and the imaging range control.

Output display standard (*us*) The standard for real-time display of thermal and mechanical acoustic output indices on diagnostic ultrasound equipment.

■ Reference: AIUM/NEMA, 1996.

over diagnosis (*clin*) The tendency for screening to identify borderline abnormalities as disease even though they make lack true significance.

over framing (*image*) *See* **exact framing.**

oversampling (frequency and phase) (*mri*) Frequency oversampling: doubling the sampling points in the **frequency encoding** direction without extending the measurement time. Phase oversampling: data acquisition beyond the **FOV** in **phase-encoding** direction. Increases **SNR**. Measurement times are increased but prevents aliasing artefacts.

overscan (*ct*) Acquisition of more than the full 360° range during a single slice scan; the additional data range of approximately 10 to 40° is used to minimize inconsistencies which can occur between data acquired at the start and at the end of the scan, e.g. by averaging.

oxidation state (^{99m}Tc) (*nmed*) This is related to the valency state of an ion which influences chemical combination. Technetium has seven oxidation states:

Tc[I]	In certain organic complexes (MIBI)
Tc[II]	Not important
Tc[III]	May be the active form of HIDA
Tc[IV]	The most common reduced state in labelled kit preparation
Tc[V]	Modified reduction in [V]-DMSA
Tc[VI]	Not important
Tc[VII]	The most stable oxidation state. Eluted material as pertechnetate[VII]

oxidation number (*chem*) *See* **oxidation state.**

oxidation reduction (*chem*) Previously described as a reaction with oxygen, the converse being reduction: the loss of oxygen. A more general idea of oxidation and reduction was developed in which oxidation was loss of electrons and reduction was gain of electrons. This latter definition embraced those reactions that did not involve oxygen. An oxidation number consists of a sign, which indicates an increase (negative) or decrease (positive). An integer which gives the number of electrons involved. The oxidation number is used in naming inorganic compounds such as technetium (Tc(IV to VII). Compounds that readily undergo reduction are oxidizing agents and those that undergo oxidation are reducing agents (see oxidation state (^{99m}Tc)).

oxidronate (*nmed*) Oxidronate sodium forms an unknown complex with ^{99m}Tc to form ^{99m}Tc-HDP, a diagnostic skeletal agent for demonstrating abnormal osteogenesis. Rapid blood clearance.

Oxilan$^"$ (*cm*) Commercial preparation of ioxilan introduced by Guerbet in 1995.

Compound	Viscosity (cP)	Osmolality mOsm/kg	Iodine mg I/mL
Oxilan 300	9.4 @ 20° 5.1 @ 37°	585	300
Oxilan 350	16.3 @ 20° 8.1 @ 37°	695	350

oxiquinoline (*nmed*) Oxine; see ^{111}In oxyquinoline (*see* tropolone).

oxygen O (*elem*)

Atomic number (Z)	8
Relative atomic mass (A$_r$)	16.0
Density (ρ) kg/m³	1.33
Melting point (K)	54.7

(*nmed*) Positron emitting radionuclide

Production (cyclotron)	$^{14}_{7}$N(d,n)$^{15}_{8}$O
Decay scheme (β+) ^{15}O	^{15}O (β+, 2γ 511 keV) → ^{15}N stable
Half life	2 minutes
Half value layer	4.1 mmPb (511 keV γ)
Uses	Nuclide for PET imaging.

P

pacemaker effect (*mri*) Implanted electronic devices are susceptible to magnetic fields. Static magnetic field, RF fields and pulsed gradients can induce voltages in circuits. Transcutaneous control and/or adjustment of pacing rate frequently uses reed switches activated by an external magnet to open/close the switch. Others use rotation of an external magnet. The fringe field around an MR magnet can activate these switches or controls. Areas with fields higher than 0.5 mT (5 G) commonly have restricted access and/or are posted as being a risk to persons with pacemakers.

packet (*comp*) Data and associated information, including source address and destination address, formatted for transmitting from one node to another. A unit of data, which is typically a part of a file, that has been prepared for transmission across a network. When a large block of data is to be sent over a network, it is broken into several packets, transmitted and then reassembled at the other end. Packets often include checksum codes to detect transmission errors. The exact coding is determined by the protocol and network architecture being used. A typical coding of information that includes a header (containing information like address destination) and, in most cases, user data (*see* token ring).

packet analyser (*comp*) A network diagnostic tool that connects into a LAN and analyses its traffic, capable of capturing a packet, examining it and breaking it down into its component parts of destination, origin, protocol, data, etc.

packing factor (*ct*) This influences the patient dosimetry for multislice CT, the packing factor (p) allows distribution of radiation density evenly over the volume of investigation when the slices are not contiguous. For a series of N slices, each of thickness T, and with a couch increment I such that the total scan length is L then the packing factor p is:

$$p = \frac{TN}{I(N-1)+T} = \frac{TN}{L}$$

where $p = 1$ for contiguous slices; $p > 1$ for overlapping slices; $p < 1$ for gaps between slices.

PACS (*comp*) Picture archiving and communication systems. The central design of a filmless digital image radiology department, enabling electronic picture archiving on bulk digital storage media (magnetic and optical disks or tape) and networking image workstations (local area and wide area networks). Teleradiology and teleconferencing have also been introduced to the available procedures.

pair production (*phys*) The formation of a positron and electron from the collision with a nucleus of a photon whose energy exceeds $2\,mc^2$ (equals 1.638×10^{-13} J or 1.022 MeV).

Mass–Energy equivalence
Total rest mass electron/positron = $9.1 \times 10^{-31} \times 2$ or 1.82×10^{-30} and $c^2 = 9 \times 10^{16}\,ms^{-1}$ then $E = mc^2 = 1.63 \times 10^{-13}$ J or 1.022 MeV (1 J = 6.24×10^{18} eV). This energy is emitted as two opposed 0.511 MeV gamma photons. Conversely, a gamma photon with $E \geqslant 1.022$ MeV in a nuclear field may undergo conversion into a positron and electron since $m = E/c^2$ yielding an electron/positron rest masses of 9.1×10^{-31} kg each.

PAL (*image*) Phase alternation line. A television transmission standard developed in Europe as the alternative to the colour NTSC signal. It provides 625 lines at 50 fps.

palladium (Pd) (*elem*) *Relevant details:*

Atomic number (Z)	46
Atomic mass (A_r)	106.4
Density (ρ) kg/m³	12000
Melting point (K)	1825
K-edge (keV)	24.3
Relevance to radiology: a K-edge filter metal in mammography	

¹⁰⁹Palladium (*nmed*) Beta emitting nuclide, used as an antibody therapeutic agent.

Decay scheme (β−) ¹⁰⁹Pd	¹⁰⁹Pd (β−) → ¹⁰⁹Ag stable
Half life	13.4 hours

pancreatic arteriography (*clin*) Pancreatic arteriography intravenous contrast medium administration used for enhancing difference between abnormal (tumour) and the normal parenchyma.

papillotomy (*clin*) An incision into the major duodenal papilla associated with biliary stenting and endoscopic retrograde choledochopancreatography.

parabolic flow (*phys*) Laminar flow with a parabolic profile.

paradigm (*mri*) Planned sequence for functional measurement (i.e. BOLD imaging), where, for instance, 10 baseline images, 10 active images, 2 ignored images are collected.

parallel beam (*xray*) A parallel beam of x-rays is approximated when the FFD is large (>2 m).

parallel hole collimator (*nmed*) A multiple-hole collimator with holes that are parallel to one another and perpendicular to the plane of the camera crystal. The common design for a gamma camera collimator. Produces a 'same-size' image without distortion at depth. High resolution and high sensitivity versions exist (*see* converging collimator, diverging collimator).

parallel imaging (*mri*) Use of multiple receiver coils collecting different portions of the image in physical space simultaneously, or different data points in k-space, which are then used to reconstruct collected images. Increases data collection and so decreases total imaging time, with some loss in signal-to-noise and longer post-acquisition reconstruction times. Parallel imaging examples include vendor-specific methods such as sensitivity-encoding (SENSE, mSENSE), simultaneous acquisition of spatial harmonics (SMASH), generalized auto-calibrating partially parallel acquisition (GRAPPA), integrated parallel acquisition techniques (iPAT).

parallel port (*comp*) A connection to the computer for input/output that can transfer a complete byte of data at a time. A typical parallel device would be a printer or film formatter. Transfers one byte of data at a time at speeds up to 100 KBps (kilobytes per second).

parallel saturation (*mri*) Saturating areas parallel to the slice plane but outside the slice of interest, so blood flowing to the measurement area produces almost no signal at the beginning of the measurement, thus eliminating the intraluminal vascular signal and preventing ghosting. This presaturation process can be performed on both sides of the slice.

paralyzable dead-time (*nmed*) A characteristic of a scintillation detector system in which its counting efficiency decreases and eventually falls to zero beyond the point at which it has achieved a maximum counting rate (*see* dead time).

paramagnetic (*mri*) A substance with a small but positive magnetic permeability. The addition of a small amount of paramagnetic substance may greatly reduce the relaxation times of water. Typical paramagnetic substances usually possess unpaired electrons in their outer orbital shells, particularly atoms or ions of transition elements (i.e. gadolinium, manganese), rare earth elements (lanthanides), some metals and some molecules,
including molecular oxygen and free radicals. They are considered promising as paramagnetic contrast agents MR imaging (*see* diamagnetic).

paramagnetic contrast agents (*cm*) Are water soluble, consisting of a metal ion and a chelating agent (i.e. DTPA); they are presented for intravenous injection. The best paramagnetic metal ions are those with an unpaired electron that exist in their outer orbital shell. This is seen in the elements of the lanthanide and transitional metal series of the periodic table. Metal ions from these series include gadolinium (Gd^{3+}) and manganese (Mn^{2+}). Gadolinium is the best since it has seven unpaired electrons, which allows it to demonstrate the largest paramagnetic moment, and is the most sufficient in exchanging the relaxation of hydrogen protons of the water molecule. These MRI contrast agents contain magnetic centres that create magnetic fields many orders of magnitude higher than those corresponding to water protons. They have their strongest effect on the T1, by increasing T1 signal ntensity in tissues where they have accumulated.

parameter (*math*) A quantity to which a value can be given in expressing performance or for use in a calculation. Examples would be exposure/dose, optical density and acoustic impedance. These quantities would take values that depended on circumstances so would not be fixed. Physiological measurements of flow, respiratory rate, gas washout are also parameters.

parametric (functional) image (*image*) An image display where the colour or grey scale no longer represents count or signal density but its scale represents a varying parameter such as blood flow (colour Doppler) or metabolic activity (PET).

parametric test (*stats*) Pertaining to exact measurement (count density, weights, temperature etc.). Tests of significance that assume a normal population distribution and involve parameters of mean, standard deviation and covariance. Examples are t-Test, correlation coefficient, F-Test. Non-parametric measurements are scores or ranks. Anova can be parametric or non-parametric (*see* non-parametric tests).

partial Fourier imaging (*mri*) An image reconstruction method where incomplete phase encoding data (as few as half the total) are used for generating the entire image. Reconstruction of an image from an MR data set comprising an asymmetric sampling of k-space. A complete image can be reconstructed since *k*-space is

P

symmetrical: an opposing value at a mirror image location in the matrix can be computed knowing the single value; conjugate symmetry. This method can be used for either shortening image acquisition time, by reducing the number of phase encoding steps required, or to shorten the echo time (TE) by moving the echo off centre in the acquisition window. In either case the signal-to-noise ratio is reduced (see half Fourier).

partial saturation (PS) (*mri*) Repeated RF pulses applied in time periods shorter than T1. Giving a decreased signal amplitude but delivering images with increased contrast between regions with different relaxation times. Signals due to variations in the interpulse time, TR, can be used for calculating the regional T1. Partial saturation is sometimes referred to as saturation recovery but should specify a particular case of partial saturation where recovery after each excitation effectively takes place from true saturation.

partial saturation spin echo (PSSE) (*mri*) Partial saturation in which the signal is detected as a spin echo. Even though a spin echo is used, there will not necessarily be a significant contribution of the T2 relaxation time to image contrast, unless the echo time TE is of the order of or longer than T2.

partial scan reconstruction (*ct*) Image reconstruction algorithm utilizing data from a projection angle range less than 360°; the minimum data range being 180°. Partial scan reconstruction enables shorter scan times so increasing temporal resolution for fluoroscopic CT or cardiac CT.

partial volume artefact (*ct*) Artefact caused by sharp material inhomogeneities (bone/soft tissue) within the beam. The mean value of the incident intensity within the detector element is not equivalent to an average of the linear attenuation coefficient itself, which is a source of nonlinear errors and thereby inconsistencies for attenuation measurements along different directions; partial volume artefacts occur within the slice and increase with slice thickness. Since spiral CT increases the width of the slice profile, the partial volume effect will also increase. (*mri*) Loss of contrast between neighbouring tissue types in an image due to insufficient resolution so that more than one tissue type occupies the same voxel (or pixel). Unsharp images are also caused by averaging different tissue types in the voxel from an MRI data set. (*nmed*) An object containing a high radioactive concentration that is smaller

than the volume that can be resolved. The object appears larger on the display (e.g. point source, phaeochromocytoma, small bone nidus). This impairs activity– volume quantitation.

particle (*phys*) A charged entity rather than part of the electromagnetic spectrum. Positive and negative beta events are particles, also alpha 'radiation', neutrons and protons. Ionization in gas causes particle formation: electrons and ions (H^- H^+).

particle acceleration (*phys*) Charged particles can be accelerated over distance by applying high voltages. This technique first developed by Cockroft and Walton is the basis of all linacs and cyclotrons.

particle fluence, Φ (*dose*) The quotient of dN by da, where dN is the number of particles incident on a small sphere of cross-sectional area da:

$$\Phi = \frac{dN}{da}$$

particle motion (*us*) Back-and-forth movement of particles in a medium (gas, liquid, solid) as a sound wave travels through.

particle velocity (*phys*) Typically $3.5 \, cm \, s^{-1}$ displacement to and fro from the rest position.

partition (*comp*) A segment of memory or storage memory, most commonly describing a section of a hard drive. A portion of a hard disk that the operating system treats as if it were an entirely different drive. Separating a disk into several partitions can speed up data transfer. When formatting a hard drive, the number of partitions can be assigned. The computer will then recognize each partition as a separate drive, and will show up as different drives under most operating systems, such as C:, D:, E: etc.

partitions (*mri*) 3D imaging application where whole volumes are excited, instead of individual slices. A 3D slab comprises multiple partitions in sequence without gaps. The number of partitions corresponds to the number of slices for a 2D measurement.

partition/distribution coefficient (*cm*) Since n–butanol does not mix with water, it is possible to assess the relative degree of lipophilicity of a contrast medium by adding equal parts of water and n–butanol to a small sample. The solvents are allowed to separate into two layers and the ratio of contrast medium dissolved in each layer is measured; this is termed the partition coefficient, which is therefore high for compounds of high lipophilicity and low for compounds of lower lipophilicity (high hydrophilicity). A measure of the relative hydrophobicity/hydrophilicity of a compound. The relative hydrophilicity of a contrast medium is estimated from its distribution between a solvent which is not miscible with water (e.g. n-butanol) and an aqueous buffer (e.g. water or saline) at varying pH. For example, a partition (or distribution) coefficient of 0.2 means that the compound is distributed with 20% in the solvent and 80% in the aqueous solution.

partition thickness (*mri*) The effective slice thickness of individual partitions in a 3D slab; the slab thickness divided by the number of partitions.

parts per million (ppm) (*mri*) The range of chemical shifts in magnetic resonance spectroscopy differs for each type of nucleus and is very small compared to the main frequency (expressed in MHz); chemical shift is given in hertz and this varies with the main magnet field intensity so comparison using frequency alone is difficult between two machines having slightly different magnetic field strengths. Measurement using parts per million or ppm is independent of field strength. Although the term parts per million in this application is not a measure of chemical concentration, it is related since the chemical shift can be changed by chemical dilution. Chemical shift tables give chemical shift ranges for various compounds.

Signal reference measurement

The frequency difference Δf between water and tetramethylsilane (a reference compound used as a standard frequency) for two field strengths: 1.5 T and 2.0 T are:

For 1.5 T (where ω_o is 63 MHz), $\Delta f = 334$ Hz
For 2.0 T (where ω_o is 84 MHz), $\Delta f = 445$ Hz

The chemical shift (ppm) is:

For 1.5 T: $334/63 \times 10^6 = 5.3 \times 10^{-6}$ = **5.3 ppm**
For 2.0 T: $445/84 \times 10^6$ = **5.3 ppm**.

The chemical shift between water and lipids if typically 3 and 3.5 ppm.

pascal (Pa) (*phys*) The SI unit for pressure measured in Nm^{-2} and 1 mmHg $= 1.33 \times 10^2$ Pa. Atmospheric pressure is 100 kPa equivalent to 1 bar. 1 millibar is 100 Pa.

Pasche, Otto Swiss radiologist who introduced moving slit exposures in 1903.

pass-band (*image*) The band of frequencies that is transmitted through a filter with maximum strength (*see* filtering (signal)).

passive shielding (*mri*) Magnetic shielding through the use of high permeability material (*see* magnetic shielding, self shielding and room shielding).

passive shimming (*mri*) Shimming by adjusting the position of suitable pieces of ferromagnetic metal within or around the main magnet of an NMR system.

passive transport (*nmed*) Passage of an agent (radiopharmaceutical) across a cell membrane by by diffusion and not involving any energy dependent metabolic process (^{99m}Tc diffusion across the blood–brain barrier) (see active transport).

patient radiation dose (*ct*) Factors influencing dose include beam energy, filtration, collimation (slice thickness), slice number and slice spacing (MSAD), desired image quality (noise) and scan pitch.

pattern (*image*) A vector of features, expressing a meaningful regularity characterizing members of a class, which can be measured and used to classify objects.

pattern classification (*image*) Process of categorizing input data into identifiable classes via the extraction of significant features from a background of irrelevant detail.

pattern recognition (*image*) The detection, measurement and classification of objects in an image by automatic or semi-automatic means.

Pauli, Wolfgang (1900–1958) Theoretical physicist born in Austria but became a Swiss citizen in 1928. Proposed a fourth spin quantum number where electrons could have $+\frac{1}{2}$ (up) or $-\frac{1}{2}$ (down) spin. Pauli's exclusion principle states that no two electrons can have exactly the same state. Pauli suggested in 1931 that the energy expended during beta decay could be shared by a massless particle (later discovered to be the neutrino) so preserving energy conservation; this idea was further developed by Fermi. Pauli was awarded the Nobel Prize in 1945.

PBP (*mri*) Percentage of baseline at peak.

PC (*comp*) Personal computer. Generally refers to computers running Windows® with a Pentium® processor. The competing design is the Apple Macintosh® which has a different architecture and operating system. Recent Intel® Macintosh computers can now run PC software including Windows®. (*mri*) Phase contrast signal variations in flow caused by phase changes; an MRA method exploiting this phenomenon.

PCA (*mri*) Phase contrast angiography.

PC board (*comp*) Printed circuit board. A board printed or etched with a circuit and processors.

Power supplies, information storage devices, can be attached. This usually forms the motherboard.

PCI (*comp*) Peripheral component interconnect. This is a standard bus design for computer motherboards and expansion slots that can transfer 32 or 64 bits of data at one time. Its expansion slots are compatible with ISA cards.

PCL (*comp*) Printer control language. A language developed by Hewlett Packard to control its LaserJet printers and supported by virtually all printer manufacturers. It consists of commands called 'escape sequences' that programs use to tell the printer about the number of copies to print, the resolution and page formatting; current release being PCL 6.

PCM (*comp*) Pulse code modulation. Audio–stereo quality audio that allows the user to record in either 12-bit or 16-bit audio. In 12-bit, two sets of stereo audio tracks are available, useful for dubbing onto an existing recording. In 16-bit, only one set of stereo audio tracks is available for recording (*see* modulation (pulse code)).

PDA (*comp*) Personal digital assistant. A hand-held computer that can store daily appointments, phone numbers, addresses and other important information. Most PDAs link to a desktop or laptop computer to download or upload information.

PDF (*comp*) Portable document format. A format presented by Adobe Acrobat® that allows documents to be shared over a variety of operating systems. Documents can contain words and pictures and be formatted to have electronic links to other parts of the document or to places on the web.

peak rarefactional pressure/peak negative pressure (*us*) Maximum of the modulus of the negative instantaneous acoustic pressure in an acoustic field during an acoustic repetition period. The unit is the megapascal, MPa.

PE (*mri*) *See* Phase encoding.

PEAR (*mri*) Phase-encoded artefact reduction Philips. Respiratory ordered phase encoding (*see* RESCOMP, RSPE, FREEZE).

peer to peer (*comp*) A network design linking computers together without a central server. This design is only efficient linking small numbers of computers. Each user can decide what resources on their workstation they wish to share. This design is only efficient for linking small numbers of computers.

pelvic aortography (*clin*) Visualization of the pelvic structures and organs. Transfemoral

percutaneous catheterization is the method used, advancing the catheter just proximal to the aortic bifurcation.

pelvic venography (*clin*) (Iliocavography). Angiography of the iliac veins and inferior vena cava, usually performed by puncturing one or both femoral veins and injecting contrast material through an angiographic cannula or a short catheter with sideholes. The main indications are thromboembolic disease, usually in connection with deep venous thrombosis (DVT), and evaluation of venous external compression or invasion by tumour masses.

penetration depth (*us*) Ultrasound attenuation increases with increasing frequency. Soft tissue attenuation is approximately 0.5 dB/cm/MHz. High frequencies have less penetration than low frequencies. After the transmission pulse all echo signals are received before a second pulse is transmitted (PRF). Frame rate (f_R), number of focuses (f_N) and lines per frame (f_L) all influence penetration depth. Propagation speed for soft tissue is approximately $15 \times 10^4 \mathrm{cm\,s^{-1}}$ (7.7×10^4 being half this) then the relationship: penetration $\times f_N \times f_L \times f_R$ l$_{\mathrm{eq}}$;7.7×10^4.

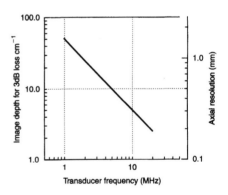

Transducer frequency (MHz)

(*see* pulse repetition frequency (PRF)).

PentaCis^{x} (*nmed*) Preparation of DTPA for $^{99\mathrm{m}}$Tc labelling (CIS/Schering).

pentetreotide (*nmed*) A DTPA conjugate of octreotide as an analogue of human somatostatin. ^{111}In pentetreotide (Octreoscan®) for the scintigraphic localization of primary and metastatic neuroendocrine tumours bearing somatostatin receptor sites.

Pentium™ (*comp*) One of Intel® family of microprocessors; introduced in 1993: a fast processor with a 32-bit bus. The Pentium MMX (multimedia) uses extra instructions and a 32k-bit cache. The Pentium-Pro (discontinued) has a 256k-bit cache designed for full 32-bit operating systems like Windows NT (since discontinued). Pentium II currently is the standard model CPU with clock speeds exceeding 400 MHz incorporating all MMX functions. The evolution of this processor is:

- Pentium® I (1993) 60 MHz, bus speeds of 66 MHz and a 64 kB cache;
- Pentium Pro® (1995) with speeds in the 166 to 266 MHz range. has a 256 k-bit cache designed for full 32-bit operating systems like Windows NT;
- Pentium® II (1997) series which began at 233 to 450 MHz with bus speeds of 100 MHz and an L2 cache of 512 kB;
- Pentium Xeon® (1998) a revised XEON version was made in 1999 in Pentium III configuration with speeds in the 800+ MHz range.
- Pentium® III series (1999), from 450 MHz to >1 GHz speed, 133 MHz bus with a 512 kB to 2 MB L2 cache with full speed capability;
- Pentium® IV (2000) 1.5 GHz. The P4 has a 2.2 to 3.6 Ghz version. A P4 Xeon® has been produced. Intel® Xeon® processor family uses hyper threading (HT) technology;
- The Pentium Celeron® was designed to lower the overall cost of computers that did not need ultra high performance. The Celeron® has a slower bus, smaller cache and less efficient (slower) decision-making path.

The Pentium series CPUs were designed to run Windows but will run ot her operating systems such as Linux (see multicore).

penumbra (xray) A point source projects a sharp shadow (umbra) onto a screen. The diagram demonstrates that with a line source (focal spot) then image unsharpness causes shadowing; the penumbra. The size of the penumbra depends on the focal spot size f and its position relative to the object and image plane. The parameters i and o in the diagram determine the penumbra dimension p (unsharpness) so that:

$$p = \frac{i \times f}{O}$$

Umbra and penumbra effects are produced by the x-ray tube fine and broad focal spots.

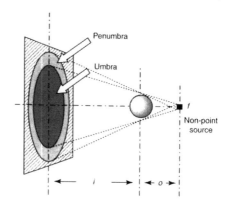

percentage collective dose (dose) See collective dose.

percentile (stats) A location parameter for the normal curve. Given a set of observations x_1, x_2, x_3, ... x_n the pth percentile P is a value such that $p\%$ of the observations are less than P and $(100-p)\%$ are greater than P. The 10th percentile is designated P_{10}, the median is P_{50}. If a set of readings for the radiation dose (in mGy) are:

Minimum:	0.63
25th percentile:	1.03
Mean:	1.24
75th percentile:	1.47
Maximum:	2.60

then for the 25th percentile 25% of the readings are below 1.03 mGy and 75% are above. For the 75th percentile 75% of the readings are below 1.47 mGy and 25% above.

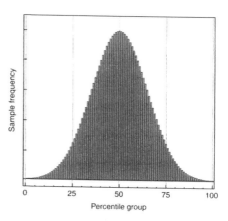

percutaneous abdominal aortography (clin) Catheteriztion is the preferred procedure for aortography. The entry sites available are transfemoral, transaxillary, translumbar and transjugular approach, depending on the type of study. Percutaneous transfemoral catheterization is most commonly employed.

percutaneous cholangiography (*clin*) Radiographic examination of the bile ducts after introduction of contrast media using a needle through the skin inferior to the right costal margin, inserting it into the liver or gall bladder.

percutaneous nephrostomy (*clin*) Drainage by collecting system via catheter inserted through the skin of the flank, under fluoroscopic viewing.

percutaneous splenoportography (PSP) (*clin*) Radiography of the splenic and portal veins by direct needle puncture of the spleen (direct splenoportography). This has an advantage over indirect splenoportography since portal pressures can be measured through the intra-splenic catheter or needle. These techniques have been replaced with the advances in non-invasive techniques (Doppler ultrasound and magnetic resonance angiography (MRA)).

percutaneous transhepatic cholangiography (PTCH) (*clin*) Radiographic examination injecting contrast medium percutaneously through a needle placed into the intrahepatic bile ducts; contrast medium opacification of the biliary duct system via direct puncture of a biliary duct. For evaluating biliary obstruction followed by subsequent transhepatic biliary drainage and for stent placement in the palliative management of obstructive jaundice. PTC has mostly been replaced by the less invasive endoscopic retrograde choledochography ERC or magnetic resonance cholangiopancreaticography (MRCP).

percutaneous transluminal angioplasty (PTA) (*clin*) A general term describing procedures used for the percutaneous approach treating the narrowing and occlusion of arteries; enlarging a stenosed vessel region by balloon inflation and withdrawing through the stenotic lesion. May involve placement of intravascular stent.

percutaneous transluminal (coronary) angioplasty PT(C)A (*clin*) Opening the stenosis of narrow coronary vessel segment by means of a balloon catheter. In addition to the dilation of the stenosis, a stent may be inserted.

perfusion imaging (*mri*) A percentage of baseline at peak image can be reconstructed for the slice. The grey scale displays the signal change relative to a basic image prior to contrast agent administration.

perfusion-weighted imaging (*mri*) Acquisition methods that highlight blood moving through arteries, veins and capillaries.

period (T) (*math*) The period of a waveform is the time for a complete wavelength which is the inverse of the frequency. Period = $1/f$. For a 50 Hz frequency this is 20 ms; for a 60 Hz frequency the period is 16.6 ms. (*us*) Time per cycle. Range 0.1 to 0.5 μs. $T = 1/f$ (*see* sine wave).

periodic table (*phys*) When the elements are grouped in ascending order according to atomic number; members of a particular family occur at regular intervals obeying a periodic law. The families generally run vertically downwards. These families fall into alkali metals (e.g. sodium potassium), halogens (e.g. chlorine, iodine bromine), inert gases (e.g. helium, argon, radon). The elements in the middle of the table are classified as transition elements. The rare earth elements are usually separated from the main body of the table as the lanthanoids, as are the uranium series as actinoids. Metallic elements tend toward the left-hand side and non-metals on the right-hand side.

peripheral angiography (*clin*) Visualization of the limb vessels (extremities) using iodine contrast material. Gd-enhanced MRI is replacing conventional x-ray angiography for imaging peripheral vascular disease. MR angiography of the peripheral vascular system has special requirements: Arterial flow is often pulsating: Large volumes are measured and images must clearly distinguish between arteries and veins. 3D gradient echo protocols with contrast agent are used most frequently.

peripheral aortography (clin) Investigation of the peripheral vascular disease of the lower limbs, visualization of the abdominal aorta, iliac arteries and arteries of both legs.

peripheral arteriography (*clin*) Lower extremity arteriography visualizing the peripheral arterial circulation in arterial occlusive disease, aneurysms, trauma, vascular malformation and occasionally for musculoskeletal tumours in the legs. The peripheral (arm, leg) imaging of the subclavian artery or femoral artery and its branches requires very high spatial resolution in order to visualize collateral and tumour vessels.

peripheral venography (arm, leg) (*clin*) For upper extremity venography, the contrast medium examination investigates venous drainage of the arm and their communicators with the superior vena cava. For ascending venography; visualization of the lower limb veins from the level of the foot to the lower vena cava using contrast media. Only veins draining blood mixed with contrast are visualized so the deep femoral and the internal iliac veins are sometimes not seen (*see* isometric venography, intra-osseus venography).

permanent magnet (*mri*) *See* magnet (permanent).

permeability (magnetic) (μ) (*phys, mri*) Tendency of a substance to concentrate a magnetic field. Absolute permeability (μ) is the ratio of magnetic flux density (B in tesla) in a material to the external magnetic field strength (H in A m^{-1}) inducing it, so $\mu = B/H$. The SI unit is henry per metre Hm^{-1}, equivalent to NA^{-2} and TmA^{-1} so the 'permeability of free space' or the magnetic constant μ_o is determined from the definition of the ampere (A) to be exactly:

- $4\pi \times 10^{-7}$ Hm^{-1}; or
- 1.256637×10^{-6} Hm^{-1};
- $\mu_o/_{4\pi} = 1 \times 10^{-7}$ Hm^{-1} exactly.

Then B = $\mu_o \cdot$ H (**tesla**) which has a magnitude dependent on the medium. The relative permeability (μ_r) is the ratio μ/μ_o and has no units. Permeability can also be expressed as magnetic susceptibility χ_m where $\chi_m = \mu_r - 1$; this is dimensionless. For most substances μ_r has a constant value that does not vary with field strength. For a vacuum and air $\mu_o = \mu_r$ approximately. If μ_r is less than unity (<1.0) the material is diamagnetic; if μ_r exceeds unity (>1.0) it is paramagnetic. Ferromagnetic materials have high permeabilities, which are not constant but vary with the field strength and the conditions under which it is measured must be stated. Some radiologically important materials are:

Material	μ_r	χm	Property
Vacuum/air	1.00000		
Water	0.99999		
Bismuth	0.999985	-1.5×10^{-5}	diamagnetic
Sodium	0.9999976	-2.4×10^{-6}	diamagnetic
Oxygen	1.0000021	$+2.1 \times 10^{-6}$	paramagnetic
Platinum	1.0003	$+3.0 \times 10^{-4}$	paramagnetic
Mn^{+2}	1.001435	$+1.44 \times 10^{-3}$	paramagnetic
Gd^{3+}	1.0028	$+2.8 \times 10^{-3}$	paramagnetic
Iron	5500		ferromagnetic
Nickel	600		ferromagnetic
Mu-metal	80 000		ferromagnetic

permeability of free space, μ_o (*phys*) The magnetic constant having a value of $4\pi \times 10^{-7}$ Hm^{-1} or 1.256637×10^{-6} NA^{-2}.

permendur (*phys*) A ferromagnetic alloy used for magnetic shielding and transformer cores. Has a very high relative permeability Consists of 50% Fe; 50% Co (*see* magnetic permeability).

perpendicular incidence (*us*) Sound wave perpendicular to a media boundary.

personal dose equivalent (H$_p$d) (*dose ICRU*) The dose equivalent in soft tissue below a specified point on the body at depth *d*. For weakly penetrating radiation a depth of 0.07 mm for the skin and 3 mm for the eye are employed; for strongly penetrating radiation a depth of 10 mm is employed.

Perspex™/Lucite™ (PMMA) (*material*) *See* PMMA.

pertechnetate (*nmed*) The $^{99\,m}$TcO$_4$ anion as eluted from the ^{99}Mo/$^{99\,m}$Tc generator.

PET (*nmed*) *See* Positron emission tomography.

PET detectors (*nmed*) The detection of 511 KeV photons for PET scanners require:

- high coincidence photopeak efficiency (41%);
- good timing resolution (approximately 3 nsec);
- good energy resolution (approximately 13% FWHM); and
- fast scintillation decay constant (better than 300 nsec).

The commonly used scintillation materials are: bismuth germinate (BiGeO$_4$ or BGO), cerium activated lutetium oxyorthosilicate (Lu$_2$OSiO$_4$:Ce or LSO), cerium activated gadolinium oxyorthosilicate (Gd$_2$OSiO$_4$:Ce or GSO) and thallium activated sodium iodide (NaI:Tl)

Property	Characteristic	Desired value
Density and effective atomic number	Defines detection efficiency of detector and scanner sensitivity	High
Decay time	Defines detector dead time and randoms rejection	Low
Relative light output (%)	Impacts spatial and energy resolution	High
Energy resolution (%)	Influences scatter rejection	Low
Nonhygroscopic	Simplifies manufacturing, improves reliability	Yes
Rugged ness	Reduces service costs	Yes

Bismuth germanate (BGO) and lutetium orthosilicate (LSO) are currently the preferred

P

scintillation-detector materials in PET scanners because their higher density and atomic number make them more sensitive than NaI(Tl) to higher energy 511-keV gamma photons. The attenuation length for 511-keV photons in both BGO and LSO crystals is approximately 10 mm. The scintillation light yield of BGO (14%) is significantly less than that of NaI(Tl), but is sufficient for high-energy photon detection; LSO has an improved light yield (75%); both are non-hygroscopic, permitting the material to be cut into small sections and packed tightly into element arrays without a metal hermetic seal.

PET (scanning detector) (*nmed*) Current PET scanners have large fields of view, built in attenuation correction and computerized whole body techniques that allow images of the entire body to be acquired in approximately 30 minutes. The specification for a current PET scanner would be:

Item	Scanner A
No. detector rings	32
Total detectors	10 000 to 20 000
Detector ring diameter	800–1020 mm
Axial FOV	108 mm
Image planes	31–90
Sensitivity	3000–20 000 cps/kBq/cm³

The detector system itself would have a typical specification of:

Detector ring	Specification
No. of rings	32
Block detectors	288
PMT per block	4
PMT total	1152
Segments	8 × 8
Size (mm)	4.05 × 4.39 × 30
Coincidence time resolution	6 ns

petabyte (*comp*) A measure of memory or storage capacity and is approximately a thousand tera-bytes (10^{15} bytes). Common storage capacities are giga-byte (1 GB = 10^9 bytes), tera-byte (1 TB = 10^{12} bytes) and peta-byte (1 PB = 10^{15} bytes) (*see* **byte**).

petaflop (*comp*) A theoretical measure of a computer's speed and can be expressed as a thousand-trillion (10^{15}) floating-point operations per second (*see* **flop**).

Pfahler, George E. (1874–1957) American radiotherapist who first filtered x-ray beams in 1905 with shoe leather.

PFI (*mri*) Partial flip imaging, general sequence Toshiba (*see* **FFE, GRE, MPGR, GRECO, FE, GE, Turbo-FLASH, TFF, SMASH, SHORT, STAGE**).

pH scale (*chemistry*) A measurement of the concentration of hydrogen ions in a solution, by using a logarithmic scale for expressing the acidity or alkalinity of a solution simply expressed as

$$pH = -\log_{10}H^+$$

where H^+ denotes the activity of H^+ ions in solution; the pH measurement is dimensionless. pH means 'potential of hydrogen'. The pH scale was first introduced by the Swedish chemist Sørensen in 1909.

Substance	pH
HCl (0.01N)	2.0
Gastric juice	2.5
Urine	6.2
Saliva	6.5
Water	7.0
Bile	7.15
NaHCO₃ (0.1N)	8.4

PHA (*nmed*) *See* pulse height analyser.

phagocytosis (*nmed*) Physical trapping of colloidal particles by Kupffer cells in the reticuloendothelial system. The main process for trapping radiopharmaceuticals targeted at the reticuloendothelial system (liver, marrow).

phantom (*qc*) Test object, often a **PMMA**-block with various embedded measuring devices. A configuration of absorber materials used for either monitoring resolution and contrast or (with defined absorption properties) an estimation of surface and depth dose. (*us*) A tissue-equivalent device that has some characteristics that are representative of tissues (e.g. scattering or attenuation properties). The most popular is the American Institute of Ultrasound in Medicine (AIUM) standard phantoms. (*xray*) Carefully constructed item with known dimensions (length, diameter) and material characteristics (tissue equivalent plastic, etc.). Usually a fluid-filled container with built-in plastic structures of various sizes and shapes. Phantoms are used to test the system and quality features of imaging systems and sometimes either radiation dose or SAR values. (*ct*) Object usually made from tissue equivalent material (PMMA), simulating the geometrical body shape. There are also physical phantoms for testing high and low contrast detection purposes (bar or line test pattern) (*see* high contrast, low contrast).

phantom, anthromorphic (*dose*) A standard phantom used by the MIRD committee for calculations of the absorbed fraction.

pharmacokinetics (contrast medium) (*clin*) Features influencing pharamacokinetics are: high hydrophilicity, low plasma binding, renal excretion, elimination T½ of 1½ to 2 hours, minimal extra-renal elimination, distribution/elimination linear or proportional to dose, zero biotransformation, zero enterohepatic circulation, minimal blood–brain barrier or placental transport, minimal central absorption.

phase (*phys*) The measure of the difference between two oscillating systems with respect to time. Phase is measured as an angle, each oscillation (one wavelength) being 360° or 2π radians. Two systems are in phase when they are at the same stage of oscillation. The second oscillation is 90° out of phase when it starts at the $\pi/2$ or 90° point on the *x*-axis with reference to the first oscillation.

phase angle (*phys*) The fraction of a cycle passed by an oscillating system (sine wave) given as an angle. The formula for a sine-wave is: $A\sin(\omega_0 t + \varphi)$, where A is the amplitude, ω_0 the angular frequency and φ the phase angle. For a complete cycle φ is 360° or 2π radians; a half cycle is 180° or π radians.

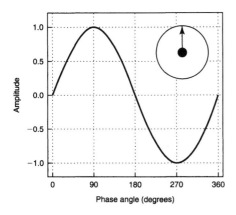

(*see* phase difference).

phase contrast angiography (*mri*) The blood contrast in the image is proportional to the local blood velocity. Method for displaying vascular angiography in terms of velocity. The phase change of the spins in flowing blood distinguishes the blood from stationary tissue where only flowing spins contribute to the signal. This technique can also be the basis for flow measurements.

phase contrast imaging (*xray*) Developed for mammography where tissue differences are displayed according to the slight differences in phase between tissue types imparted on a monochromatic x-ray source.

phase correction (*mri*) Either (i) corrective processing of the spectrum so that spectral lines at different frequencies all have the absorption-made phase or (ii) in imaging, adjustment of the signal indifferent parts of the image to have a consistent phase.

phase cycling (*mri*) Techniques of signal excitation in which the phases of the exciting or refocusing RF pulses are systematically varied and the resulting signals are then suitably combined in order to reduce or eliminate certain artefacts.

phase difference (*phys*) The graph shows two sine-waves with the same frequency but with a 90° ($\pi/2$) phase difference in time. Phase differences are measured by reference to a standard waveform.

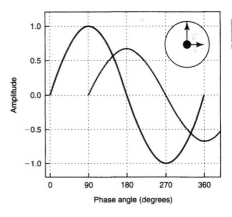

phase elimination (*mri*) Fat and water protons have only slightly different resonant frequency, resulting in phase cycling; fat and water spins switch in and out of phase after the application of an RF pulse. The strength of the oscillation depends on the relative proportion of fat and water protons in the tissue. Occurs primarily with gradient echo sequences, where the signal intensity of a voxel containing fat and water oscillates with an increasing echo time.

phase encoding (*mri*) Encoding the distribution of sources of MR signals along a direction in space with different phases by applying a pulsed magnetic field gradient along that direction prior to detection of the signal. The amplitude of the phase-encoding gradient changes incrementally from excitation to excitation. For this reason, each row of raw data has different phase information. The pulsed magnetic field gradient changes frequency for a short time so that after this pulse the nuclei resume their original frequency but now with phase differences. It is necessary to acquire a set of signals with a suitable set of different phase-encoding gradient pulses in order to reconstruct the distribution of the sources along the encoded direction. Phase-encoding steps are required to fully scan the slice, the number depending on the matrix size. The applied Fourier transform can allocate the various phases to the respective rows.

phase encoding order (*mri*) The timing in which the phase encoding gradient pulses are applied. The order can be sequential, centric, reverse centric, random, etc.

phase gradient vectors (*mri*) Matrix of the phases of the matrix of gradient vectors.

phase image (*mri*) Phase images can be reconstructed from the raw data measured. In the magnitude image, the grey scale of the pixel corresponds to the MR signal magnitude at that location. In the phase image, each pixel grey scale represents the respective phasing between −180° and +180°. Stationary spins have the same phasing, moving spins have differing phasing depending on blood velocity.

phase oversampling (*mri*) *See* oversampling.

phase quadrature (*phys*) Two signals differing by a quarter cycle.

phase reordering (*mri*) Phase reordering Hitachi. Respiratory ordered phase encoding (*see* RESCOMP, RSPE, PEAR, FREEZE).

phase shift (*mri*) Loss of phase coherence in precessing spins (signal reduction). In most situations, vascular spins move at variable velocities; faster flowing spins undergo a stronger phase shift than slower flowing spins.

phase sensitive detector (*mri*) A method for detecting and distinguishing the phase of a signal by reference to the phase of a reference signal (*see* quadrature detector).

phase transfer function (PTF) (*mri*) The phase of the optical transfer function, represents the phase shift, expressed as a function of spatial frequency, of an output corresponding to a sinusoidal input.

phased array (*us*) An array that steers and focuses the beam electronically (with short time delays). A transducer where the elements are pulsed together using signal delays to steer the beam in a sector scan.

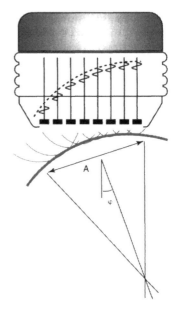

The principle of the phased array is shown in the figure above. The transmit pulses are applied to each element via a delay which gives a swivelled (angled) wave-front. The degree of swivel (±45°) requires very narrow elements of approximately ½λ dimensions. The effective aperture A' is $A \cdot \cos \varphi$ where A is the total aperture or array length without the swivel. During receive mode, the same pulse delays are used. The phased array can produce directional and focused beams giving electronic dynamic focusing in conjunction with beam steering. Unlike the linear sequenced array, all the elements are pulsed at the same time during transmission and reception and the phased array image formation is achieved by using polar co-ordinates and not rectilinear.

phased array coils (*mri*) Multiple linked surface coils served by separate amplifiers. A typical design consisting of six coils which can be used separately or combined for 3D data collection.

A large field of view can be obtained with high signal to noise ratio.

phased linear array (*us*) Linear array with phased focusing added; linear array with phased steering of pulses to produce a parallelogram-shaped display.

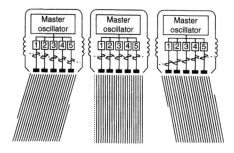

phasors (*math*) These represent voltage strength V in phase angles Φ as $V \angle \phi$ as a circular diagram where Φ is measured in radians. The fixed length of the phasor either represents maximum voltage or the root mean square voltage. The mathematics of phasors resembles that of vectors.

phlebography (*clin*) Radiography of the vein using contrast medium (*see* venography).

phosphates (*chem*) Salts based on phosphorus(V) oxoacids and in particular salts of phosphoric acid. A large number of polymeric phosphates exist, containing P-O-P bridges. Linear polyphosphates, cyclic polyphosphates and cross-linked polyphosphates or ultraphosphates are known. These are used in bone seeking radiopharmaceuticals and bone therapy agents (*see* MDP, HMDP, pyrophosphate (PYP)).

Phosphocol⁰ (*nmed*) Chromic ^{32}phosphate (Mallinckrodt Inc) (*see* ^{32}Phosphorus).

phosphor (*image*) A compound exhibiting luminescence (fluorescence, phosphorescence and thermoluminesence). Fluorescent phosphors are used for intensifying screens and scintillation detectors. The common types are:

Phosphor	Application
CaWO$_4$	Early intensifying screen
Gd$_2$O$_2$:Tb	Terbium doped gadolinium intensifying screen
La$_2$OBr:Tm	Thulium doped lanthanum intensifying screen
Y$_2$O$_2$S:Tb	Terbium doped non-rare earth intensifying screen
YTaO$_4$	Ultraviolet light intensifying screen (DuPont Ultravison®)

Phosphorescent phosphors are most often seen as output screens in image intensifiers and display monitors (generally of the form ZnCdS:Ag). Special phosphors having matched light output have been developed P45 and P4. Thermoluminescent phosphors are used in radiology as dosimeters or as image-plate detectors:

Phosphor	Application
LiF	Tissue equivalent personal TLD
CaF2:Mn	Environmental, high dose TLD
CaSO$_4$:Dy	Environmental TLD
BaFCl:Eu	Image plate phosphor
BaFBr:Eu	Image plate phosphor

phosphorescence (*phys*) The term phosphorescence is often incorrectly considered synonymous with luminescence. If the luminescence continues after the radiation causing it has stopped, then it is known as phosphorescence. Philipp Lenard first advanced a theory for its action. A phosphor material emits light which persists after the exciting source is removed, unlike fluorescence where de-excitation of the electrons is almost instantaneous. The material is excited to a metastable state from which a transition to the initial state is forbidden. Emission can occur when thermal energy raises the electron to a state from which it can de-excite so phosphorescence is temperature dependent. Light output can continue for some time after stimulation since electrons trapped in the forbidden zone are periodically excited into the conduction band. A summary of events is:

- The phosphor has empty traps before stimulation.
- After stimulation electrons from the valency band are ejected into the conduction band.
- Conduction band electrons fall into traps in the forbidden zone.
- Intrinsic energy lifts some trapped electrons into the conduction band.
- Electrons fall into valency band emitting broad continuous light spectrum.

Its value is found in CRT and flat-panel displays and film intensifying screens, however phosphorescence produces an unwanted afterglow in these applications. Impurities or doping of the phosphor material plays an important part by serving as activators or coactivators of the phosphorescent phenomenon (*see* energy bands, fluorescence, thermo-luminescence).

phosphorus (P) (*elem*)

Atomic number (Z)	15
Relative atomic mass (A_r)	30.97
Density (ρ) kg/m^3	2200(r)
	1800(y)
Melting point (K)	317.2
K-edge (keV)	2.14

^{32}Phosphorus (*nmed*) Therapy agent for poly-cythaemia rubra vera and also used for bone pain therapy.

Production	$^{32}_{16}$S(n,p)$^{32}_{15}$P
Decay scheme (β^-) ^{32}P	^{32}P T½ 14.3 d ($\beta-$ mean energy 694.9 keV) $\rightarrow$ ^{32}S stable
Decay constant	0.04846 d^{-1}

Days	Fraction remaining
1	0.953
5	0.785
10	0.616
15	0.483
20	0.379
30	0.233

Uses in radiology: ^{32}P is a pure beta therapy isotope (*see* Phosphocol®).

Phosphotec (*nmed*) A kit for the preparation of ^{99m}Tc-pyrophosphate (PYP) (Bracco).

phot (*phys*) A non-SI measure for illuminance equivalent to 1 lumen cm^{-2}.

photocathode (*xray*) Directly applied to the glass envelope window of the photomultiplier tube or placed immediately behind, and in contact with, the very thin (500 μm) input phosphor of the image intensifier and transforms the intensity distribution of the x-ray image into an electron flux density. The photocathode of the image intensifier is in optical contact with the input phosphor transforming light quanta into an electron flux density distribution. The electrons are accelerated onto an output phosphor screen. The photocathode is a complex antimony/caesium (cesium) compound SbCs$_3$. The electron flux from the large photocathode area is focused onto a much smaller output screen area; luminous flux is not increased but luminance is, so providing minification gain. Quantum efficiency varies between the various transformation stages of an image intensifier; the photocathode demonstrates one of the best quantum efficiencies.

photoconductive detectors (*rad*) Used as an x-ray detector; a common example being amorphous selenium (α-Se). Unlike crystalline selenium which is a semiconductor, amorphous selenium has a very high electrical resistance but on exposure to light or ionizing radiation it becomes a photoconductor. Sensitivity depends on the x-ray absorption efficiency of the selenium layer, the surface charge neutralized per unit energy absorbed. Efficiency is quite high at low photon energies due to the density (4810 kg m^{-3}) and thickness of the plate and having a Z = 34, however, efficiency falls off rapidly as the photon energy increases. The K-edge and fluorescent yield of selenium (12.66 keV and 0.56, respectively) are fairly low and the energy absorption efficiency does not show large changes in efficiency associated with the K-edge of materials of higher atomic number.

photoconductor (*phys*) The forbidden energy band in some semiconductors is relatively small, consequently only a small amount of energy can move valence electrons into the conduction band. In photoconductors such as selenium and silicon this energy can be supplied by incident electromagnetic radiation (light, heat x-rays, etc.). Electrons are then elevated into the conduction band and an electric current can flow under the influence of an applied voltage.

Material	Band gap (eV)
Silicon	1.11
Germanium	0.67
Cadmium telluride	1.58
Selenium	1.3–1.9

(*see* luminescence, direct radiography).

photo-diode (*elec*) Light energy falling on the depletion layer of a reversed biased p-n junction produces electron hole pairs. Visible light of 550 nm has a photon energy of 2.3 eV; greater than the ionization energy of silicon of 1.1 eV.

photoelectric effect (*phys*) The complete absorption of a photon by interaction with a bound electron (K or L-shell). The photon interacts with the electron and gives it its entire energy, the photon disappearing in the process. This only occurs if the photon energy can overcome the binding energy E_b of the electron. The kinetic energy of the electron equals $E_1 - E_b$, the vacancy in the K or L shell is filled by an electron cascade yielding characteristic fluorescent x-rays; Auger electrons can also be ejected in this process. The photoelectric effect involves bound electrons since it cannot give all its energy to a free electron. Photoelectric absorption involves the atom as a whole, the atom undergoing recoil simultaneously. The photoelectron is important in radiation detection and dose (*see* Compton scatter, linear absorption coefficient, mass absorption coefficient, K-edge).

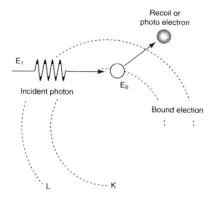

Recoil or photo electron

E_1

Incident photon

E_B

Bound election

L   K

photoelectron (*phys*) Electron ejected from K or L-shell as the result of a photoelectric effect.

photometric quantity (*phys*) An indication of light levels spectrally weighted by the standard photometric visibility curve, peaking at 550 nm. Photometric quantities such as luminance (cd m^{-2}) and illuminance (lux) are hybrid quantities defined by the visible light spectrum (non-linear eye response).

photomultiplier tube (*phys*) A light sensitive device for amplifying very small light signals. It is a vacuum tube device with a photocathode and accelerating dynodes steering the accelerating electrons onto a positively charged collector. The output signal represents a $\times 10^6$-fold amplification of the photon fluence.

photon (*phys*) A quantum of electro-magnetic radiation having zero rest mass is called a photon (a term first used by G.N. Lewis in 1926); it possesses energy related as $E = hf$ where h is Planck's constant and f is the frequency. The energy can be expressed as joule seconds where $h = 6.62 \times 10^{-34}$ Js. The relationship derived by Einstein is $E = hf = mc^2$ which becomes $mc = E/c$ or hf/c where mc is the photon momentum (related to frequency). Momentum and wavelength are related as $mc = h/\lambda$ (de Broglie); energy and wavelength are related as $E = hc/\lambda$.

Substituting the constants for h and c yields 1.986×10^{-25} J; since 1 keV is equivalent to 1.6×10^{-16} J then $hc = 1.2412$ keV. The conversion formula $E = 1.2412/\lambda$ or $\lambda = 1.2412/E$ allowing wavelength (nm) and energy (keV) conversion, e.g. an 80 keV photon will have a wavelength of 0.0155 nm.

photon energy (*phys*) Measured in electron volts where 1 eV is equivalent to 1.6×10^{-19} J. Visible wavelengths have an eV of 2 to 3, x-rays from 25 to 150 keV and gamma radiation overlaps x-radiation and extends to beyond 1 GeV.

Photon fluence and photon flux

A red laser (wavelength 760 nm) has an output of 1 mW (1.0×10^{-3} W) and a beam diameter of 1 mm. Radiation frequency ($f = c/\lambda$) is 3.95×10^{14} Hz.

The energy of each photon ($E = hf$), where h is Planck's constant, is:

6.626×10^{-34} (J Hz^{-1}) $\times 3.95 \times 10^{14}$ (Hz) $= 2.62 \times 10^{-19}$ J

Photon fluence:

$$\frac{1.0 \times 10^{-3} \text{ W}}{2.62 \times 10^{-19} \text{ J}} = 3.82 \times 10^{15} \text{ photons s}^{-1}$$

Photon flux: (for a 1 mm diameter laser):

$$(\text{area } 0.786 \times 10^{-6} \text{ m}^2 = \frac{3.82 \times 10^{15} \text{ photons s}^{-1}}{0.786 \times 10^{-6} \text{ m}^2}$$

$$= 4.86 \times 10^{21} \text{ photons s}^{-1} \text{m}^{-2}$$

Laser energy: *photon flux* $\times$ *photon energy*
$= 4.86 \times 10^{21} \times 2.62 \times 10^{-19}$ J
$= 1273.3$ W (1.27 kW m^{-2})

---

photon exposure (*xray*) This is measured as either photon fluence (photons cm^2) or photon flux (photons cm^2 s^{-1}). The number of x-ray photons from an exposure can be calculated knowing kV, efficiency of x-ray production and mAs. From this basic calculation the photon fluence and photon flux can be calculated.

Standard radiograph

For a standard radiograph exposure of 60 kV (0.06 MeV) at 100 mA at 0.05 s (5 mAs), the photon fluence for 5 mAs = 5×10^{-3} coulombs where the electron charge is 1.6×10^{-19} C.

Then the number of electrons is:

$5 \times 10^{-3}/1.6 \times 10^{-19} = 3.3 \times 10^{16}$.

Allowing x-ray production of 0.5% efficiency then **1.5×10^{14}** x-ray photons will be available.

---

photon fluence (Φ) (*xray*) A measure of photon intensity per unit area. For N photons of energy E incident on a surface area A for time t then:

$$\Phi = \frac{N}{A} \text{ photons cm}^{-2} \text{ or m}^{-2}$$

X-ray photon fluence
From the photon number 1.5×10^{14} (calculated from photon exposure) the x-ray photon fluence over a chosen 1500 cm^2 area is:

$$\Phi = \frac{N}{A} = \frac{1.5 \times 10^{14} \text{ photons}}{1.5 \times 10^3 \text{ cm}^2}$$
$$= 1.0 \times 10^{11} \text{ photons cm}^{-2}$$

---

photon fluence (energy) Ψ (*xray*) Photon energy (E) deposited per square centimetre. For a mono-energetic beam this is expressed as $\Psi = \frac{NE}{A}$ or ΦE which is measured in joules as $J m^{-2}$ or more conveniently as $J cm^{-2}$.

X-ray photon energy fluence
From the photon fluence of **1.0×10^{11} photons cm^{-2}** then for a single energy photon beam the photon energy fluence is:

$$\phi = \frac{\Phi}{t} = \frac{1.0 \times 10^{11}}{0.5}$$
$$= 2.0 \times 10^{12} \text{ photons cm}^{-2} \text{ s}^{-1}$$

(φ) (*xray*) The photon fluence per unit time t is:

$$\phi = \frac{N}{A \cdot t} = \frac{\Phi}{t} \text{ photons cm}^{-2} \text{ s}^{-1} \text{ or m}^{-2} \text{ s}^{-1}$$

X-ray photon flux
From the standard radiograph giving **1.5×10^{14} x-ray photons** the x-ray photon fluence of 1.0×10^{11} photons cm^{-2} the photon flux is:

$$\phi = \frac{\Phi}{t} = \phi = \frac{\Phi}{t} = \frac{1.0 \times 10^{11}}{0.05}$$
$$= 2.0 \times 10^{12} \text{ photons cm}^{-2} \text{ s}^{-1}$$

---

photon flux (energy) ψ (*xray*) For a mono-energetic beam this is simply photon flux $\frac{NE}{A \cdot t}$ or ΦE.

X-ray photon energy flux
From the standard radiograph having an x-ray photon flux of 2.0×10^{12} photons cm^{-2} s^{-1} the photon energy flux is:

$$\phi E = 2.0 \times 10^{12} \times 0.06 \text{ MeV cm}^{-1} \text{ s}^{-1}$$

$$\psi = 1.2 \times 10^{11} \text{ MeV cm}^{-2} \text{ s}^{-1}$$

For a poly-energetic beam the proportion of each energy per unit time (E_i) gives the energy flux density which is the sum of all the different energy components:

$$\psi = \sum (\phi \times E_i) \text{MeV cm}^{-2} \text{ s}^{-1}$$

Energy flux density depends on the anode material, tube current and applied kilovoltage so that as already seen in $\psi \propto Z \times I \times E^2$, where Z is the atomic number, I the tube current and E the applied kilovoltage. A change in tube kilovoltage has a much greater effect on intensity than a change in tube current. From the above formula, increasing the kV by 10 kV from 60 to 70 has the same effect on energy flux density as increasing the tube current by roughly $\times 1.5$.

photopeak (*nmed*) The part of the gamma spectrum which identifies the photoelectric event. This represents the peak gamma energy. The peak in an energy spectrum (e.g. scintillation detector) corresponding to complete photoelectric absorption.

photopenia (*image*) Areas on an image that have decreased density due to either lack of radioactivity or x-ray photons. Examples would be liver metastases and breast micro-calcifications.

photopic (*clin*) Visual response associated with cones are the principal receptors. The illumination intensity is high in order to record colour information (*see* scotopic).

photostimulated luminescence (*phys*) Light emitted by phosphor plate when stimulated by infrared laser (*see* image plate).

physical half-life (*nmed*) *See* half-life (physical).

physiologic imaging (*image*) Detects blood flow within tumours (*see* molecular imaging).

PhytaCis * (*nmed*) Commercial preparation of phytate for labelling with ^{99m}Tc.

phytate (*nmed*) A radiopharmaceutical as sodium phytate labelled with ^{99m}Tc for imaging liver, spleen and bone marrow (RES).

Picker, Harvey (1915–2008) American physicist, inventor and businessman. Produced first commercially available machines for radiotherapy and nuclear imaging.

pie chart (*stats*) A 360° display of data; typically the entire 360° representing 100% and sections or slices representing the individual percentages. The example shows a 3D pie chart for diagnostic imaging collective dose. The importance of each can be seen at a glance.

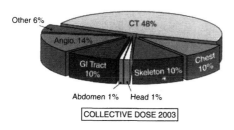

COLLECTIVE DOSE 2003

piezoelectric (*phys*) The property of certain crystals that causes them to oscillate when subjected to electrical pressure (voltage). The piezoelectric effect shown by a material whose dimensions change with electric charge. Mechanical deformation produces an electrical charge.

piezoelectric effect/piezoelectricity (*us*) Shown by a material whose dimensions change with electric charge. Mechanical deformation produces an electrical charge.

pigment inks (*image*) While conventional inks are essentially oil-based dyes, pigment inks consist of tiny chunks of solid pigment suspended in a liquid solution. According to their proponents, such as HP which uses them for its inkjet range, pigment inks offer richer, deeper colours and have less of a tendency to run, bleed or feather.

pile-up (*phys*) Pulse pile up in a detector due to detector or ADC dead-time; an inability to process fast count rates so information is lost.

pincushion distortion (*xray*) Display distortion (*see* barrel distortion).

PIN diode (*phys*) A semiconductor device having an intrinsic layer interposed between the p- and n-type layers. Its RF resistance varies in proportion to an applied DC bias current. PIN diodes are used in RF coils for rapid switching between transmit and receive modes and for coil decoupling.

pinhole collimator (*nmed*) A single-hole collimator used to magnify images of a patient's thyroid gland.

PIOPED (*nmed*) Prospective investigation of pulmonary embolism diagnosis. A set of criteria for judging the probability of pulmonary embolism from the results of nuclear medicine ventilation perfusion (V/Q) images, including normal, low, intermediate and high probability. Other finer categories also exist. In general:

Ventilation	Perfusion	Chest x-ray	Probability for PE
Normal	Normal	Normal	V. low
Normal	Small defect	Normal	Low
Defect	Medium defect	Abnormal	Fair + also COAD
Normal	Large defect	Abnormal	High

PIOPED was endorsed as a method for judging nuclear medicine lung scans by the American Medical Association in 1990.

pitch (*ct*) Ratio of table feed (*T*) per 360° rotation and the total slice collimation (slice width *d*).

Single detector

$$\text{pitch} = \frac{\text{table travel per rotation}}{\text{slice width}}$$

Manufacturers use a variety of pitch definitions; however the generally accepted definition of pitch should be in agreement with IEC 60601 regulations for computed tomography. Multislice CT systems use two different definitions of pitch. The terminology $pitch_z$ (x-ray beam width or z-dimension) and $pitch_d$ (detector width) differentiates between the two definitions. $Pitch_z$ is determined by x-ray collimation which defines the number of active detectors in a multislice machine, while $pitch_d$ will depend on the individual detector dimensions:

$$\text{pitch}_z = \frac{\text{table travel per rotation}}{\text{x-ray beam collimation}}$$

$$\text{pitch}_d = \frac{\text{table travel per rotation}}{\text{single slice detector aperture}}$$

so: $\text{pitch}_d = \text{pitch}_z \times$ number of slices per rotation

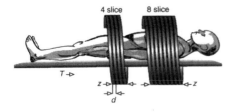

4 slice   8 slice

■ Reference: WA Kalender, 2000.

pitch factor (*ct*) The ratio of the patient couch travel in horizontal direction per rotation of the x-ray tube divided by the product of the number of tomographic sections produced by a single rotation of the x-ray tube times the nominal tomographic slice thickness (*see* couch/travel increment). This ratio of table feed to total slice width is generally termed the pitch factor:

$$\text{pitch factor} = \frac{\text{table feed}}{\text{number of slices} \times \text{slice width}}$$

For a four or eight-slice CT design with a nominal slice width of 1 mm and a table feed of 4–8 mm per rotation respectively, gives a pitch factor of 1.0. The generally accepted definition of pitch according to the equation is in agreement with the IEC 60601 regulations for computed tomography. Choice of pitch factor is mostly determined by clinical requirements depending on examination time and a given scan range.

pixel (*image, ct*) The abbreviation for representing the individual picture element/cell of a two-dimentional digital image. Pixel size is determined by the field of view area and the number of elements in the display matrix. Pixel depth determines the gray/grey or color/colour scale. In CT the pixel represents the sampled (windowed) voxel within the scanned slice.

pixel noise (*ct*) Statistical variation in CT number reconstructed for a single pixel within the image matrix due to projection noise (variation in voxel position) within the measured attenuation profiles. The level of pixel noise depends on the geometrical resolution and the convolution kernel: pixel noise increases with increasing resolution.

pixel size (*mri*) *See* spatial resolution.

pixels per inch (ppi) (*image*) *See* dot pitch.

pixilation (*image*) The matrix pixels become visible on a low resolution digital image.

placentography (*clin*) Radiography of placenta following intrauterine injection of contrast medium. via a catheter placed proximal to the aortic bifurcation. Entirely replaced by ultrasound techniques.

planar imaging (*nmed, mri*) Acquiring the volume activity image of an organ either as a static or dynamic sequence.

planar spin imaging (*mri*) One particular technique of planar imaging that creates an MR image of a plane from one excitation sequence by selectively exciting a grid of points within the plane and then applying a magnetic field gradient so that each point has a different Larmor frequency Fourier transformation of the FID can be used to separate the signals from each selected point and create the image.

Planck's constant (h) (*phys*) A constant which allows the energy of the photon in terms of either joule seconds $(6.626205 \times 10^{-34} \text{J} \cdot \text{s}$ $(\text{J Hz}^{-1}))$ or eV seconds $(4.136 \times 10^{-15} \text{eV} \cdot \text{s}$ $(\text{eV Hz}^{-1}))$ to be calculated from its frequency. The rationalized Planck constant or Dirac constant symbol $\bar{h} = h/2\pi$ is 1.054589×10^{-34} J · s (*see* Compton scattering).

plasma proteins (*clin*) A mixture of dissolved proteins in blood plasma which carry out a number of different functions. The most common plasma protein is albumin, and its main function is to transport other substances, particularly waste products and foreign substances (drugs and some contrast media) to the liver for destruction and/or to the kidneys for elimination. Contrast media with a high degree of binding to plasma proteins (and albumin in particular) is seen as a sign of chemotoxicity; the higher the degree of protein binding, the more likely a substance may cause adverse reactions.

plasma volume (plasmacrit) (clin) *See* blood volume.

plaster (barium) (*shld*) Barium plaster having a typical density of 3200 kg m^{-3}. The measurements are:

Thickness (mm)	Weight (kg m^{-2})	Pb-equivalent (mm Pb)
10	32	1.0
21	64	2.0

plaster (gypsum) (*shld*) Hydrated calcium sulphate/sulphate (CaSO$_4$.H$_2$O), having a typical density of 840 kgm^{-3} plaster board thickness includes the thick paper covering. Typical equivalents are:

Thickness (mm)	Weight kg m^{-2}	Pb-equivalent (mm Pb)
9.5	6.5	0.5
12.5	8.5	
15.0	10.0	
17.0	14	1.0
38.0	28	2.0

plastic (acrylic-lead) (*dose*) *See* Clear-Pb, shielding (glass).

Thickness (mm)	Pb equivalent (mm-Pb)	Weight (kg m^{-2})
8	0.3	12
12	0.5	19
18	0.8	29
22	1.1	35
35	1.5	56
46	2.2	74
70	3.0	112

platform (*comp*) The operating system, such as UNIX®, Macintosh®, Windows®, on which a computer is based.

platinum (Pt) (*elem*)

Atomic number (Z)	78
Relative atomic mass (A$_r$)	195.09
Density (ρ) kg/m^3	21450
Melting point (K)	2042
Specific heat capacity J kg^{-1} K^{-1}	130
Thermal conductivity W m^{-1} K^{-1}	71.6
K-edge (keV)	78.3
Relevance to radiology: occasionally used as a K-edge filter. Used in QC equipment to give narrow slits for focal spot cameras.	

plug flow (*us*) Fluid portions traveling with the same flow speed and direction.

Plumbicon (*elec*) A type of vacuum video camera with higher sensitivity than the basic vidicon and low lag time.

plutonium (Pu) (*elem*)

Atomic number (Z)	94
Relative atomic mass (A$_r$)	244
Density (ρ) kg/m^3	19740
Melting point (K)	914
K-edge (keV)	–
Relevance to radiology: Contaminant in reactor produced generators	

^{239}Plutonium

Nuclear data	Emission
Half life	2.4×10^4y
Decay mode	α
Decay constant	2.88E–5y^{-1}
Photons	γ (very weak)

Seen sometimes as a contaminant in reactor prepared radionuclides.

plymax (*radpro*) A shielding material consisting of wood layers (plywood) which acts as a support for sheet lead of various thicknesses. Useful for partitions or doors in radiology and nuclear medicine departments.

PMMA (*dose*) The synthetic material polymethylmethacrylate, a plastic material used for manufacturing tissue equivalent absorbers. Also known as Lucite, Perspex or Plexiglas.

Effective atomic number (Z$_{eff}$)	6.56
Density (ρ) kg/m^3	1190
Melting point (K)	350

PMT (*rad*) *See* photomultiplier tube.

Pochin, Edward Sir (1910–1990) Clinician who investigated thyroid disease and its radiation dosimetry. Chairman of ICRP 1962 and UNSCEAR.

point imaging (*mri*) *See* sequential point imaging.

point scanning (*mri*) *See* sequential point imaging.

point source (*image*) An infinitesimal point emitting light, gamma or x-radiation used for assessing the resolution of an imaging system as a point spread function. The practical limitations associated with a point source concern its dimensions, which should be two to three times smaller than the system resolution. For conventional x-ray imaging this requires a 10 micrometre hole drilled in platinum. A 100 μm hole is usually sufficient for CT measurements and a 2 mm hole in thick lead sheet for gamma camera measurements. Long imaging times are required to accumulate sufficient photons to give a dense spot.

point spread function (PSF) (*image*) The count profile through a displayed point source, obtained from an infinitesimal point object or point source:

$$PSF(x, y) = \delta(x)\delta(y)$$

where δ (x) and δ (y) are delta (Dirac) functions in the x and y planes for a shift invariant system (ICRU, 1986). (*ct*) The image of a point source or

P

circular object with infinitely small diameter (in comparison to the machine resolution) oriented orthogonal to the image plane. The PSF of a CT scanner can be measured using a thin wire (tungsten) aligned parallel to the z-axis; the wire's diameter is smaller than the expected FWHM of the PSF (*see* line spread function, modulation transfer function (MTF)).

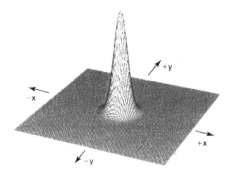

poise (*phys*) Unit of viscosity where 1 poise = $0.1 \ N.s.m^{-2} = 0.1 \ Pa.s$.

Poiseuille flow (*phys*) *See* flow.

Poiseuille's Law (*phys*) Describing the dependence of volume flow rate on pressure, vessel length and vessel radius together with fluid viscosity (J.L. Poiseuille 1799–1869 French physiologist) (*see* Hagen–Poiseuille's Law).

polar co-ordinates (*us*) The positional geometry used by a phased array transducer producing a sector scan.

polarization transfer (*mri*) Polarization transfer from hyperpolarized gas to ^1H, ^{13}C, and other atomic nuclei, holds promise for sensitivity enhancement of solution-state NMR and low signal to noise imaging using hyperpolarized, supercritical xenon. Detection of Overhauser enhancement of solute proton magnetization by factors of 3 to 7 confirms the intimate contact between ^{129}Xe and ^1H.

■ Reference: Leawoods *et al.*, 2000..

pole piece (*mri*) High permeability material used to shape the uniformity of the useful volume of a magnet, especially a permanent magnet.

polycarbonate (*material*) A thermoplastic polymer with high density and impact resistance making it useful for engineering construction.

Density (ρ) kg/m^3	1200–1220
Melting point (K)	540

polychromatic radiation (*ct*) X-ray beam with a broad spectral distribution of the photon energy (see Bremsstrahlung, monochromatic radiation).

polyester (*chem*) A synthetic polymer made from terephthalic acid and glycol. Can be manufactured in sheet form (used as a film base) or as filaments which can be woven as Terylene® or Dacron®.

polyethylene (*material*) A thermoplastic polymer with tissue equivalence so useful for tissue phantom construction. Low melting point.

Density (ρ) kg/m^3	920 (high density) 955
Melting point (K)	410

polymethylmethacrylate (PMMA) (*chem*) *See* PMMA.

polynomial functions (*image*) The standard equation for a straight line is $y = a + bx$, a linear polynomial (first degree) containing two constants a and b. The constant b multiplied by a variable x is a coefficient. This basic formula can be elaborated by adding further coefficients: $y = a + bx + cx^2$ describes a quadratic (second degree), $y = a + bx + cx^2 + dx^3$ describes a cubic (third degree) and so on (quartic, quintic etc.). The series are polynomial functions and are used for close approximation curve fitting to analogue signals.

polypropylene (*material*) A thermoplastic polymer with good resistance to fatigue (bending).

Density (ρ) kg/m^3	900
Melting point (K)	450

polystyrene (*material*) A thermoplastic polymer with good transparency.

Effective atomic number (Z_{eff})	5.74
Density (ρ) kg/m^3	1050
Melting point (K)	510

polyvinylidene fluoride (*us*) A piezoelectric thin-film material.

POMP (*mri*) Phase-offset multi-planar RF multiplexing technique (GE Medical) to acquire multiple slices simultaneously.

pooled analysis (*dose*) Epidemiology study, original data from several sources analysed in parallel.

PoP (*web*) Point of presence. Location of the nearest node for an ISP. Used for connection to the Internet.

population dose (*dose*) The whole body exposure to a population group is measured as the collective effective dose. A community of 40 000 people receiving 2 mSv and 20 000 receiving 4 mSv both receive a collective effective dose of 80 man-sieverts (man-Sv), which on present estimates would cause one cancer.

POPUMET (*dose*) *See* Ionising Radiation (Protection of Persons Undergoing Medical Examination or Treatment) Regulations.

positive predictive accuracy (*stats*) *See* predictive accuracy.

positron (*phys*) β^+, the anti-particle to β^- or negatron (electron). The two mutually annihilate producing 180° opposed 0.511 MeV gamma photons. Proton decay in the nucleus yields the positron:

$$^1_1p_0 \rightarrow {}^1_0n_1 + e^+$$

$$^A_Z X \rightarrow {}^A_{z-1}Y + {}^0_{+1}e + {}^0_0 v$$

A continuous β^+ spectrum is produced since there is a simultaneous emission of a neutrino (v). This compares with a β^- decay with simultaneous emission of an anti-neutrino ($\bar{v}$):

$$^{13}_7 N \rightarrow {}^{13}_6 C + \beta^+ \ (\beta^+ \rightarrow 2 \times 0.511 \text{ keV } \gamma\text{'s}$$

(*see* electron capture).

positron emission tomography (PET) (*nmed*) An imaging technique using radio-isotopes that undergo positron decay and emit positrons (positively charged electrons), whose annihilation photons (opposed 511 keV gamma photons) are imaged in coincidence to form tomographic views of the body. The gamma photons are detected by either a modified gamma camera or dedicated PET scanner. Because of the short half-life of the nuclides, they are produced on site. Some positron generators are available (*see* radionuclides (positron), radionuclides (generator produced)).

positron (radionuclides) (*nmed*) *See* radionuclides (positron).

positron energy (*nmed*) The mean distance travelled by a positron before annihilation with a free electron is an important factor which determines the positional resolution in tomography (*see* event location (PET)).

positron (labelled compounds) (*nmed*) Some applications for clinically active agents labelled with positron emitters are given in the table with estimated patient dose:

Positron emitter	Labelled compounds	Dose(H_E) mSv/40MBq	Clinical use
^{11}Carbon	^{11}CO $^{11}CO_2$ ^{11}CN-$^{11}CH_3I$ $H^{11}CHO$	0.05–0.2	Dopamine sites. Opiate receptor sites. Amino acid metabolism Cellular proliferation Methionine and receptor binding agents
^{13}Nitrogen	^{13}N-N_2 $^{13}NH_3$	0.002–0.05	Blood flow Myocardial perfusion
^{15}Oxygen	^{15}O-O_2 $H_2^{15}O$ $C^{15}O$ $C^{15}O_2$	0.02–0.2	Metabolic Activity Cerebral blood flow
^{18}Fluorine	^{18}F-F_2 $H^{18}F$ ^{18}F- ^{18}FDG	0.5	Glucose metabolism Dopamine storage Cellular proliferation

Compound	Application
[^{15}O]–O_2	Cerebral oxygen extraction and metabolism
[^{15}O]–CO_2	Cerebral blood volume
[^{15}O]–CO_2	Myocardial blood volume
[^{15}O]–H_2O, [^{11}C]-n-butanol	Cerebral blood flow
[^{15}O]–H_2O, [$^{13}NH_3$], [^{82}Rb]	Myocardial blood flow
[^{11}C]–glucose, [^{18}F]-FDG	Cerebral glucose metabolism
[^{11}C]–palmitate, [^{11}C]-acetate	Myocardial metabolism
[^{18}F]–FDG	Myocardial glucose metabolism
[^{18}F]–FDG	Tumour glucose metabolism
[^{18}F]–spiperone, [^{18}F]-N-methyl-spiperone	Dopamine receptor binding
[^{18}F]–16α-fluoro-17β-oestradiol	Oestrogen receptor binding
[^{68}Ga]–citrate	Plasma volume

positron range (*nmed*) *See* event localization (PET)

POST (*comp*) Power-on self test. The first process a PC runs when it is switched on which checks that memory, processor, graphics, etc., are all functioning.

post-injection (*nmed*) Injecting a further aliquot of radionuclide. Example would be [201]Thallium rest study after exercise (or vice versa) and [99m]Tc *in-vivo* labelling of red cells using an earlier injection of cold (unlabelled) pyrophosphate.

posterior probability (*stats*) The situation where new data are added to a set of observations. The updated probability of the disease or event after new information has been received; where event A occurs if it is already known that independent event B has occurred (*see* prior probability, Bayes' theorem).

   ■ Reference: Armitage P, Matthews JNS, Berry G, 2001.

PostScript (*comp*) A printer control language developed by Adobe Systems that describes each page as a collection of geometric shapes, rather than telling the printer where to place each dot of ink or toner. It is more suited to graphics printing than PCL as it can produce better output quality at higher print resolutions. While PostScript is generally used by laser printers, it is also common in high-end inkjet models.

potassium (K) (*elem*)

Atomic number (Z)	19
Relative atomic mass (A_r)	39.10
Density (ρ) kg/m^3	860
Melting point (K)	336.8
K-edge (keV)	3.6

[40]Potassium

Half life	1.3×10^9y
Decay mode (mixed)	$\beta^-\beta^-$
Decay constant	5.33E–10 y^{-1}
Photon	1.461 MeV

Natural isotope of potassium, comprising 0.0118% abundance. A measure for body composition when using a whole body counter. Delivers an average effective dose of 0.3 mSv per year (*see* specific activity).

potassium chlorate (*clin, dose*) In purified form used as a suppressant of thyroid activity preventing the organification of iodine. Protects the thyroid from accidental ingestion of radioactive iodine.

potential difference (PD) (*units*) The unit is the volt (V) where $1 V = 1 J C^{-1}$ $1 V = 1 W A^{-1}$.

potential energy (*phys*) The energy of a body due to its condition or state. Forms of potential energy are **electrical energy, chemical energy** and **nuclear energy**. The amount of potential energy is measured by the **work** the system performs until the energy source reaches its ground state.

potential exposure (*dose*) Radiation exposure that is unlikely but may result from an accident at a source or owing to an event or sequence of events including equipment failure and operating error and spills.

potential recoverability correction factor (PRCF) (*dose*) Factors that consider the probability of different germ line mutations will show differing degrees of recoverability in the offspring, such as differing capacities for completion of embryonic foetal development.

Potter H.E. (1880–1964) American radiologist who in 1917 introduced a focused grid that was moved transversely. The Potter–Bucky grid was marketed in 1921 (*see* **Bucky**).

pound (*phys*) An imperial measure of weight. The common (avoirdupois) pound is equivalent to 0.45359237 kg exactly, or approximately 453.6 g. The troy and apothecary pounds are both approximately equivalent to 373.236 g.

power (*phys*) The rate of doing work or the time taken to do an amount of work (SI unit is the watt (W) and $1 J = 1 W s$). This is defined as the rate of doing work (spending energy) per second:

$$\text{Power} = \frac{\text{work done}}{\text{time taken}}$$

It is measured in joules per second, the SI unit being watts W where $1 W = 1 J s^{-1}$ and 1 joule is 1 watt-second. Electrical energy is measured in joules and electrical power in watts.

Units of power

S.I. units	
1 W s^{-1}	1 J
watt (W)	$1 W = 1 J s^{-1} = 1 N m s^{-1} = 1 m^2\ kg\ s^{-1}$
1 Wh	3600 J
kW hour	$10^3 W \times (3.6 \times 10^3 s) = 3.6 \times 10^6 J$
c.g.s. units	
CGS erg s^{-1}	$1 W = 1 \times 10^7\ erg\ s^{-1}$

power (ultrasonic) (*us*) The amount of ultrasound energy emitted by the transducer per unit time. A quantity describing the rate at which acoustic energy travels per unit time in the direction of propagation. Unless stated otherwise, all references to power measurements in this standard will be to temporal-average values; work done per unit time Js^{-1}. Symbol: *Wo*. Units: Watts, W

power density (*phys*) The power per unit cross sectional area in an electromagnetic field. The unit is watts per square metre: Wm^{-2}

power Doppler (*us*) Colour-flow display in which colour scale is assigned according to the strength (amplitude, power, intensity, energy) of the Doppler-shifted echoes (*see* Doppler (power)).

power law (*math*) A function giving a straight-line when plotted on log–log axes.

PowerPC (*comp*) A family of RISC chips which is a collaboration between IBM, Apple and Motorola. Used on all Apple Macintosh computers and many IBM workstations. Apple has currently installed Intel® processors.

power rating (*phys*) A measure of power dissipation in an electrical machine or component.

power spectral density (*image*) Spectral decomposition can be obtained from auto-correlation for random signals without harmonic components. A Fourier series analysis will give peak amplitudes in the frequency domain. The power spectral density of the signal in the presence of noise containing several strong periodic components such as chromatography or magnetic resonance spectroscopy.

power spectrum (*image*) *See* cepstrum, autocorrelation.

ppi (pixels per inch) (*image*) *See* dot pitch.

ppm (*mri*) *See* parts per million.

PPP (*comp*) Point to point protocol; communications program.

practices (ICRP) (*dose*) Activities that cause an increase in a person's overall exposure to radiation by introducing new sources, pathways, etc. These would include medical and occupational practices. These practices are controlled by justification, optimzation and dose limits (*see* intervention (ICRP)).

praseodymium (Pr) (*elem*)

Atomic number (Z)	59
Relative atomic mass (A_r)	140.91
Density (ρ) kg/m³	6800
Melting point (K)	1208
K-edge (keV)	41.9

Relevance to radiology: sometimes used as a dopant in phosphors.

preamplifier (*elec*) An analogue circuit, connected to the input signal source, whose main function is to establish the correct input impedance or fixed gain before signal processing. A device that amplifies very low-level signals. A preamplifier is generally placed close to its signal source and has a very low noise figure as it is the principal determinant of electronic noise within the system.

precession (*mri*) The rotation axis of a spinning body about another line intersecting it. The movement of a spinning body which traces out a conical shape. The magnetic moment of a proton with spin will precess at an angle to the magnetic field precessing at the Larmor frequency.

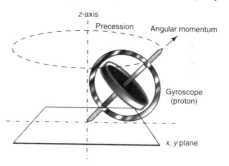

precession frequency (*mri*) *See* Larmor frequency.

precision (*math*) The variation (usually relative standard deviation) in observed values. (*math*) A measure of incremental size.

Precision

A kVp meter suitable for mammography should have a precision of ±0.1 kV. The display has three digits, which cover readings from 25 to 40 kV. Since there is an uncertainty of 10% in the least significant digit, this instrument cannot guarantee a precision of 0.1 kV so a four digit kVp meter is chosen.

Dependent on the number of significant figures and decimal places. A value of 13.6428 has six significant figures and is accurate to four decimal places; its least significant figure is eight, giving a rounded value of 13.643. A radiation meter able to give a maximum reading of 19.99 mGy is more precise than one giving a maximum of 999 mGy although not necessarily as useful if readings above 20 mGy are required (*see* truncation).

predictive accuracy (negative) (*stats*) The negative diagnostic predictive accuracy is a measure of the likelihood of a patient with a negative test actually being normal or not having the disease. It is expressed as:

$$NPA = \frac{TN}{TN + FN} \times 100\%$$

From the results of the **diagnostic accuracy** data: (300 + 56950)/60000 = 95.4%.

predictive accuracy (positive) (*stats*) (diagnostic) This is a measure of the likelihood of a patient with a positive test actually having the disease. It is expressed as:

$$PPA = \frac{TP}{TP + FP} \times 100\%$$

From the results of **diagnostic accuracy**: 300/(300 + 2700) = 10%

pre-emphasis (*mri*) Means of compensating for the non-ideal response of a system such as the magnetic field gradient system by modifying the input function.

pre-emptive multitasking (*comp*) A feature of the hardware and operating system that allows the CPU to share processing time with all the running programs. Gives the appearance that all programs are running simultaneously as opposed to round-robin multitasking when each program can control the CPU for as long as it needs it (*see* multitasking).

pre-heating (*xray*) A preparatory step when making an x-ray exposure. The filament is pre-heated by a low current prior to the full operating current. This extends filament life.

Premac[x] **lead acrylic** (*shld*) Transparent substitute for lead glass (Wardray Premise (UK) plc). A lead loaded acrylic copolymer resin can be used in the production of glove boxes, windows, mammography screens, laboratory ware, cabinets and bench shields.

PRESAT (*mri*) Pre-saturation, Picker Medical Inc., Siemens, Toshiba motion artefact reduction techniques. spatial pre-saturation to reduce MR signal intensity in specific locations (*see* SAT, REST, EFAST, SATURATION).

pre-saturation (*mri*) Frequency-selective pre-saturation (fat saturation, water saturation), pre-saturation with inversion pulses (**dark fluid imaging**). Regional pre-saturation can be used to reduce the signal from undesired tissue which minimizes artefacts caused by movement of the chest. An additional saturation pulse is applied at the beginning of the pulse sequence to saturate the spins within the saturation slice. The saturated region produces almost no signal and appears black in the image (*see* PRESAT, saturation).

PRESS (*mri*) Point resolved spectroscopy. Similar application to STEAM but uses a 90° section select pulse followed by two mutually orthogonal 180° section select refocusing pulses. Like STEAM, only spins that have experienced all three RF pulses can form a spin echo so signals inside the slice but outside the delineated voxel are suppressed with spoiler gradients. Useful for long TEs and has a larger signal to noise ratio (*see* ISIS).

pressure (*phys*) The weight of material pressing on its surface or by collisions of atoms or molecules of gas within a container (i.e. gas radiation detectors), it acts in all directions. The SI unit is the pascal (after B. Pascal 1623–62: French mathematician) which is related to the kelvin as 1 pascal (Pa) = 1 N m^{-2}. Atmospheric pressure is approximately 1.01×10^5 Pa or approximately 10^5 Nm^{-2}. The non-SI unit mmHg extensively used in medicine is retained by agreement and is related: 1 mmHg = 1.33×10^2 Pa. Standard atmospheric pressure previously given as 760 mmHg is now taken as 105 Pa. Pressure P is defined as the force per unit area:

$$P = \frac{\text{total force on surface } F}{\text{area of surface } A} \text{ Nm}^{-2}$$

Hence, pressure is not the same as force and the result is measured in newtons per square metre (Nm^{-2}). This is true for incompressible substances solids and liquids.

1 millibar	10^2Pa
1 atm	$\approx 10^5$Pa
1 mm Hg	1333.32 Pa = 1.00 torr
Standard pressure	1 atm or 760 torr
1 lb in^{-2} (1 psi)	6.89×10^3 Pa
Conversion	
mmHg to KPa	divide by 7.5
cm H$_2$O to mmHg	divide by 1.34
cm H$_2$O to KPa	divide by 10

(*us*) *See* acoustic pressure.

prevalence (*stats*) The total number in a population with the disease. The prevalence of a disease A gives the unconditional probability of the disease as P(A) or:

$$\frac{\text{number of incidences of the disease}}{\text{total population at the time}}$$

For example, if there are 330 000 incidences of breast cancer in a population of 3 million women, then the prevalence is 11%.

prevalent screen (*clin*) The first screening investigation which will detect all the prevalent disease which would have accumulated up to that time.

pre-whitening matched filter (PWMF) (*mri*) Observers which whiten, i.e. remove spatial correlations (or colour), from image noise before analysing the image. The ideal observer acts as a pre-whitening matched filter.

PRF (*us*) Pulse repetition frequency.

PRFT (*mri*) Partially relaxed Fourier transform.

primary barrier (*shld*) Protection from the primary x-ray beam must be incorporated into any part of the ceiling, floor, walls and control area that the primary beam can be directed toward. The information necessary for the calculation of the primary barrier:

- yearly dose limit under constraint (P);
- workload in mA min per week (W);
- maximum likely kilovoltage;
- occupancy factor (T);
- use factor (U).

The allowable transmission B for maintaining radiation levels:

$$B = \frac{P \times d^2}{W \times U \times T \times 52}$$

primary radiation (*shld*) Measured in the collimated x-ray beam.

Primovist[*] (*cm*) Commercial (Schering) preparation of disodium gadoxetic acid (181.43 mg mL^{-1} gadoteridol) for MR imaging.

print server (*comp*) An application-specific computer that manages printers and requests for print services; allows multiple users to share a network printer.

print spooler (*comp*) A software application, typically installed on a LAN server, that manages multiple print requests.

print through (*film*) See halation, separation.

prior probability (*stats*) The situation where the probability of an event A occurs with respect to another independent event B; the outcome of B is not known at the time (*see* posterior probability, Bayes' Theorem).

probability (*stats*) A measure of the relative frequency or likelihood of a disease (*see* posterior probability).

probability density function (*stats*) For continuous variables the theoretical probability distribution or probability density function. This is represented by a continuous curve; the *y*-axis representing the density for a given value and the *x*-axis the frequency. The probability distribution graph is a smooth curve with the area under the curve scaled to 1.0; this is the probability density function *f*(*x*). The area of the probability for the segment *a* and *b* is selected in the graph.

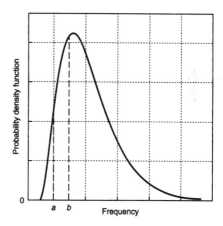

■ Reference: Sokal and Rohlf, 1995 (*see* noise (*image*)).

probe (*nm*) A single detector (typically a scintillation detector) used for detecting *in-vivo* dispersed radionuclide in a selected organ (thyroid, stomach, kidney) using tight collimation in order to reduce background interference.

product (*math*) The result of multiplying two numbers or quantities.

profile of CT numbers (*ct*) Representation of the CT numbers of the pixels along a specified direction in a CT image.

progenitor cell (*dose*) Undifferentiated cell capable of limited proliferation.

program/programming language (*comp*) A series of instructions written by a programmer according to a given set of rules or conventions ('syntax'). High-level programming languages are independent of the device on which the application (or program) will eventually run; low-level languages are specific to each program or platform. Programming language instructions are converted into language specific to a particular machine or operating system ('machine language') so that the computer can interpret and carry out the instructions. Some common programming languages are BASIC, C, C++, dBASE, FORTRAN.

progressive saturation (*mri*) *See* saturation recovery.

progressive scanning (*imaging*) A non-interlaced video display giving higher definition and less flicker (*see* interlacing).

Prohance[x] (*cm*) Commercial preparation of non-ionic gadoteridol (Bracco Diagnostics) for MR imaging.

Compound	Concentration mg mL^{-1}	Viscosity cP	Osmolality mOsm/kg
Gadoteridol	279.3	2.0 @ 20°	630
Gd-HP-DOTA		1.3 @ 37°	

projected dose (*dose*) The expected radiation if a specified countermeasure, set of countermeasures or zero countermeasures are taken.

projection (*ct*) Synonymous with the 1D or 2D attenuation profile.

projection angle (*ct*) Angular position at which the x-ray source is located when measuring an attenuation profile.

projection noise (*ct*) Noise within the ray projections measured in a CT axial scan. The main sources for projection noise are quantum noise (varying photon flux) and electronic noise caused by the A/D conversion; the image reconstruction algorithm also contributes to the noise figure.

projection profile (*mri*) Spectrum of NMR signal whose frequency components are broadened by a magnetic field gradient. In the simplest case (negligible line width. no relaxation effects, and no effects of prior gradients), it corresponds to a 1D projection of the spin density along the direction of the gradient: in this form it is used in projection-reconstruction imaging.

projection-reconstruction imaging (*mri*) Imaging technique in which a set of projection body profiles are obtained by using suitable corresponding sets of magnetic field gradients. Images are then reconstructed using techniques similar to conventional computed tomography (e.g. filtered back projection). It can be used for volume imaging or with plane selection techniques. for sequential plane imaging.

propagation period (*us*) Equal to reciprocal frequency as $1/f$ in microseconds μs.

propagation velocity (*us*) Speed of sound displacement through the medium. Typical value $1540\,\mathrm{m\ s^{-1}}$ for soft tissue.

Tissue	Propagation velocity (m s^{-1})
Water	1492
Brain	1530
Blood	1570
Liver	1549
Bone	4080

proportional counter (*phys*) An ionization chamber where the applied voltage is kept stable at approximately 1000 V. The secondary electron events are then proportional to the primary events. The dead time is of the order of microseconds and so the counter can be operated in pulse mode. Proportional counters are used as accurate radiation dose monitors.

protection quantities (*dose*) ICRP dose quantities developed for radiological protection that allow quantification of exposure to ionizing radiation from both whole and partial body external irradiation and from intakes of radionuclides.

prospective synchronization (*mri*) *See* synchronization (prospective).

ProstaScint[x] (*nmed*) A kit for the preparation of [111]Indium-Capromab Pendetide (Cytogen Corp) a murine monoclonal antibody, 7E11-C5.3, conjugated to glycyl-tyrosyl-(N,diethylene-triamine-penta-acetic acid)-lysine hydrochloride (GYK-DTPA-HCl). An antibody directed against a glycoprotein expressed by prostate epithelium known as prostate specific membrane antigen (PSMA) (*see* capromab pendetide).

protein-binding (*cm*) Cholegraphic contrast material are excreted and concentrated in the bile, rather than eliminated by the kidneys, due to their very high protein-binding. The cholegraphic contrast agents, therefore being ionic, have a higher chemotoxicity than urographic contrast material. A low partition coefficient is an advantage in contrast media since a high hydrophilicity contributes to low protein binding. Gallium-67 citrate (a radiopharmaceutical agent) binds to plasma proteins and then localizes in tissues, particularly the liver, spleen, bone marrow and skeleton.

protocol (*comp*) Any defined set of procedures, conventions or methods that, when adhered to, allow two devices to inter-operate; used to implement LAN services.

proton (*phys*) A nuclear particle having a charge equal and opposite to an electron, its rest mass is 1.672×10^{-27}kg and rest energy 938.2 MeV (slightly smaller than the neutron).

proton density (*mri*) Number of hydrogen protons per unit of volume (spin density).

proton density image (*mri*) In a proton density-weighted MR image, contrast is affected primarily by the proton density of the tissue to be displayed.

proxy server (*comp*) A server that sits between the browser and a web server, the proxy server intercepts all requests and checks if the requested web page is already stored on the hard disk. Proxy servers speed up Internet access for large numbers of users, and can also be used by companies to filter out requests for unsuitable web pages.

PSIF (*mri*) Time inverted (mirrored) FISP steady-state GRE sequence with sampling of the SP/STE component used by Siemens producing strong T2-weighted contrast in a short measurement time. Commonly used for imaging of cerebrospinal fluid (*see* SSFP, DE-FGR, CE-FAST, True-FISP, ROAST, T2-FEE, E-SHORT, STERE).

pseudo-gating (*mri*) Obtained with a TR corresponding to the R-R interval in the cardiac cycle. Prevents flow artefacts (assuming a stable heart rate).

PS (*mri*) *See* partial saturation.

PSSE (*mri*) *See* partial saturation spin echo.

PTCA (*clin*) Percutaneous transluminal coronary angioplasty. Dilatation of narrow vessel segment by using balloon catheters. By positioning a dilatation balloon at the narrow vessel segment, inflation of the balloon will dilate the vessel lumen. The damage to the vessel wall during dilatation will depend on the degree of atherosclerosis.

public area (*shld*) Areas immediately outside the radiology zones (controlled area, supervised area), where dose constraint levels of 0.3 mSv y^{-1} prevail (ICRP60, NCRP 116) (*see* public dose limits).

public (exposure levels) (*dose*) Individuals of the population, excluding exposed or designated workers or students during their working hours. Nurses and administrative staff in hospitals should be treated as members of the public, along with patients' visitors.

public dose limits (*dose*) There are differences between ICRP and NRCP as:

	ICRP60 (1991a)	NCRP 116 (1993)
Stochastic effects	Annual average over 5 years not to exceed 1 mSv	1 mSv annual effective dose limit for continuous exposure or 5 mSv for infrequent exposure
Deterministic effects	15 mSv annual equivalent dose limit to lens of eye; 50 mSv to skin and extremities	50 mSv annual equivalent dose to lens, skin and extremities
Embryo/foetus	2 mSv equivalent dose on declared pregnancy	0.5 mSv equivalent dose per month on declared pregnancy.
Negligible individual	–	0.01 mSv annual effective dose per source dose (NID)

PUGWASH (*dose*) Series of conferences held to discuss the implications of nuclear developments on the world population. First held in Pugwash, Nova Scotia 1957.

PulmoCis [*] (*nmed*) Preparation of MAA by CIS/Schering.

pulmonary angiography (*clin*) Angiography demonstrating the pulmonary arteries and veins by using a catheter passed into the trunk of the pulmonary artery. Generally, a femoral approach is used, but alternatively the internal jugular vein or the median cubital vein may be approached.

pulsatile flow (*us*) Flow pattern that accelerates and decelerates with each cardiac cycle.

pulsatility index (*us*) Description of the relationship between peak-systolic and end-diastolic flow speeds or Doppler shifts.

pulse (*elec*) The simple pulse is a single electrical, RF, sound or fluid/gas disturbance, increasing from zero to a maximum value in a short time period. Undamped pulses have a large overshoot, ringing and undershoot. Critically damped pulses are designed to reduce these factors. A short burst of RF or sound energy consisting of two to three wavelengths used in

MRI or ultrasound. An x-ray pulse is a very short exposure (<1 ms) from a **grid controlled** x-ray tube (*see* **cathode cup**).

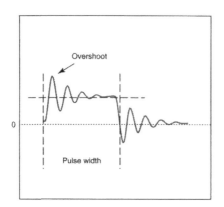

pulse 90° (π/2 pulse) (*mri*) An RF pulse which rotates M_z (macroscopic magnetization vector) into the transverse plane M_{xy}. RF pulse designed to rotate the 90° in space as referred to the rotating frame of reference, usually about an axis at right angles to the main magnetic field. If the spins are initially aligned with the magnetic field, this pulse will produce transverse magnetization and an FID signal.

pulse 180° (π pulse) (*mri*) RF pulse which inverts the magnetization vector as $-M_z$. RF pulse designed to rotate the macroscopic magnetization vector 180° in space as referred to the rotating frame of reference, usually about an axis at right angles to the main magnetic field. If the spins are initially aligned with the magnetic field, this pulse will produce inversion.

pulse average intensity (I_{PA}) (*us*) Average intensity over repetition period. The ratio of the **pulse intensity integral** (energy fluence per pulse) to the **pulse duration** as:

$$I_{PA} = \frac{TA}{\text{duty cycle}}$$

The unit is Watt per square-centimetre, W cm^{-2}. Typical values are given under **ultrasound (intensity)**.

pulse bandwidth (*mri*) The transmitter bandwidth or the range of frequencies in the excitation pulse and the **gradient strength** defines the slice thickness. Narrow RF bandwidths correspond to thinner slices. The receiver bandwidth defines the pixel size, defined as: N_{pf}/t_s where N_{pf} is the number of phase or frequency **encoding**

steps and t_s is the sampling time. Also since noise content increases with bandwidth:

$$\text{Signal to noise} = \frac{1}{\sqrt{\text{bandwidth}}}$$

(*us*) The bandwidth of an ultrasound pulse, the number of frequencies in the pulse, is specified between ±6 dB points. Bandwidth is inversely related to **spatial pulse length**. Fractional bandwidth is bandwidth divided by operating frequency. The **quality factor** is:

- Operating frequency/bandwidth; or
- 1/fractional bandwidth (see **pulse**).

pulse duration (period) (PD) (*us*) The time for 2–3 wavelengths, a typical pulse duration is 0.5–3 μs.

$$PD = \frac{\text{cycles} \times \text{period or cycles}}{\text{frequency}}$$

1.25 times the interval between the time when the time integral of **intensity** in an acoustic pulse at a point reaches 10% and when it reaches 90% of the **pulse intensity integral**.

Pulse duration (PD) = n/f micro-seconds (μs) (*see* **spatial pulse length**).

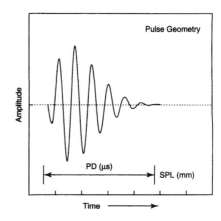

pulse, gradient (*mri*) *See* **gradient pulse**.

pulse height analyser (*nmed*) An electronic circuit that can threshold the lower and upper limits of the photopeak energy and accept signals just within these limits.

pulse, gradient (*mri*) *See* **gradient pulse**.

pulse intensity integral (PII) (*us*) The time integral of instantaneous intensity, for any specific point and pulse, integrated over the time in which the envelope of acoustic pressure or hydrophone signal for the specific pulse is nonzero. It is equal to the energy fluence per pulse. For a transducer assembly operating in a non-autoscanning mode, it is equal to the product of temporal-average intensity and pulse repetition period. Unit: J cm^{-2}.

pulse length (*mri*) Time duration of a pulse. For an RF pulse near the Larmor frequency, the longer the pulse length, the greater the angle of rotation of the macroscopic magnetization vector; also the narrower the equivalent range of frequencies in the pulse will be (narrower the bandwidth). (*us*) *See* pulse duration

pulse NMR (*mri*) NMR techniques that use RF pulses and Fourier transformation of the NMR signal have largely replaced the older continuous wave techniques.

pulse pile up (*nmed*) A cause of acquired data loss due to the slow response of pulse handling electronics at high count rates. Mainly associated with the ADC and its sample and hold circuit. A form of pulse pile up is seen in nuclear detectors when their dead time prevents each single event from being distinguished.

pulse power (*us*) Each ultrasound pulse transfers power measured in watts (or mW). The energy emitted per unit time or the average transmitted power (A): $A =$ pulse energy $\times$ PRF, where PRF is pulse repetition frequency. The total energy is this value multiplied by the transducer on time (time of study) (*see* duty cycle).

pulse programmer (*mri*) Part of the spectrometer or interface that controls the timing, duration, phase and amplitude of the pulses (RF or gradient).

pulse repetition frequency (PRF) (*us*) For a pulsed waveform, the number of pulses generated per second. Determines the distance or depth from where the echoes are collected. A chain of timed transmission pulses delivered to the transducer. $PRF = 1/PRP$ which is typically 2–10 kHz. A lower PRF increases image depth (see table below). The timing between the transmission pulses, the pulse repetition period (PRP), is critical for each transducer type since this determines the rate of image formation or frame rate. If a 1 μsec transmission pulse is followed by a waiting period of 200 μs (receive period) this will give a pulse repetition frequency as:

$$10^6 = 200 = 5000\,\text{Hz}(5\,\text{kHz})$$

Typical PRF values range from 2 to 10 kHz for diagnostic imaging. Pulse duration is typically 1 μs compared to a pulse repetition period of 200 μs. The pulse repetition period (PRP) is matched to the image depth or scan line length, otherwise echo pulses may clash with transmission pulses if the PRP is too short.

PRF (kHz)	PRP (μs)	Depth (cm)
5	200	15.4
8	125	9.6
12.5	80	6.0
15	66	5.0
20	50	3.8

pulse repetition period (PRP) (*us*) Time to repeat ultrasound pulse; the time from one pulse to the next. $PRP = 1/PRF$ which has a typical range 0.1 to 0.5 ms. Pulse repitition period (PRP), the time between pulses or waiting time for echo collection typically 200 μs.

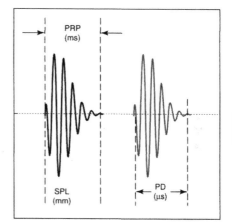

pulse, RF (*mri*) *See* RF pulse.

pulse sequences (*mri*) Set of RF pulses and/or gradient magnetic field changes and time periods between these pulses, synchronized with magnetic field gradients and NMR signal reception to produce NMR images. Recommended shorthand of interpulse times used to generate a particular image is to list the repetition time (TR), echo time (TE); if using inversion-recovery, the inversion time (TI) is given in milliseconds. A 2500/30/1000 sequence would indicate an inversion-recovery pulse sequence with TR of 2500 ms, TE of 30 ms and TI of 1000 ms; with a multiple spin echo sequence (e.g. CPMG) the number of spin echoes should be stated.

pulse triggering (*mri*) Pulse triggering suppresses motion and flow artefacts as a result of pulsating blood and fluid. The pulse wave obtained with a finger sensor is used as the trigger.

pulse wavelength (*us*) This is derived as *c/f* mm.

pulse width (*us*) The pulse period or pulse duration measured in microseconds.

pulsed Doppler (*us*) A Doppler device that uses pulsed-wave ultrasound.

pulsed mode (*us*) Mode of operation in which pulsed ultrasound is used.

pulsed ultrasound (*us*) Ultrasound produced in pulsed form by applying electric pulses or voltages of a few cycles to the transducer.

pulsed wave (*us*) A wave consisting of a series of pulses, each containing a few cycles of ultrasound; not continuous.

purity (radiochemical) (*nmed*) *See* high performance liquid chromatograph.

PVDF (*us*) Polyvinylidene fluoride, a piezoelectric thin-film material.

PW (*us*) Pulsed wave.

pyelography (*clin*) Radiography of the kidneys, ureters and often the bladder by either injecting contrast medium intravenously or via a ureteral or nephrostomy catheter. Also performed percutaneously. Also known as pelvi-ureterography, pyelo-ureterography or uretero-pyelography.

Retrograde pyelography (urography) is the radiographic examination of the renal pelvis and ureter by means of contrast medium counterflow injection using a ureteric catheter (*see* urography (retrograde)).

pyrogens (*nmed*) Substances that induce a febrile reaction (*see* limulus test).

pyrophosphate (PYP) (*nmed*) As sodium pyrophosphate; its structure is condensed phosphate radicals forming chains of -P-O-P- units. A bone seeking radiopharmaceutical labelled with ^{99m}Tc. A radiopharmaceutical previously used for skeletal imaging but now used for labelling red blood cells, *in vivo* or *in vitro*. ^{99m}Tc-PYP uptake is a function of blood flow to the bone and the bone efficiency in extracting the complex. The complex also reacts with mitochondrial calcium compounds within infarcted myocardial cells.

Generic name	^{99m}Tc - pyrophosphate
Commercial names	Phosphotec® – (Bracco)
	Pyrolite® (CIS)
	Technescan® PYP
	Amersham PYP®
Imaging category	*In-vivo* / *in-vitro* RBC
	Blood pool labelling

(*see* MDP, HMDP).

PyTest^{℞} (*nmed*) *See* ^{14}Carbon (labelled urea).

PZT (*us*) *See* lead zirconate titanate.

Q

QCSI (*mri*) Quantitative chemical shift imaging.

Q-factor (*phys*) *See* quality factor.

QMRI (*mri*) Quantitative magnetic resonance imaging.

quad core processor (*comp*) Quad core chips feature two separate duo core processors enabling it to perform four separate tasks simultaneously instead of two. A typical specification would be 4×2.93 GHz duo cores with a total of 2×4 MB L2 cache per 65 nm core. Multi-threading programmes can be operated efficiency. Typically, each duo core has a cache memory of 4 MB. The quad-core chip commonly features a heat spreader which diffuses the CPU's heat over a larger surface area.

Quadramet (*nmed*) Commercial preparation of ^{153}Samarium (Schering Inc.) (*see* samarium).

quadrapole moment (*phys, mri*) Measure of the non-spherical distribution of electrical charge possessed by nuclei with a nuclear spin nuclear spin greater than $^1/_2$. The resulting interaction with electric field gradients in the molecule can lead to a shortening of relaxation times and a broadening of spectral lines.

quadrature (*mri*) Two periodic quantities (sine-wave) having the same frequency are in quadrature when they differ in phase by 90°.

quadrature coil (*mri*) A coil that produces an RF field with circular polarization by providing RF feed points that are out of phase by 90°. When used as a transmitter coil, a factor of two power reduction over a linear coil results: as a receiver an increase in SNR of up to a factor of $\sqrt{2}$ can be achieved.

quadrature demodulator (*mri*) An electronic circuit part of the quadrature detector, sensitive to phase and frequency differences which analyses the signal from coils having quadrature or circularly polarized features.

quadrature detector (*mri*) *See* quadrature phase detector.

quadrature phase detector (*mri*) A phase sensitive detector or demodulator (also called circularly polarized detector), either an analogue or digital electronic circuit, that detects the proportion of a signal in phase with a reference signal and 90° out of phase with the reference. By joining a pair of coils at 90° and driving them during the transmit cycle through a power divider and phase shifter, a rotating field

can be produced that only requires half the RF power. Single phase detection uses only one reference frequency. A phase sensitive **quadrature** (circularly polarized) detector uses two reference signals in quadrature, and since two signals are being obtained the SNR is improved by $\sqrt{2}$ or 1.4. Patient motion will reduce this benefit. Both positive and negative phase differences can be detected. Any poor adjustment of the phase shift will give a ghost image artefact; this can be eliminated by adjusting phase and gain of the receiver minimizing the quadrature peak in an off-resonance signal.

quality (*xray*) *See* beam quality.

quality assurance QA (*dose*) A protocol set up to serve purchase specifications, commissioning and quality control of diagnostic imaging equipment together with ancillary equipment (dosimeters, dose calibrators and contamination monitors). Defined by WHO as 'All those planned and systematic actions necessary to provide adequate confidence that a structure, system or component will perform satisfactorily in service' (ISO 62 15-1980). Satisfactory performance in service implies the optimum quality of the entire diagnostic process (the consistent production of adequate diagnostic information with minimum exposure of both patients and personnel). (*ct*) *See* acceptance tests and quality control.

quality control (*qc*) Defined by WHO as 'The set of operations (programming, coordinating, carrying out) intended to maintain or to improve equipment (ISO 3534-1977). As applied to a diagnostic procedure, it covers monitoring, evaluation and maintenance at optimum levels of all characteristics of performance that can be defined, measured and controlled'. (*xray*) After purchase and commissioning, the equipment performance is monitored so that it remains within original specifications and radiation safety levels are maintained. This is carried out on a daily (e.g. film processors, gamma camera uniformity), weekly, monthly (e.g. personal dosimetry, resolution/contrast, film cassettes) or yearly (e.g. focal spot, beam quality) basis. A standard of precision and accuracy for the QC instrumentation is required for testing reproducibility. An error of <5% and precision of 0.1 kV is necessary for mammography kVp meters.

quality control (radiopharmaceuticals) (*nmed*) The study of radiochemical purity (RCP) defined as the fraction of the radionuclide which is in the correct chemical form. The major analytical techniques routinely used are:

- Chromatography (thin layer and paper (TLC/PC));
- Chromatography (high performance liquid (HPLC));
- Electrophoresis.

These procedures are designed to separate precursors, impurities and decomposition products as well as to identify the desired product. Simple chromatographic techniques employ gel paper and either alcohol or acetone as the solvent. The solvent front advances along a strip of absorbent gel (thin layer chromatography strips): an activity profile is taken through the active areas on the strip. The quality control result gives a measure of:

- bound ^{99m}Tc;
- free ^{99m}Tc (TcO_4);
- hydrolyzed ^{99m}Tc (TcO_2).

quality factor Q or w_R (*dose*) *See* weighting factor (radiation), weighting factor (tissue).

quality factor Q (*phys*) This applies to any resonant circuit and is a measure of the quality of a resonating system (ultrasound transducers and MRI coils) indicating the sensitivity of the system at resonance. It is defined as:

$$Q = \frac{f_R}{f_2 - f_1}$$

where f_R is the frequency giving maximum response, which is the resonant frequency; f_1 and f_2 the frequencies either side of resonance (f_R) where the response falls to 0.707 of maximum ($\sqrt{2} \times 0.5$). The ratio of the resonance frequency f_R, to the band-width f_2-f_1 is the Q factor of the transducer. The Q factor describes the sharpness of the frequency response curve: The undamped curve shows a narrow frequency range and a distinct peak at the resonance frequency. Alternatively, the damped curve has a frequency response that is broader and not so sharply peaked at the resonance frequency. Q is inversely related (1/Q) to selectivity, the range of frequencies over which the system will show resonance and the ability of the system to select a given frequency within narrow limits. The quality factor affects the SNR since both transmitted and detected signal in ultrasound in MRI increases proportionally to Q

whereas the noise increases as $\sqrt{Q}$. The Q of a coil in MRI will be affected by external influences (patient volume and tissue type). Two systems are plotted in the graph example showing high and low Q values. A high Q ultrasound transducer produces a pure single frequency with a long duration (Doppler waveform); a low Q transducer producing a short duration mixed frequency pulse.

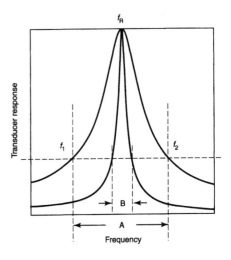

(*mri*) Applies to the coil(s) and determines the overall efficiency. Inversely related to the fraction of the energy in an oscillating system and also inversely related to the range of frequency over which the system will exhibit resonance. It affects the signal-to-noise ratio, because the detected signal increases proportionally to Q while the noise is proportional to $\sqrt{Q}$. The Q of a coil will depend on the circumstances under which it is measured; 'unloaded' (no patient) or 'loaded' (patient). (*us*) Describes the sharpness of the frequency response curve. The curve for the undamped transducer displays a narrow frequency range and shows a distinct peak at the resonance frequency f_R. Alternatively, in the damped transducer, due to increased absorption the frequency response is broader and not so sharply peaked at the resonance frequency. Points f_1 and f_2 on the undamped (sharp) curve represent frequencies on either side of the resonance frequency where the response has diminished to half (−3 dB). The ratio of the resonance frequency f_R, to

Q

the bandwidth f_2-f_1 is the Q factor of the transducer.

quantile (*stats*) General name for the values of a variable which divide its distribution into equal groups (*see* quartile, normal curve).

quantitative computed tomography (QCT) (*ct*) The use of CT images and the corresponding CT numbers for quantitative characterization of organs or tissues. QCT is most widely used in relation to the determination of bone mineral content and treatment planning in radiotherapy.

quantization noise (*image*) The uncertainty introduced into a digital image matrix by allocating random photon events on a surface (film) into the regular pixel pattern of a digital image degrades image information; this is the noise associated with quantization of the image signal. It is reduced by employing high bit number analogue to digital converters along with finer matrices but this then introduces quantum noise (*see* digitization noise).

quantum efficiency (*phys*) The efficiency of converting photons to electrons (photocathode) or vice versa (scintillation detector). The detector response to electromagnetic radiation. Since the photon carries energy $h\,f$ and the quantum of electric charge is e (the elementary charge) then quantum efficiency η is the ratio of induced elementary charge N_e and the number of incident photons (the fluence) Φ as $\eta = N_e/\Phi$.

quantum mechanics (*phys*) Newton's laws cannot be used for describing events on the atomic scale. The English polymath James Young (1773–1829) perhaps sparked off the concept of wave/particle duality with his experiments using slit light sources. The quantum theory grew later from observations made by Planck and Einstein on photon events, developed further by the work of Schrödinger and Dirac (wave mechanics), then Born and Heisenberg (matrix mechanics).

quantum mottle (*film, image*) Random noise exhibited by a display system (*see* quantum noise).

quantum noise (*stats*) Determined by the number of quanta or photons responsible in forming the image; also referred to as quantum mottle. Poisson statistics are obeyed so the standard deviation of the photon density N follows $\sqrt{N}$.

Quantum noise

If each unit area of surface receives:

100 photons, then $\sqrt{100} = 10$, so there will be 10% variation or quantum noise.

1000 photons, then $\sqrt{1000} = 30$, so there will be 3% variation or quantum noise.

1×10^6 photons then $\sqrt{1} \times 10^6 = 1000$, so there will be 0.1% variation or quantum noise. (*ct*) Noise contribution due to the random processes and the statistical nature of x-ray generation, attenuation and detection; Since efficient image detectors are used in low dose (exposure) imaging these are prone to show quantum noise (*see* projection noise).

quantum sink (*phys*) The point loss of signal data. The quantum sink in an image intensifier is the photon detector surface (caesium iodide). Every absorbed x-ray quantum generates several thousand light quanta of which only a small fraction reach the photocathode leading to the emission of photoelectrons with a quantum yield of a few percent.

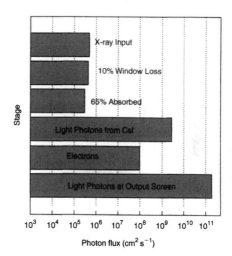

quartile (*stats*) The value of a variable below which three-quarters (first or upper quartile) or one-quarter (3rd or lower quartile) of a distribution lie. The median divides a distribution in two halves. The three quartiles cut the distribution at 25, 50 and 75% at points dividing the distribution into 1st, 2nd, 3rd and 4th quarters by area. The second quartile is the median (*see* percentile).

quasi-ideal observer (*stats*) Model observers whose performance is lower than that of the

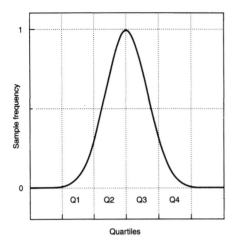

Quartiles

ideal observer, e.g. Hotelling observer and the NPWMF, but whose performance may be measurable in circumstances where the use of the ideal observer is not appropriate.

quasi-threshold dose D_q (*dose*) An extrapolation point on the exponential portion of a multi-target dose-response survival curve (*see* survival curve).

quench (*mri*) Sudden loss of superconductivity by a local temperature increase in the magnet. The cryogen used for superconductivity (liquid helium) evaporates rapidly and the magnetic field strength is reduced. As the magnet becomes resistive, heat will be released that can result in rapid evaporation of liquid helium in the cryostat. This may present a hazard if not properly planned for.

quenching (*phys*) A form of signal loss in the gas Geiger detector.

QUEST (*mri*) Quick echo split imaging technique. FSE variant using multiple unequally spaced RF pulses and collecting STEs and SEs

QuickTime ˣ (*comp*) Audio–visual software that allows cine-delivery via the Internet and e-mail. QuickTime mages are viewed on a monitor.

Quimby, Edith Hinkley (1891–1982) American medical physicist. Pioneer in nuclear medicine and exact measurement of radiation dose.

quotient (*math*) The result of the division of one number or quantity by another. A ratio of two numbers or quantities to be divided.

R

R1 (*mri*) Longitudinal relaxation rate equal to reciprocal of relaxation time (R1 = 1/T1).

R2 (*mri*) Longitudinal relaxation rate equal to reiprocal of relaxation time (R2 = 1/T2).

RACE (*mri*) Real time acquisition and velocity evaluation. A single dimension velocity measurement.

rad (*dose*) The non-SI unit of dose superseded by the gray (Gy):

* 1 rad = 100 ergs g^{-1};
* 1 rad = 10 mGy = 1 cGy;
* 100 rads = 1 Gy;
* 1 mrad = 10 µGy;
* 1 Gy = 1 J kg^{-1}.

(*see* kerma, sievert).

radian (*unit*) A supplementary SI unit for the plane angle (rad). The angle which as the central area of a circle radius 1 m cuts an arc 1 m out of the circumference. 1 rad = ≈57.295°. It is used for describing the 2π geometric efficiency of a flat detector surface (*see* degree, geometry, steradian).

radiance (*phys*) The flux per unit projected area per unit solid angle leaving a source or surface. Radiance is the combined (integral) of the spectral radiances from a surface. It is a measure of the power given by an emitting or reflecting surface detected by an optical system (eye) looking at the surface from the solid angle (steradian) subtended by the eye. Radiance and luminance are both used for describing the 'brightness' of a source. Radiance has the SI units W sr^{-1} m^{-2} or m Wsr^{-1} cm^{-2} This measure is used for hazard and safety analysis.

Quantity	SI unit	Abbr.
Radiant flux	Watt	W
Irradiance	Watt per square metre	W × m^{-2}
Radiant intensity	Watt per steradian	W × sr^{-1}
Radiance	Watt per steradian per square metre	W × sr^{-1} × m^{-2}

Source	Radiance
Fluorescent lamp	2.5 mW cm^{-2} sr^{-1}
1 kW tungsten/halogen lamp	58 W cm^{-2} sr^{-1}

radiant density (*phys*) The radiant energy per unit volume of the radiation field. The unit is J m^{-3} (*see* photon energy).

radiant energy fluence rate (*phys*) The radiant power incident on a small sphere divided by the cross sectional area of the sphere. The unit is Wm^{-2} (*see* photon energy fluence).

radiant energy Q (*phys*) The total energy in a radiation field or the total energy delivered by such a radiation field. The unit is the joule (J) (*see* photon energy).

radiant exitance (*phys*) The flux per unit area leaving the surface of a source of radiation. The unit is Wm^{-2} (*see* photon flux).

radiant exposure (*phys*) Energy per unit area received on a surface. The unit is J m^{-2} (*see* photon exposure).

radiant intensity (*phys*) The flux per unit solid angle emitted by a source in a given direction. The unit is W sr^{-1} (*see* photon energy).

radiant power (*phys*) (radiant flux). The rate at which radiant energy is transferred from one region to another by the radiation field. The unit is the watt (W).

radiating cross-sectional area (S) (*us*) The area of the surface at and parallel to the face of the active transducer element(s) and consisting of all points where the acoustic pressure is greater than −12 dB of the maximum acoustic pressure in that surface. The area of the active element(s) of the transducer assembly may be taken as an approximation for the radiating cross-sectional area. The unit is cm^2.

radiation (*phys*) The emission of energy as waves or particles in the case of electromagnetic radiation or as pressure changes in a medium (air) in the case of sound radiation.

radiation (ionizing) (*dose*) Radiation having sufficiently high energy (greater than 13.6 eV) which causes ionization of the absorbing material (e.g. air, water, soft tissue, etc.). It can be electromagnetic (photons) or particulate (alpha, beta, neutrons, etc.). Ionization is defined as the formation of free radicals and does not apply to simple dissociation of molecules into ions seen in other non-radiation events (e.g. NaCl → Na$^+$ and Cl$^-$). When ionization occurs in air, an average of 34 eV is dissipated (probably less in liquids and solids).

radiation (non-ionizing) (*phys*) This describes that part of the electromagnetic spectrum with energies less than x- and gamma radiation.

The threshold energy is taken as 13.6 eV. It includes ultraviolet light, visible light, infrared and radio waves. Electromechanical radiation (ultrasound) is sometimes considered. Since no ionization is caused in their interactions, the terms associated with ionizing radiation (specific ionization, LET, etc.) do not apply, however non-ionizing radiation undergoes attenuation and absorption and the rate at which energy is deposited is described as the specific absorption rate (SAR).

radiation (thermal) (*phys*) The transfer of heat by conduction and convection requires a material medium, either solid, liquid or gas, for its transport but heat can be transmitted through a vacuum by radiation (infrared). The radiation from an x-ray tube anode depends on the nature of its surface, temperature T and surface area A. So that intensity I of radiation emitted by a body: $I \propto AT^4$. So a doubling of temperature increases the heat intensity by 2^4 or $\times 16$. Conversely, a reduction of surface temperature from 1000 to 500°C reduces heat radiated to 6% of the original.

radiation area (USA) (*dose*) Defined (USA) as an area accessible to staff where radiation levels could approach $50 \mu Svh^{-1}$ at 30 cm ($50 \mu Sv$ or 5 mrem), either from the source itself or any surface that the radiation penetrates. A high radiation area is where radiation levels to staff could approach $1 mSvh^{-1}$ at 30 cm.

radiation chemistry (*nmed*) The study of the chemical effects of radiation on matter.

radiation detriment (*dose*) Assumed to be a stochastic effect. The detriment (e.g. radiation induced cancer) is never certain to occur but has a certain probability of occurrence proportional to radiation exposure. It is defined by ICRP to have several factors, including incidence of radiation-related cancer or hereditary defects, lethality of these conditions, quality of life and years of life lost due to these conditions.

radiation dose (acute) (*dose*) Doses greater than 40 Gy cause vascular system damage and cerebral oedema leading to death within 48 hours. Doses of 10–40 Gy cause less severe vascular damage with fluid and electrolyte loss through the intestinal wall, causing death within 5–10 days. Doses of 2–10 Gy cause bone marrow damage leading to infection; death occurs within

4 to 5 weeks. LD_{50} is approximately 3–3.5 Gy to the bone marrow.

radiation dose (late effects) (*dose*) Mostly secondary effects from vascular damage. Significant increases in leukaemia, thyroid, lung and breast tumours are mainly seen in populations exposed to doses greater than 1 Gy (*see* erythema).

radiation energy (*phys*) *See* photon.

radiation exposure (mAs) (*xray*) *See* exposure, mAs product, workload, radiographic exposure.

radiation output (*xray*) The air kerma measured free-in-air (without backscatter) per unit of tube loading at a specified distance from the x-ray tube focus and at stated radiographic exposure factors. Free air exposure 1 m from the focal spot at 80 kVp with 2.5 mm total filtration. Expected values from current machines are:

- 30–45 μGy (3.0–4.5 mR) per mAs for single phase;
- 50–100 μGy (5–10 mR) per mAs for constant potential.

At 30 kVp using a 0.3 mm focal spot at 65 cm, a typical value for digital mammography could be $100 \mu GymAs^{-1}$.

radiation protection adviser (RPA) (*dose*) A qualified (postgraduate) and experienced physicist (typically 5 years) appointed in accordance with national ionizing radiation regulations to advise an employer on compliance with the national regulations and on radiation safety matters (equipment QC).

radiation protection survey (*nmed*) Evaluation of the radiation hazards incidental to the production, use or presence of radioactive materials or other source of radiation. Such evaluation includes measurement of the dose rates of radiation being emitted from the material.

radiation quality (*xray*) A measure of the penetrating power of an x-ray beam, usually characterized by a statement of the tube potential and the half-value layer (*see* kerma).

radiation weighting factor (*dose*) (ICRP60) *See* weighting factor (radiation).

radioactive concentration (*nmed*) The ratio of activity of a radionuclide to the total mass of the material or volume of solution. Usually expressed in Bq g^{-1} or Bq cm^{-3}.

radioactive (transport) (*nmed*) Certain conditions have been defined by the International Atomic Energy Authority (IAEA) for the packaging and transport of radioactive material. Transport indices are indicated on the three types of package label:

Category label	Surface dose μSv hr^{-1}	Transport index
I White: Low level	5	0
II Yellow: Moderate level	5–500	<1
III Yellow: High level	500–2000	1–10

radioactive waste (*nmed*) Radioactive waste for disposal may be identified as:

- decayed sealed sources;
- spent radionuclide generators (^{99m}Tc, ^{81m}Kr, ^{185m}Au etc.);
- laboratory solutions of low activity;
- low activity liquid washings from vials;
- liquid scintillants immiscible with water;
- biologically contaminated solid waste, i.e. syringes, vials;
- radioactive gases.

Classification	No control	Controlled
GROUP 1	Not used	Not used
GROUP 2 ^{125}I, ^{131}I	5 × 10^4 Bq (1.4 μCi) (USA 1.0 μCi)	1 × 10^7 Bq (270 μCi) (USA10.0 μCi)
GROUP 3 ^{201}Tl, ^{32}P, ^{67}Ga, ^{51}Cr, ^{111}In, ^{57}Co, ^{58}Co, ^{99}Mo	5 × 10^5 × Bq (14 μCi) (USA10.0 μCi)	5 × 10^6 Bq (140 μCi) (USA 100 μCi)
GROUP 4 ^{99m}Tc, ^{133}Xe	5 × 10^6 Bq (140 μCi) (USA 100 μCi)	5 × 10^7 Bq (1.4 mCi) (USA 1 mCi)

radioactivity (*unit*) *See* bequerel (Bq).

radiochemical (*nmed*) A radioactive chemical suitable for *in vitro* studies, but unsuitable for administration to humans.

radiochemistry (*nmed*) The study and production of radionuclides and compounds.

radiofrequency (RF) pulse (*mri*) Oscillating magnetic field (B) typically of relatively short duration, produced by an RF coil. In MR imaging, RF pulses are applied to excite a selected slice of tissue.

radiofrequency radiation (RF) (*phys*) The section of the electromagnetic spectrum used for telecommunication. The range of frequencies between 3 kHz and 300 GHz. The subdivisions are: very low frequency, low frequency, medium frequency, high frequency, very high frequency, ultra high frequency, super high and extremely high frequency.

radiographic exposure (*xray*) Product of tube current and exposure time mA × s = mAs.

radioimmunoassay (RIA) (*nmed*) An *in vitro* test in which very small quantities of certain substances in blood, urine, etc. can be measured by using specific antibodies or other agents which have been labelled with radioactive tracers. Since the patient does not receive the radioactive material, there is no patient radiation exposure involved.

radioisotope (*nmed*) An unstable atom having the same atomic number but a different number of neutrons in the nucleus than the comparable stable element.

radiometric quantity (*phys*) A set of light measurement quantities used to describe the brightness of a source (radiance) and irradiance levels on a surface.

radionuclide (*nmed*) An unstable nuclide.

radionuclides (cyclotron produced) (*nmed*) Reaction mechanisms and reaction dynamics follow

$$A_t = NF\alpha(1 - e^{-\lambda t}).$$

A_t is the number of activated atoms at time t per unit volume, N the number of target atoms per unit volume, F the cyclotron beam flux, and α the activation cross section for the specific neutron energy with λ the decay constant of the product nuclide. The irradiation time is approximately three to four half-lives of the product. The particle ion beam is commonly derived from a light gas. Cyclotron produced radionuclides have a proton excess. Decay is by positron emission or electron capture. Since the nuclides tend to be relatively neutron deficient, in order to gain a stable neutron : proton ratio they decay by creating a neutron from a proton by one of two reactions:

Positron emission (β^+) by proton decay:

$$p \rightarrow n + e^+ + neutrino$$

Orbital electron capture by a nuclear proton:

$$p + e^- \rightarrow n + anti\text{-}neutrino$$

The most common reaction for the small cyclotron using a proton beam is (p, n), one

R

neutron is lost. Typical small current (p, n) reactions are ^{15}O, ^{13}N and ^{18}F (see radionuclides (positron)). The commonly produced radionuclides from small and medium sized cyclotrons are:

Target	Reaction	Nuclide	Beam energy MeV
^{14}N	(d, n)	^{15}O	3
^{18}O	(p, n)	^{18}F	10
^{12}C	(d, n)	^{13}N	10
^{10}B	(d, n)	^{11}C	10
^{68}Zn	(p, 2n)	^{67}Ga	20–30
^{203}Tl	(p, 3n)	^{201}Tl	20–30
^{112}Cd	(p, 2n)	^{111}In	20–30
^{82}Kr	(d, 3n)	^{81}Rb (^{81m}Kr)	20–30
^{124}Xe	(p, pn)	^{123}Xe ... ^{123}I	20–30
^{127}I	(d, 2n)	^{127}Xe	20–30

If the target is bombarded with energic deuterons then two neutrons are emitted in a (d, 2n) reaction. With higher energy deuterons (d, 3n) reactions can be achieved. Typical large current reactions. Many more reactions are theoretically possible but cost plays an important part.

radionuclides (generator produced) (*nmed*) Radioactive decay can lead to the formation of an intermediate or metastable state, which decays by isomeric transition usually yielding a pure gamma or positron emitting radionuclide. Metastable states can exist for periods of seconds (^{81m}Kr and ^{185m}Au) to hours (^{99m}Tc and ^{113m}In). Metastable products form useful imaging nuclides if their parent isotope has a sufficiently long half-life to allow for generator construction and shipment. As the parent decays the activity of the daughter rises. The carrier free daughter is then eluted from the generator by passing a solvent over the column. Clinically useful generators showing parent (*pt*) and daughter (*dt*) properties are:

pt : dt	Production	Pt T½	Dt T½	γ-Energy
^{81}Rb → ^{81m}Kr	Cyclotron	4.6 h	13 s	190 keV
^{99}Mo → ^{99m}Tc	Reactor	66 h	6.0 h	140 keV
^{113}Sn → ^{113m}In	Reactor	115 d	99 m	390 keV
^{62}Zn → ^{62}Cu	Cyclotron	9.3 h	9.7 m	511 keV (β$^+$)
^{68}Ge → ^{68}Ga	Cyclotron	270 d	68 m	511 keV (β$^+$)
^{82}Sr → ^{82}Rb	Cyclotron	25 d	1.3 m	511 keV (β$^+$)
^{178}W → ^{178}Ta	Cyclotron	21 d	9.3 m	93 keV
^{191}Os → ^{191m}Ir	Reactor	15 d	5 s	130 keV
^{195m}Hg → ^{195m}Au	Cyclotron	41 h	30 s	190 keV

(*see* Bateman equation).

radionuclides (positron) (*nmed*) The most common positron radionuclides and their properties and typical applications are:

Nuclide	T½ (minutes)	β$^+$ yield (%)	β$^+$ energy (MeV)
Cyclotron produced			
^{15}O	2.0	99.9	0.735
^{13}N	9.9	99.8	0.491
^{11}C	20.4	99.8	0.385
^{18}F	109.8	96.9	0.242
Generator produced			
^{68}Ga	68.1	89	0.740
^{82}Rb	76.4	95	1.409
^{62}Cu	9.7	97	1.280
^{122}I	3.6	77	1.087

Nuclide	Application
^{11}C	Metabolic and pharmacological studies
^{13}N	Metabolic and pharmacological studies
^{15}O	Blood flow, blood volume and metabolic studies
^{18}F	Labelled glucose analogues for regional cerebral blood flow and myocardial metabolism
^{68}Ga	Transmission source, tumour imaging
^{82}Rb	Myocardial perfusion
^{62}Cu	Myocardial perfusion
^{122}I	Thyroid metastases

(*see* positron (labelled compounds), radionuclides (generator produced).

radionuclide production (*nmed*) Three methods are available for producing nuclear medicine radionuclides:

- Bombardment of stable elements with charged beams (cyclotron).
- Irradiation of stable elements with neutrons in a nuclear reactor.
- Generator production.

The first two procedures mentioned above obey the same basic equation for the rate of isotope production:

$$A = C(1 - e^{-\lambda t})$$

where A is the amount of activity and C is a saturation constant, since it is the maximum amount of activity that can be produced for the given conditions; t is the irradiation time and λ the decay coefficient for the nuclide. At a certain time, during irradiation, a production limit is reached: the number of atoms being produced is balanced by those decaying. This point is the saturation limit. The factor C for reactor irradiation is calculated as:

$$C = 1.6 \times 10^{-8} \frac{w \times \phi \times \sigma}{\text{Atomic weight}}$$

where w is the sample weight in grams, ϕ is the neutron flux and σ is the cross-section for the nuclear reaction in barns.

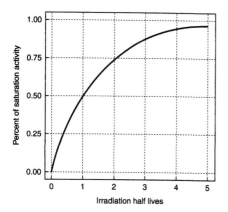

Irradiation half lives

radionuclides (reactor) (*nmed*) Some commonly produced radionuclides from neutron irradiation using the (n,γ) reaction or as fission products are:

Radionuclide	Use
^{99}Molybdenum	^{99}Mo/^{99m}Tc generator
^{125}Iodine	Radio-immunoassay and thyroid therapy
^{131}Iodine	Thyroid therapy and some scintigraphy
^{32}Phosphorus	Therapy
^{133}Xenon	Ventilation imaging
^{51}Chromium	Red blood cell labelling
^{60}Cobalt	Therapy and calibration
^{57}Cobalt	Reference

radionuclide therapy (*nmed*) Radiation therapy from a radiopharmaceutical given directly to the patient (e.g. 131 J for hyperthyroidism).

radiopharmaceutical (*nmed*) A radiolabelled compound administered for the purpose of diagnosis or therapy. Conforming to a recognized standard of clinical purity. These compounds do not elicit physiologic effects on the body because of the carrier-free nature of the radionuclide and the inherent safety of most radiopharmaceuticals. A radiopharmaceutical contains two parts, the radionuclide and the pharmaceutical, e.g. ^{99m}Tc DTPA.

radiopharmacy (*nmed*) The design requirements for laboratories where radionuclides are to be dispensed for clinical use should comply with national legislation. The degrees of usage are categorized into low, medium and high levels.

Radiotoxicity	Low	Medium	High
Group 2 ^{89}Sr, ^{125}I, ^{131}I	<500 kBq	500 kBq to 500 MBq	500 MBq to 5 GBq
Group 3 ^{51}Cr, ^{57}Co, ^{99}Mo, ^{111}In	<5 MBq	5 Bq to 5 GBq	5 to 500 GBq
Group 4 ^{99m}Tc	<500 MBq	500 MBq to 500 GBq	500 GBq to 50 TBq

The radiopharmacy must comply with controlled/supervised area restrictions of access.

■ Reference: Frier *et al.*, 1988.

radio-resistive (*dose*) Tissues that have a higher resistance to radiation damage than others due to their relatively low rate of cell division. ICRP60 places vascular and connective tissue as intermediate and CNS the slowest to respond.

radiosensitive (*dose*) Tissues that have a higher sensitivity to radiation damage than others. It is essentially the processes of cell division that are radiosensitive and the cell populations with the higher rate of cell division show the earlier response to radiation. ICRP60 places gonads, bone marrow and intestine high on the scale. Breast tissue was ranked high in the ICRP26 report but has been downgraded since both male and female tissue is ranked together in ICRP60 (*see* weighting factor (tissue w_T)).

radio waves (*phys*) Radio waves are a form of electromagnetic radiation produced by oscillating electrons in an inductor (coil). The waves are transferred to an aerial which at low frequencies can be a short length of wire but at higher frequencies a system of conductors is necessary to shape the transmitted beam or increase the ability to detect radiowaves of a certain frequency band. Very high frequency (VHF) radio waves (20–80 MHz) are within the RF spectrum of magnetic resonance imaging signals. At these frequencies it is essential to maintain impedance matching otherwise the signal strength will be reduced.

radium (Ra) (*elem*)

Atomic number (Z)	88
Relative atomic mass (A$_r$)	226
Density (ρ) kg/m³	5000
Melting point (K)	970
K-edge (keV)	103.9
Relevance to radiology: abandoned as a therapy agent in favour of other nuclides.	

^{226}Radium

Half life	1600y
Decay mode	alpha
Decay constant	0.000433 y^{-1}
Photons/particles	α 4.5–7.6 MeV
	β– 0.42–3.2 MeV
	γ 0.29–1.7 MeV

radon (Rn) (*elem*)

Atomic number (Z)	86
Relative atomic mass (A$_r$)	222
Density (ρ) kg/m^3	9.73
Melting point (K)	202
K-edge (keV)	98.4

Of the 20 known isotopes only two are significant in radiation protection:

- ^{220}Rn (thoron) a decay product of ^{232}Th;
- ^{222}Rn (radon) a decay product of ^{238}U.

The uranium series starts with ^{238}U and ends with stable ^{206}Pb. The mass number 238 is divisible by 4 with a remainder of 2 so this series is known as the '4n+2' series, where n is an integer between 51 and 59. Similarly, ^{220}Rn starts with ^{232}Th and ends with stable ^{208}Pb; this is the '4n series'.

^{220}Rn

Half life	55.6s
Decay mode	alpha

A short lived radionuclide decaying to astatine and polonium each giving an alpha emission:

$$^{232}_{90}\text{Th} \rightarrow {}^{220}_{86}\text{Rn}(\alpha) \rightarrow {}^{218}_{85}\text{At}(\alpha)$$
$$\rightarrow {}^{216}_{84}\text{Po}(\alpha) \rightarrow \ldots {}^{208}_{82}\text{Pb } stable.$$

^{222}Radon

Half life	3.8 d
Decay mode	Complex
Decay constant	0.1823 d^{-1}
Photons/particles	Complex emissions starting with ^{238}U

The ^{222}Rn decays further in the lung tissue to ^{218}polonium and ^{214}lead, each giving an alpha emission:

$$^{238}_{92}\text{U} \rightarrow \ldots {}^{222}_{86}\text{Rn}(\alpha) \rightarrow {}^{218}_{84}\text{Po}(\alpha)$$
$$\rightarrow {}^{214}_{82}\text{Pb}(\alpha) \rightarrow \ldots {}^{206}_{82}\text{Pb } stable.$$

Of the 20 known isotopes only three occur in nature: ^{222}Rn (radon: T½ 3.8 d) a decay product of ^{238}U; ^{220}Rn (thoron: T½ 54 s) a decay product of ^{232}Th and ^{219}Rn (actinon: T½ 3.9 s) a decay product of ^{235}U. ^{222}Rn is an important contaminant of buildings, giving higher radiation exposure to some hospital staff than x-rays. Polonium-218 and 214, as radon daughters, deliver an alpha dose to lung tissue. From ICRP65 the annual effective dose of 10 mSv can be maintained by applying the following constraint levels:

Situation	Constraint (Bq m^{-3})
Domestic dwellings	600
Workplaces	1500

An action level is set below these figures, typically 200 and 400 Bq m^{-3} for domestic and workplaces respectively (*see* alpha decay).

radon concentration (*dose*) The indoor concentration depends on the composition of the underlying rock formation. The mean radon concentration from an NRPB survey was 20.5 Bq m^{-3} implying a mean effective dose of 1 mSv y^{-1}. Typical values in Bq m^{-3} from some localities are:

Switzerland	150
UK (Cornwall)	110
Ireland	80
USA	60
Germany	50
Austria	15
Japan	10

radon dose (*dose*) The mean radon concentration from an NRPB survey was 20.5 Bq m^{-3} implying a mean effective dose of 1 mSv y^{-1}. In high radon concentrations (Cornwall) effective dose levels exceed 50 mSv in 6% of houses and a yearly effective dose rate of 20 mSv is common. Action levels recommended by most national institutions is 200 Bq m^{-3} with schools having a lower action level of 150 Bq m^{-3}.

Radon transform (*ct*) In 1917 an Austrian mathematician working on gravitational theory showed theoretically that an object can be reconstructed from the infinite set of all its projections. The first reconstructed images using a type of Radon transform were obtained in radioastronomy.

RAGE (*mri*) Gradient echo.

RAID (*comp*) Redundant array of inexpensive/independent disks. A method of spreading information across several disks set up to act as a unit, using two different techniques, stores information across several disks or with disk mirroring: simultaneously storing a copy of information on another disk so that the information can be recovered if the main disk crashes. Speed of access and reliability are improved. Levels of access are available from immediate (most recent cases) to less immediate (cases older than a certain time period: e.g. weeks, months).

RAM (*comp*) Random access memory where data can be written to and read from. One of two basic types of memory. Portions of programs are stored in RAM when the program is launched so that the program will run faster. Only portions of RAM will be accessed by the computer at any given time. Also called memory. Stored data are lost when power is removed (computer switched off).

RAMBUS (*comp*) A form of RAM which processes instructions 16 bits at a time, rather than 5 bits, making the process twice as fast as standard RAM.

RAM disk (*comp*) A simulated disk drive created and maintained by a special driver that stores data in the main memory. Very fast access for disk intensive application programs since they operate at memory speed. The data stored are lost when power is removed.

RAM-FAST (*mri*) Rapidly acquired magnetization prepared Fourier acquired steady state. Reduced acquisition matrix FASTTurbo-FLASH-like sequence (Picker Medical Inc.).

ramping (*mri*) Changing the strength of the magnetic field of a magnet.

ramp time (*mri*) Time required for a change in the magnetic field strength, shown in the graph. Usually measured in $mT\,min^{-1}$: depends on construction of the magnet and design of the magnet power supply. Typical values are from 1 to $10\,mT\,min^{-1}$ but for dast sequences such as EPI, rise times of 0.2 ms are required (*see* slew rate).

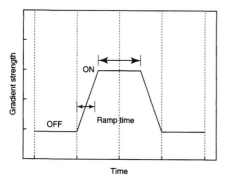

Time

random events (*nmed*) For coincident counting in PET, simple probability provides that given singles rates S_1 and S_2 for a pair of detectors and a coincidence window of width 2τ then events will be found in coincidence due to random occurrence with a rate:

$$R = 2\tau * S_1 * S_2$$

These coincidences occur at random within the coincidence window. Since the detector's 'singles' rate is proportional to the imaged activity, then the 'random' rate is proportional to the square of the activity. This contrasts with the 'true' coincident events, which are only proportional to the activity. Random coincident events become a limiting factor at higher activities and may limit the activity which may usefully by imaged. As the real coincidence count rate increases, the proportion of randoms also increases, eventually becoming unacceptable; this is particularly serious when the detector efficiency is low.

random error (*stats*) These errors may vary in a non-reproducible way but can be treated statistically by using probability methods.

random labelling (*nmed*) Red blood cell (RBC) labelling using either ^{51}Cr as chromate or ^{99m}Tc labelling pyrophosphate either being incorporated into the globin portion of haemoglobin by randomly aged cells.

range (*math*) The absolute or relative difference of minimum and maximum values of measured quantities.

range ambiguity (*us*) The artefact produced when echoes are placed too close to the transducer because a second pulse was emitted before they were received.

range equation (*us*) The relationship between round-trip pulse-travel time, propagation speed, and distance to a reflector.

range gating (*us*) A selection of the depth from which echoes are accepted based on echo arrival time.

rapid-excitation MRI (*mri*) An approach for speeding up the MRI data acquisition process by repeating the excitation RF pulses in times short compared to T1, using small flip angles and gradient echo refocusing. When TR is equal to or shorter than T2, the repeated RF pulses will tend to refocus transverse magnetization remaining from prior excitations, setting up a condition of steady state free precession and a dependence of signal strength (and image contrast) on both T1 and T2 which can be modified commonly by either:

- Spoiling the tendency to build up a steady state by reducing coherence between excitations;
- By variation of the phase or timing of consecutive RF pulses or of the strength of spoiler gradient pulses. Thus increasing the relative dependence of signal strength on TI; or
- Acquire the signal when it is refocusing immediately prior to the next RF pulse, thus increasing the relative dependence of signal strength on T2.

RARE (*mri*) Rapid acquisition with relaxation enhancement. The original fast spin echo acquiring multiple RF echoes with different phase encoding steps. A very rapid scan technique that consists of a train of individually phase-encoded spin-echoes and gave rise to TurboSE. Data acquired from the image acquisition, organized as a two-dimensional matrix with points along the horizontal axis representing individual frequency-encoding samples and points along the vertical axis representing individual phase-encoding lines. Shows bright fat; prone to ghosts and edge artefacts. High specific absorption rate.

rare earth elements (lanthanides/lanthanoids) (*elem*) A series of 15 elements in the periodic table from atomic number 58 (cerium) to 71 (lutetium); to include:

Z	Element		Use
57	lanthanum	La	Phosphor; Blue light intensifying screen
58	cerium	Ce	Phosphor dopant
59	praseodymium	Pr	Laser dopant
60	neodymium	Nd	Laser dopant
61	promethium	Pm	–
62	samarium	Sm	Permanent magnet alloys
63	europium	Eu	Phosphor doping; image plate dopant
64	gadolinium	Gd	Green/yellow light intensifying screen; paramagnetic MRI contrast agent
65	terbium	Tb	Phosphor doping; intensifying screen dopant
66	dysprosium	Dy	TLD dopant
67	holmium	Ho	K-edge filter
68	erbium	Er	K-edge filter
69	thulium	Tm	Phosphor/intensify screen dopant
70	ytterbium	Yb	–
71	lutetium	Lu	Phosphor

(*see* phosphor).

rarefaction (*us*) Region of low density and pressure in a compressional wave.

rarefaction pressure (*us*) The amplitude of a negative instantaneous ultrasonic pressure in an ultrasound beam.

rasterize (*image*) Breaking down an image into individual scan lines. Most graphics monitors and printers are raster based.

Räth, Curt German chemist who first patented a pyridine derived intravenous urographic x-ray contrast agent in 1927 (Uroselectan). Developed its clinical application with Binz.

rating (*xray*) The energy rating for x-ray anodes range from 250 kJ to 3.5 MJ. Heat dissipation is given in watts (W) or joules per second. The table shows some heat ratings for typical x-ray tubes, anode heat capacity and anode heat dissipation are shown in heat units, joules per minute and watts.

Use	Anode heat capacity	Anode heat dissipation	Anode diameter
Conventional	300 kHU 210 kJ	60 kHU/min 44.4 kJ/min 740 W	80 mm
CT	6.3 MHU 4.7 MJ	840 kHU/min 621.6 kJ/min 10.3 kW	120 mm
Fluoroscopy	300 kHU 210 kJ	908 kHU/min 672 kJ/min 11.2 kW	200 mm

(*see* cooling curve).

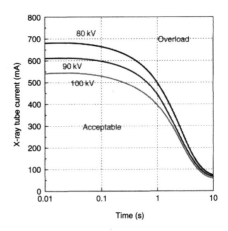

ratio (iodine) (*cm*) One of the physical descriptions of an iodine contrast agent measuring its ability to attenuate x-rays and its tendency for inducing side-effects (osmotoxicity). Measured as a ratio of the number of iodine atoms per volume contrast medium by the number of particles (contrast medium ions or contrast medium molecules) per volume contrast medium solution.

rational number (*math*) Any number that can be written as x/y where x and y express the ratio of two integers. Examples of rational numbers are 0.5 (1/2), 1.5 (3/2) and 0.33333... (1/3). Compare an irrational number π or e where the number cannot be represented as a ratio.

RAW (*image*) These are image files that are not yet processed. Normally the RAW image file will be processed before conversion into RGB, TIFF or JPEG file format for storage or hardcopy. There is no standard RAW format and they can be similar or radically different between manufacturers.

raw data (*ct*) The values of x-ray detector response from all views and rays within a scan. These data are convolved with the convolution filter and undergo back projection to produce a CT image.

raw data pre-processing (*ct*) A processing step that is applied to the measured attenuation profiles in order to correct for the beam harden-ing. Variation in detector sensitivity and dis-tances between detector channels, along with other sources of measurement errors. These essential corrections must be performed before image reconstruction (*see* data post-processing).

ray (*ct*) The collimated narrow beam of x-rays from the tube window incident on a single detector within a detector array, giving rise to the detector signal. Each view or projection is composed of numerous rays (*see* ray sum).

ray sum (*ct*) The total absorption figure for a row of values constituting a projected line across the object. The ray sums then undergo back projec-tion in order to find the separate matrix values.

rayl (*us*) Unit of acoustic impedance. The m.k.s. (SI) value measured as $N \times s \times m^{-2}$ ($kg\,m^{-2}\,s^{-1}$); the c.g.s. value is dyne $\times s \times cm^{-3}$ or $10\,N \times s \times m^{-3}$ ($g\,cm^{-2}\,s^{-1}$).

Rayleigh noise (*image*) A distribution describing the magnitude of the noise amplitude following a Gaussian distribution. The mean value of this distribution is roughly $1.25\,\sigma$, where σ is the standard deviation of the original Gaussian dis-tribution (*see* probability density distribution).

reactor (*nmed*) *See* nuclear reactor.

reactor (nuclear) (*nmed*) A critical assembly of fissionable material (^{235}U, ^{238}U, ^{239}Pu) and mod-erator (carbon or heavy water). The nuclear reactor is used for thermal energy production and also as a source of neutrons for radionu-clide production by either neutron irradiation of a prepared sample or from products of nuclear fission.

readout delay (*mri*) *See* TE.

real focal spot (*xray*) The rectangular area on the anode, bombarded by the electron beam. The area and angle of the real focal spot determines the **effective focal spot**. Single filaments are used in x-ray tubes having a single anode target; dual sized focal spots can be obtained by alter-ing the electron beam size. Dual filaments, oper-ated in parallel on a single focal spot, are used in mammography tubes to overcome the space charge limitations; these are operated as the sin-gle filament (above) to obtain dual focal spot sizes. Separate dual focal spots are also used (fluoroscopy) but operated independently and focused on separate differently angled targets to give dual focal spots. Focal spots can be moved to slightly different positions on the tar-get surface by control coils which surround the x-ray tube; used in some CT machines as 'fly-ing' focal spots to increase image resolution (*see* focal spot (effective), filament, line focus principle).

real signal (*mri*) In-phase component of signal detected with a quadrature detector.

real-time (*us*) Imaging with a rapid-frame-sequence display.

real-time display (*us*) Employing a sufficient frame rate that the display appears to image moving structures or a changing scan plane continuously.

receiver (*mri*) Portion of the MR apparatus that detects and amplifies RF signals picked up by the receiving coil includes a preamplifier, amplifier and demodulator.

receiver bandwidth (*mri*) Describes the fre-quency content of the pixel in MRI and depends on the number of phase/frequency encoding steps N and signal sampling time t which decides matrix dimensions:

Bandwidth = N/t

receiver coil (*mri*) A coil or antenna which picks up the MR signal.

receiver dead time (*mri*) Time after exciting. RF pulse during which FID is not detectable due to saturation of receiver electronics.

receiver gate (*us*) A device that allows only echoes from a selected depth (arrival time) to pass.

receiver operating characteristic (ROC) (*image*) A method for analysing data that takes note of the operator's skill or bias. It is a plot of the conditional probability of deciding that an observed data set (e.g. image) was generated by a specified state (e.g. that a specified disease was present) when that state was in fact present (true positive; TP) versus the conditional probability of deciding that the data were generated by the specified state when, in fact, it was absent (false positive; FP). This is equivalent to a plot of the 'sensitivity' of a diagnostic test versus one minus the 'specificity' of the test. Observers report findings with a range of responses from definitely abnormal through various grades of equivocal findings to definitely normal. The sensitivity and specificity of an imaging system encompassing this range can be described visually by applying ROC analysis. Different points on the ROC curve (i.e. different compromises between TP and FP or between 'sensitivity' and 'specificity') are achieved by adopting different settings of the critical value of the decision variable that distinguishes 'negative' decisions from 'positive' ones, i.e. the decision criterion.

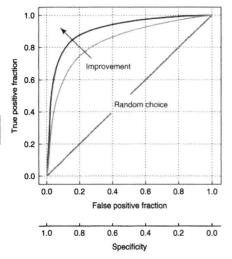

■ Reference: Metz CE, 1986 (*see* contrast detail diagram).

receptor binding (*nmed*) A mechanism by which the radiopharmaceutical binds to receptor sites on tumours (e.g. imaging of a wide variety of tumours containing somatostatin receptor sites using mm OctreoScan, a somatostatin analogue).

receptor site (PET) (*nmed*) Regions in the central nervous system that are associated with drug localization (morphine, DOPA, etc.). Achieving a specific activity of 10^5 to 10^7 mCi (4 to 40 TBq) per mole, it has been estimated that tissue concentrations can be imaged having 10^{-11} to 10^{-13} mole per gram or 0.04 to 4.0 ng per gram of material. (*see* neurotransmitters (PET), metabolites (PET)).

recessive (*dose*) In genetics, a trait that does not manifest itself in the presence of traits that are dominant to it.

recoil electron (*phys, nm, dose*) The path taken by the free electron after a Compton interaction (*see* linear scatter coefficient).

reconstruction algorithm (*ct*) Mathematical procedure used to convert raw data into an image. Different algorithms are used to emphasize, enhance or improve certain aspects of the data.

reconstruction increment (*ct*) The spacing of images reconstructed from spiral CT data sets along the *z*-axis.

reconstruction matrix (*ct*) The array of rows and columns of pixels in the reconstructed image.

rectifier/rectification (*phys*) Conversion from an alternating current (reversing) to a direct current (one-way) supply. AC rectification is achieved by using one-way current devices (diodes) which, in early machines used thermionic emission but in present day equipment use semiconductors. These rectifiers only allow passage of current in one direction so their output has a single polarity. A half wave rectifier uses a single diode and is 50% efficient since it does not utilize the negative half of the AC waveform. A full-wave rectifier uses four diodes and is 100% effective in utilizing all the AC power.

rectilinear co-ordinates Position geometry used by a linear sequenced array.

recursive filter (*di*) The output from a recursive digital filter depends on one or more previous output values as well as on inputs; it involves feedback (*see* averaging filter).

reduced matrix (*mri*) Measurement time is saved by not acquiring the high spatial frequencies (high resolution) raw data lines. Rows that are not measured are filled with zeroes prior to the image calculation (zero filling); corresponding to an interpolation in the phase-encoding direction, so a square image is still displayed on screen.

reference cassette (*qc*) The identified cassette that is used for the QC tests.

reference compound (*mri*) Used as a standard reference spectral line when defining chemical shifts for a given nucleus. For ^1H the reference is tetramethylsilane (TMS) and for ^{31}P it is phosphoric acid. For some biological applications, water and PCr have been used as secondary references for hydrogen or phosphorus spectroscopy, respectively. The reference compound can be in a capsule outside the subject (external) or can be in the subject (internal): internal references are generally preferable where possible.

reference date (generator) (*nmed*) Radionuclide generators are sized according to their activity on a specified reference or calibration day. This is always quoted with the generator specification. From the calibration graph, activity levels at elution are known and a specific generator reference activity on a specified day can be chosen (e.g. 11, 15, 30 GBq on Monday or Thursday) to suit requirements over the working week.

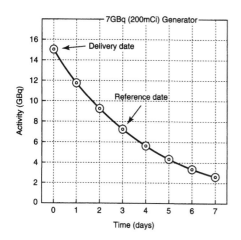

reference exposure (*qc*) The exposure of the phantom to provide an image at the reference optical density.

reference image (*mri*) Post-processing template for defining reconstruction methods, i.e. MIP or MPR.

reference individual (*dose*) An idealized human with characteristics defined by the ICRP for the purpose of radiological protection.

reference man (*nmed*) A model with the anatomical and physiological characteristics of an adult male as defined in ICRP Publication 23 (ICRP Publication 23, 1975) (*see* standard man).

reference optical density (*qc*) The optical density of 1.0 OD, base and fog excluded, measured in the reference point.

reference person (*dose*) A person with the anatomical and physiological characteristics defined in the report of the ICRP Task Group on Reference Man (Publication 89; ICRP Publication 89, 2001).

reference phantom (*qc*) A phantom similar to the standard phantom, but of a different stated thickness.

reference point (*mamm*) A measurement position in the plane occupied by the entrance surface of a 45 mm thick phantom, 60 mm perpendicular to the chest wall edge of the table and centered laterally.

reference value (*dose*) The value of a quantity obtained for patients which may be used as a guide to the acceptability of a result (used in CEC 1990). In the 1995 version of the Quality Criteria Document it is stated that the reference value can be taken as a ceiling from which progress should be pursued to lower dose values in line with the ALARA principle. This objective is also stated to be in line with the recommendation in paragraph 180 of ICRP Publication 60 that consideration be given to the use of 'dose constraints or investigation levels' for application in some common diagnostic procedures. Reference values may be specified to a greater degree of precision than that which would be chosen to reflect the certainty with which the value is known, in order to avoid the accumulation of rounding errors in a calculation.

reflection (non-specular) (*us*) Reflection of ultrasound from a rough surface.

reflection (specular) (*us*) Reflection of ultrasound from a smooth surface (*see* angle of reflection).

reflection angle (*us*) Angle between the reflected sound direction and a line perpendicular to the media boundary.

reflector (*us*) Medium boundary that produces a reflection; reflecting surface.

reflector speed (Doppler) (*us*) See Doppler (reflector speed).

refocusing (*mri*) See spin echo.

refraction (*us*) The change in the direction of a wave front when passing from one medium to another (*see* Snell's Law).

refractive index (*us*) The product of the sine of angle of incidence to the sine of the angle of refraction (*see* Snell's Law).

refresh rate (*comp*) An indication of how fast the graphics card will refresh the computer video display; the rate at which video monitors/displays are refreshed to prevent image fading. Measured in Hz. Typical values are from 56 to over 100 Hz. A minimum of 75 Hz is required to minimize display flicker. Rates above 80 Hz are preferable.

refrigeration (refrigerator) (*mri*) System for actively cooling structures in a superconducting magnet. If only cryoshields are cooled (two-stage refrigerator), no liquid nitrogen will be needed and He boil-off will be reduced. If, additionally, the superconducting coil support is actively cooled (three-stage refrigeration) the helium consumption can be essentially reduced to zero.

region of interest (ROI) (*ct*) A circular, rectangular region, operator selected, identifying an area of measurement of of anatomical interest. Based on the ROI local statistical information can be calculated from the CT numbers. (*nmed*) Used for identifying whole organs (kidneys) or specific regions (lung transit studies). Having selected a single or series of ROIs, a total count over these regions for all the frames collected in the study is made. The results are then presented as a time/activity curve which is the renogram in the case of kidney studies.

registered images (*image*) Two or more images of the same scene that have been positioned with respect to one another so that the objects in the scene occupy the same positions.

regression (*stats*) A test which calculates the best fit for a straight line through a set of points on a graph when y is the dependent variable and x the independent (*see* least squares).

rejection (*us*) Elimination of small-amplitude voltage pulses.

relative atomic mass (r.a.m.) (*phys*) Replaces atomic weight. The relative mass of an atom depends on the isotope mix. For gadolinium with eight stable isotopes the average value is 157.25; for aluminium with only a single stable isotope it is exactly 27.

relative biological effectiveness (RBE) (*dose*) The relationships between different ionizing radiations to produce the same biological effect depends on the subjective measurement or ranking of the precise effect itself (LD_{50}, DNA damage, cell transformation, etc.). An attempt to give an accurate scaling factor to the radiation was the RBE. It compares the absorbed doses of different ionizing radiations required to give the same biological damage. The RBE is now called the radiation weighting factor (w_R) in ICRP60 (*see* weighting factor (radiation)).

relative density (*unit*) Relative mass density (*see* relative volumic mass).

relative life lost (*dose*) Ratio of the proportion of observed years of life lost in an exposed population dying of disease to the corresponding proportion in a similar control population without the exposure.

relative molecular mass (r.m.m.) (*unit*) Formally called molecular weight. The ratio of the mass per molecule of an element or compound to one twelfth of the mass of one atom of ^{12}C. For naturally occurring forms of the material, usually involving a mixture of isotopes, the ratio applies to the average mass per molecule (see relative atomic mass (r.a.m.)).

relative permeability (*phys*) See permeability.

relative risk (*stats*) *See* risk (relative).

relative survival (*dose*) Ratio of the proportion of cancer patients who survive for a specified number of years (typically 5 years) following diagnosis to the proportion in a control set of cancer-free individuals.

relative volumic mass (*unit*) (also relative density, relative mass density) The dimensionless ratio of the mass of a volume of an object.

relaxation frequencies (*us, mri*) Frequency of maximum absorption in a medium.

relaxation rates (*mri*) Reciprocals of relaxation times T1 and T2 (R1 = 1/T1; R2 = 1/T2). There is often a linear relation between concentration of MR contrast agents and the resulting change in relaxation rate.

relaxation times (*mri*) After excitation by the RF pulse, net nuclear spins M will tend to return to their equilibrium state where transverse magnetization M_{xy} is zero and longitudinal magnetization M_z is maximum and in the direction of the magnetic field orientation. The transverse magnetization relaxation decays toward zero (time constant T2) and longitudinal relaxation returns to equilibrium with time constant T1.

rem (*dose*) (roentgen equivalent man) The non-SI dose equivalent. The absorbed dose in rads multiplied by the radiation quality factor. The SI unit is the sievert where 100 rem = 1 Sv; 100 mrem ≡ 1 mSv or 1 mrem ≡ 10 μSv.

remote boot (*comp*) A firmware-based program in a network adapter that asks to have the workstation's operating system downloaded from a boot server on the network; used by networked diskless workstations.

remote execution (*comp*) The ability to run programs on remote systems; exporting time consuming processes to other systems frees up the local workstation. An example would be an image array processor.

renal (contrast medium) (*cm*) Intravenous urography using non-ionic dimer iodixanol, non-ionic monomer iohexol.

renal insufflation (*clin*) Obsolete technique using air or carbon dioxide to give negative contrast for visualizing the adrenal glands.

Reno-60[x] (*cm*) Commercial preparation (Bracco) of ionic salt meglumine diatrizoate.

Compound	Viscosity (cP)	Osmolality mOsm/kg	Iodine mg I/mL
Meglumine diatrizoate 60%	6.4 @ 20° 4.3 @ 37°	1404	282

Renocal[x] (*cm*) (Bracco) A mixture of meglumine diatrizoate and sodium diatrizoate; 66% and 10%.

Compound	Viscosity (cP)	Osmolality mOsm/kg	Iodine mg I/mL
Meglumine diatrizoate	15.0 @ 20° 9.1 @ 37°	1870	370

RenoCis[x] (*nm*) Commercial preparation (Schering) of DMSA.

Reno-DIP[x] (*cm*) Commercial preparation (Bracco) of ionic salt meglumine diatrizoate.

Compound	Viscosity (cP)	Osmolality mOsm/kg	Iodine mg I/mL
Meglumine diatrizoate	2.0 @ 20° 1.5 @ 37°	607	141

Renografin[x] (*cm*) Commercial preparation (Bracco) of ionic salt and sodium/meglumine diatrizoate, 52%:8%.

Compound	Viscosity (cP)	Osmolality mOsm/kg	Iodine mg I/mL
Diatrizoate-Na-meglumine 52%	6.2 @ 20° 4.2 @ 37°	1450	292

renogram (*nmed*) An example of a dynamic study using multi-phase acquisition where (for instance) the vascular phase is collected as 30 frames at 0.5 s, GFR phase as 30 at 1 s and excretion phase as 30 at 20 s.

repeater (*comp*) A device that regenerates and amplifies signals to create long-distance networks.

repetition time (TR) (*mri*) The time between two excitation pulses. In the case of the spin echo sequence it is the time between the 90° pulses. Within the TR interval, signals may be acquired with one or more echo times, or one or more phase-encodings (depending on the measurement technique). TR is one of the measurement parameters that determines contrast, largely influencing T1 contrast (*see* echo time, T1 weighting).

rephasing (*mri*) Reversal from dephasing; the spins go back into phase. Achieved through a 180° pulse that creates a spin echo, or a gradient pulse in the opposite direction.

rephasing gradient (*mri*) Magnetic field gradient applied for a short period after a selective excitation pulse opposing the direction of the selective excitation gradient; a magnetic field gradient pulse applied to reverse the spatial variation of phase of transverse magnetization caused by a dephasing gradient. The gradient reversal rephases the spins forming a gradient echo. The result of the gradient reversal is a rephasing of the spins (which would have become out of phase with each other along the direction of the selection gradient).

reproducibility (*math*) or consistency. The reliability expressed as accuracy of measurement. Several readings are taken at timed intervals from a constant source and the percentage error between the readings calculated. The results are expressed as a percentage error for a single machine or if a number of machines are being assessed the error range is given as percentiles (25th, mean, 75th). (*qc*) Indicates the reliability of a measuring method or tested equipment. The results under identical conditions should be constant (*see* precision).

RESCOMP (*mri*) Respiratory compensation GE. Respiratory ordered phase encoding (*see* RSPE, PEAR, FREEZE).

residual dose (*dose*) Applied to chronic exposure. The dose expected to be incurred in the future after intervention has been terminated (or a decision has been taken not to intervene).

resistance, φ (*phys*) Defined by the proportionality between the voltage across a conductor and the current flowing in it: $V = IR$. The unit of resistance is the ohm ϕ. One ohm maintains a current of one amp at one volt so that: $R = V/I$. Variations of this basic formula are: $I = V/R$ and $V = IR$. If a is the cross sectional area of a conductor then providing the length L is constant its resistance is proportional to cross-sectional area. So that:

$$R \propto \frac{L}{a^2}$$

If the diameter of the wire is doubled (increasing the area a) then resistance decreases by ¼. Also it determines the power, P, consumed as heat in the conductor, $P = IV$. In NMR, magnets and resistance of the windings limit the current they carry and thereby the strength of the B field they can produce.

resistance (flow) (*us*) Pressure difference divided by volume flow rate for steady flow.

resistive magnet (*mri*) *See* magnet (resistive).

resolution (*ct*) *See* geometrical resolution, high contrast resolution, low-contrast resolution.

resolution (axial) (*us*) *See* ultrasound (resolution).

resolution (display) (*comp*) *See* flat panel display, line pairs.

resolution element (*mri*) The smallest spatially resolved image element. It may be isotropic (the same x, y and z dimension), or anisotropic where x and y dimensions are different; the slice thickness z does not match one or other of the x, y dimensions. The resolution element may be larger than the pixel or voxel and is dependent on sampling theory.

resolution (energy) (*phys*) The FWHM dimension of a photopeak, the energy spread at this level expressed as a percentage of the peak energy. Typical value for a single NaI(Tl) detector would be 8% for most current gamma cameras (140 keV gamma). (*us*) The FWHM dimension of a photopeak, the energy spread at this level expressed as a percentage of the peak energy. Typical value for a single NaI(Tl) detector would be 8%. A gamma camera value would be 11%.

resolution (extrinsic) (*nmed*) This is a measure of the camera system resolution with the collimator in place, frequently referred to as the system resolution R_s, this combines the effects of intrinsic resolution (R_i), selected collimator resolution (R_c), image magnification (M), so that:

$$R_S = \sqrt{R_C^2 + (R_i/M)^2}$$

Measured in mm. Typical high resolution collimator gives 5 mm FWHM.

resolution (intrinsic) (*nmed*) The resolving power of the gamma camera system without any collimation is obtained by exposing the uncovered crystal to a point or line source of activity. In practice, the crystal is covered by a lead-sheet in which fine points or a thin single line has been cut. Intrinsic resolution is quoted with count rate; typical values are 5 mm at 75 k cps and 5.7 mm at 150 k cps.

resolution (lateral) (*us*) Resolving power across the beam. Depends on focal dimensions of the beam influenced by aperture size and electronic focusing.

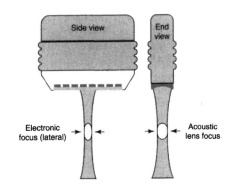

Lateral resolution $\dfrac{R\lambda}{a}$

the minimum distance required by a display to resolve two point sources.

Frequency	Image depth	Axial res.	Lateral res.
2.0	30	0.7	3.0
3.5	17	0.4	1.7
5.0	12	0.3	1.2
7.5	8	0.2	0.8
10.0	6	0.15	0.6

resolution (spatial) (*image*) *See* spatial resolution.

resolution (system) R_s (*nmed*) This combines the effects of intrinsic resolution (R_i), selected collimator resolution (R_c), image magnification (M), so that:

$$R_S = \sqrt{R_C^2 + (R_i/M)^2}$$

resolution (temporal) (*math*) The ability to separate to events in time. This depends on image matrix size and storage speed for each image frame.

resolution (visible) (*image*) Maximum visual resolution is approximately $30 \, \text{Lp} \, \text{mm}^{-1}$ but at distance this is reduced to $15 \, \text{Lp} \, \text{mm}^{-1}$. The acuity of scotopic vision is highest approximately 20° from the fovea, where the density of rods is greatest; for photopic vision it is highest on the fovea where the cones are most dense. Photopic acuity is always greater than scotopic. The human eye is most sensitive to variation in the intensity of objects with a spatial frequency of between 6 and $10 \, \text{Lp} \, \text{mm}^{-1}$.

resolution element (*mri*) The smallest spatially resolved image element. It may be isotropic (the same x, y and z dimension), or anisotropic where x and y dimensions are different, or the slice thickness z does not match one or other of the x, y dimensions. The resolution element may be larger than the pixel or voxel and is dependent on sampling theory.

resonance (*phys*) The frequency of the undamped waveform or the system's natural frequency. When the input or forcing frequency is equal to the natural frequency of the system then resonance occurs producing the greatest power output. Of practical use in radiology where an oscillating system (e.g. ultrasound transducer crystal or tuned MRI inductive circuit) has the same frequency as that of the driving force (electrical pulse). Considerable energy is absorbed at resonant frequency from the system supplying the external force. The two resonance signals in the graph show a strong undamped resonant signal together with a slightly damped signal of lower amplitude.

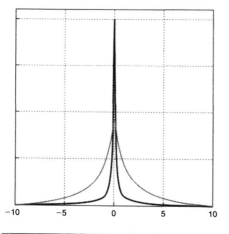

resonant frequency (*phys*) The frequency at which resonance will occur. Determined by mechanical size in ultrasound, by conductance and inductance components of an electronic circuit or given by the Larmor equation in NMR.

Resovist [x] (*cm*) Ferrous based MRI agent (Schering) containing 28 mg iron as ferucarbotran, a superparamagnetic iron oxide in the form of nanoparticles coated with carboxydextran.

respiratory gating (*mri*) Synchronization of patient's breathing with data acquisition. Technique for reducing respiratory artefacts. A respiratory signal acquired with suitable sensors or MR methods (navigator echo) is used as the trigger signal.

respiratory ordering of phase encoding (*mri*) Respiratory synchronization that acquires image data at regular times independent of the respiratory cycle, but chooses the sequence of phase encoding data acquisition so as to minimize the respiratory motion–induced artefacts in the resulting image. For example, choosing the sequence of phase encoding such that adjacent samples in the final full data set have minimal differences in respiratory phase will minimize the spacing of ghost artefacts in the final image.

RE spoiled (*mri*) FAST RE spoiled Fourier-acquired steady-state technique rapid gradient-echo imaging techniques T1-weighted contrast (Picker Medical Inc.) (*see* FLASH, SPGR, FSPGR, HFGR, 3D-ME-RAGE, T1-FEE, STAGE-T1W).

REST (*mri*) Regional saturation technique Philips, motion artefact reduction techniques, spatial pre-saturation to reduce MR signal intensity in specific locations (*see* SAT, PRE-SAT, PRESAT, EFAST, SATURATION).

responsivity (R) (*image*) This is a measure of the sensitivity of a detector to radiation and is the ratio between the radiative flux ϕ incident on the detector area and the resulting signal s, so that $s = R\phi$. A good detector shows a constant responsivity, R, over a wide flux range so that the signal output is proportional to the input flux.

reproducibility (*qc*) Indicates the reliability of a measuring method or tested equipment. The results under identical conditions should be constant.

restricted area (*dose*) A limited access area where exposure to individuals may occur. The limits are stated in national and local radiation safety rules.

retrograde (*clin*) Counter or backflow.

retrograde angiography (*clin*) Imaging sections of blood vessels lying upstream of the injection or catheterization point and introducing contrast medium in a direction counter to the blood flow.

retrograde pyelography (*clin*) or cystoscopic urography. *See* retrograde urography.

retrograde urography (*clin*) Radiography of the urinary tract following injection of contrast medium directly into the bladder, ureter or renal pelvis.

retrospective gating/synchronization (*mri*) Simultaneous acquisition of untriggered data and the ECG signal. The ECG signal is used during subsequent post-processing to assign the images to the correct phase in the cardiac cycle. Can also be used for pulsatile flow (*see* synchronization, retrospective).

Reynold's number (Re) (*us*) A dimensionless value used as an indication of laminar flow. Mean fluid velocity (*v*), vessel radius (*r*), density (*ρ*) and viscosity (*η*).

$$Re = \frac{I \cdot \nu \cdot \rho}{\eta}$$

This formula indicates whether flow will be laminar or turbulent. Typically, values above 1200 indicate turbulent flow.

Reynolds number (critical) The Reynolds number above which turbulence occurs.

RF antenna (*mri*) *See* RF coils.

RF coils (*mri*) These act as antennas which transmit RF pulses and/or receive MRI signals. Transmitter coils should excite the protons/nuclei in the volume of interest. Receiver coils should receive the MRI signal with a high Q. The signal strength depends on the excited volume measured in the coil and its distance to the measurement object. Noise depends primarily on the coil size.

RF (radiofrequency) pulse (*mri*) An impulse comprising 2–3 wavelengths of radiofrequency delivered by an RF transmitter. If the RF pulse is at or near the Larmor frequency it will rotate the macroscopic magnetization vector into the rotating frame of reference (transverse plane). The amount of rotation depends on the strength and duration of the pulse. A 90° pulse (π/2) and 180° pulse (π) are used together with intermediate flip angles.

RF-FAST (*mri*) RF spoiled Fourier acquired steady state.

RF shield (*mri*) Efficient shielding against radio-frequency interference from:

* computers and their display units;
* radio-pagers;
* radiotransmitters;
* television transmitters.

Harmonic frequencies from these sources may be a problem even though their primary transmit frequency is above the bandwidth of interest.

RF spoiling (*mri*) Preventing a steady state precession occurring in rapid excitation sequencing by using varying phase or timing of the RF pulses.

rhenium (Re) (*elem*)

Atomic number (Z)	75
Relative atomic mass (A_r)	186.2
Density (ρ) kg/m³	20 500
Melting point (K)	3450
Specific heat capacity J kg^{-1} K^{-1}	137
Thermal conductivity W m^{-1} K^{-1}	47.9
K-edge (keV)	71.6
Relevance to radiology: used as an alloy with tungsten for x-ray anodes.	

^{186}Rhenium

Decay scheme	^{186}Re (β− 1.0 MeV, γ137 kev) →
(β⁻) **^{186}Re**	^{186}W stable
Half life	3.7 days
Decay mode	β− 1.07 MeV
Decay constant	0.1872 d^{-1}
Emission	β− 1070 keV (max) γ 137 keV
Uses: Rhenium [^{186}Re] sulphide used as a therapy/palliative agent in cases of synovectomy.	

rhodium (Rh) (*elem*)

Atomic number (Z)	45
Relative atomic mass (A_r)	102.91
Density (ρ) kg/m³	12 440
Melting point (K)	2230
Specific heat capacity J kg^{-1} K^{-1}	242
Thermal conductivity W m^{-1} K^{-1}	150
K-edge (keV)	23.2
Relevance to radiology: as a target and K-edge filter material for mammography	

RICE (*mri*) Rapid imaging using composite echo, the FSE/RARE technique used by Toshiba.

RIMM (*comp*) RAMBUS inline memory module. Also known as RDRAM, this is the latest type of memory that has the potential to run at up to 800 MHz as opposed to SDRAM's 100 MHz. Speed is also increased by processing instructions 16 bits at a time.

ring artefacts (*ct*) Circular artefacts, usually found in third-generation scanners, caused by faulty calibration or a defect in detector function. (*nmed*) Or bullseye artefact A concentric ring artefact in SPECT of alternating high- and low-count densities that results from a gamma camera with inadequate field uniformity.

ring detector (*ct*) Fan beam scanner (4th generation) with detector elements positioned on a full circle and only the x-ray tube rotating around the object.

ring-down artefact (*us*) An artefact resulting from a continuous stream of sound emanating from an anatomic site.

ring topology (*comp*) A network cabling configuration in which each system is connected in a series, forming a closed loop.

ripple (*xray*) A superimposed AC waveform (typically 50 or 60 cycles) on the rectified DC power supply. Seen as maximum interference in single phase half-wave rectified supplies and at a minimum (<1%) in constant potential or high frequency supplies.

RISA (*nmed*) Radio-iodated human serum albumin as ^{125}I-RISA for plasma volume estimation. Available as Isojex®.

RISC (*comp*) Reduced instruction set computer. A type of CPU which can reduce to a minimum the number of instructions that are processed simultaneously which increases the CPU efficiency.

rise rate (*mri*) See slew rate.

rise time (*mri*) The time required for the gradient field to rise from zero to the maximum value.

risk (*dose*) The probability of injury, harm or damage from a hazard; usually radiation.

risk (assessment) (*dose*) The risk of cancer per unit dose is calculated by comparing an irradiated population group with an identical unexposed group then:

$$\text{Risk factor} = \frac{\text{increased cancer incidence}}{\text{population} \times \text{dose}}$$

Risk assessment

If 500 000 people are exposed to 500 mSv over their lifetime and show a increased cancer incidence of 5000 then the risk is:

$$\frac{5000}{500000 \times 0.5} = 0.02 = 2 \times 10^{-2} \; \frac{1}{2} \text{Sv}^{-1}$$

This cancer increase of 1 in 50 is due to radiation at this level. There is an expected natural cancer incidence of 1:7 of this population.

The population size studied increases as the square of the reduction in dose. A 5 mSv exposure study would require 5×10^8 people, however, the response is assumed to be linear so 5 mSv will give a risk of 1 : 4000 (*see* risk (nominal), relative risk).

risk (nominal) (*dose*) Since there is still uncertainty in the risk estimates given in ICRP60, the probability of a fatal radiation induced cancer is termed the nominal risk coefficient. The nominal risk for an adult is:

$$4 \times 10^{-2} \; \text{Sv}^{-1} \; (1{:}20) \text{ or } 1{:}25000 \, \text{mSv}^{-1}$$

For the whole population (of all ages):

$$5 \times 10^{-2} \; \text{Sv}^{-1} \; (1{:}20) \text{ or } 1{:}20000 \, \text{mSv}^{-1}$$

Support for these risk factors comes from the National Registry for Radiation Workers (UK) which covers 95 000 occupationally exposed workers (*see* risk (assessment), relative risk).

risk factor (*dose*) The probability of cancer or hereditary damage per unit equivalent dose or effective dose. The risk factor is measured as per Sievert, Sv^{-1} (*see* risk (nominal), relative risk).

risk (relative) (*dose*) Cancer risk may relate to the spontaneous risk or natural incidence of cancer in a given population. The absolute risk model where the additional risk associated with radiation exposure is independent of the spontaneous/natural risk, contrasted with the relative risk model where the additional risk is proportional or related to the spontaneous risk.

RMS (*math*) See root mean square.

road mapping (*xray*) Subtraction of a contrast filled reference image continuously from the display to reveal catheter placement (*see* digital subtraction angiography (DSA)).

ROAST (*mri*) Resonant offset averaging in the steady state. Steady-state free precession commonly used for imaging of cerebrospinal fluid, Siemens (*see*: SSFP, DE-FGR, CE-FAST, True-FISP, PSIF, T2-FEE, E-SHORT, STERE).

Roberts, John Eric (1907–1998) British medical physicist. Pioneer of medical dosimetry. Founder member of the British Hospital Physicists' Association.

ROC (*di*) See receiver operating characteristic.

rod artefacts (*ct*) If a spiral scan of a cylinder or rod is made, angulated with respect to the scan plane, while the table holding the rod is moved during acquisition the rod in the scan plane changes. Every subsequent projection locates the rod at a different position. Without table movement, i.e. in a conventional scan, the image would show an ellipse. With table movement, the variation in the registered position of the rod, together with the interpolation scheme, gives a distortion of the ellipse. These rod artefacts are especially seen in the liver in the area of the ribs.

ROI (*di*) Region of interest. A defined area, either by the operator or automatically, of a region on a digital image for subsequent detailed analysis (time/activity curve etc.).

Rollins, William Herbert (1852–1929) American clinician/dentist who first advocated the use of collimating diaphragms and shielded x-ray tube housings in 1898. Introduced the concept of radiation protection for diagnostic radiology. He also introduced the idea of double intensifying screens to increase sensitivity. He suggested a pulsed supply to the x-ray tube in order to reduce dose during fluoroscopy and also selective beam filtration before Pfahler published the idea.

ROM (*comp*) Read only memory. A part of memory containing a permanent program sequence (typically in the form of special chips) for essential start-up procedures (boot-up and disk read routines). ROM contains only permanent information put there by the manufacturer. Information in ROM cannot be altered, nor can the memory be dynamically allocated by the computer or its operator. These data are not lost when the computer is switched off.

Röntgen/Roentgen, Wilhelm, Konrad (1845–1923) German physicist who in 1895 discovered a form of electromagnetic radiation he called x-rays. Awarded the first Nobel prize in physics in 1901.

röntgen/roentgen (R) (*dose*) The non-SI unit of exposure mainly applied to x-rays defined as 2.58×10^{-4} coulombs kg^{-1} of air. Replaced by the gray (Gy). The energy absorbed in tissue from 1 R is 0.0095 J kg^{-1}; equivalent to approximately 0.87 rad or 8.7 mGy; 1 mR = 8.7 μGy.

room shielding (*mri*) See magnetic shielding. (dose) See shielding.

root mean square (RMS) (*image*) The value of alternating current or voltage which would dissipate heat at the same rate in a given resistance which for direct current is given by: $W = I^2 \times R \times t$. For an AC waveform the electrical energy is not converted into heat energy at a constant rate. The sine wave for a mains supply shows maximum energy when the current is maximum and zero when the current is zero. Then a mean value is derived called the root mean square (RMS) value. The RMS value of an AC power source, restating the above definition, is simply that value of DC which produces the same power or heating effect. For any sinusoidal waveform the RMS value is:

$$\frac{\text{peak value}}{\sqrt{2}}$$

Alternating supply (mains a.c.) is quoted as an r.m.s. value, so 220 V a.c. has a peak voltage of 311 V and 115 V a.c. a peak of 162 V. The quoted mains supply is always given as its RMS value, the peak voltages are obtained by multiplying by $\sqrt{2}$ (or 1.414).

RMS value	Peak value
115	162 (USA)
220	311 (Europe)
240	339 (UK)

ROPE (*mri*) Respiratory ordered phase encoding. Respiratory compensation technique during MRI data collection.

rotating anode (*xray*) An x-ray tube having a circular rotating anode usually angled at the periphery. The periphery acts as the x-ray target, so the position of the focal spot on the target surface changes continuously (*see* target (x-ray)). Since the target area is bombarded by the electron beam during a small time window the tube loading can be significantly higher than that for stationary targets.

rotating frame of reference (*mri*) A frame of reference (with corresponding coordinate systems) that is rotating about the axis of the static magnetic field Bo (with respect to a stationary frame of reference) at a frequency equal to that of the applied RF magnetic field B1 (RF pulse). Although B1 is a rotating vector, it appears stationary in the rotating frame, leading to simpler mathematical formulations.

rotating frame zeugmatography (*mri*) Technique of MR imaging that uses a gradient of the RF excitation field (to give a corresponding variation of the flip angle along the gradient as a means of encoding the spatial location of spins in the direction of the RF field gradient) in conjunction with a static magnetic field gradient (to give spatial encoding in an orthogonal direction). It can be considered to be a form of Fourier transform imaging.

rotation time (*ct*) This is defined as the time taken for the tube/detector system to rotate 360° around the patient. This can be selected between 0.8, 1.0, 1.5, 2.0 and 3.0 seconds in modern scanners. If rotation time is decreased, spiral coverage/body length, increases and vice versa. With shorter rotation times, thinner slices, for the same volume, can be acquired in the same amount of time. Selecting a 100 mm anatomical range using a 10 mm slice, pitch 1 (10 mm feed/rotation); and a rotation time of 1 s, will take a scan time of 10 s. Decreasing the rotation time to 0.8 s will reduce this to 8 s to cover the same range. Shorter rotation times are chosen with thinner slice collimation, since the same range can be covered in the same time; however, x-ray tube current may need to be increased to maintain the same mAs and maintain image quality (noise).

rotor (*xray*) An integral part of the anode stem making up the induction motor. Made from copper it is attached to the anode by a molybdenum stem. This revolves about a central axle which forms the positive electrode (+75 kV). The axle bearing consists of either ball-races, lubricated by a silver paste, or sleeve bearings also lubricated by a high temperature paste. Excessive heat transfer along the anode stem is restricted since molybdenum has relatively poor heat conductivity. Additionally, sleeve bearings have an oil circulation path which passes along the axle. Larger disc diameters require better support and the anode stem in these tubes is carried forward and supported by its own bearing, giving support both front and rear.

round-off error (*di*) Computational inaccuracy independent of truncation error where unwieldy numbers (e.g. π taken as 3.142 to four significant figures or three decimal places) are restricted in size. The numbers will be inexact even if the formula is precise (*see* truncation).

router (*comp*) A device used to link multiple LANs together; connects two networks at the network layer (Layer 3) of the OSI model. Operates like a bridge but also can choose routes through a network. It examines packets of data from the Internet and sends them to their appropriate destination. More effective when multiple paths are available as it can read the destination address of each packet of data and determine the best path for it to take. In a packet-switching network, such as the Internet, a router is a device which examines packets of data and sends them on to their appropriate destinations.

routine exposure (*xray*) The exposure of the phantom under the conditions that would normally be used to produce a mammogram. It is used to determine image quality and dose under clinical conditions.

rows (*mri*) The phase-encoded portion of the measurement matrix. Often also a row in the displayed image (*see* Columns).

RS (*mri*) Rapid scan.

RS-232C (*comp*) Recommended standard 232C. A standard specifying the connector, pin functions and voltages used to connect a DTE and DCE. V.42: An error detection and correction standard used by modems that specifies both LAPM and MNP 4.

RSPE (*mri*) Respiratory-sorted phase encoding GE. Respiratory ordered phase encoding (*see* RESCOMP, PEAR, FREEZE).

rubidium (Rb) (*elem*)

Atomic number (Z)	37
Relative atomic mass (A$_r$)	85.47
Density (ρ) kg/m³	1530
Melting point (K)	312
K-edge (keV)	15.2

^{81}Rubidium

Production (cyclotron)	
Half life	4.6 h
Decay mode	e.c. and β+
Decay constant	0.150 h^{-1}
Photon (decays to ^{81m}Kr)	Multiple (190 keV)
Uses: The parent for ^{81m}Kr generators	

^{82}Rubidium (*nmed*) Generator derived positron nuclide. 82Sr/82Rb (as CardioGen-82®). For the elution of ^{82}Rb chloride. After intravenous injection clears from the blood and is extracted by the myocardium.

Production (generator)	^{82}Sr (e.c.) $\rightarrow$ ^{82}Rb
Decay scheme (β+) **^{82}Rb**	^{82}Rb T½ 76s (β+ 1.4 MeV, 2γ 511 kev) $\rightarrow$ ^{82}Kr stable
Eluent	0.9% (normal) saline
Decay constant	0.00911 s^{-1}
Half life	1.25 minutes
Half value layer	4.1 mm Pb (511 keV)

R

Rubratope˟ (*nmed*) ^{57}Cyanocobalamine preparation for Schilling Test (Bracco).

RUFIS (*mri*) Rotating ultra-fast imaging sequence.

run length encoding (*comp*) This algorithm is based on the observation that image areas which contain little detail have neighbouring pixels with the same value, so these locations can be stored as a pixel value and pixel range – a 'run length'. Storage area for the image can be considerably reduced since radiographs contain large areas of black background which can be omitted (*see* compression (image)).

ruthenium (Ru) (*elem*)

Atomic number (Z)	44
Relative atomic mass (A$_r$)	101.07
Density (ρ) kg/m^3	12400
Melting point (K)	2520
K-edge (keV)	22.11

Rutherford, Ernest (1871–1937) New Zealand born physicist who in 1895 started work at the Cavendish Laboratory, Cambridge University, UK, where he discovered the three types of uranium radiations, alpha, beta and gamma. In 1898 he became professor of Physics at McGill University, Montreal where he formulated the theory of atomic disintegration. In 1907 he became Professor of Physics at Manchester where, with Geiger and Marsden, he investigated the nucleus by bombarding gold foil with alpha particles and derived the orbital model for the atom. He also discovered that alpha bombardments of nitrogen liberated hydrogen nuclei. In 1919 he was appointed to the Cavendish Laboratory, suceeding J.J. Thomson. He predicted the existence of the neutron later discovered by Chadwick. He was awarded the Nobel Prize for Chemistry in 1908.

R

S

S-value (*dose*) MIRD parameter describing the mean dose per unit cumulated activity. Most dose calculations using MIRD techniques use tabulated values of the S-value.

SAAV (*mri*) Simultaneous acquisition of artery and vein.

saddle coil (*mri*) RF coil design commonly used when the static magnetic field is coaxial with the axis of the coil along the long axis of the body (e.g. superconducting magnets and most resistive magnets) as opposed to solenoid or surface coil.

safety (*mri*) Safety concerns in MR include magnetic field strength, RF heating induced currents due to rapidly varying magnetic fields (dB/dt) effects on implanted devices such as pacemakers, magnetic torque effects on in dwelling metal such as clips and possible missile effect of magnetic forces and acoustic noise (*see* SAR).

safety (ultrasound) (*us*) *See* ultrasound (safety).

sagittal plane (*ct*) Anatomical plane oriented parallel to the symmetry (median) plane of the human body, orthogonal to the transverse and the coronal plane; in the CT coordinate system the sagittal plane is usually oriented parallel to the y/z-plane.

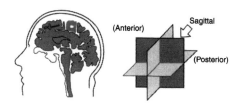

(*see* coronal plane).

saline (*clin*) *See* isotonic saline.

Saloman, Albert German surgeon who first radiographed the breast in 1913.

salpingography (*clin*) *See* hysterosalpinography.

samarium (Sm) (*elem*)

Atomic number (Z)	62
Relative atomic mass (A_r)	150.35
Density (ρ) kg/m^3	7500
Melting point (K)	1345
K-edge (keV)	46.8

^{153}**Samarium** (*nmed*) Chelated with EDTMP (ethylene-diamine-tetramethylene-phosphonate)

as a bone seeking agent. Beta emission provides palliative properties and the gamma emission allows scintigraphy.

Production	$^{235}_{92}$U(n,f) $^{153}_{62}$Sm(+$^{80}_{30}$ Zn +3n)
Decay scheme	^{153}Sm T½ 46.8 hr ($\beta-$ 803,
($\beta-$) ^{153}Sm	γ 103 keV) → ^{153}Eu stable
Half life	46.8 hours
Decay constant	0.01474 h^{-1}
Photons (abundance)	$\beta-$ 803 (0.2)
	700 (0.53)
	630 (0.26)
γ	70 (0.34)
	103 (0.77)

Generic name	^{153}Sm-EDTMP
Commercial names	Quadramet
Non-imaging category	palliative treatment of bone pain
Uses: Palliative therapy for bony metastases.	

sample size (*stats*) The population number to be included in a trial or investigation. The known variance, the population mean and the normal deviate should be assessed.

sample volume (*us*) The anatomic region from which pulsed-Doppler echoes are accepted.

sampling (*elect*) Conversion of the continuous (analogue) signal to a series of discrete (digital) values by measurement at a set of particular times: this utilizes the analogue to digital converter. If the rate of sampling is less than twice the highest frequency in the signal, abasing will occur. The duration of sampling determines how small a difference of frequencies can be separated.

sampling distance (*ct*) Distance between equidistant points at which a continuous function is sampled for measurement (*see* sampling frequency).

sampling frequency (*ct*) Expressed as the reciprocal value of the sampling distance; group of parameters (detector spacing etc.) which determine projection geometry and distance during the CT scan; the most important parameters are the distance between single detector channels (sampling distance), detector quarter shift; effective width of the detector elements and the angular increment between successive projections.

sampling theorem (*math, ct*) Defined by Shannon sampling theory, stating that a continuous, bandlimited function can be completely recovered from a finite number of measured values, if this function does not contain spatial frequencies above the Nyquist frequency (*see* sampling frequency, aliasing).

sampling time (*mri*) Duration over which the MR signal is measured. Longer sampling time results in higher image signal-to-noise.

sampling window (*comp*) *See* acquisition window.

SA (*us*) *See* spatial average intensity.

SAPA (*us*) *See* spatial average/pulse average.

SAR (*mri*) *See* specific absorption rate.

SAT (*mri*) A regional saturation pulse sequence for spatial presaturation to reduce the MR signal intensity in specific locations. A motion artefact reduction technique applied to blood flow imaging. Motion artefact reduction techniques. Spatial presaturation to reduce MR signal intensity in specific locations (*see* REST, PRE-SAT, PRESAT, EFAST, SATURATION).

SATA (*us*) *See* spatial average/temporal average.

satumomab pendetide (*nmed*) A murine monoclonal antibody of the immunoglobulin subclass IgG 1, satumomab (MAb B72.3), localizes or binds specifically to a tumour-associated glycoprotein (TAG-72), a cell surface antigen expressed at high levels on nearly all colorectal and ovarian adenocarcinomas (*see* OncoScint®).

saturation (*image*) The purity of a colour's hue on a scale from grey to primary colour. (*mri*) A non-equilibrium state where equal numbers of spins are aligned against and with the main magnetic field; zero net magnetization. Produced by repeated short interval RF pulses compared to T1; repeat 90° RF pulses with short TR times (*see* SAT, REST, PRE-SAT, PRESAT, EFAST, SATURATION).

saturation constant (*nmed*) *See* radionuclide production, saturation limit.

saturation limit (*nmed*) At a certain time, during irradiation, a production (saturation) limit is reached: the number of atoms being produced is balanced by those decaying.

saturation pulses (*mri*) A sequence of either 90° or gradient pulses so timed to produce saturation. Usually accompanied by a spoiler pulse. Used for reducing the signals from flowing blood by saturating regions upstream from region being imaged. A sequence of RF or gradient pulses designed to produce saturation, typically in a selected region or set of regions most often by the use of selective excitation followed by a spoiler pulse.

saturation recovery (*mri*) A partial saturation pulse sequence where after an RF saturation pulse the timing allows some net magnetization to establish. A particular type of partial saturation pulse sequence in which the preceding pulses leave the spins in a state of saturation, so that recovery at the time of the next pulse has taken place from an initial condition of no magnetization. A method for generating primarily T1 dependent contrast through a series of 90° excitation pulses. Immediately after the first pulse, longitudinal magnetization is zero because the tissue is saturated. The next 90° pulse is not applied until longitudinal magnetization has recovered. The repetition time (TR) depends on the T1 constant of the tissue.

saturation slice (*mri*) Regional presaturation to suppress undesired signals for specific areas, either within the slice or parallel to it.

saturation transfer (or inversion transfer) (*mri*) Nuclei retaining their magnetic orientation through a chemical reaction. When RF energy is given to the spins at the chemical shift frequency of the nuclei in one chemical state producing saturation or inversion; then any subsequent chemical reactions transform the nuclei into another chemical state with a different chemical shift. The NMR spectrum can show the effects of the saturation or inversion. Used to study reaction kinetics/chemical transformations of suitable molecules.

scalars (*math*) Quantities that are fully specified by a statement of purely size. Examples are mass, distance, speed, work and energy (*see* vectors).

scale (*image*) In wavelet analysis, a term meaning the same as scale in geographical maps, very large scales mean global views, while very small scales mean detailed views.

scan converter (*elec*) A device that stores imaging information in one format and reads it out for display in another.

scan cross-sectional area (*us*) For auto-scanning systems the surface within the beam cross-sectional area during the scan. Measured as centimetre squared, cm^2.

scan line (*us*) A line produced on a display that represents the echoes from a pulse. The signal line produced by a transducer element whose length defines image depth.

scan projection radiograph (SPR) .(*ct*) Generic name for the digital image obtained by linearly translating the patient through the gantry aperture during an x-ray exposure while the x-ray tube remains stationary. The SPR has a similar appearance to a plain radiograph and is used primarily for localizing the required region of scanning. Synonymous terms include radiographic mode and localizer image, together with the proprietary names Pilot scan, Scanogram, Scanoscope, Scoutview, Surview and Topogram.

scandium (Sc) (*elem*)

Atomic number (Z)	21
Relative atomic mass (A$_r$)	44.96
Density (ρ) kg/m^3	3000
Melting point (K)	1812
K-edge (keV)	4.4

scanhead (*us*) Transducer assembly.

scanner (*comp*) An electronic device that uses light-sensing equipment to scan paper or film images such as text, photos and illustrations and translate the images into signals that the computer can then store, modify or distribute.

scanner (film) (*image*) A mechanical/optical device for digitizing film or paper records. It consists of an intense linear light source, which travels over the film or paper surface. Its mirrored reflected signal is superimposed on a linear CCD array having more than 2000 cells. For black and white images a single light source is employed; for colour information red, green, blue light sources are used. The resolution offered by current radiography scanning devices is approximately $3\,Lp\,mm^{-1}$ on a $35 \times 43\,cm$ $(14 \times 17'')$ film. Laser film imagers can achieve a pixel size of 0.08 mm giving a resolution of $1/(2 \times 0.08) = 6\,Lp\,mm^{-1}$ for this film size and 35 mm film scanners give a pixel size of 0.0128 mm which delivers $38\,Lp\,mm^{-1}$ for this small format (*see* charge coupled device, film formatter).

scanner geometry (*ct*) Geometrical arrangement of the x-ray tube and detector array with respect to the axis of rotation.

scanogram (*ct*) *See* scan projection radiograph.

scan plane (*ct*) The *x*/*y*-plane of the coordinate system forming the axial image; the scan plane contains the central trajectory and is consequently in

the plane of rotation of the CT gantry. The gantry tilt alters the scan plane but in most cases the scan plane coincides with the transverse plane.

scan time (*ct*) The time interval between the beginning and the end of the acquisition of attenuation data for a single exposure. For some CT scanners, this may be longer than the exposure time due to the pulsing of x-ray emission.

SCART (*comp*) An audio/video connector used in consumer equipment, especially in Europe. The SCART connector's 21 pins has two audio in and out channels, in and out video channels, RGB signals, ground and some additional control signals.

scatter radiation (*phys*) A general term describing both elastic and in-elastic (Compton) events within an absorber. The primary photon is deflected from its path and in the case of Compton scattering loses energy to a free electron. (*ct*) Radiation scattered from the main section (SSP) produced by interaction of the primary beam with a material medium. The interaction can be characterized by a reduction in radiation energy and/or by a change in the direction of the radiation. (*xray*) Radiation scattered from the main beam (x-ray or gamma) produced in the interaction of the original radiation with a material medium. The interaction can be characterized by a reduction in radiation energy and/or by a change in the direction of the radiation. (*us*) *See* ultrasound (scatter), linear scatter coefficient, back-scatter.

scatter coincidence events (*nmed*) A scatter coincidence in positron emission tomography (PET) occurs when one or both γ-photons from an annihilation event are scattered but both are detected within a single detector ring. Scatter coincidences are seen as true coincidence events, so the correction for accidental coincidences does not compensate for them. Annihilation radiations may undergo scattering while passing through the body tissue, and because of the high energy (511 keV), most of these scattered radiations move in the forward direction without much loss of energy to be accepted within the energy window of 511 keV and therefore be counted as true coincidences. The position information of the event is lost. In practice, scattered events constitute a significant fraction of the events detected by the system (10–20% of total counts in a '2D system' and 40–60% of total counts in a '3D system'). PET machines using **septal collimator** rings markedly reduce scatter events from being collected, due to improved geometric efficiency.

scattered photon (*phys*) The path taken by the incident photon after a Compton interaction (*see* **Compton scatter**).

scatterer (*us*) An object that scatters sound because of its small size or its surface roughness.

scattering (*us*) Redirection of sound in several directions upon encountering a particle suspension or a rough surface (*see* **specular reflection**).

Schilling test (*nmed*) This, combined with a test for the intrinsic factor, indicates malabsorption of vitamin B_{12}. ^{58}Co-labelled B12 given orally after a fasting period. A flushing dose of non-radioactive (cold) vitamin B_{12} is then injected. A complete urine collection is made. A dual radionuclide modification ^{58}Co-labelled B12 and ^{57}Co-labelled B_{12} attached to intrinsic factor (**Dicopac Test**, Amersham/ GE Healthcare Inc) distinguishes malabsorption of B_{12} due to lack of intrinsic factor and that due to a lesion of small intestine.

scientific notation (*math*) A numerical form similar to floating point: $a \times 10^n$ or aEn where a is a number 1 to 10 and n is a whole number as before, e.g. 5.64E–2 or 0.0564.

scintigraphy (*nm*) General term for imaging a radionuclide distribution usually applied to gamma camera studies.

scintillation detector (*phys*) Radiation detectors consisting of inorganic or organic crystals have valency/forbidden/conduction bands. A scintillator coupled to either a **photomultiplier** or **photodiode** which gives an electrical signal whose amplitude corresponds with the energy of the radiation (particulate or photon). Electromagnetic radiation or particulate energy (electron beam) allows transition between bands. These form the basis of **luminescence** which includes **fluorescence**, **phosphorescence** and **thermoluminescence** (*see* **semiconductor**).

scintillator (*phys*) An inorganic crystal, organic compound (plastic) or liquid capable of demonstrating **fluorescence** when bombarded by particle or photon radiation. (*ct*) Substance that emits visible light when exposed to radiation; used in the construction of solid state detectors (*see* **ceramic detector, luminescence, phosphor**).

scotopic (*clin*) Visual process associated with rods as the principle receptors and used particularly with low light levels; colours cannot be identified (*see* **photopic**).

ScoutView (*ct*) *See* **scan projection radiograph (SPR)**.

screen activators (*phys*) Mainly rare earth trace elements added to phosphors to increase efficiency of emission.

screen pigment (*film*) Pigment added to intensifying screen to prevent light diffusion.

screening (population) (*clin*) Screening a population for hidden disease (e.g. tuberculosis, breast cancer, cervical cancer, prostate cancer, heart disease, etc.). Normally certain criteria are considered before organizing a screening programme:

- The disease is common enough in the population.
- The disease has a serious early mortality.
- Early detection and intervention will significantly improve life expectancy or quality of life.
- The aetiology of the disease is understood.
- The screening interval can be maintained shorter than cancer appearance.
- The screening test is accurate and safe.
- Proven, acceptable and effective treatment can be readily organized (*see* **lead time bias, predictive accuracy**).

SCSI (*comp*) Small computer systems interface. A method for connecting devices to a PC. A single SCSI adapter can handle a mix of up to eight different devices such as hard drives, CD-ROMs and scanners. The most recent Ultra3 SCSI supports up to 16 devices (including the SCSI adapter card or chip) and has transfer rates of 160 MBbps (megabytes per second).

SDRAM (*comp*) Synchronous DRAM. A type of memory that synchronizes itself with the speed of the CPUs bus and can run at 100 MHz. It is about twice as fast as EDO RAM and the latest SDRAM can run at 133 MHz on PCs that support this speed.

SE (*mri*) Spin echo pulse sequence.

Seaborg, Glen T (1912–1999) American nuclear physicist who synthesized plutonium and discovered the fissile nature of Uranium-235 achieving the first chain reaction with Fermi in December 1942. He synthesized americium and curium in 1944, then berkelium and californium in 1950. His team later synthesized einsteinium, fermium and mendelevium. In 1951 Seaborg shared the Nobel Prize for Chemistry with McMillan.

sealed source (*nmed*) Radioactive material permanently bonded or fixed within a capsule or matrix designed to prevent release and dispersal

S

of the radioactive material under the most severe conditions likely to be encountered in normal use and handling.

SECAM (*image*) Système électronique couleur avec mémoire. Television transmission standard developed in France providing 625 lines at 50 fps.

second (*phys*) The SI unit of time defined as the duration of an exact number of periods corresponding to the transition between two hyperfine states in ^{133}Cs. The standard time periods commonly used are:

	Second	Minute	Hour	Day
Seconds	1	60	3600	86 400
Minutes		1	60	1 440
Hours			1	24

secondary barrier (*shld*) Any surface receiving scatter or leakage radiation and not subjected to potential exposure from the primary beam (*see* primary barrier).

secondary radiation (*shld*) or scattered radiation. Depends on the volume of the patient or object being exposed to the primary beam.

secondary reconstruction (*ct*) Image recalculated from a series of raw reconstructed, adjacent or overlapping CT images; usually a secondary reconstruction is oriented orthogonal to the slice plane (*see* sagittal plane, coronal plane).

SE-CSI (*mri*) Spectroscopy hybrid procedure based on spin echo.

section thickness (*ct*) The narrowest or focal point of a section or slice; thickness of the scanned tissue volume perpendicular to the scan plane; also called slice thickness. (*us*) The narrowest or focal point of a section or slice. section thickness. thickness of the scanned tissue volume perpendicular to the scan plane; also called slice thickness.

sector. (*us*) A geometric figure bounded by two radii and the arc of a circle included between them.

sector scan (*us*) Produced by a phased or annular ultrasound transducer.

secular equilibrium (*nmed*) A parent:daughter decay series where decay constant $\lambda_d > \lambda_p$. The decay constant for ^{81}Rb parent is 0.000042 and ^{81m}Kr is 0.0533. There is almost an instantaneous growth of daughter activity and continuous elution is possible (steady state studies ^{81m}Kr).

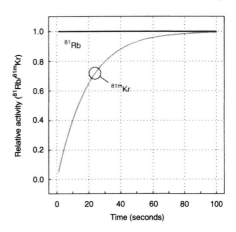

(*see* transient equilibrium).

segmented HASTE (*mri*) Variant of standard HASTE technique where half the image information is acquired after the first excitation pulse, and half after the second. The acquired raw data are then interleaved into a raw data matrix. Long repetition time (TR) is selected which allows the spin system to recover between excitation pulses. As a consequence the length of the multi-echo pulse train halved. HASTE sequences may also be divided into more than two segments.

segmented k-space data acquisition (*mri*) A set of k-space lines collected in a specified order but not constituting a complete coverage of k-space. Several segmental acquisitions are needed for complete coverage of k-space.

SeHCAT * (*nmed*) Taura-23-selena-25-homocholic acid. A ^{75}Se-labelled agent used for following bile acid absorption (Nycomed-Amersham/GE Healthcare). A non-imaging technique; maximum administered activity typically 400 kBq.

selection bias (*clin*) The tendency for people who elect to be screened to differ from the general population (more health conscious, so tend to be fitter).

selective excitation (*mri*) A specific region of tissue excited by controlling frequency bandwidth of an RF pulse while applying a magnetic field gradient. Originally used to excite all but a desired region but more commonly used to select only a desired region, such as a plane, for excitation.

selective irradiation (*mri*) *See* selective excitation.

selectivity (*mri*) The ability of an RF receiver to distinguish between selected and unwanted signals. Measured as FWHM of the pass band. Influenced by aerial (coil) design and placement.

selenium (Se) (*elem*)

Atomic number (Z)	34
Relative atomic mass (A$_r$)	78.96
Density (ρ) kg/m^3	4810
Melting point (K)	490
K-edge (keV)	12.6

Relevance to radiology: an imaging plate detector for x-rays.

^{75}Selenium (*nmed*) Adrenal gland and pancreas imaging.

Production	$^{74}_{34}$Se (n,γ) $^{75}_{34}$Se
Decay scheme (e.c.)	^{75}Se T½ 120 d (γ 136, 265, ^{75}Se 280 keV) : ^{75}As stable
Gamma ray constant	5.6 × 10^{-2} mSv hr^{-1} MBq^{-1} @ 1 m
Half life	120 days
Decay constant	0.005784 d^{-1}
Photons (abundance)	121 keV (0.171)
	136 keV (0.588)
	265 keV (0.590)
	280 keV (0.252)
	401 keV (0.115)

Uses: combined with nor-cholesterol to image the adrenals, combined with methionine to image the pancreas and with taurocholic acid for tracer studies of bile acid loss.

^{75}Se–homocholic acid taurine (*nmed*) *See* SeHCAT®.

^{75}Se–seleno-cholesterol (*nmed*) Has limited role in adrenal imaging. Discontinued.

^{75}Se–selenomethionine (*nmed*) Early agent for imaging hepatomas. Discontinued.

^{75}Se–selenomethyl-19-norcholesterol (*nmed*) An imaging agent (Scintadren®) that has been used for the adrenal cortex.

self-shielding (*mri*) Magnetic shielding by attaching a high permeability yoke to the magnet (passive shielding) or by incorporating additional magnetic field-generating coils designed to reduce the external field (active shielding) (*see* magnetic shielding).

semiconductor (*phys*) A material (element or compound) whose conductivity can be influenced by adding impurities. The pure materials produce relatively few 'free' electrons at normal temperatures. The valency and conduction bands in an intrinsic semiconductor are very close in energy so an appreciable number of electrons will have enough thermal energy to enter the conduction band. These electrons (negative charge) and the corresponding 'holes' left in the conduction band by absent electrons (positive charge) are freely mobile. An intrinsic semiconductor such as silicon or germanium can therefore conduct electric current under certain conditions. Semiconductors such as germanium, silicon, selenium and a variety of complex compounds are manufactured in very pure crystalline form and have very small levels of impurities added (doping); these impurities produce defects in the crystalline structures and function as localized electron donors just below the conduction band so the energy required to lift an electron into the conduction band is much smaller. Doping creates *n* and *p* type semiconductors. '*n*-type' where the *n* depicts conduction due to negative charges (electrons) and '*p*-type' when doping leaves positively charged electron vacancies or 'holes' in the valence bands, which are highly mobile and can conduct an electrical current. Semiconductors are used in signal and power rectifying devices (diodes), RF and AF amplifying devices (transistors) and switching devices (thyristors, triacs, transistors). They can be assembled as integrated microcircuits. Semiconductors as photoconductors can be used as radiation detectors and imaging surfaces (selenium, silicon). Hyperpure germanium (HpGe) and lithium drifted silicon is used as a cooled detector giving excellent energy resolution, the latter for lower photon energies.

semiconductor detector (*ct*) X-ray detector made completely of a semi-conducting material; the incident radiation causes ionization within the material which is directly transformed into an electrical (current or voltage) output signal (*see* solid state detector).

seminal vesiculography (*clin*) Seminal vesicle identified by ultrasound them imaged using non-ionic contrast material.

■ Reference: Jones *et al.*, 1997.

sensitive plane (*mri*) Technique of selecting a plane (or sequential plane) imaging by using an oscillating magnetic field gradient and filtering out the corresponding time-dependent part of the NMR signal. The gradient used is at right angles to the desired plane and the magnitude of the oscillating magnetic field gradient is equal to zero only in the desired plane.

sensitive point (*mri*) Technique of selecting out a point for sequential point imaging by applying three orthogonal oscillating magnetic field gradients such that the local magnetic field is time-dependent everywhere except at the desired point. and then filtering out the corresponding time-dependent portion of the NMR signal.

sensitive volume (*mri*) The region of the tissue or organ from which the NMR signal will preferentially be acquired because of strong magnetic field inhomogeneity elsewhere. Achieved by altering the bandwidth of the RF pulse and applying oscillating magnetic gradient fields. Effect can be enhanced by use of a shaped RF field that is strongest in the sensitive region.

sensitivity (*phys*) The response of a detector to different photon energies. (*stats*) *See* sensitivity (diagnostic). (*us*) Ability of an imaging system to detect weak echoes. (*mri*) Atomic nuclei must have a nuclear spin; this excludes all atomic nuclei with an even number of protons and neutrons. Because the hydrogen isotopes are the most sensitive, it is set as a reference to all other atomic nuclei and has the relative sensitivity of 1 (or 100%).

Nucleus	Relative sensitivity
^{1}H	1.0
^{19}F	8.3×10^{-1}
^{23}Na	9.3×10^{-2}
^{31}P	6.6×10^{-2}
^{13}C	1.6×10^{-2}

(*nmed*) *See* sensitivity (system).

sensitivity (diagnostic) (*stats*) A measure of the performance of a diagnostic test which detects the presence of disease in a selected population group. Calculated from an analysis of diagnostic accuracy, representing the proportion of people with the disease that will be detected by the imaging method used. For a clinical test series (i.e. screening results), the results can be listed according to true positive (TP), false positive (FP):

Test result	Expected+	Test−	Total
Positive test	TP	FP	TP + FP
Negative test	FN	TN	FN + TN
Total	TP + FN	FP + TN	TP + FP + FN + TN

Sensitivity is measured as the ratio of true positive (TP) to the sum of true positive and false negative (FN):

$$\frac{TP}{(TP + FN)} \times 100\%$$

For the results presented in diagnostic accuracy the sensitivity is 300/350 = 85%. **Selectivity** is measured as:

$$\frac{TN}{TN + FP} \times 100\%$$

Overall accuracy is measured as:

$$\frac{TP + TN}{\text{Grand total}} \times 100\%$$

(*see* Bayes' theorem, predictive accuracy).

sensitivity (system) (*nmed*) The response of a gamma camera to a known activity A with a chosen collimator. The counts registered by the camera are noted using a 20% window C so C/A cps MBq^{-1} is a measure of the sensitivity. Typical values for ^{99m}Tc are:

- *H R collimator* 85 to 115 cps MBq^{-1};
- *General purpose* 150 to 200 cps MBq^{-1}.

Excessive count rates approaching the camera dead time should not be used. The conversion between counts per second per megabecquerel (MBq) and counts per minute per microcurie (μCi) where the conversion is:

cps MBq$^{-1} \times 2.22 =$ cpm μCi^{-1}

cpm μCi$^{-1} \times 0.45 =$ cps MBq^{-1}

(*see* resolution (system)).

sensitivity analysis (*dose*) Aims to quantify how the results from a model depend upon the different variables included in it.

sensitivity centres (*film*) (*see* emulsion ripening).

sensitivity profile (*ct*) Relative response of a system for CT as a function of position along a line perpendicular to the tomographic plane.

sensitometer (*film*) A calibrated light source for exposing a stepped grey-scale.

separation (*film*) Loss of definition due to separation of the intensifying screen and film surface by dirt or distortion.

sEPI (*mri*) spiral EPI.

septa (*ct*) Thin metal plates separating adjacent detectors in an array: the septa are oriented parallel to the incident x-rays and parallel to the axis of fan beam rotation.

septal collimator rings (*nmed*) PET machines using these markedly reduce scatter events from being collected, due to improved geometric efficiency. If an annihilation occurs within a

S

particular detector ring then, if either of the photons scatters, it is most likely that the new trajectory of the photon will cause it to miss the detector ring, thereby preventing a scatter coincidence event.

sequence time (*mri*) or repetition time TR. The period between repeating an identical pulse sequence.

sequential CT (*ct*) Conventional CT scanning technique in which each slice is measured at a fixed *z*-position followed by an appropriate transport of the patient in the *z*-direction. Sequential CT has been replaced by spiral CT involving multiple detector rows.

sequential line imaging (line scanning; line imaging) (*mri*) Imaging techniques in which the image is built up from successive lines through the object. In various schemes, the lines are isolated by oscillating magnetic field gradients or selective excitation, and then the NMR signals from the selected line are encoded for position by detecting the FID or spin echo in the presence of a magnetic field gradient along the line: the Fourier transform of the detected signal then yields the distribution of emitted NMR signal along the line.

sequential multislice (*mri*) Slices in the imaging area under examination (ROI) are measured sequentially. The slices desired are selected using suitable gradients (selective excitation).

sequential plane imaging (planar imaging) (*mri*) Imaging technique in which the image of an object is built up from successive planes in the object in various schemes, the planes are selected by oscillating magnetic field gradients or selective excitation.

sequential point imaging (point scanning) (*mri*) Imaging techniques in which the image is built from successive point positions in the object. The points are isolated by oscillating magnetic field gradients (sensitive point) or shaped magnetic fields.

serial port (*comp*) A connection to the computer that transfers one bit of information at a time data queues up 'in line'. This is much slower than the parallel port but is more universal between computer types (*see* RS232, USB).

server (*comp*) A central computer in a network responsible for holding data and program files and serving workstations that are clients.

sestamibi (*nmed*) A ^{99m}Tc complex containing isonitrile ligands for a myocardial perfusion

agent. Commercial (DuPont Pharma: Bristol Myers Squibb) kit as Cardiolite® or Miraluma® for the preparation of ^{99m}Tc-sestamibi. ^{99m}Tc-(MIBI)$^+_6$ (as (Sestamibi or 2-methoxy-isobutyl-isonitrile) Cu(I) tetrafluoroborate) (*see* Myoview, thallium).

SFP (*mri*) *See* steady state free precession.

shadowing (*us*) Reduction in echo amplitude from reflectors that lie behind a strongly reflecting or attenuating structure.

shallow dose equivalent (H$_s$) (*dose*) The external exposure to the skin is the dose equivalent at a tissue depth of 0.007 cm averaged over an area of 1 cm^2 (*see* deep dose equivalent).

Shannon, Claude (1916–2001) American electrical engineer and mathematician. Created the concept of information theory influencing digital communications and information storage. Developed a mathematical theory of communication in 1948, deriving his Shannon equations.

Shannon equations (*image*) Transmission of information and the theory of communication is described by two equations presented by Shannon in 1948. The first is $I = -p \log_2 p$; which describes the signal content (*I*) (in bits) required to transmit certain information; *p* being the system probability. A simple application would be for alphabetical messages requiring 26 characters; 5 bits gives 2^5 or 32 possible characters. An alphanumeric message (36 characters) would require 6 bits. The second equation called the Shannon Limit describes data transmission *C* in bits per second for a given bandwidth and signal to noise ratio S/N as $C = W \log_2(1 + S/N)$ showing that a restricted bandwidth requires a low noise transmission system (*see* Nyquist frequency).

■ Reference: Shannon, 1948.

shaped pulse (*mri*) *See* tailored pulse.

shelf-life (*nmed*) A measure of radionuclide storage, related to half-life. ^{123}I has a poor shelf-life (T½ 13 hr) whereas ^{201}Tl has a good shelf-life (T½ 3.0 d).

Shepp–Logan filter (*image*) CT, SPECT and PET image reconstruction using simple back-projection gives a blurred image. Low pass filtering is applied to the back-projection data to obtain an accurate representation of the original object. There are a number of low pass filters, the simplest being the ramp filter but this is very sensitive to noise. Other filters do not have this disadvantage, the most common being the Shepp–Logan filter, which combines a sinc-function with the ramp filter. The Shepp–Logan filter gives a small amount of blurring, but is much less sensitive to noise.

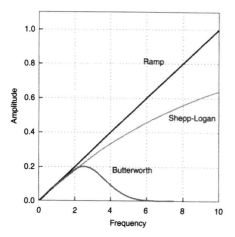

shielding (*mri*) *See* magnetic shielding, cryo-shielding, RF shielding, Faraday shield.

shielded gradient coils (*mri*) Using secondary active coils inductively coupled to the gradient coils inside the magnet cryostat reducing the gradient fringe field. The shielding can be accomplished by secondary actively driven coils or by passive screens which are inductively coupled to the gradient coils. In both cases eddy current interference will be reduced.

shielding (brick) (*dose*) *See* brick (shielding).

shielding (concrete) (*dose*) *See* concrete (shielding).

shielding (generator) (*nmed*) *See* generator (shielding).

shielding (lead) (*dose*) *See* lead (shielding).

shielding (lead-glass) (*dose*) *See* lead glass.

shielding (legislation) (*shld*) NCRP report 147.

shielding (plaster barium) (*dose*) *See* plaster (barium).

shielding (plaster gypsum) (*dose*) *See* plaster (gypsum).

shielding (steel) (*dose*) *See* steel (shielding).

shielding (syringe/vial) (*nmed*) *See* syringe/vial shielding.

shift invariant (*img*) A linear system is shift invariant if the impulse response function (point spread function) is the same for all input points (*see* space invariant).

shift reagents (*mri*) Paramagnetic compounds designed to induce a shift in the resonance frequency of nuclei with which they interact. Many rare earths have been used as shift reagents for positive metal ions such as sodium and potassium.

shim (*mri*) The correction of magnetic field inhomogeneities caused by the magnet itself, ferromagnetic objects, or the patient's body. Passive shim usually involves the introduction of small iron pieces in the magnet. The patient-related fine shim is software-controlled and performed using active shimming with coils (*see* global shim, interactive shim, local shim, 3D shim).

shim coils (*mri*) Coils carrying a relatively small current that are used to provide auxiliary magnetic fields in order to compensate for inhomogeneities in the main magnetic field of an NMR system. Shim coils can be either resistive or superconducting and typically up to 18 in number.

shimming (*mri*) Correction of magnet inhomogeneity; 'active' using shim coils, 'passive' using iron sheets. Process of maximizing the homogeneity of the static magnetic field. Active shimming techniques use current carrying coils within the magnet bore, while passive shimming places sheets of iron at various locations within the magnet.

shock-excited mode (*us*) Excitation of a transducer by a brief driving voltage impulse.

SHORT (*mri*) Short repetition technique pulse sequence (*see* FFE, GRE, MPGR, GRECO, FE, PFI, GE, TFF, SMASH, STAGE).

shoulder (*film*) The non-linear region of saturated exposure typically showing an optical density greater than 3.0.

sialography (*clin*) Radiography of salivary glands by using contrast medium in the ducts. Imaging the ducts and acini of a salivary gland. Usually for the parotid or submandibular gland.

SI units (*phys*) (*see* Système International).

SI prefixes (*units*)

	Prefix	Symbol
10^{15}	peta	P
10^{12}	tera	T
10^{9}	giga	G
10^{6}	mega	M
10^{3}	kilo	k
10^{2}	hector	h
10^{1}	deca	da
10^{-1}	deci	d
10^{-2}	centi	c
10^{-3}	milli	m
10^{-6}	micro	μ
10^{-9}	nano	n
10^{-12}	pico	p
10^{-15}	femto	f
10^{-18}	atto	a

side lobe (*image*) A product of non-recursive filter design. Used for low pass filtering or smoothing. Simple moving average filters can have unwanted side lobes which are sometimes >20% of the main lobe. (*us*) Minor sound beams travelling at an angle from the main beam given by a single element.

siemens (S) (*phys*) The reciprocal ohm (1/Ω or Ω^{-1}) so 1 S = 0.1 Ω; previously called the mho. Adopted as an SI unit.

Material	Siemens m^{-1}
Conductor	10^9
Semiconductor	10^9 to 10^{-7}
Insulator	10^{-15}

Sievert, Rolf Maximilian (1896–1966) Swedish radiologist giving his name to the SI unit for equivalent dose.

sievert (Sv) (*dose*) The unit of effective dose and equivalent dose, 1 Sv = 1 J kg^{-1}. Obtained as the product of absorbed dose and radiation weighting factor: gray × (Q or w_R) (*see* gray).

sigma function (*math*) A curve approximating to $1/(1 + e^{-x})$ which simulates the film characteristic curve and dose response from low to high exposure levels and dose/mortality curves.

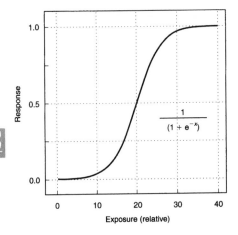

sigma value (*stats*) *See* standard deviation.

signal averaging (*image*) Multiple signals acquired under identical conditions (RF frequency, gradient field strength) and averaged to reduce noise; combining signals from identical acquisition procedures to reduce signal noise Usually four repeat signals are averaged to reduce noise by $\sqrt{N}$. (*mri*) Taking the average

of a signal's parameter (amplitude, frequency, etc.) acquired under the same or similar conditions so as to suppress the effects of random variations or random artefacts. The number of signals averaged together can be abbreviated to NSA (*see* signal to noise ratio).

signal decay (*ct*) The falling output signal from a detector or signal amplifier as a function of time after the incident x-ray flux or the electrical input signal has been switched off (*see* sodium iodide).

signal elimination (*mri*) Areas in the image without signal (displays as black). Caused by: metal items, susceptibility artefacts, flow and saturation effects. Flow voids can occur with fast flows when using spin echo sequences if the bolus flows out of the slice between the 90 and 180° pulses. No spin echo is produced, and blood appears black in the image.

signal suppression (*mri*) Elimination or reduction of a selected signal by applying a narrow band frequency-selective pre-pulse centred on the resonant frequency of the signal. Can also be achieved by using an inversion recovery technique to null the signal as it recovers its longitudinal magnetization.

signal to noise ratio (SNR) (*phys*) The displayed signal divided by the standard deviation of signal noise. In the diagram:

$$SNR = \frac{D2 - D1}{\sigma}$$

definitions of the SNR vary. In the context of signal detection theory, the SNR is generally proportional to a ratio of:

- The magnitude of the difference between the mean values of some quantity under two conditions that are to be distinguished; to
- a measure of the magnitude of statistical variation in that difference.

The ratio of the strength of the signal for information content in the image to the noise level (the standard deviation of the signal).

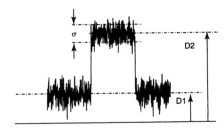

Ways to improve SNR in radiology and particularly MRI include:

- increasing the number of averagings;
- increasing the measurement volume (although spatial resolution degrades);
- using special coils and local coils;
- smaller bandwidth;
- shorter echo time;
- thicker slices.

(*see* noise, DQE, NEQ).

significance (*math*) A probability of rejecting the null hypothesis. $p = 0.05$ borderline significance, $p = 0.01$ significant, $p = 0.001$ highly significant.

significant figures (*math*) The number of significant figures in a given number is the number of digits from the left ignoring leading zeroes but counting final zeroes. It is the number of *meaningful* digits, e.g. 1.2345, 123.45, 0.0012345 and 12345.0 all have five significant figures. The number 12345000 has at least five significant figures but without more precision it is not known whether more figures are significant (*see* least significant figure).

silicon (Si) (*elem*)

Atomic number (Z)	14
Relative atomic mass (A$_r$)	28.09
Density (ρ) kg/m^3	2300
Melting point (K)	1680
K-edge (keV)	1.83

Relevance to radiology: as a low energy detector with a very narrow energy resolution. The depletion layer is increased by doping with lithium Si(Li).

silver (Ag) (*elem*)

Atomic number (Z)	47
Relative atomic mass (A$_r$)	107.87
Density (ρ) kg/m^3	10 500
Melting point (K)	1234
Specific heat capacity J kg^{-1}K^{-1}	232
Thermal conductivity W m^{-1}K^{-1}	429
K-edge (keV)	25.5

Relevance to radiology: Silver halides used exclusively as photosensitive compounds in film emulsions.

silver halides (*image*) Film emulsion components of silver iodide, bromide and chloride.

SIMM (*comp*) Single in-line memory module. A small circuit board holding a row of memory chips and has a 72-pin connector and uses a 32 bit-wide bus. Forms the basis of the RAM memory. As Pentium processors have a 64-bit bus, SIMM must be installed in pairs.

simple diffusion (*nmed*) A mechanism of localization in which a radiopharmaceutical diffuses across a cell membrane and is absorbed by the bloodstream (e.g. inhaled ^{133}Xe gas appears in the peripheral circulation).

simultaneous volume imaging (*mri*) *See* volume imaging.

SIMUSIM (*mri*) Simultaneous multi-slice imaging.

sinc function (*di*) The Fourier representation of a square wave in the time domain:

$$\sin c(x) = \frac{\sin(\pi x)}{\pi x}$$

This is a pulse shape with tails stretching to infinity. In practice, these undergo truncation which gives an imperfect square wave. The sinc function shapes the RF pulse in MRI; truncation errors (too much foreshortening) leads to slice overlap.

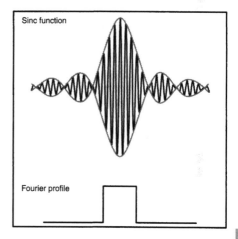

Sinc function

Fourier profile

sinc interpolation (*mri*) Interpolating image data by zero filling the high spatial-frequency components of the raw data so that after Fourier transformation the image matrix size has been increased.

sine wave (*math*) A continuous sinusoidal signal described by the equation $f(t) = A \sin(\omega t + \phi)$ where A is the signal amplitude and ω is the angular frequency $2\omega f$, where f is the frequency of the waveform and ϕ the phase angle in radians or the amount the wave is time shifted (*see* oscillation).

Sinerem$^\chi$ (*cm*) Guerbet MRI agent; the brand name for colloidal ferromagnetic iron oxide to detect metastatic disease in lymph nodes.

Single photon emission computed tomography (SPECT) (*nmed*) Single or dual head rotating gamma camera 180 or 360° around the patient or a set of fixed detectors in a 360° array. Axial tomographic images acquired and reconstructing multiple slices according to the camera field of view. The gamma camera heads take a series of images at equal angular spacing called projections during its rotational movement. 3D distribution of a radionuclide obtained by sampling with a rotating gamma camera (1, 2 or 3 heads) to obtain a series of ray sums (emission) and by filtered back-production reconstructing matrix as a voxel matrix depending on activity concentrations. Attenuation correction is also applied. Coronal and sagittal slices can be obtained from the axial information. SPECT images were obtained in the early 1960s using separate scanning detectors (David Kuhl, USA).

single-shot technique (*mri*) All image information acquired in a single excitation pulse. Magnetization of a fully relaxed spin system is used. Each of the subsequent echoes is given a different phase encoding relationship between the intensity of signal and noise. Only slightly more than half the raw data are acquired. The image is obtained using Half Fourier reconstruction. Single shot techniques include EPI, RARE and HASTE.

single volume spectroscopy (SVS) (*mri*) Mapping the metabolic information from the VOI in a spectrum. Single volume techniques are advantageous in case of pathological changes that cannot spatially be limited to a few VOIs: local inhomogeneity in the magnetic field can be compensated to a large extent using a local volume-sensitive shim. Clinical spectroscopy currently uses single volume techniques based on spin echoes (SE) or stimulated echoes (STEAM).

Sinografin[x] (*cm*) Bracco version of meglumine diatrizoate and meglumine iodipamide with an iodine content of 380 mg I mL^{-1} indicated for hysterosalpingography.

sinograms (*ct,nmed*) Constructed by combining information from several lines-of-response (LORs) and representing these as projected points on a sine wave. In PET line-of-response, coincident events for all projection rays are commonly sorted and stored this way, so organizing the data so that it can be examined more readily. The LOR has a certain angular inclination and a radial distance from the central axis so it is convenient to adopt a cylindrical coordinate system for storing other tomographic image data. The collection of many such views can be presented as a 2D plot or image; each is a one-dimensional profile of measured attenuation as a function of position, corresponding to a particular angle. The sinogram of a 2D slice is a collection representing the entire image; the phase and amplitude of the sine wave is unique to the source location in the tomographic plane and the intensity (amplitude) of the sine wave indicates source strength. Sinograms are transferred to the array processor and used for transaxial image reconstruction using filtered back projection or iterative reconstruction with a standard spatial filter (Shepp–Logan, Butterworth, Hann, Hamming, a simple ramp filter or a specific user defined filter).

SIP (*mri*) Saturation inversion projection.

skew (*stats*) A distribution where mean (Mn), mode (Mo) and median (Me) do not coincide as they do in the normal distribution.

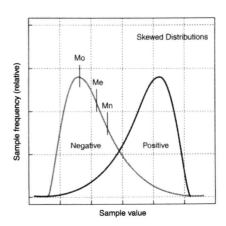

skin depth (*mri*) Time-dependent electromagnetic fields are significantly attenuated by conducting media (including the human body): the skin depth gives a measure of the average depth of penetration of the RF field. It may be a limiting factor in MRI at very high frequencies (high magnetic fields). The skin depth also affects the Q of the coils.

slew rate (*mri*) Gradient field increase by unit time:

$$\text{Slew rate} = \frac{\text{gradient strength}}{\text{rise time}}$$

Measured in tesla m^{-1} s^{-1}. The magnetic gradient speed represented by the slope of the linear ramp; also known as **ramp time**. Defined as the maximum gradient rise time to maximum amplitude. Influences minimum TR and TE values. Typical values 20 to $60\,Tm\,s^{-1}$ although this figure can reach $200\,Tm\,s^{-1}$ for 3T machines (*see* magnetic field gradient).

slice (*ct*) Tomographic section (defined by position and thickness) of a test phantom or patient under investigation during a single CT exposure in serial scanning.

slice distance (*mri*) The separation between the centre planes of two sequential slices or 3D slabs.

slice dose profile (SDP) (*ct*) Represents the dose as a function of the position along the z-axis resulting; due to x-ray scatter the slice dose profile (SDP) is always broader than the slice sensitivity profile (SSP) in spite of detector collimation.

slice gaps (*mri*) The gap between the nearest edges of two adjacent slices. Not to be confused with the slice distance.

slice orientation (*mri*) Orthogonal planes are available for use as the basic slice orientation:

- sagittal;
- coronal;
- transverse.

An oblique or double-oblique slice is obtained by rotating the slice out of the basic orientation.

slice plane (*ct*) A plane oriented orthogonal to the axis of rotation and located centrally within the slice of the object shown in the reconstructed and displayed image. Altered by the gantry tilt.

slice position (*mri*) The position of the slice to be measured within the area under examination. Graphical positioning of the slices/saturation slices to be measured in a basic image.

slice profile (*mri*) The spatial distribution of sensitivity of the imaging acquisition in the direction perpendicular to the plane of the slice (z-axis). When the profile deviates appreciably from rectangular, the slice thickness alone may not provide an adequate description (*see* slice sensitivity profile, SDP).

slice selection (*mri*) For orthogonal slices, a magnetic field gradient is applied perpendicular to the desired slice plane (slice-selection gradient). Oblique and double-oblique slices are excited by simultaneously applying two or three gradient fields.

slice sensitivity profile (SSP) (*ct*) Relative response of a system for CT as a function of position along a line perpendicular to the tomographic plane. The slice sensitivity profile is an important factor of a CT machine since it determines the image quality. The steeper the profile slope the less interference from adjacent slices that would cause partial volume artefacts. The perfect sensitivity profile would be rectangular and for a point source of x-rays this could be achieved by simple collimation. In practice, where the focal spot has a finite size, geometrical unsharpness causes penumbra effects and tight collimation at the detector entrance is necessary. When opposing beam shapes are super-imposed (seen in a full 360° data collection) the two diverging beams give a slice section that departs from a true rectangle. The middle of the slice is thicker than the periphery; particularly noticeable for thin slices.

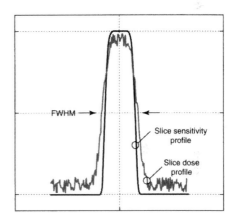

(*see* slice dose profile (SDP)).

slice sequence (*mri*) Parameter for multi-slice measurements, the excitation sequence can be selected as desired:

- ascending $(1, 2, 3, \ldots, n)$;
- descending $(n, n-1, \ldots, 3, 2, 1)$;
- interleaved $(1, 3, 5, \ldots, 2,4, 6, \ldots)$;
- or freely defined.

slice shift (*mri*) Distance between the centre of a slice group and the centre of the magnetic field (FOV) in slice-selection direction.

slice thickness (*ct*) Effective thickness of the tomographic section; the nominal slice thickness (width) is the full width at half maximum of the slice sensitivity profile. This is usually meant by the term slice thickness. Selection of a particular section thickness causes:

- movement of the pre- and post-patient collimators; and
- selection of detector rows.

Activating or deactivating the detector elements creates all available section thicknesses for the linear detector design. For unequal-width **adaptive detector** designs, post patient **collimation** is not needed for wider section thicknesses (5.0 and 2.5 mm); however, narrower section thicknesses (1.0 and 0.5 mm) require precise post patient collimation to cover portions of the detectors, which are exposed to radiation in the **penumbra**. Any nominal slice thickness can be reconstructed after acquisition providing that it is thicker than the original single detector configuration (scanned nominal slice thickness). The reconstruction of thicker slices than originally obtained reduces the number of images to be viewed and decreases **image noise**. (*us*) *See* **focus** (ultrasound).

slice width (*ct*) *See* **slice thickness**.

SLIP/PPP (*comp*) Serial line interface protocol/point to point protocol. These are standards for connecting directly to the **Internet** rather than simply logging on to it via a host computer.

slip-ring (*ct*) A method for uninterrupted power supply and data collection. Single slice or multi-slice spiral acquisition is a continuously rotating fan beam assembly. A conductive ring usually coated and lubricated copper, allows continuous contact between the x-ray tube (for its electrical supply) and detectors (for signal collection). Continuous data collection can then be obtained without rewinding the fan-beam assembly. Slip rings operate at either:

- low voltages (200–300 volts), when the generator and x-ray tube must rotate together (tank unit); or
- high voltages (up to 140 kV) supplying just the x-ray tube alone.

Both low and high voltage techniques have their advantages and disadvantages. Low-voltage connectors require a lightweight high-voltage generator rotating with the fan beam (the **tank unit** contains the high frequency transformers and control electronics); this adds additional mass to the rotating fan assembly. **Centrifugal forces** are therefore an important consideration in helical scanners capable of subsecond rotation

speeds. High voltage designs locate the generator externally away from the fan beam assembly, reducing weight but requiring substantial insulation for the slip rings.

slope (*math*) The straight-line portion of a curve (the film characteristic).

small bowel enema (enteroclysis) (*clin*) Radiographic examination of small intestine by retrograde filling from barium contrast filled large bowel; barium contrast examination of the small bowel after duodenal intubation. Distension of the small intestine by the contrast infusion provides detail and characterization of lesions. The contrast medium examination may be performed as a single-contrast or a double-contrast study.

SMART (*comp*) Self monitoring analysis and reporting technology or a feature of EIDE (on motherboards that support it) where the BIOS can receive data about hard disk performance and warn a user if it predicts a failure is likely to occur. (*mri*) Simultaneous multi-slice acquisition with arterial-flow tagging (Shimadzu). Reduction of motion-induced phase shifts during TE (*see* **GMR, GMN, FLOW-COMP, CFAST, MAST, FLAG, GMC, FC, STILL, GR**).

SMASH (*mri*) Short minimum-angle shot (subsecond imaging), general sequence, Shimadzu (*see* **FFE, GRE, MPGR, GRECO, FE, PFI, GE, TFF, SHORT, STAGE**).

smearing artefact (*mri*) With non-periodic movement (such as eye movement), the excited spins may be at a different locations in the gradient field at the echo time, resulting in wrong phase-encoding. The object is smeared in the phase-encoding direction. These artefacts are more discrete for periodic movements.

SMI (*mri*) Simultaneous multislice imaging.

smoothing (*di*) *See* **filtering** (spatial).

SMPTE (*comp*) Society for Motion Picture and TV Engineers. Provides standard test patterns for radiology video display quality.

SMTP (*comp*) Simple mail transport protocol. A high-level protocol for exchanging mail messages on the Internet. An extension of this is the Post Office Protocol (POP) to serve mail that are not permanently available on the Internet (turned off overnight).

Snapshot FLASH (*mri*) A very rapid FLASH sequence (scan time 200–500 ms) using a low flip angle (approximately 5°) to produce proton density-weighted scans. Contrast can be manipulated by

S

suitable preparation of the magnetization prior to the scan (*see* TurboFLASH).

Snell's Law (*us*) Describes the extent of the relationship between angles of incidence and refraction. The angles of incidence θ_i, reflection θ_r and refraction θ_t (of the transmitted beam) are related by the following laws for specular reflection:

- the directions of incident, refracted and reflected beams are all in one plane, which is normal to the surface of the two media;
- for specular reflection: $\theta_i = \theta_r$;
- considering the respective velocities in the incident and refractive medium (c_i and c_t respectively) then:

$$\frac{\sin \theta_i}{\sin \theta_t} = \frac{c_i}{c_t} = k$$

This last statement is Snell's Law and the constant k is the index of refraction of medium Z_2 with respect to medium Z_1. When $k < 1$ there is an angle of incidence where $\sin \theta_i = k$ then the above equation gives $\theta_t = 1$ or $90°$ and the refracted beam is parallel to the surface; θ_i is then the critical angle (θ_λ) which depends only on the velocity of ultrasound in the two media Z_1 and Z_2. If $\theta_i > \theta_\lambda$ or $\sin \theta_i > k$ then $\sin \theta_t > 1$ which is not possible so no refracted beam exists only a reflected one. The total reflection factor is important to fibre optics (*see* angle of reflection, sound (refraction)).

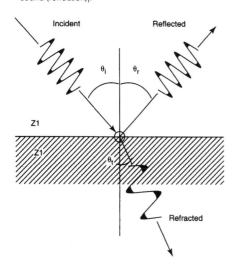

Incident   Reflected

θ_i θ_r

Z1

Z1

θ_t

Refracted

Snell, Willebrord (**1580–1626**) Dutch mathematician at Leyden University described reflection

and refraction of light in 1621 as Snell's Law which also applies to ultrasound.

SNMP (*comp*) Simple network management protocol; a standard for managing network devices, including adapters, switches, routers, servers and workstations.

SNR (*image*) *See* signal-to-noise ratio.

Soddy, Frederick (**1877–1956**) British radiochemist who shared the discovery of atomic disintegration with Rutherford and discovered with Ramsay helium production from alpha particles. He is best known for the discovery of isotopes. Awarded Nobel Prize for chemistry in 1921.

sodium (Na) (*elem*)

Atomic number (Z)	11
Relative atomic mass (A_r)	22.99
Density (ρ) kg/m³	970
Melting point (K)	371
Specific heat capacity $J\,kg^{-1}K^{-1}$	1230
Thermal conductivity $W\,m^{-1}K^{-1}$	141
K-edge (keV)	1.0

^{22}**Sodium** (*nmed*) Used as a calibration source for positron tomography.

Production	$^{23}_{11}Na\,(n,2n)\,^{22}_{11}Na$
Decay scheme ($\beta+$)	
^{22}Na	^{22}Na T½ 2.6 yr ($\beta+$ 1.82 MeV, 2γ 511 kev) → ^{22}Ne stable
Half life	2.6 years
Half value layer	4.1 mm Pb
Uses	A calibration source for positron emission detectors.

sodium iodide (*rad*) Sodium iodide (thallium-doped NaI(Tl)). This detector material has a relatively low stopping power compared to other detectors, it demonstrates very good energy resolution (11%) and has excellent light yield. The better energy resolution permits lower energy thresholds approaching 435 keV (rather than 350 keV) to limit scattered events without reducing true events (the window has an upper threshold of 665 keV). The coincidence time window is typically 8 ns which is an improvement on bismuth germinate (BGO) systems. A shorter coincidence time window should improve counting characteristics. The system has a long crystal decay time (230 ns) compared to lutetium oxy-orthosilicate (LSO) systems (40 ns), but this is shorter than the decay time for BGO (300 ns).

soft tissue (muscle) (*material*)

Effective atomic number (Z_{eff})	7.64
Density (ρ) kg/m^3	1040

soft tissue thermal index (TIS) (*us*) A thermal index for thermal exposure caused by an ultrasound beam heating soft tissue and bone interfaces (*see* ultrasound (heating)).

software (*comp*) The set of instructions. or computer program, that controls the activities of the computer. Programs may be written in machine language (sequences of numbers directly interpretable by the computer). assembly language, or higher level languages such as BASIC, C or FORTRAN. The software includes overall supervising 'executive' programs, data acquisition programs, data processing programs (including image reconstruction) and display programs (*see* macros).

solenoid coil (*mri*) A coil of wire wound in the form of a long cylinder. When a current is passed through the coil. the magnetic field within the coil is relatively uniform. Solenoid RF coils are commonly used when the static magnetic field is perpendicular to the long axis of the body.

solid state detector (*ct*) A photon detector can be a pure semiconductor device, ceramic or crystal scintillator in combination with a light sensitive semiconductor diode.

Solutrast^x (*clin*) Generic name iopamidol. A non-ionic monomeric radiographic contrast medium manufactured by Bracco.

solvent suppression (*mri*) *See* suppression.

somatic effects (*dose*) Pertaining to all cells except reproductive cells. Radiation effects induced in the person irradiated (*see* genetic effects).

somatostatin analogues (*nmed*) Somatostatin is a neuropeptide exerting an inhibitory effect on growth hormone secretion. Naturally occurring somatostatin has a short biological half-life. It is found in endocrine cell neurons with the highest density in the brain, peripheral neurones, endocrine pancreas, gastrointestinal tract and in smaller amounts in glands such as the thyroid. Synthetic derivatives of somatostatin analogues have prolonged survival in the circulation. Octreotide® is used for imaging tumours expressing somatostatin receptors,

SonoVue^x (*cm*) Bracco ultrasound agent using sulphur hexafluoride microbubbles.

sound (*phys*) Sound is a longitudinal wave made up of areas in a material (air, tissue, water, etc.) where the density and pressure are higher (compression) or lower (rarefaction) than normal.

The amplitude of the wave corresponds to denser compression events. High frequency is represented by denser packing of the compression and rarefaction events.

sound (conduction) (*phys*) *See* conduction (sound).

sound (intensity) (*phys*) Measured as sound power per unit area and proportional to pressure squared: $I \propto P^2$; measured as $J s^{-1} m^{-2}$ or $W m^{-2}$. Normal conversation has an intensity of 10^{-7} to $10^{-4} W m^{-2}$ and the threshold of hearing is $10^{-12} W m^{-2}$. The ultrasound unit is $10^{-3} W m^{-2}$ ($mW cm^{-2}$). Average intensity obeys the inverse square law from the point source. So the intensity of a spherical wave decreases as $1/r^2$. The amplitude A decreases with distance as $1/r$ since:

$$A_2 = A_1 \left[\frac{I_1}{I_2} \right]$$

(*see* ultrasound (intensity)).

sound (reflection) (*phys*) Sound is reflected from a smooth surface. Smooth is defined as any unevenness in the surface is much less than the wavelength; this gives specular reflection. A rough surface will give non-specular reflection.

sound (refraction) (*phys*) The transmitted wave will change direction depending on material composition. The beam is refracted and is due to the fact that the speed of sound is different in the two materials. The frequency of the sound will not change but the wavelength will. This will be less in the material in which the wave travels more slowly. The angle between the refracted wave and the normal is the angle of refraction. The sine of the incident angle divided by the sine of the angle of refraction is a constant. This constant is the refractive index:

$$\text{refractive index} = \frac{\sin\theta_i}{\sin\theta_t}$$

(see Snell's Law).

sound (velocity) (*phys*) As gas density (ρ) is proportional to pressure then sound velocity is independent of pressure changes. From Charles' Law at constant pressure $V \propto T$; since $V \propto 1/\rho$ then $1/\rho \propto T$. Therefore, at constant pressure, sound velocity is proportional to $\sqrt{T}$. A list of sound velocities ($m s^{-1}$) is shown where the velocity of sound in air is approximately $330 m s^{-1}$ being independent of pressure but proportional to $\sqrt{T}$ as stated above.

Material	Velocity
Air	330
Helium	1000
Water	1540
Soft tissue	1540
Bone	4080
Aluminium	6400

space charge (*xray*) Accumulation of an electron cloud around a filament. More pronounced at low kV.

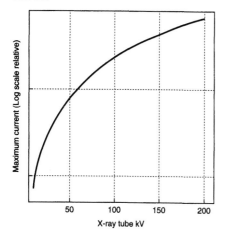

space invariant (*image*) If the image of a point source has the same functional form in all positions of the *x*, *y* plane, space variant distribution would consider all four spatial co-ordinates (*x*, *y* and −*x*,−*y*).

SPAMM (*mri*) Spatial modulation of magnetization.

spatial average intensity (*I$_{SA}$*) (*us*) Average intensity over transducer area.

spatial average/pulse average (*I$_{SAPA}$*) (*us*) A measure of ultrasound intensity at the face of the transducer divided by the duty cycle, given in mW cm^{-2} derived as:

$$I_{SAPA} = \frac{I_{SATA}}{\text{duty cycle}}$$

a measure of sound intensity given in mW cm^{-2} (*see* spatial peak/temporal average).

spatial average/temporal average intensity (*I$_{SATA}$*) (*us*) For non-autoscanning systems, the temporal-average intensity averaged over the beam cross-sectional area (may be approximated as the ratio of ultrasonic power to the beam cross-sectional area) as:

$$I_{SATA} = \frac{TA}{a^2}$$

For autoscanning ultrasound systems, the temporal-average intensity averaged over the scan cross-sectional area on a surface specified; it may be taken as the ratio of ultrasonic power to the scan cross-sectional area or as the mean value of that ratio if it is not the same for each scan. It is greatest at the mechanical focal point of the transducer. For non-autoscanning systems, the temporal-average intensity averaged over the beam cross-sectional area may be taken as the ratio of ultrasonic power to the beam cross-sectional area. *I$_{SATA}$* is frequently quoted by manufacturers and is the lowest intensity measurement. A complete family of intensity values can be derived from *I$_{SATA}$*. Typical values are given under ultrasound (intensity). Unit: mW cm^{-2}.

spatial average/temporal peak (*I$_{SATP}$*) (*us*) The peak intensity over the transducer face. An infrequently used measurement for ultrasound transducer intensity which combines spatial and temporal intensity. Unit: W cm^{-2}.

spatial distortion (*nmed*) The misregistration of an image event on the display so that its true position on the crystal is distorted. This is commonly due to unmatched PM tubes or variation over the face of the PM tube itself.

spatial frequency (*mri*) A dimension of the Fourier transform space (*k*-space), having units of inverse distance. Higher values of spatial frequencies correspond to finer detail in the image. (*ct*) The reciprocal value of the wave length of a periodic structure.

spatial intensity (*us*) *See* ultrasound (intensity).

spatial linearity (*nmed*) Establishing the image deviation from an ideal grid of line sources.

spatial non-uniformity (*nmed*) Irregular response to radiation across the input field of view.

spatial-peak intensity (*I$_{SP}$*) (*us*) Highest intensity in the ultrasound beam.

spatial-peak/pulse average, intensity (*I$_{SPPA}$*) (*us*) The value of the pulse average intensity at the point in the acoustic field where the pulse average intensity is a maximum or is a local maximum within a specified region. The measurement is derived from the duty cycle as:

$$I_{SPPA} = \frac{I_{SPTA}}{\text{duty cycle}}$$

This is the maximum power given by the full ultrasound pulse from the transducer. It is a good indicator for cavitation and other mechanical

S

bio-effects. Typical values are given under ultrasound (intensity).

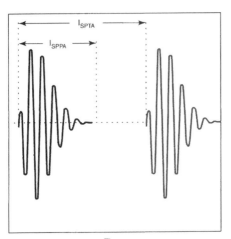

Time

Both I_{SPTA} and I_{SPPA} are required by FDA for acceptance and registration of new ultrasound equipment. Unit: $W\,cm^{-2}$.

spatial-peak/temporal-average,   intensity (I_{SPTA}) (us) The value of the temporal-average intensity at the point in the acoustic field where the temporal-average intensity is a maximum, or is a local maximum within a specified region. This is the sound intensity as the time averaged power, commonly quoted in ultrasound specifications and relates peak power to the pulse width and the duty factor; a higher pulse repetition frequency (PRF) will increase the I_{SPTA} value. It is derived as:

$$I_{SPTA} = I_{SATA} \times \frac{SP}{SA}$$

For a peak power of $1\,W\,cm^{-2}$ and a duty factor of 0.1, the I_{SPTA} value would be $100\,mW\,cm^{-2}$; it can also be derived as:

$$I_{SPTA} = I_{SPPA} \times \frac{\text{pulse length}}{PRP}$$

where the pulse repetition period (PRP) $=1/PRF$. Highest values of I_{SPTA} are seen in pulsed Doppler and CW Doppler and indicates heating effects. Both I_{SPTA} and I_{SPPA} are required by FDA for acceptance and registration of new ultrasound equipment. Typical values are given under ultrasound (intensity). Unit: $mW\,cm^{-2}$.

spatial peak/temporal peak (I_{SPTP}) (us) A measurement of maximum (peak) intensity within the ultrasound beam at any instant. It is obtained from the highest value of the pulse amplitude and is a good indicator for cavitation effects. Measured as:

$$I_{SPTP} = \frac{I_{SPTA}}{\text{duty cycle}}$$

A useful indicator for cavitation effects. Spatial peak/temporal peak pressure, measured in MPa, is similar to I_{SPTP} but refers to the peak pressure in the beam at any instant.

spatial pulse length (SPL) (us) Length of a single pulse which is (*wavelength × number of cycles*). Calculated as:

$$\frac{\text{cycles in pulse} \times \text{propagation speed}}{\text{frequency}}$$

and is related to wavelength as:

$$SPL = \lambda \times \text{number of cycles (mm)}$$

The pulses are damped to give 2–3 complete cycles. Dimensions are typically between 0.45 and 2.25 mm for a diagnostic imaging range.

Frequency (MHz)	SPL (mm)	PD (µs)
2.5	1.8	1.2
5.0	0.9	0.6
7.5	0.6	0.4
10.0	0.45	0.3

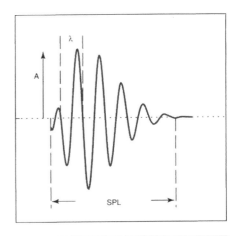

spatial registration (multi window) (*nmed*) A source of activity whose nuclide has more than one gamma energy imaged at all separate energies. Using radionuclides with multiple energies ([67]Ga 93, 185, 300 keV; [111]In 171, 245 keV) events should be collected using two or three energy windows in order to avoid loss of sensitivity and resolution. A ^{67}Ga source is usually placed at the centre of the UFOV and images collected for each energy window. Maximum registration error is then determined by combining all images.

spatial resolution (or high contrast resolution) (*image*) The displayed resolution described as high contrast (measured in line pairs) or low contrast (measured in grey level separation). (*ct*) The ability to resolve different objects in the displayed CT image, when the difference in attenuation between the objects and the background is large compared to noise. Spatial resolution in the scan plane is referred to as the axial spatial resolution. Resolution in the coordinate perpendicular to the scan plane (the z-axis) referred to as the longitudinal spatial resolution. Axial spatial resolution is principally determined by the distances between the x-ray tube, the centre of rotation and the detector, as well as by the width of the focus and the detector elements, and the number of measurements made per rotation. These factors are determined by the construction of the scanner. Longitudinal spatial resolution is principally determined by the dimension of the cone beam angle and the selected protocol. In conventional CT, the longitudinal spatial resolution is entirely determined by the slice thickness.

spatially localized spectroscopy (*mri*) Process by which regions of tissue are selectively sampled to produce spectra from defined volumes in space. These methods may be employed to sample a single region in space (single voxel method) or multiple regions simultaneously (multi-voxel methods). The spatial selectivity can be achieved by several methods including surface coils, surface coils in conjunction with RF gradient methods or RF pulses in combination with switched magnetic field gradients (volume-selective excitation). An indirect method of achieving spatial selectivity is the destruction of coherence of the magnetization in regions that lie outside the region of interest.

A variety of spatial encoding schemes have been employed for multi-voxel localization (*see* chemical shift imaging).

spatial resolution (intrinsic) (*nmed*) Measured by using a multiple line source. Values are given for both the central and useful field of view (CFOV, UFOV). The line spread function in both the x and y directions yield the FWHM for the spatial resolution of the camera. Typical values would be 3–4 mm. Full width tenth maximum (FWTM) measures the degree of light scatter within the detector.

spatial resolution (system) R_s (*nmed*) *See* resolution (extrinsic). This is a function of the particular collimator used and the distance from the collimator face. A line source similar to the one used for the intrinsic measurements gives FWHM values for CFOV and UFOV so:

$$R_s = \sqrt{R_c^2 + \left(\frac{R_i}{M}\right)^2}$$

where R_c is the collimator resolution, M the matrix size and R_i the intrinsic resolution. If R_s and R_i are obtained then a value for R_c (the collimator alone) can be derived independent of camera performance.

SPDIF (*comp*) Sony/Phillips digital interface. Was the most common digital audio interface between external digital audio recorders and the computer. The advent of optical connection has meant most high-end sound cards include both type of connection.

specific absorbed fraction (*dose*) The fraction of energy emitted as a specified radiation type in a source tissue which is absorbed in 1 kg of a target tissue.

specific absorption rate (SAR) (*phys*) A safety reference for measuring energy deposited in tissue by non-ionizing radiation. The rate at which energy (electromagnetic RF or sound) is absorbed by a unit mass of tissue as watt per kilogram (W kg^{-1}). (*mri*) RF energy absorbed per unit time. Time varying electromagnetic fields deposit energy in tissues; mostly in the form of heat which is considered the primary mechanism of biological effect. As a measure of heat transfer it is an important value for establishing safety thresholds. The SAR estimates RF heating effects which increase with field strength, duty cycle, flip-angle squared, coil type and patient geometry. Inhomogeneity of the RF fields leads to a local exposure where most of the power that is absorbed is applied to one body region rather than the entire person (local SAR). Averaging over the whole body leads to the global SAR where safety thresholds avoid thermoregulation or cardiac stress. The SAR is proportional to the product of tissue geometry (r as radius), field strength (B), flip angle (α), and duty cycle (D). Coil type also plays a part, as:

$$SAR \propto r^2 \cdot B^2 \cdot \alpha^2 \cdot D \, W\,kg^{-1}$$

High field strengths (3T) impart far greater energy than low strength magnets and inversion pulses (180°) deposit four times more energy than 90° pulses. Current FDA guidelines recommend SAR does not exceed $0.4\,W\,kg^{-1}$ whole body or $3.2\,W\,kg^{-1}$ to the head.

specific activity (unit) (*nmed*) The activity of a radionuclide contained in a sample, divided by the mass of the sample. The unit is $Bq\,kg^{-1}$.

specific activity (concentration) (*dose*) Radiochemical purity of the ^{99m}Tc eluate can be calculated from the decay constants of the participating radionuclides.

Specific activity, concentration

The decay chain is ^{99m}Tc (T½ 6h) → ^{99}Tc (T½ 2.1×10^5y). The chemical concentration of ^{99}Tc will increase on storage (in generator and eluate).

$$Mole\ fraction = \frac{0.86\lambda_1 \times (e^{-\lambda t} - e^{-\lambda_1 t})}{(\lambda_2 - \lambda_1) \times (e^{-\lambda_1 t})}$$

where λ_1 and λ_2 are decay constants for ^{99}Mo and ^{99m}Tc. If the time between elutions is >10h, then the chemical concentration (mole fraction) of ^{99}Tc exceeds ^{99m}Tc.

---

specific activity (dispensing) (*dose*) Reconstituting radiopharmaceuticals to give a total activity, sufficient for a fixed number of patients, so that a known volume (typically 1 mL) contains the required activity. The example shows a high specific activity dose but low specific activity doses can be calculated using the same procedure. Volume dispensing, instead of dispensing a measured activity, reduces hand dose.

Specific activity, dispensing

Adult patient dose is 600 MBq.
Vial reconstituted to give 10 doses (Total vial volume 10 mL). Total vial activity is $600 \times 10 = 6000$ MBq or 6 GBq; so 6 GBq is required in 10 mL for vial reconstitution. Eluted activity is 20 GBq in 10 mL giving 20/10 or 2.0 GBq per mL. Volume of eluate required (using GBq values) is:

$$\frac{Total\ vial\ activity\ (GBq)}{Eluate\ activity\ (GBq/ml)}\ \frac{6}{2.0} = 3.0\ mL$$

So 3.0 mL of generator eluate is made up to a total volume of 10 mL in a syringe to give a total vial activity of 6 GBq and added to the vial contents. Therefore, 1 mL gives a single adult patient dose of approximately 600 MBq.

---

specific activity (intrinsic) (*nmed*) Each radioactive species has an intrinsic specific activity which is the activity of a unit mass of the pure material. It depends on the decay constant and the nuclear mass of the nuclide.

Specific activity, intrinsic

The specific activity of a 4 mg sample containing ^{60}Co (T½ 5.26y) is 14×10^6 dps or 14 MBq representing $14/4 = 3.5$ MBq mg^{-1}. The intrinsic specific activity of 1 mg.

$$Number\ of\ nuclei\ (N) = \frac{Avogadro's\ number}{At.\ Wt.}$$

$$= 1 \times 10^9\ nuclei\ per\ mg.$$

The decay rate = $\lambda N = 4.18 \times 10^{-9} \times N = 4.18 \times 10^{10}$s^{-1} or 41 800 MBq mg^{-1} or 41.8 GBq mg^{-1}.
The given 4 mg sample of ^{60}Co is obviously a much-diluted source and is not carrier free.

---

specific activity (volume) (*nmed*) Using the basic formula $At = Ao \times e^{-\lambda t}$

Specific activity, volume

A solution of thallous (^{201}Tl) chloride has an activity of 200 MBq on day 1 (T½ 73h). The volume required for an 80 MBq study on day 3 (48h later) is: $200 \times e^{-\lambda t} = 127$ MBq, where λ is 0.693/73. A volume of 1.25 mL will contain approximately 80 MBq.

---

specific activity (weight) (*nmed*) The weight of radionuclide in a given activity is calculated from the formula: $W = {(M \times N)}/k$, where M is the atomic mass; N the number of radioactive atoms per gram of material of activity A (in becquerels) so $A = \lambda N$ and $N = A/\lambda$. k is Avogadro's constant.

Specific activity, weight

The weight of iodine in a 550 MBq ^{131}Iodine therapy dose. T½ 8 d (7 × 10⁵ s). $\lambda = 0.693/T½ = 10 \times 10^{-7}$. The number of atoms N in 550 MBq ^{131}I is:

$N = (550 \times 10^6)/(10 \times 10^{-7}) = 5.5 \times 10^{14}$
$W = 1.2 \times 10^{-7}$ g or about 120 nanograms.

The activity from naturally occurring ^{40}K in the human body (75 kg). Standard man contains 140 g of potassium of which 0.0168 g is ^{40}K (0.012% abundance). Since:

$$W = \frac{M \times (A/\lambda)}{k} \quad \text{then}$$

$$A = \frac{W \times k \times \lambda}{M} = 4366 \, Bq$$

---

specific gamma ray constant Γ *(nmed)* This is an early measure of the exposure rate as equivalent dose per unit activity at a certain distance from a point source. This has been replaced by the dose rate constant according to ICRU33, although the two terms are not identical. The SI unit for the specific gamma ray constant is $C kg^{-1} s^{-1} Bq^{-1}$ at 1 m. The practical measure being $mSv h^{-1} GBq^{-1}$ at 1 m or $\mu Sv h^{-1} MBq^{-1}$ at 1 m. The original values are calculated in non-SI units were $R h^{-1} Ci^{-1}$ at 1 m (known as Rhm, pronounced 'rum') or alternatively $R hr^{-1} mCi^{-1}$ at 1 cm. Converting from $mSv h^{-1} MBq^{-1}$ to $mrem h^{-1} \mu Ci^{-1}$ multiply by 3.7. Values for unshielded point sources in $mSv h^{-1} GBq^{-1}$ at 1 m (SI) and $R hr^{-1} mCi^{-1}$ at 1 cm (non-SI) are:

Nuclide	Gamma energy (keV)	Dose rate (SI)	Dose rate (non-SI)
^{99m}Tc	140	0.017	0.78
^{131}I	364	0.057	2.2
^{111}In	171, 245	0.084	3.21
^{137}Cs	662	0.087	3.3
^{60}Co	1.173, 1.333 MeV	0.360	13.2

In order to convert from R/hr/mCi at 1 cm to mSv/hr/GBq at 1 m, multiply by 0.235.

specific heat (specific heat capacity) *(phys)* This is the heat capacity per kg of the substance. Specific heat capacities are expressed in $J kg^{-1} K^{-1}$. The specific heat of a substance is the heat required to increase the temperature of 1 kg by 1 K (or °C^{-1}). So 42 J of heat raises:

2 gm water	by 5°C
2 gm aluminium	by 20°C
2 gm copper	by 50°C

Specific heat capacity and melting points (°C) of some common materials:

Substance	Specific heat capacity (J kg^{-1}K^{-1})	Melting point °C
Water	4200	
Oil	2130	
Aluminium	910	660
Graphite	711	≈3550
Titanium	523	1660
Copper	386	1083
Zirconium	280	1852
Molybdenum	246	2607
Rhenium	138	3180
Tungsten	136	3377
Glass	67	1127

Water and oil for heating and cooling liquids are chosen since their capacity to both store and transport heat is good. Water is a good reservoir for excess heat or a good cooling medium whereas aluminium and copper take up heat rapidly and since they are also good heat conductors, are able to conduct it away rapidly. The specific heat of gases varies according to pressure.

specificity (diagnostic) *(stats)* Calculated from an analysis of diagnostic accuracy, representing the proportion of the population without the disease that will be shown by the test to be free of disease. It is the ratio of true negative (*TN*) to the sum of true negative and false positive (*FP*):

$TN/(TN + FP) \times 100\%$.

For the results presented in diagnostic accuracy, the sensitivity is 56950/59650 = 95.5%.

speckle *(us)* The granular appearance of images and spectral displays that is caused by the interference of echoes from the distribution of scatterers in tissue.

speckle reduction imaging (SRI) *(us)* A technique introduced by GE Healthcare which reduces speckle noise in ultrasound by classifying the image content by comparing neighbouring pixels for expected greyscale trend or sharp changes; the latter most probably due to noise.

SPECT *(nmed)* See single photon emission tomography.

spectral analysis *(us)* Separation of frequencies in a Doppler signal for display as a Doppler spectrum.

spectral broadening *(us)* The widening of the Doppler shift spectrum; that is, the increase of the range of Doppler shift frequencies present that occurs because of a broadened range of

S

---

flow velocities encountered by the sound beam; this occurs for disturbed and turbulent flow.

spectral display (*us*) Visual display of a doppler spectrum.

spectral editing (*mri*) Methods of selectively enhancing or suppressing the signal from a particular molecular substance by using its spin properties, typically through spin–spin coupling (*see* J modulation).

spectral line-particular (*mri*) Distinct frequency or narrow band of frequencies at which resonance occurs corresponding to a particular chemical shift.

spectral maps (*mri*) Mapping a CSI spectral matrix to an anatomical image using magnetic resonance spectroscopy. Regional changes in metabolites can be superimposed on contours.

spectral width (*mri*) The overall width in hertz needed to observe a particular NMR spectrum. This width is generally set using the Nyquist limit, namely, that the temporal sampling rate must be equal to twice the maximum spread in frequencies.

spectrometer (*mri*) The portions of the NMR apparatus that actually produce the NMR phenomenon and acquire the signals, including the magnet, the probe, the RE circuitry, the gradient coils, etc. The spectrometer is controlled by the computer via the interface under the direction of the software.

spectroscopy (MRS) (*mri*) Magnetic resonance spectroscopy. Provides an estimation of cellular metabolic chemistry. The signal peak intensity is proportional to the concentration of metabolites. MR spectroscopy can be an important method for *in-vitro* and *in-vivo* examination of tissue and organs (*see* gamma spectrum, magnetic resonance spectroscopy).

spectrum (*mri*) The frequency plot of the MRS signal. The signal intensity is displayed as a function of the chemical shift (as ppm). Nuclei with different resonant frequencies appear as separate peaks in the spectrum (*see* MR spectroscopy).

spectrum (power) (*us*) Range of frequencies (*see* power spectrum).

spectrum analyser (*us*) A device that derives a frequency spectrum from a complex signal.

specular reflection (*us*) Reflection from a large (relative to wavelength), flat, smooth boundary; also mirror reflection; reflection at a smooth border where the surface unevenness is much less than the wavelength. For specular reflection the

angle of incidence is equal to the angle of reflection. The angle of incidence θ_i between the direction of motion of the incident wave and the normal (perpendicular from the surface) is equal to the angle of reflection θ_r. The sound wave may be partially reflected and the remaining wave front travelling through the new medium. The transmitted wave will change direction depending on material composition, undergoing refraction (*see* angle of reflection, Snell's Law, non-specular reflection).

speed (*film*) *See* film sensitometry.

speed error (*us*) A propagation speed that is different from the assumed value.

SPGR (*mri*) Spoiled gradient recalled rapid gradient-echo imaging techniques; T1-weighted contrast GE Healthcare (*see* FLASH, FSPGR, HFGR, RE Spoiled, 3D-ME-RAGE, T1-FEE, STAGE-T1W).

spherical aberration (*phys*) If a wide parallel beam is incident on a lens, not all the rays are brought to the same focus causing image distortion. Restricting the light beam to the centre of the lens by an iris diaphragm reduces effect. A distortion sometimes seen in fluoroscopy with large iris apertures.

SPI (*mri*) Selective population inversion; population inversion of a selected region in MR spectroscopy and imaging. By using as a driving function a complex radiofrequency (r.f.) pulse magnetization can be accurately inverted over a very sharply defined bandwidth, while outside that region, magnetization is returned to its initial position, and population is unaffected.

■ Reference: Silver *et al.*, 1984.

spin (*mri*) The intrinsic angular momentum of an elementary particle, or system of particles such as a nucleus, that is also responsible for the magnetic moment. The spins of nuclei have characteristic fixed values. Pairs of neutrons and protons align to cancel out spins. Nuclei with an odd number of neutrons and/or protons will have a net nonzero rotational component characterized by an integer or half integer quantum nuclear spin number.

spin density (*mri*) The number of resonant spins in a set region or locality which determines the strength of the NMR signal. The SI unit is mole m^3. For water this is 1.1×10^5 moles H per m^3. One of the principal determinants of the strength of the NMR signal from the region. True spin density is not imaged directly but must be calculated from signals received with different interpulse times.

spin echo (*mri*) Reappearance of an NMR signal after the FID has decayed as a result of the effective reversal of the **dephasing** of the spins (refocusing) by techniques such as specific RF pulse sequences (e.g. **Hahn** echo, or pairs of magnetic field gradient pulses (**gradient echo**) applied in times shorter than or on the order of T2). Gradient echoes will not refocus phase differences due chemical shifts or inhomogeneities of the magnetic field (unlike RF spin echoes).

spin echo imaging (*mri*) Any of many MR imaging techniques in which the spin echo is used rather than the FID. Can be used to create images that depend strongly on T2 if TE has a value on the order of or greater than T2 of the relevant image details. Spin echo imaging does not directly produce an image of T2 distribution. The spin echoes can be produced as a train of multiple echoes by using the CPMG pulse sequence.

spin echo sequence (*mri*) An RF pulse series having 90° followed by 180° gives the Carr–Purcell sequence, depends strongly on T2.

spin-lattice relaxation (*mri*) T1 relaxation time, also known as the longitudinal or thermal relaxation time. Regrowth of T1 relaxation which requires net transfer of energy from the nuclear spin system to the compound lattice (crystalline lattice). T1 relaxation only occurs when a proton encounters another micro-magnetic field at or near the **Larmor frequency**; it is a dipole–dipole interaction (*see* **spin–spin relaxation**).

spin number (nuclear) (*mri*) *See* **spin quantum number**.

spin quantum number (I) (*mri*) Property of all nuclei related to the largest measurable component of the nuclear **angular momentum**. Non-zero values of nuclear angular momentum are quantized (fixed) as integral or half-integral multiples of $(h/2\pi)$ where h is **Planck's constant**. The number of possible energy levels for a given nucleus in a fixed magnetic field is equal to $2I + 1$. Similarly, an unpaired electron has a spin of ½ and two possible energy levels.

spin tagging (*mri*) Nuclei will retain their magnetic orientation for a time on the order of T1 even in the presence of motion. Thus, if the nuclei in a given region have their spin orientation changed, the altered spins will serve as a tag to trace the motion for a time on the order of T1 of any fluid that may have been in the tagged region.

spin warp imaging (*mri*) A form of Fourier transform imaging in which phase-encoding gradient pulses are applied for a constant duration but with varying amplitude. The spin warp method, as other Fourier imaging techniques, is relatively tolerant of non-uniformities (inhomogeneities) in the magnetic fields.

spin–spin coupling (*mri*) Some spectral lines may consist of groups of lines or multiplets; multiplet structure of spectral lines are due to interaction between nuclei that split the NMR energy levels and result in the observation of multiple allowed transitions separated by an amount of energy related to J (the **spin–spin coupling** constant); the interactions are due to spin–spin coupling.

spin–spin relaxation (*mri*) T2 relaxation time or transverse relaxation time. May take place with or without energy dissipation and may occur without T1 relaxation. The numerical value of T2 is always less or equal to T1. T2 relaxation is the result of loss of coherence between adjacent spins (*see* **spin-lattice relaxation**).

spinal angiography (*clin*) *See* **vertebral angiography**.

spinal venography (*clin*) Rarely used procedure but may be indicated when others (myelography, spinal arteriography) have failed. Can be used for observing obstruction of the drainage into the epidural venous system.

SPIR (*mri*) Spectral presaturation with inversion recovery (Philips). Spectral presaturation to reduce MR signal intensity of fat (*see* **FATSAT**, **ChemSat**).

spiral (*ct*) *See* **helical/spiral**.

spiral artefact (*ct*) The interpolation algorithm is meant to overcome artefacts due to data inconsistency. This is only successful to some extent. The remaining effects can be divided in two groups: **cone beam artefacts** and **rod artefacts**.

spiral/helical acquisition (*ct*) Continuous fan beam rotation and simultaneous continuous object translation (couch/bed movement) in the z-direction, contrasting with **sequential** CT scan where the bed is stationary during fan beam rotation. This enables continuous acquisition of CT image data (single or multi-slice acquisition) using a machine with **slip-rings**. Detector signals can be collected by slip-rings or optical means. The CT axial sections have a helical geometry, which is corrected during the reconstruction process. Very fast subsecond scan times are obtained so that breath-hold techniques or bolus chasing can be performed. Spiral acquisition also allows a complete data set to be built up and multi-sectional displays, e.g. sagittal, coronal and oblique as well as 3D displays for angiography (*see* **pitch**).

SPL (*us*) Spatial pulse length = cycles × wavelength.

splenic arteriography (*clin*) Selective splenic arteriography (or coeliaco-arteriography) performed preoperatively to ascertain vascular anatomy prior to slenectomy or post traumatic procedures. Demonstration of the splenic artery is mostly performed by indirect splenoportography. The procedure has been largely replaced by CT and MRI techniques.

splenoportography (*clin*) Imaging splenic and portal veins. Radiography of portal vessel of the portal circulation by introducing contrast material into the spleen. Injection of iodine contrast material into the spleen to demonstrate the splenic vein, portal vein and oesophageal varices; as direct splenoportography where portal pressure can be measured at the same time and indirect splenoportography performed via a simultaneous selective contrast medium injection into the splenic artery (coeliac trunk) and superior mesenteric artery (*see* percutaneous splenoportography, PSP).

spline fit (*di*) A smoothly joined piece-wise polynomial. It resembles the position that a draftsman's spline (thin flexible ruler) would occupy if it were constrained to pass through the points. Cubic spline interpolation is a useful method for fitting the data points and smoothing discontinuities. It is an improvement on polynomial interpolation when the number of data points increases.

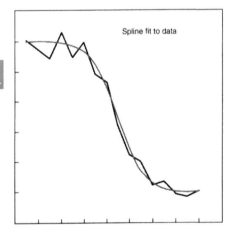

Spline fit to data

spoiler (*mri*) Gradient pulse or RF pulse applied to eliminate transverse magnetization that persists after the readout period.

spoiler gradient (*mri*) A gradient of sufficient amplitude and/or duration to fully dephase a signal. Often placed symmetrically about refocusing pulses so that they have no effect on the refocused signal but eliminate any signal originating at the refocusing pulse.

spoiler gradient pulse (homospoil pulse) (*mri*) A reverse magnetic field gradient to eliminate residual magnetization in the nucleus, removing remnants of transverse magnetization. Magnetic field gradient pulse applied to reduce/remove transverse magnetization by producing a rapid variation of its phase along the direction of the gradient, used to remove the unwanted signal after an imperfect 180° refocusing RF pulse, a corresponding compensating gradient pulse may be applied prior to the refocusing RF pulse in order to avoid spoiling the desired transverse magnetization resulting from the initial excitation (*see* FLASH).

SPPA (*us*) *See* spatial peak/pulse average.

SPT (*mri*) Selective population transfer. A pulse sequence for determination of coupling in small- and medium-sized organic compounds. The method uses a combination of the double pulsed field gradient spin-echo (DPFGSE) and the selective population transfer (SPT) techniques and is shown to be useful in magnetic resonance spectroscopy with many overlapped signals.

■ Reference: Uzawa and Yoshida, 2004.

SPTA (*us*) *See* spatial peak/temporal average.

SPTP (*us*) *See* spatial peak/temporal peak.

spreadsheet (*comp*) Primarily accounting software that allows calculation in a format that is similar to pages in a conventional ledger (*see* Excel).

SQL (*comp*) Structured query language. An IBM developed language used in client/server networks to enable microcomputers to access databases. SQL is data and device independent. There are several competing versions.

square wave modulation transfer function (square wave MTF) (*image*) Image contrast of a rectangular modulation as a function of the spatial frequency of the modulation of the object with constant contrast; the square wave modulation transfer function can be obtained directly from imaging a bar test pattern and can be used to calculate the sinusoidal MTF; because the area below a half wave of a rectangular modulation is larger than for a sinusoidal modulation. The square wave MTF yields better figures for spatial resolution than sinusoidal MTF; comparisons of

S

two MTFs is therefore valid only if they are of the same kind.

SR (*mri*) *See* saturation recovery.

SRAM (*comp*) Static RAM. This retains information until the power is switched off. Is slower and more expensive than DRAM.

SS (*mri*) Slice select gradient.

SSD (*image*) Shaded surface display.

SSFP (*mri*) Steady-state free precession (Shimadzu). Enhanced intensity rewinding of phase-encoding and no intentional spoiling; method of NMR excitation in which strings of RF pulses are applied rapidly and repeatedly with inter-pulse intervals short compared to both TI and T2. The strength of the FID will depend on the time between pulses (TR), the TI of the tissue and the flip angle of the pulse. With the use of appropriate dephasing gradients, the signal can be observed as a frequency-encoded gradient echo either shortly before the RF pulse or after it (*see* GRASS, FGR, FISP, FAST, GFEC, F-SHORT, DE-FGR, CE-FAST, True-FISP, PSIF, ROAST, T2-FEE, E-SHORT, STERE).

stability (*ct*) The maintenance over time of constancy of CT numbers and uniformity.

STAGE (*mri*) Small-tip-angle gradient echo (Shimadzu) (*see* FFE, GRE, MPGR, GRECO, FE, PFI, GE, TFF, SMASH, SHORT).

STAGE:T1W (*mri*) Small-tip-angle gradient echo. T1-weighted rapid gradient-echo imaging techniques, T1-weighted contrast (Shimadzu) (*see* FLASH, SPGR, FSPGR, HFGR, RE Spoiled, 3D-ME-RAGE, T1-FEE).

stainless steel (18Cr/8Ni) (*material*) High tensile strength metal alloy with magnetic properties consisting of cobalt, nickel and steel in various ratios. In general use for syringe needles and surgical instruments as well as machine construction.

Composition	(18Cr/8Ni)
Tensile strength	600
Density (ρ) kg/m³	7930
Melting point (K)	1800

standard breast (*mamm*) A model used for calculations of glandular dose consisting of a 40 mm thick central region comprising a 50 : 50 mixture by weight of adipose tissue and glandular tissue surrounded by a 5 mm thick superficial layer of adipose tissue. The standard breast is semicircular with a radius >80 mm and has a total thickness of 50 mm.

standard deviation σ (*stats*) A measure of sample dispersion. Square root of the variance. The first σ occupies an area 34% of the normal distribution, the second σ occupies 13% and the third σ 3%. Calculating the standard deviation is confused by two different formulas; the first using the divisor $n - 1$ and the second using the divisor n:

$$\sigma = \sqrt{\frac{1}{n-1}\Sigma(x - \bar{x})^2}$$

$$\sigma = \sqrt{\frac{1}{n}\Sigma(x - \bar{x})^2}$$

The formula using $n - 1$ is the most common.

standard error (*stats*) Also called the standard error of the mean. Due to random sampling error, chance variations cause the sample mean to be different from the population mean. The standard error σ_n is a measure of uncertainty of the mean figure, where:

$$\sigma_n = \frac{\sigma}{\sqrt{n}}$$

Standard error

From a large collection of mammograms 100 are measured for mean optical density (OD) which is 1.8 OD with a standard deviation of 0.5 OD. The degree of uncertainty is $0.5/\sqrt{100} = 0.05$. Two standard deviations would be $2 \times 0.05 = 0.1$ OD. So the true result would suggest that the population (complete collection) did not vary more than 0.1 OD from the mean.

---

standard ion dose J_s (*dose*) The ion dose produced in air by photon irradiation under conditions of electron equilibrium. The ICRU definition of exposure (*see* ion dose, cavity ion dose).

standard man (*dose*) The chemical composition of a standard 75 kg man has been estimated to be:

Element	Mass (kg)	Percent
Oxygen	45.5	65.0
Carbon	12.6	18.0
Hydrogen	7.0	10.0
Nitrogen	2.1	3.0
Calcium	1.05	1.5
Phosphorus	0.7	1.0
Sulphur	0.175	0.25
Potassium	0.140	0.2
Sodium	0.105	0.15
Chlorine	0.105	0.15
Magnesium	0.035	0.05
Iron	0.004	0.006
Copper	0.0001	0.0001
Iodine	0.00003	0.00004

The proportion of organ mass is:

Organ	Weight (kg)
Muscles	30.0
Skeleton	7.0
Marrow (red)	1.5
Marrow (yellow)	1.5
Blood	5.4
Gut	2.0
Fat	10.0
Lungs	1.0
Liver	1.7
Kidneys	0.3
Spleen	0.15
Pancreas	70 g
Thyroid	20 g
Testes	40 g
Heart	0.3
Lymph	0.7
Brain	1.5
Skin	6.1
Bladder	0.15
Other tissues	2184 g

These values are used for estimating organ dose (*see* MIRD schema).

standard phantom (*mamm*) A PMMA phantom to represent approximately the average breast (although not an exact tissue-substitute) so that the x-ray machine operates correctly under automatic exposure control and the dosemeter readings may be converted into dose to glandular tissue. The thickness is $45 \pm 0.5\,mm$ and the remaining dimensions are either rectangular $>150\,mm \times 100 \times mm$ or semicircular with a radius of $>100\,mm$.

standard temperature/pressure (*phys*) (STP) In order to make comparisons (i.e. relative density) many measurements are made at standard temperature and pressure (STP). The standard temperature is $298.15\,K$ ($25°C$) and the pressure is $10^5\,Pa$ (approximately $760\,mmHg$) (*see* temperature).

stannous chloride ($SnCl_2$) (*nmed*) A strong reducing agent used in most radiopharmaceutical labelling procedures involving ^{99m}Tc. Reducing Tc[VII] to Tc[IV] with the reaction:

$$Tc[VII] + Sn{+}{+} \rightarrow Tc[IV] + Sn{+}{+}{+}$$

star network (*comp*) Each networked PC is connected to a central controller, or hub, with its own piece of cable. Unlike bus networks, if a cable fails it will only affect the attached PC rather than the entire network.

star topology (*comp*) A network cabling configuration that uses a central connection point (called a hub), through which all communication must pass.

statistical efficiency (*stats*) When comparing different statistical methods for computing the same parameter, the method returning the lowest variance is judged to be the most efficient. To compare two analytical designs, the relative efficiency of one design compared to the other is a ratio (usually as a percentage) of the variances resulting from the two designs.

stator (*xray*) The external winding surrounding the rotor section which completes the induction motor (*see* rotor).

STD bus (*comp*) A small rugged bus design, originally 8 bits but has been increased to 16 and 32 bits.

STE (*mri*) Stimulated echo. generic term steady state develops for both transverse and longitudinal components of magnetization to refer to this sequence when the SE/STE is sampled (GE Medical).

steady state (*nmed*) Maintaining a constant delivery of tracer material (liquid or gas) in order to represent the dynamic function of an organ in a single image. The material must be prevented from recirculating so that background activity is kept as near zero as practical. This is achieved by using nuclides with a very short half life. ^{81m}Krypton (T½ 13 s) for steady state lung studies and in aqueous solution for cardiac studies; ^{195m}Au (T½ 30 s) for venous flow.

steady state free precession (SSFP) (*mri*) A technique for excitation where strings of RF pulses are applied with short TR times. The strength of the FID will depend on TR, the T1 of the tissue and the flip angle. Signal strength will also depend on the tissue T2. To avoid SSFP it may be necessary to use RF spoiling.

STEAM (*mri*) Stimulated echo acquisition mode. A single voxel MR spectroscopy pulse train consisting of three mutually orthogonal 90° section-select pulses. The sequence of choice for short TE spectroscopy.

steel (shielding) (*chem*) Mild steel sheet with 1% carbon can be used for shielding having a density of $7900\,kg\,m^{-3}$. Old steel (manufactured prior to 1945) is not contaminated with tiny quantities of radionuclide (^{60}Co) used in the quality control processes of modern steel manufacture. This old

S

steel can be used in low background counting systems:

Thickness (mm)	Weight (kg m⁻²)	Pb-equivalent (mm Pb)
11	87	1.0
23	182	2.0

(see stainless steel).

stem cells (*dose*) Cells capable of self renewal and of differentiation to produce all the cells in a particular lineage (white and red blood cells). Non-differentiated, pluripotent cell, capable of unlimited cell division.

STEP (*mri*) Stimulated echo progressive imaging. TI-weighted variant of RARE.

step and shoot (*nmed*) As opposed to continuous rotation where the camera stops at each angular projection and acquires data. The gamma camera indexes around the patient, (stops to collect counts over a fixed time), then moves to the next projection and collects count data. It progresses around the patient until a full 360° (or 180°) data set has been collected.

step response (*di*) A companion to the impulse response. The step response displays characteristic of the bandpass filter then settles to a d.c. value. Useful for characterizing a system.

steradian (*unit*) The solid angle of a cone (Ω) defined as the ratio of the area F of the surface of a sphere cut by a cone whose apex coincides with the centre M of the sphere to the square of the radius. $\Omega = F/r^2$. Its value describes the efficiency of a 4π detector (dose calibrator) or the isotropic dispersion of radiation from a point source (see radian, geometry 4π).

STERE (*mri*) Steady-state technique with refocused free induction decay steady-state free precession commonly used for imaging cerebrospinal fluid (Shimadzu) (see SSFP, DE-FGR, CE-FAST, True-FISP, PSIF, ROAST, T2-FEE, E-SHORT).

STERF (*mri*) Steady-state refocused free induction decay (Shimadzu); resembling PSIF.

sterility (*dose*) A deterministic effect in the male. Temporary sterility is observed for a single exposure of approximately 150 mGy. Permanent sterility for a dose between 3.5 and 6 Gy.

stiffness (*us*) Property of a medium; applied pressure divided by the fractional volume change produced by the pressure. The resistance of a material to compression. Sound propogation in a solid medium increases with stiffness.

STILL (*mri*) Flow/motion compensation Elscint. Reduction of motion-induced phase shifts during TE (see GMR, GMN, FLOW-COMP, CFAST, MAST, FLAG, GMC, FC, SMART, GR).

stimulated echo (*mri*) A form of spin echo produced by three-pulse RF sequences, consisting of two RF pulses following an initial exciting RF pulse. The stimulated echo appears at a time after the third pulse which equals the interval between the first two pulses. Commonly produced with 90° RF pulses others can produce a stimulated echo (except 180°). The echo signal strength is associated with T1 relaxation time since the excitation is stored as longitudinal magnetization between the second and third RF pulses. The use of stimulated echoes with spatially selective excitation with orthogonal magnetic field gradients permits volume-selective excitation for spectroscopic localization.

STIR (*mri*) Short TI inversion recovery. A pulse sequence to eliminate the fat signal using differences in T1 (T-one). It uses a modified IR sequence, the fat signal (having a short T1) can be maintained at the zero crossing point and so is not visible (see FATSAT, inversion recovery).

stochastic (*stats*) An entirely random process. There is no threshold, having a linear response to the incidence of damage (cancer induction) for all radiation exposures and giving a normal distribution.

stochastic effect (*dose*) (*ICRP60*) A linear or curvilinear response to low doses of radiation where the incidence of cellular transformation to radiation has no threshold. The probability of which, rather than their severity, is a function of radiation dose without threshold. Examples would be leukaemia, breast and colon cancer. Somatic or hereditary effects which may start from a single cell. Excess number of malignancies in a population has been observed above 200 mSv with a probable increase at 50 mSv (see deterministic effect (tissue reactions)).

stokes (*unit*) A non-SI (c.g.s.) unit of kinematic viscosity.

Stokes, Sir George Gabriel (1819–1903) An Irish physicist and mathematician. Work on light spectroscopy, identified x-rays as electromagnetic rays, formulated Stokes' Law for the frictional force moving in a viscous medium. He also established a law describing that the radiation emitted in fluorescence is always greater than the input (exciting) radiation.

S

stop-band filter (*image*) The stop band filter the frequencies should be suppressed with a maximum amplitude of δ2. A signal filter which rejects a narrow band of frequencies. Examples would be rejection of interference from mains supply frequency. The width of the transition in the diagram determines how fast the filter changes. In the pass-band the transfer function should be one within a tolerance of δ1 (*see* Kaiser window).

storage (bulk) (*comp*) Refers to storage devices other than the computer main memory where high speed access is not required. Usually magnetic disk, optical disk or magnetic tape. These can be fixed or removable devices.

Storage device	Capacity (M-bytes)	Access time	Data transfer (byte s^{-1})
Hard disk	100 GB–1 TB	10–20 ms	2.4 MBps
Flash	4–64 GB	100–450 ms	10–60 MBps (375 MBps)
Optical	400–650	150 ms	V. slow
DVD	17 GB	150 ms	V. slow
DAT	4 GB	Slowest	Slowest
RAM	120–300	15–100 ns	10–250 MBps

STP (*comp*) Shielded twisted pair. A thin-diameter network wire, wrapped with a metal sheath for extra protection against electrical interference. Most installations use a superior data-grade. Shielded twisted pair (STP) wiring is wrapped in an extra layer of sheathing for better shielding against electrical noise, offering high-speed transmission. Category 5 wire supports 100 Mbps data over UTP and STP; Category 4 wire supports 20 Mbps data over UTP and STP; and Category 3 wire supports 16 Mbps data over UTP and STP.

STREAM (*mri*) Suppressed tissue with refreshment angiography method.

stress relieved anode (*xray*) Large anode disc diameters increase the heat capacity and also the area radiating heat, however, there is potential mechanical damage due to localized expansion. This is prevented by cutting radial slots into the anode; these are stress relieved anodes.

strontium (Sr) (*elem*)

Atomic number (Z)	38
Relative atomic mass (A_r)	87.62
Density (ρ) kg/m^3	2600
Melting point (K)	1042
K-edge (keV)	16.1

^{82}Strontium (*nmed*) The parent nuclide for generating ^{82}Rubidium, a positron emitter for positron emission tomography (PET).

Production (cyclotron)	$^{80}_{36}$Kr (d, 3pn) $^{82}_{38}$Sr
Decay scheme (e.c.)	^{82}Sr → ^{82}Rb T½ 75 s
^{82}Sr/^{82}Rb Generator	(β+) → ^{82}Kr stable
Half life	25 days
Half value layer	7 mm Pb

Days	Fraction remaining
1	0.973
5	0.871
10	0.758
15	0.660
20	0.574

^{85}Strontium (*nmed*) 514 keV T½ 64.7 days
^{89}Strontium (*nmed*)

Production	$^{88}_{38}$Sr(n,γ)$^{89}_{38}$Sr
Decay scheme (β$^-$)	
^{89}Sr	^{89}Sr T½ 51d (β−583, γ 909 keV) → ^{89}Y stable
Decay constant	0.01372 d^{-1}
Photons	pure β− 1.46 MeV

Generic name	^{89}Strontium
Commercial names	Metastron
Non-imaging category	Palliative treatment of bone pain

^{90}Strontium (*nmed*)

Production	^{235}U (n,f)^{90}Sr
Decay scheme (β$^-$)	
^{90}Sr	^{90}Sr (b2) → ^{90}Y T½ 2.7d (b2) ^{90}Zr stable
Decay constant	0.02423 y^{-1}
Photons	Pure β− 546 keV
Uses: Palliative therapy of bony metastases.	

structured noise artefact (*ct*) The main components of structured noise are due mostly to partial volume artefact and beam hardening. Both display streaking artefacts which are seen in regions of high contrast when a sharp discontinuity in object density, (air-tissue, tissue-bone or metal-tissue boundaries). Structured noise artefact will also arise from mechanical misalignment within the scanner and patient movement; it is also seen when using high-density contrast media.

stunned myocardium (*clin*) *See* myocardium (stunned).

subject contrast (*image*) Factors influencing the emerging x-ray beam and film exposure. The x-axis on the film characteristic.

subtraction (DSA) (*image*) The essential requirement for DSA is that the contrast signal corresponds linearly with the concentration of the contrast material. Direct subtraction will produce an image dependant on overlying structures (bone) so non-linear subtraction methods are available:

- logarithmic;
- hybrid/dual energy.

Logarithmic subtraction ensures an artery of uniform diameter traversing regions of mixed tissue type of varying thickness, appears with uniform contrast. It relies on the Beer–Lambert law for radiation absorption. The logarithm of the signals is obtained prior to subtraction so:

$$I_t = I_o \cdot e^{-\mu_t \cdot x_t} \quad \text{and} \quad I_c = I_o \cdot e^{-(\mu_t \cdot x_t + \mu_v \cdot x_v)}$$

where I_o is incident fluence; I_t is transmitted intensity before contrast; I_c is transmitted intensity after contrast; μ_t is tissue attenuation coefficient; x_t is tissue thickness; μ_v is iodine attenuation coefficient; and x_v is vessel thickness. Direct subtraction of the transmitted intensities I_s is not independent of overlying tissue but dependent on incident fluence I_o thus:

$$I_s = I_c - I_t = I_o \cdot e^{-(\mu_t \cdot x_t + \mu_v \cdot x_v)} - e^{-\mu_t \cdot x_t}$$

However, subtracting the logarithms of the transmission:

$$I_s = \log(I_c) - \log(I_t)$$
$$= -(\mu_t \cdot x_t + \mu_v \cdot x_v) - (-\mu_t \cdot x_t) = \mu_t \cdot x_t$$

The logarithmic subtraction does not retain stationary anatomical information. The display is not influenced by patient size or tissue type and only shows thickness and attenuation coefficient of the contrast medium. Hybrid/dual energy: Artefacts caused by involuntary motion (gut peristalsis or cardiac motion) can be suppressed by dual energy subtraction since μ differences of gas or soft tissue change little between energies. The decrease for bone is much greater between energies (typically 60 and 110 kVp).

		Bone	Tissue	Iodine
Mask				
M_L	kV_{low}	++	+	zero
M_H	kV_{high}	+	+	zero
Contrast image				
C_L	kV_{low}	++	+	++
C_H	kV_{high}	+	+	++

Subtracting low and high kV masks leaves a pre-contrast mask: $M_L - M_H \rightarrow M_B$ (bone image). During the contrast phase low and high kV images are subtracted to yield:

$$C_L - C_H \rightarrow C_{(B+V)}$$

Finally, the dual energy mask is subtracted to give the iodine contrast vessels alone:

$$C_{(B+V)} - M_B \rightarrow C_{(V)}$$

Hybrid subtraction combines dual energy and temporal subtraction to remove overlying bone together with movement artefacts.

succimer (DMSA) (*nmed*) *See* DMSA.

Sulesomab (*nmed*) Monoclonal antibody LeucoScan® (Immunomedics).

sulphur/sulfur (S) (*elem*)

Atomic number (Z)	16
Relative atomic mass (A$_r$)	32.06
Density (ρ) kg/m^3	2070
Melting point (K)	386
K-edge (keV)	2.4

[35]**Sulphur/sulfur** (*elem*) As a tracer label for proteins in autoradiography.

Production (reactor)	^{34}S (n,γ) ^{35}S
Half life	87 d
Decay mode	β− 167 keV
Decay constant	0.00796 d^{-1}
Photons	Pure beta decay

sulphur/sulfur colloid (*nmed*) *See* colloid.

sulphur/sulfur hexafluoride (*cm*) Inert gas used as an ultrasound contrast agent.

sum peak (*nmed*) A photopeak-like feature of a PMT pulse-height spectrum that corresponds to the simultaneous photoelectric absorption in a scintillation detector crystal of two or more primary unscattered, gamma emissions of a radionuclide.

SUP/PPP (*comp*) Serial line interface protocol/point to point protocol. These are both standards for connecting directly to the Internet, as opposed to having to log on to it via a host computer.

superconductor (*mri*) A substance whose electrical resistance essentially disappears at temperatures near absolute zero. A commonly used superconductor in NMR imaging system magnets is niobium-titanium, embedded in a copper matrix to help protect the superconductor from quenching.

superconducting magnet (*mri*) *See* magnet (superconducting).

super-paramagnetic (*mri*) T2 or T2* contrast agents; have unpaired electrons in their outer orbital shell, which gives them magnetic susceptibility. When these compounds are placed in an applied magnetic field, a positive magnetic moment is induced resulting in an attractive force. Originally ferromagnetic substances which have a very small size and thus have lost their permanent magnetism. Also known as bulk susceptibility agents.

super scan (*nmed*) Applied to bone scintiscans where there is a diffuse and uniform increase in ^{99m}Tc-bone agent (HMDP, MDP) throughout the skeleton. There is generally a lack of focal activity.

superficial (*us*) (as used with the musculoskeletal application) Structures located at a depth of 1.5 cm or less.

superior mesenteric arteriography (*clin*) Radiography of the superior mesenteric artery demonstrating the vascular supply to the small bowel and the right side of the large bowel.

superior vena cavography (*clin*) Angiography of the superior vena cava performed either by femoral venous approach into the proximal superior vena cava or by contrast medium injection into one or both median cubital arm veins.

supervised area (*dose*) (*ICRP73*) The control of occupational exposure in medicine can be simplified by the designation of workplaces into controlled areas and supervised areas. A supervised area is one where the working conditions are reviewed but special procedures are not normally needed and there is very little danger of exposure. Commonly defined in the department's local rules as an area where dose rates exceed 1/10 but are less than 3/10 of any maximum.

suppression (*mri*) One of a number of techniques designed to minimize the contribution of a particular component of the object to the detected signal. For example, commonly used to suppress the strong signal from water in order to detect spectral Tine from other components.

surface area (body) (*clin*) The surface area of a disk is: $2\pi r \times (h + r)$ where r is disk radius and h is disk height; its volume is $\pi r^2 h$ so surface area varies in proportion with volume. The surface area of a sphere is $4\pi r^2$ whereas its volume is $4/3\pi r^3$ so surface area and volume alters disproportionately. This is variation is incorporated into the formula for body surface area where W is body weight and H height: $W^{0.425} \times H^{0.725} \times 0.0072 \, m^2$ (*see* body surface area).

surface coil (*mri*) A localized receiver coil that does not surround the body. Placed close to the surface over a region of interest having a selectivity for a volume approximately subtended by the coil circumference and one radius deep. Used to restrict the region of the body contributing to the detected signal. Only the region close to the surface coil will contribute to the noise, there will be an improvement in the signal-to-noise ratio for regions close to the coil compared to the use of general receiver coils that surround the body. A surface coil used for localization measurements of chemical shift spectra and blood flow studies.

surface rendered (*image*) or surfaced shaded reconstruction. A method of 3D image reconstruction that simulates reflected light/shade, so conveying depth relationships. Threshold dependent. Does not give attenuation information or depict calcification (*see* maximum intensity projection).

surface-shaded reconstruction (SSR) (*image*) or surface rendered. A method of 3D image reconstruction that simulates reflected light/shade, so conveying depth relationships. Threshold dependent. Does not give attenuation information or depict calcification; the most commonly used 3D images are surface-shaded reconstructions (SSR) and maximum-intensity projection (MIP). These have differing features. Generally, several 3D reconstructions are made at regular angular increments around a given axis. These can then be viewed in sequence to give more information, for example about vessel origins:

- simulates reflected light/shade;
- conveys depth relationships;

- threshold dependent;
- does not give attenuation;
- does not depict calcification;
- editing not always necessary.

surge protector (*comp*) A filter that protects a computer from surge spikes and smoothes variations in voltage (*see* UPS).

survey (*nmed*) (*see* radiation protection survey). Survey meter: a device for monitoring the dose rate in an area.

survey meter (*nmed*) Ionization chamber used to survey the exposure rate in radiation areas.

survey radiograph (*ct*) *See* scan projection radiograph.

survival curve *See* dose survival curve.

susceptibility (*mri*) *See* magnetic susceptibility.

susceptibility artefact (*mri*) At interfaces between tissues of different magnetic susceptibility (e.g. tissue and air) the local magnetic field becomes inhomogeneous setting up a local field gradient causing signal dephasing (signal loss) and spatial misregistration. FLASH and FISP sequences frequently show this in different muscle groups and air voids in temporal bone.

SVS procedure (*mri*) *See* Single volume spectroscopy (SVS).

swap file (*comp*) Also known as virtual memory. A part of the hard disk is used exclusively as cache memory (Windows) to speed up transfers between memory and disk.

swept gain (*us*) *See* time gain compensation (TGC)

Swick, M. American physician who first published a series of intravenous urograms in 1929 using iodides of pyridine for excretory urography, leading to the development of Hypaque, Renografin and Conray.

switch (*comp*) An intelligent hub that reads the destination addresses of incoming data packets and only sends them to the port where the recipient is physically attached.

switchable coil (*mri*) An RF array coil consisting of several separately resonant elements, any one of which can be selected as the receiver coil at a particular time. Coils not in use are decoupled. Applications of switchable coils include imaging the whole spine without patient repositioning (where the coil elements may collectively be known as a ladder coil), imaging of bilateral structures, such as TMJ or orbit using separate coils. or imaging using a coil with selectable field-of-view.

switching (*comp*) The process by which packets are received, stored and transmitted to the appropriate destination port.

synchronization (cardiac) (*mri*) Acquiring images of particular phases of the cardiac cycle, through either retrospective or prospective synchronization. Also sometimes called cardiac gating.

synchronization (prospective) (*mri*) Controlling the timing or sequence of image data acquisition according to the phase of respiratory or cardiac cycles.

synchronization (retrospective) (*mri*) Sorting and possibly adjusting image data acquired asynchronously with the cardiac or respiratory cycle, according to the phase of the cycle at which it was acquired so as to reconstruct a set of images corresponding to different phases of the cycle.

synchronization (respiratory) (*mri*) The respiratory phase can be used to control imaging either by only acquiring the image data during a particular portion of the respiratory cycle (which increases image acquisition time) or by adjusting the sequence of image data collection according to the phase of the respiratory cycle in such a way as to minimize motion-induced artefacts in the reconstructed image.

synchronous transmission (*comp*) Data transmission between stations in synchrony. Data are transmitted in continuous stream (*see* asynchronous transmission).

synthetic aperture (*us*) Digital beam former technology used to improve spatial resolution by synthetically enlarging the receiving aperture. Optimal lateral focus in echo signals originating from deep regions is obtained by using the full width of the transducer array. Synthetic aperture technology is applied to the total area of the transducer array which is divided into sub-apertures processed sequentially. Synthetically enlarged apertures increase transducer sensitivity and lateral resolution in deep body regions but at reduced frame rates.

syringe/vial shielding (*nmed*) A cylinder made of lead-containing glass absorbs radiation emitted from radioactive material in a syringe, thereby reducing the radiation dose to personnel. Lead or tungsten syringe shields of approximately 3 mm thickness reduce finger and body doses by approximately $\times 200$ from syringe activities. The dose rate from an unshielded vial containing 4 GBq (100 mCi) ^{99m}Tc would be 800 μSv h^{-1}

S

at 30 cm; the suggested shielding is based on an HVL of 0.25 mm Pb (140 keV). Maintaining a surface dose level of 7.5 μSv h⁻¹ would require 1.67 mm Pb. A typical vial lead-pot supplies 3 to 10 mm.

system characteristic curve (*image*) Curve that relates a system input value to the corresponding system output value (e.g. an optical density versus exposure curve for a film detector, or a grey level versus optical density curve for a digitizer).

system (*comp*) Anything that accepts an input and produces an output in response.

system axis (*ct*) *See* axis of rotation.

system resolution (*nmed*) *See* resolution (extrinsic).

Système International (SI) (*phys*) The 10th and 14th General Conference on Weights and Measures (1954, 1971) agreed seven independent base units for:

Quantity	Dimensions
Length	metre (m)
Mass	kilogram (kg)
Time	second (s)
Electric current intensity	ampere (A)
Thermodynamic temp	kelvin (K)
Amount of substance	mole (mol)
Luminous intensity	candela (cd)

Derived SI units are formed by combination of powers of base units, e.g. the SI unit of energy as $m^2 kg\, s^{-2}$ is the joule (J), the newton metre (Nm) or the volt ampere second (VAs). Supplementary units are the plane angle as the radian (rad) and the solid angle as the steradian (sr).

Derived units (SI)	Dimensions	non-SI unit
Area	m^2	cm^2
Volume	m^3	cm^3
Force (newton N)	$kg\,m\,s^{-2}$	dyne
Pressure (pascal P)	$N\,m^{-2}$	$dyne\,cm^{-2}$
Density (ρ)	$kg\,m^{-3}$	$g\,cm^{-3}$
Work/Energy (joule J)	$kg\,m^2 s^{-2}$	Erg
Speed (c)	$m\,s^{-1}$	
Linear velocity	$m\,s^{-1}$	$cm\,s^{-1}$
Angular velocity	$rad\,s^{-1}$	
Acceleration	$m\,s^{-2}$	$cm\,s^{-2}$
Momentum	$kg\,m\,s^{-1}$	$g\,cm\,s^{-1}$
Angular momentum	$kg\,m^2 s^{-1}$	$g\,cm^2 s^{-1}$
Moment of inertia	$kg\,m^2$	$g\,cm^2$
Electric charge (coulomb C)	$A\,s$	

Systeme International SI *(Contd.)*

Derived units (SI)	Dimensions	non-SI unit
Electric conductance	siemens	
Electric capacitance	farad	
Power (watt W)	$J\,s^{-1}$	$erg\,s^{-1}$
Voltage (volt V)	$J\,C^{-1}$	
Resistance (ohm Ω)	$V\,A^{-1}$	
Thermal conductivity	$W\,m^{-1}\,K^{-1}$	
Frequency (hertz Hz)	s^{-1}	s^{-1}
Radioactivity (bequerel Bq)	s^{-1}	curie
Luminous flux (lumen lm)	cd sr	
Illuminance (lux)	$lm\,m^{-2}$	
Magnetic flux (weber Wb)	V s	
Magnetic flux density (tesla T)	$Wb\,m^{-2}$	
Inductance (henry H)	$Wb \cdot A^{-1}$	
Radiation dose (gray (Gy))	$J\,kg^{-1}$	
Surface tension	$dyne\,cm^{-1}$	$N\,m^{-1}$
Viscosity	$kg\,m^{-1}s^{-1}$	poise

Supplementary units (dimensionless)

Plane angle (Radian)	rad
Solid angle (Steradian)	sr

system magnification (*xray*) Depends on focus-to-film distance (FFD) and object-to-film distance (OFD). Geometrical unsharpness U_g increases if the focal spot remains the same. Dual focal spot tubes overcome this (mammography tubes having 0.4 and 0.1 mm FS).

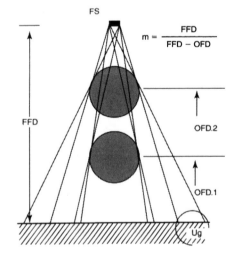

$$m = \frac{FFD}{FFD - OFD}$$

T

T-tube cholangiography (*clin*) Postoperative investigation when a T-tube is left *in situ* during surgery to exclude presence of calculi in the common bile duct.

T1 contrast (*mri*) Contrast of a T1-weighted image depends primarily on the various T1 time constants of the different tissue types.

T1 (*mri*) Longitudinal relaxation time. Returning to equilibrium after RF excitation. Also known as spin-lattice relaxation process. Measured by T1 relaxation time. T1 time is influenced by magnet field strength, spin mobility, paramagnetic agents. The standard indirect technique for measuring T1 uses a series of 90° pulses. The variation of T1 with magnet field.

Tissue	T1			T2
	0.5T	1.0T	1.5T	
Fat	210	240	260	80
Liver	350	420	500	40
Kidney	430	590	690	58
Muscle	550	730	870	45
Heart	570	750	880	57
White matter	500	680	780	90
Grey matter	650	810	900	100
CSF	1800	2160	2400	160

(*see* T2).

T1 FAST (*mri*) Fourier acquired steady state (T1-weighted).

T1–FEE (*mri*) Contrast-enhanced fast field echo rapid gradient-echo imaging techniques T1-weighted contrast (Philips) (*see* FLASH, SPGR, FSPGR, HFGR, RE spoiled, 3D-ME-RAGE, STAGE-T1W).

T1 TFE (*mri*) Contrast enhanced TFE (T1-weighted).

T1 weighting (*mri*) Pulse sequences with short TR (200–500 ms) and short TE (15–30 ms), often used to indicate an image where most of the contrast between tissues or tissue states is due to differences in tissue T1. A T1 contrast state is approached by imaging with a TR short compared to the longest tissue T1 of interest and TE short compared to tissue T2 (to reduce T2 contributions to image contrast). Due to the wide range of TI and T2, an image that is T1-weighted for some tissues may not be so for others.

Grey scale	Tissue
White	Fat
Light grey	Bone marrow
Dark grey	CSF
Black	Blood

Examples of T1-weighted pulse sequences are: FLASH, spoiled gradient recalled (SPGR) and RAGE.

T2 (*mri*) Spin-spin or transverse relaxation time, the characteristic time constant for loss of phase coherence among spins oriented at an angle to the static magnetic field due to interactions between the spins, with resulting loss of transverse magnetization and NMR signal starting from a non-zero value of the magnetization. In the xy plane, the xy magnetization will decay so that it loses 63% of its initial value in a time T2 if relaxation is characterized by a simple single exponential decay.

T2 constant (*mri*) Tissue-specific time constant. Describes the decay of transverse magnetization, taking into account the inhomogeneity in static magnetic fields and the human body. The contrast of a T2-weighted image depends primarily on the various T2 time constants of the different tissue types.

T2* (*mri*) The FID time constant influenced by loss of phase coherence among spins oriented at an angle to the static magnetic field. Influenced by a combination of magnetic field inhomogeneities and spin-spin relaxation with resultant more rapid loss in transverse magnetization and NMR signal. NMR signals can usually still be recovered as a spin echo in times less than or on the order of T2.

T2* constant (*mri*) Characteristic time constant always less than T2.

T2-FFE (*mri*) Contrast-enhanced fast field echo steady-state free precession commonly used for imaging of cerebrospinal fluid (Philips) (*see* SSFP, DE-FGR, CE-FAST, True-FISP, PSIF, ROAST, E-SHORT, STERE).

T2 PEDD (*mri*) T2 Proton electron dipole dipole interaction.

T2 PRE (*mri*) T2 Proton relaxation enhancement.

T2 weighting (*mri*) Pulse sequences that have long TR (2000–3000 ms) and long TE (100–200 ms), used to indicate an image where most of the contrast between tissues or tissue states is due to differences in tissue T2. A T2 contrast state is approached by imaging with a TR long compared to tissue T1 (to reduce T1 contribution to image contrast) and a TE between the longest and shortest tissue T2s of interest. A TR greater than 3 times the longest T1 is required for the T1 effect to be less than 5%. An image that is T2-weighted for some tissues may not be so for others.

Grey scale	Tissue
White	CSF
Light grey	Brain
Dark grey	Fat
Black	Blood

An example of a T2-weighted pulse sequence is FISP.

T2*-weighted (*mri*) The effective T2-weighting in a gradient-echo acquisition when magnetic field inhomogeneity effects are included. Short TR, 2D sequence (TR 5–10 ms) with a contrast controlling inversion-pulse preceding the usual 2D data collection, and a scan time on the order of 1 second.

table feed/increment (*ct*) The direction of the table travel between successive sequential scans or during spiral scanning; the direction of table feed coincides with the patient's longitudinal direction, and with the system's *z*-axis (if no gantry tilt is applied). For a given examination time t (s) and a given scan range R (mm) the desired table speed $T_s = R/t$ (mm per second). This can be obtained if the selected slice width S, pitch factor p, and the number of slices per rotation M are known:

$$T_s = \frac{p \cdot M \cdot S}{\text{rotation time}}$$

The capability of the most modern scanners to acquire several slices simultaneously, where M is 4 or greater, gives the advantage of being able to achieve thin slice volume date sets at high scan speeds (bolus chasing and breath hold). A larger table increment gives faster acquisition, but leads to a wider slice sensitivity profile (SSP) and consequently lowers resolution. The scan width specified by the operator is approximately equal to full width at half maximum of the SSP for one reconstructed image from the spiral volume data set.

TACE (*clin*) *See* transarterial chemoembolization.

TAD (*mri*) Duration of acquisition window (time of analogue to digital conversion).

tagging (*mri*) Spin tagging. A grid of saturation lines across the cardiac image in order to view myocardial motion. Stripe tagging: Parallel stripes for viewing myocardial motion in primary axis view or four-chamber view.

tailored excitation (*mri*) *See* selective excitation.

tailored pulse (*mri*) Shaped pulse whose magnitude (and possibly phase) is varied with time in a predetermined manner. Affects the frequency components of an RE pulse in a manner determined by the Fourier transform of the pulse.

tank unit (*ct*) Contains the high frequency transformers and control electronics small enough to be located on the rotation gantry. It receives its low voltage power supply (200–300 V) from the slip ring assembly. This construction adds considerable mass to the already heavy rotational stage, which contains the high-power-tube housing and related components (*see* centripetal acceleration).

tantalum (Ta) (*elem*)

Atomic number (Z)	73
Relative atomic mass (A$_r$)	180.95
Density (ρ) kg/m^3	16 600
Melting point (K)	3269
Specific heat capacity J kg^{-1}K^{-1}	140
Thermal conductivity W m^{-1}K^{-1}	57.5
K-edge (keV)	67.4

Relevance to radiology: as a shielding material and in the construction of collimators. Yttrium tantalate is used as scintillants for intensifying screens.

^{178}Tantalum

Production	
Half life	9 min
Decay mode	Useful x-rays
Decay constant	0.077 min^{-1}
Photon	x-rays
55–65 keV	

Uses: ^{178}W generator (T½ 28 d) produced ^{178m}Ta has been used for imaging the blood pool (low dose paediatric imaging).

target (x-ray) (*xray*) The angled periphery on the anode that is bombarded by the electron beam. Since useful x-rays originate from 100 to 500 μm of the metal surface depth; the target thickness is reduced to approximately 1 mm thick. Dual targets are placed concentrically, each having a different angle.

target OD (*mamm*) The optical density (OD) at the reference point of a routine exposure, chosen by the local staff as the optimal value, typically in the range 1.3 to 1.8 OD, including base and fog.

target organ (*dose*) The organ receiving most activity. The thyroid is the target organ for iodine radionuclides and ^{99m}Tc; for labelled complex phosphates the target organ is bone.

target region (*dose*) Region in which radiation is absorbed. This may be an organ, a tissue, the contents of the gastrointestinal tract or urinary bladder, or the surfaces of tissues as in the skeleton and the respiratory tract.

TCP/IP *(comp)* Transmission control protocol/ Internet protocol. This is the standard governing communication between all computers on the Internet. TCP/IP works by sending packets of information across multiple networks.

TD *(mri)* Difference in time of formation of RE spin echo (TER) and gradient echo (GRE).

TDMA *(comp)* Time division multiple access. A second generation European mobile cellular radio technology which has now been adopted in some 100 countries. TDMA operates by dividing a single radiofrequency into time slots allocating these to multiple calls. A single transmission frequency can support multiple simultaneous data channels. Three non-compatible mobile wireless protocols are GSM, TDMA and CDMA.

TE *(mri)* Time to echo; the time between middle of 90° RF exciting pulse and middle of spin echo production. For multiple echoes TE1 and TE2 etc. are used. When the RF spin echo and gradient echo are not coincident in time, TE refers to the time of the gradient spin echo.

TE$_{eff}$ *(mri) See* effective echo time.

teboroxime *(nmed)* Generic name ^{99m}Tc-teboroxime for Cardiotec®, a myocardial perfusion agent.

Teceos® *(nmed)* CIS/Schering preparation of DPD; a bone agent for ^{99m}Tc labelling.

Technegas® *(nmed)* A commercial radio-aerosol used for ventilation lung scintigraphy. The aerosol is manufactured by vaporizing an aliquot of ^{99m}TcO$_4$ in a graphite crucible.

TechneScan-PYP® *(nmed)* A kit for the preparation of ^{99m}Tc-pyrophosphate (Mallinckrodt); a diagnostic skeletal imaging agent used to demonstrate areas of altered osteogenesis in adults and children. Also used for cardiac imaging.

technetium (Tc) *(elem)*

Atomic number (Z)	43
Relative atomic mass (A$_r$)	99
Density (ρ) kg/m³	11 400
Melting point (K)	2500 K
K-edge (keV)	21.0

Relevance to radiology: exclusively as ^{99m}Tc metastable isotope.

^{99m}Technetium Decays by isomeric transition with a physical T½ of 6.02 hours. Widespread use in scintigraphy.

Production (generator)	^{99}Mo/^{99}Tc
Decay scheme (i.t.) ^{99m}Tc	^{99m}Tc (γ 140 keV) →^{99}Tc
	T½ 2.13 × 10^{5}y
Half life	6.02 hr
Decay constant	0.11492 h^{-1}
Photon (abundance)	18–21 keV (0.077)
	140.5 keV (0.879)
Gamma ray constant	1.7 × 10^{-2} mSv hr^{-1} GBq^{-1} @1 m
Half value layer	0.25 mm Pb
	45 mm H$_2$O

Uses: generator produced ^{99m}Tc is the most common nuclide for nuclear medicine imaging.

Radiation attenuation coefficient for 140 keV:

Shield thickness (mm Pb)	Attenuation coefficient
0.17	0.5
0.8	10^{-1}
1.6	10^{-2}
2.5	10^{-3}
3.3	10^{-4}

Physical decay for ^{99m}Tc T½ 6.02 hr:

Hours	Fraction remaining	Hours	Fraction remaining
0	1.000	8	0.398
1	0.891	9	0.355
2	0.794	10	0.316
3	0.708	11	0.282
4	0.631	12	0.251
5	0.562		
6	0.501		
7	0.447		

(see 99Mo/99mTc generator).

^{99}Technetium *(nmed)* The decay product of ^{99m}Tc; also as a reactor fission product:

Production (fission)	$^{235}_{92}$U (n,f) $^{99}_{43}$Tc (+$^{134}_{49}$In)
Decay scheme	^{99}Tc T½ 2.13 × 10^{5}y
(beta decay) ^{99}Tc	(β−292 keV) →^{99}Ru stable.
Decay constant	3.253 E−6y^{-1}
Photon	Very weak gamma β−293 keV

Technegas™ *(nmed)* A commercial radio-aerosol used for ventilation lung scintigraphy. The aerosol is manufactured by vapourizing an aliquot of ^{99m}TcO$_4$ in a graphite crucible.

Teflon™ (PTFE) *(mat)* Product registered by DuPont. Polyterafluoroethylene. Extremely low coefficient of friction.

Density (ρ) kg/m³	2200
Melting point (K)	600

Relevance to radiology: General bearing surface or insulator.

teleconferencing (*comp*) Communication by vision and sound on a LAN, WAN or Internet using a compatible modem and video camera. Image compression (MPEG) allows almost real time viewing of video movements.

Telebrix[x] (*cm*) Preparation of 66% meglumine ioxithalamate (Guerbet). Ionic monomer.

Compound	Viscosity (cP)	Osmolality (mOsm/kg)	Iodine (mg I/mL)
Meglumine ioxithalamate	5.2	@ 37° 1500	300

Telepaque[x] (*cm*) Generic name iopanoic acid. A monomeric hepatobiliary x-ray contrast material for oral use (*see* cholegraphic contrast agents).

tele-radiology (*comp*) Transmitting and receiving diagnostic images (radiographs, MRI, ultrasound etc.) between workstations that are networked by LAN or WAN. This is an important part of a PACS design and systems in the design should be DICOM compatible.

tellurium (Te) (*elem*)

Atomic number (Z)	52
Relative atomic mass (A_r)	127.60
Density (ρ) kg/m³	6240
Melting point (K)	722.6
K-edge (keV)	31.8

temperature (*phys*) The base SI unit of thermodynamic temperature is the kelvin (K) defined as the fraction 1/273.16 of the triple point of water (where solid, liquid and gaseous phases are in equilibrium). Absolute zero is 0K. The gas laws play an important academic role in the derivation of the SI scale for temperature. The increase in volume per unit volume of gas at 0°C per °C rise in temperature keeping pressure constant forms a volume coefficient a:

$$\frac{\text{Increase in volume from 0°C}}{\text{Original volume at 0°C} \times \text{Temperature rise}}$$

This is a constant whose measurement indicates that a value of 3.6609×10^{-3} or $1/273.15°C^{-1}$ for all gases. Charles' Law states that a given mass of gas increases by 1/273.15 of its volume at 0°C for every degree rise in temperature at constant pressure. The magnitude of one degree kelvin is identical with 1° Celsius. Standard temperature is the ice point of water 0°C or 273.15 K and 100°C = 373.15 K. Three temperature scales have been used for measuring change in heat output:

- Celsius or centigrade: 0°C is melting ice and 100°C is boiling water both at normal pressure $10^5\,N\,m^{-2}$;
- Fahrenheit (now discontinued in Europe);
- The kelvin is the SI unit and its derivation has been given from the gas laws stated above. Zero degrees Kelvin (0 K) is absolute zero ($-273.15°C$).

Temperature conversion from Fahrenheit T_f to Celsius Tc uses a polynomial function where:

$$T_f = \tfrac{9}{5}(T_c + 32) \text{ and } T_c = \tfrac{5}{9}(T_f - 32)$$

Since Celsius and Kelvin scales have the same magnitude, conversion is simply $T_c = T_k - 273.15$:

Physical state	¡F	¡C	K
Absolute zero	−460	−273.15	0
Freezing point water	32	0	273.15
Boiling point water	212	100	373.15

(*see* standard temperature/pressure).

temporal average intensity (I_{TA}) (*us*) Time averaged intensity for the period that the transducer is used:

duty factor × pulse average intensity

It is the intensity of the entire pulse train averaged over time. If the PRF of the transducer is high then I_{TA} will be high and vice versa. If the ultrasound is continuous (CW Doppler) then pulse average = I_{TA}. The time average of intensity at a point in space. For non-autoscan systems, the average is taken over one or more pulse repetition periods; intensity of the entire pulse train over a stated time (time of image frame) as:

$$I_{TA} = \frac{\text{total power per frame}}{\text{frame duration}}$$

For autoscan systems, the intensity is averaged over one or more scan repetition periods for a specified operating mode. For autoscan modes, the average includes contributions from adjacent lines that overlap the point of measurement. For combined modes the average includes overlapping lines, from all constituent discrete operating mode signals. The unit is milliwatt per square-centimeter, mW cm^{-2}. Typical values are given under ultrasound (intensity).

temporal peak intensity (I_{TP}) (*us*) The highest intensity of the pulse. The peak intensity within each pulse of the ultrasound imaging system is the temporal peak; the average intensity over each pulse is the pulse average (PA). Measured as Watt per square-centimeter, $W\,cm^{-2}$

temporal resolution (*image*) Ability to distinguish closely spaced events in time; improves with increased frame rate.

tensor (*math*) An extension of vector quantities into a matrix array of components (usually in orders of two or more dimensions in space); describes anisotropic distributions. A tensor of order zero is a scalar; a tensor of order 1 is a vector (*see* diffusion tensor imaging).

   ■ Reference: Daintith and Nelson, 2003.

TER (*mri*) Time of formation of RE spin echo when adjusted to be different from gradient spin echo.

terabytes (TB) (*comp*) A thousand gigabytes (10^{12} bytes), 1000 GB (*see* byte, kilobyte).

teraflop (*comp*) A measure of a computer's speed. It can be expressed as a trillion floating-point operations per second (10^{12}).

teratogenesis (*nmed*) The production of physical defects in offspring *in utero*.

terbium (Tb) (*elem*)

Atomic number (Z)	65
Relative atomic mass (A$_r$)	158.92
Density (ρ) kg/m³	8300
Melting point (K)	1629
K-edge (keV)	51.9
Relevance to radiology: as a dopant for gadolinium intensifying screens.	

terboroxime (*nmed*) Myocardial imaging agent, marketed as Cardiotec® (Bracco Diagnostics) for labelling with ^{99m}Tc (*see* Cardiolite®, sestamibi).

Tesla, Nikola (1856–1943) Croatian/American physicist and electrical engineer. Worked with both Edison and Westinghouse. Developed AC electricity as a power source obtaining patents on a poly-phase (3-phase) system and also predicted wireless communication two years before Marconi.

tesla (T) (*unit*) A magnetic field of 1T will produce a force of one newton (1 N) on each metre of conductor carrying 1 A at 90° to the field, so $1\,T = 1\,Nm^{-1}$ at 90° to the field. $10\,mTm^{-1} = 1$ gauss cm^{-1}, also $1\,T = 1\,Wb\,m^{-2}$.

Teslascan® (*cm*) (Nycomed Amersham/GE Healthcare Inc). Preparation of manganese based trisodium salt of mangafodipir; the chelating agent fodipir with manganese ion as a paramagnetic agent.

Compound	Concentration (mg mL^{-1})	Viscosity (cP)	Osmolality (mOsm/kg)
Mangafodipir	37.9	0.8@37°	298

test object (*qc*) A device without tissue-like properties that is designed to measure some characteristic of an imaging system (*see* phantom).

test phantom (*qc*) Object of particular shape, size and structure (including standardized representations of human form), used for the purposes of calibration and evaluation of performance of CT scanners (*see* CTDI, MIRD, body phantom).

tetramethylsilane (*mri*) A reference compound for measuring chemical shifts. Tetramethylsilane is assigned a value of 0 parts per million (ppm); other compounds have chemical shifts greater than 0.

tetrofosmin (*nmed*) Chemically [6,9,-bis(2-ethoxy-ethyl)-3,12-dioxa-6,9-diphosphatetradecane]. Indicated for myocardial scintigraphy at rest and exercise. The radiopharmaceutical kit consists of tetrafosmin which is reconstituted with sodium (^{99m}Tc) pertechnetate to yield ^{99m}Tc-tetrofosmin (Myoview®). Since it is concentrated in mitochondria, it has been used for imaging other mitochondria-rich sites (e.g. tumours) (*see* Cardiotec®, Cardiolite®, terboroxime, sestamibi).

texture (*image*) In image processing, an attribute representing the amplitude and spatial arrangement of the local variation of grey level in an image. It is a measure of image coarseness, smoothness and regularity.

TFE (*mri*) Turbo field echo, general sequence (Philips) (*see* FFE, GRE, MPGR, GRECO, FE, PFI, GE, SMASH, SHORT, STAGE).

TFT (*elec*) *See* thin film transistor.

TGC (*us*) *See* time gain compensation (TGC).

TGSE (*mri*) Turbo gradient spin echo.

thallium (Tl) (*elem*)

Atomic number (Z)	81
Relative atomic mass (A$_r$)	204.37
Density (ρ) kg/m³	11 860
Melting point (K)	576.6
K-edge (keV)	85.5

^{201}Thallium (*nmed*) As ^{201}Thallous chloride for myocardial perfusion and parathyroid scintigraphy. Accumulates in viable myocardium as a potassium analogue. Also localizes in parathyroid adenomas and normal skeletal muscle. Weak gamma emitter scintigraphy achieved with Hg x-rays.

Production	$^{203}_{81}$Tl(p,3n) $^{201}_{82}$Pb ($^{201}_{82}$Pb → $^{201}_{81}$Tl)
Decay scheme	^{201}Tl (γ135, 167 keV: 70–80
(e.c.) ^{201}Tl	x-rays) → ^{200}Hg stable
Decay constant	0.009480 h^{-1}
Half life	72 hr
Photons	68–82 keV (0.93) x-rays
(abundance)	135 keV (0.028) γ
	167 keV (0.106) γ
Gamma ray constant	1.2×10^{-2} mSv hr^{-1} GBq^{-1} @ 1 m
Half value layer	0.3 mm Pb
	43 mm H$_2$O

Uses: Behaves as a potassium analogue for muscle chemistry and so is used as a myocardial imaging agent.

Hours	Fraction remaining
6	0.940
18	0.84
24	0.80
36	0.71
48	0.63
72	0.51
96	0.40

Pb(mm)	Attenuation
0.006	0.5
0.15	10^{-1}
0.98	10^{-2}
2.1	10^{-3}
3.3	10^{-4}

thermal conductivity/heat loss (xray) The speed of heat measured in watts per metre per degree kelvin (or Celsius) W m^{-1} K^{-1} ($^{\circ}$C^{-1}). It is the characteristic of the material independent of size or shape.

Substance	Specific heat (J kg^{-1}K^{-1})	Therm. cond. (W m^{-1}K^{-1})
Water	4200	0.59
Oil	2130	0.15
Air	993	241
Silver	235	427
Aluminum	910	237
Graphite	711	~130
Titanium	523	23
Copper	386	401
Zirconium	280	22
Molybdenum	246	140
Rhenium	138	48
Tungsten	136	178
Glass	67	0.9–1.3

(see specific heat).

thermal equilibrium (mri) A state in which all parts of a system are at the same effective temperature, in particular where the relative alignment of the spins with the magnetic field is determined solely by the thermal energy of the system (in which case the relative numbers of spins with different alignments will be given by the Boltzmann distribution).

thermal index (TI) (us) An indicator of thermal mechanism activity (estimated temperature rise). A measure related to the potential for ultrasonic heating. The thermal index is given by the ratio of the ultrasonic power emitted by the transducer to the ultrasonic power required to raise tissue temperature by 1°C for the exposure conditions. The average ultrasonic attenuation in the model is assumed to be 0.3 dB cm^{-1} MHz^{-1} along the beam axis. The thermal index has no units and can be separated into:

- TIS where only soft tissue is exposed;
- TIB where bone is exposed at depth;
- TIC where bone is close to the surface (cranium).

For foetal exposure, TI should be limited to no more than 0.7 and the tissue temperature increase maintained below 1.5°C.

TI	Maximum exposure time (minutes)
0.7	60
1.0	30
1.5	15
2.0	4
2.5	1

■ Reference: WFUMB, 1998.

thermal neutrons (phys) Neutrons which have velocities that are approximately the same as matter in which they are diffusing – in thermal equilibrium usually at 20°C. Standard velocities are 2200 m s^{-1} with an energy of 0.025 eV. Common thermal neutron reactions are designated n, gamma (n,γ) (see radionuclides (reactor)).

thermal units (units)

Heat measurement	Units
Heat unit	1.4 J (1 J = HU × 0.7)
1 W	1 J s^{-1}
1 cal	4.186 J
1 British thermal unit	1 Btu = 1055 J
1 kWh	3.6×10^6 J
Temperature	kelvin K (0°C = 273.15 K)
Heat capacity	J K^{-1}
Specific heat	J kg^{-1}K^{-1}
Thermal conduction	W m^{-1}K^{-1}
Latent heat	J kg^{-1}

thermionic emission (*phys*) When heat is applied to a wire filament, electrons close to the surface gain energy and leave the metal due to thermionic emission, forming a cloud. The concentration of electrons causes a negative space charge which repels further electron emission. Placing a positive charged electrode (anode) above the filament will draw electrons so a current will flow. Electrons only flow from the negative cathode (filament) to the positive anode. As the filament temperature is increased, the current increases non-linearly reaching a saturation point or plateau. The saturation current level depends on the applied voltage between cathode and anode. This device is non-linear and unidirectional (a diode), allowing current to pass from cathode to anode (not vice versa) which removes the negative half of the alternating current; this is the rectification action.

thermoluminescence (*phys*) A variation of the luminescent process where the traps in the forbidden zone are empty, as in phosphorescence (*see* luminescence). These traps are well below the conduction band so the electrons require added energy (heat) in order to enter the conduction band and subsequently return to the valency band and emit light which is proportional to earlier radiation dose. Thermoluminescence differs from phosphorescence and fluorescence since the energy obtained from the radiation exposure is stored indefinitely within the crystal matrix and the output signal (light) is only emitted when the trapped electrons are dislodged by infrared energy (heat or infrared laser). Summarizing the events:

1 The phosphor has empty traps in the forbidden zone at different energy levels and during x-ray interaction electrons are ejected from the valency band into the conduction band.
2 These electrons then fall in to the empty traps where they can stay indefinitely.
3 Energy (heat) is required to eject the trapped electrons once again into the conduction band.
4 This process can be stimulated by an electric field, by infrared light, or by simply warming crystal.
5 The electrons fall back into the valency band emitting a broad light spectrum whose intensity is equivalent to the original radiation exposure in (1).

Thermoluminescent materials are used for dosimetry (TLD) and imaging.

thermoluminescent dosimeter (TLD) (*nmed*) A dosimeter containing a crystal-line solid for measuring radiation dose, plus filters (absorbers) to help characterize the types of radiation encountered. (When heated, TLD crystals that have been exposed to ionizing radiation give off light proportional to the energy they received from the radiation). Common TLD materials are:

Material	Application
LiF (Mg or Ti doped)	Personal dosimeter Tissue equivalent
$CaSO_4$ (Dy or Tm doped)	Sensitive environmental monitor. Not tissue equivalent.
Lithium borate ($Li_2B_4O_7$:Mn)	Personal dosimeter Tissue equivalent

thermoluminescent material (*phys*) A substance which having been irradiated releases light, when heated to a specific temperature, in proportion to the quantity of ionizing radiation absorbed (*see* glowcurve).

thick Ethernet (*comp*) The original Ethernet cable specification, requiring an AUI connector; noise-resistant but expensive and difficult to install (*see* thin-net).

thimble dosimeter (*dose*) The design of this small ion-chamber compensates for the difficulties of using a large standard ion-chamber by providing a solid medium surrounding a central electrode. By suitable choice of materials the thimble chamber mimics an air-equivalent device and is calibrated over the diagnostic energy range. The thimble chamber is the basis for much of the dosimetry in radiography and radiotherapy after the readings are corrected for temperature/pressure and f-factors convert for tissue type (*see* dosimetry).

thin client (*comp*) Client with small data processing capability. Most of the processing is performed by the server (*see* fat client, server/client).

thin-film transistor (TFT) (*elec*) An insulated gate field effect transistor constructed as a flat device fixed to an insulating substrate rather than as part of an integrated circuit chip. Many discrete FETs are printed on the surface since TFTs, with their companion charge detector (capacitor), can occupy a very small area. They are used in colour flat field displays for workstations and computers. Combined with an x-ray detector material (either fluorescence or photoconductor) the TFT matrix acts as a position-sensitive device and forms the basis of direct radiology (DR) flat field x-ray detectors for projection radiography, mammography and multislice CT. For a workstation/computer high quality liquid crystal **flat panel display** the TFT matrix uses between one and four transistors per pixel to control illumination. Each transistor requires very little power and has a fast response.

thin layer/paper chromatography (TLC/PC) (*nmed*) Includes reverse phase thin layer chromatography (RPTLC) and instant thin layer chromatography (ITLC), the main vehicles for determining radiochemical purity. Usually employs mixtures of commonly available solvents and chemicals but can suffer from the inability of any one system to separate out all the likely impurities. Practical quantification has made these techniques popular for the analysis of radiopharmaceuticals.

thin-net (*comp*) (thin Ethernet) A CSMA/CD network based on thin coaxial cable (also called thin Ethernet), based on the **10BASE-2** IEEE standard. Thin Ethernet suffers from a few serious disadvantages: (*i*) If a user inadvertently disconnected or damaged the cable at one node, the whole network stops, (*ii*) if a user gets reassigned to a new location, the cable must be re-routed to the user's new location.

Thompson, Silvanus P. (1851–1916) British physicist and educationalist. First president of Roentgen Society in 1897, later to become British Institute of Radiology. Awarded Fellow of the Royal Society (FRS) in 1891 (*see* Mackensie Davidson).

thoracic aortography (*clin*) Imaging the thoracic aorta and its major branches using percutaneous transfemoral catheterization (*see* aortography).

Thoravision™ (*xray*) A system developed by Philips for digital chest radiography using a selenium detector on a moving drum. The electrostatic signal is retrieved by scanning electrodes. The field size 49 × 43 cm is represented by 2000 × 2000 pixels.

thorium (Th) (*elem*)

Atomic number (Z)	90
Relative atomic mass (A_r)	232.04
Density (ρ) kg/m^3	11500
Melting point (K)	2000
K-edge (keV)	109.6

Relevance to radiology: historically naturally occurring ^{232}Th as thorium oxide was used as a contrast agent (Thorotrast); since it is an alpha emitter it was quickly replaced with barium and iodine agents.

Thorotrast (*cm*) A thorium dioxide x-ray contrast material proposed by Moniz in 1931. Serious radiation hazard from alpha activity caused it to be abandoned in the 1940–50s, but long-term retention can still be seen.

threshold contrast (*image*) The contrast that produces a just visible difference between two optical densities.

threshold dose for tissue reactions (*dose*) Dose estimated to result in only 1% incidence of tissue reactions.

threshold value (film) (*image*) The lowest density measurement above base + fog level (*see* **characteristic curve, film gamma**).

thresholding (*image*) One of the most important approaches to image segmentation. It is the process of producing a binary image from grey scale image by assigning each output pixel the value 1 if the grey level of the corresponding input pixel is at, or above, the specified threshold, and the value 0 if the input pixel is below that level. Thresholding can be applied to a property other than grey level by first using an operation that converts that property to grey level.

THRIFT (*mri*) Throughput heightened rapid increase flip T2 (Picker Medical Inc.); large flip angle SE technique

thulium™ (*elem*)

Atomic number (Z)	69
Relative atomic mass (A_r)	168.93
Density (ρ) kg/m^3	9300
Melting point (K)	1818
K-edge (keV)	59.3

Relevance to radiology: as a dopant for lanthanum and yttrium intensifying screens.

thyroid function (*clin*) By measuring a 24 hour uptake, using ^{131}iodine in capsule form and comparing thyroid activity levels with a carefully prepared reference phantom, an estimate of thyroid activity can be made. Euthyroid conditions show a 15–35% uptake; hypothyroid a 0–10% and hyperthyroid conditions 40–80%. Non-toxic goitre (endemic) shows a 40–90% uptake.

TI (*mri*) Inversion time; inversion recovery, time between the inverting 180i RF pulse and the subsequent exciting 90i pulse; detects amount of longitudinal magnetization.

TIB (*us*) Thermal index for bone.

TIC (*us*) Thermal index for cranial bone.

TIFF (*comp*) Tagged image file format. This is a tag-based file structure. Where a BMP file is built on a fixed header with fixed fields followed by the sequential data, a TIFF has a much more flexible structure which is a simple 8-byte header that points to the position of the first image file directory (IFD) tag, which can be of any length and contain any number of other tags, thus enabling completely customized headers. BMP is an important format for fast and efficient screen display, but TIFF is a better standard for print-based work. TIF image data are not stored scan line by scan line, but can be broken into tagged strips of multiple scan lines, convenient for handling large print files, allowing for easy buffering and random access.

Tim (*mri*) A Siemens term for total imaging matrix. A selection of various organ specific coils.

time (*phys*) *See* second.

time activity curve (*nmed*) A plot of increase or decreased radioactivity through an organ (e.g. kidney) or tissue (e.g. lung) with time. A kidney time activity curve is the renogram. The curve is created by collecting total count date from a series of ROIs placed over the organ of interest in a dynamic series.

time (spatial) domain (*di*) A signal whose amplitude varies with time (e.g. a sine wave, ultrasound echo or RF pulse) exists in the time domain (*see* frequency domain, Fourier transform).

time of flight (TOF) (*nmed*) Improving PET resolution by including time of detection for the coincidence gammas. TOF imaging systems have very short resolving times and coincidence localization can be obtained to within a fraction of a nanosecond, permitting improved sensitivity, signal to noise ratio. and improving image resolution. Commercial systems can resolve events less than 200 pico seconds apart (0.2 ns). (*mri*) When the local magnetization of moving tissue or fluid is selectively altered in a region, e.g. by selective excitation, it will carry the altered magnetization with it when it moves. This is the source of several flow effects. The flow of non-saturated fully relaxed blood into the slice generates a high signal, for time-of-flight angiography. Stationary spins are partially saturated and so give a lower signal intensity.

time-gain compensation TGC (*us*) Signal post processing amplification for correcting attenuation loss. The slope of the TGC curve can be altered to compensate for both low and high attenuation tissues. The maximum gain limits image depth. The gain can also be altered selectively at particular depths.

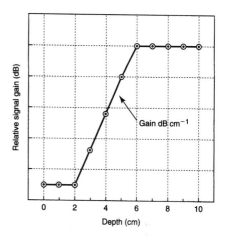

time series (TS) (*mri*) T2* images labelled with number and time position in the series.

time to peak map (TTP) (*mri*) Shows the regional distribution of the time needed to the minimum perfusion signal, either grey scale or colour coded. It is generated for the TIR sequence.

TIR (*mri*) *See* turbo inversion recovery.

TIRM sequence (*mri*) *See* turbo inversion recovery magnitude (TIRM).

tin (Sn) (*elem*)

Atomic number (Z)	50
Relative atomic mass (A_r)	118.69
Density (ρ) kg/m^3	7300
Melting point (K)	505.1
Specific heat capacity J kg^{-1}K^{-1}	228
Thermal conductivity W m^{-1}K^{-1}	66.6
K-edge (keV)	29.2

Relevance to radiology: as a lightweight shielding material for protective aprons. The K-edge makes it more effective than lead over diagnostic energies.

tip angle (*mri*) *See* flip angle.

TIPS (*clin*) Transjugular intrahepatic portosystemic shunt. The non-surgical creation of a portosystemic shunt in portal hypertension using a transjugular stented channel between an intrahepatic vein and the portal vein.

TIS_as (*us*) The soft-tissue thermal index at surface for non-autoscanning mode as:

$$TIS\_as = \frac{W_{0 \mid x \mid} \cdot f_c}{210}$$

where $W_{01\times1}$ is the bounded-square output power in mW and f_c is the centre frequency in megahertz. It has no units.

tissue characteristics (*clin*) The approximate atomic number and electron density, used in attenuation calculations. The electron density (volume) is the product of the density and electron density (weight).

Material	Z	Density (g cm^{-3})	Electron density ($\times10^{23}$ cm instant thin layer chromatography[3])
PMMA	7.4	1.19	3.87
Water	7.4	1.0	3.34
Muscle	7.4	1.04	3.45
Fat	6.1	0.91	3.08
Bone	12.7	1.66	5.25
Titanium	22	4.51	12.47

tissue equivalent (*dose*) Having the same sensitivity to photon energy as soft tissue. Applied to detectors which mimic closely the response of tissue to radiation so accurate tissue doses can be calculated. Air and lithium fluoride are tissue equivalent detectors; film emulsion is not.

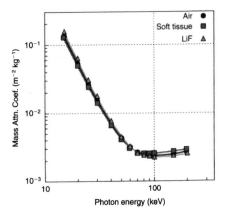

(*us*) Tissue equivalence having similar acoustic impedance to soft tissue.

tissue reactions (*dose*) Injury in populations of cells. Characterized by a threshold dose, and an increase in the severity of the reaction as the dose is increased further (*see* deterministic effect).

tissue synchronization imaging (TSI) (*us*) Analyses tissue velocity within the image for assessing delayed cardiac wall motion. The delay value produces a functional image.

tissue weighting factor w_T (*dose*) (*ICRP60*) *See* weighting factor (tissue).

titanium (Ti) (*elem*)

Atomic number (Z)	22
Relative atomic mass (A$_r$)	47.90
Density (ρ) kg/m^3	4540
Melting point (K)	1948
Specific heat capacity J kg^{-1} K^{-1}	523
Thermal conductivity W m^{-1} K^{-1}	21.9
K-edge (keV)	4.96

Relevance to radiology: very low density input window for image intensifiers. Tensile strength $\times8$ of aluminium and equal to that of stainless steel but half the density.

TLA (*clin*) Translumbar abdominal aortography.

TMR (*mri*) Topical magnetic resonance.

TMS (*mri*) Tetramethylsilane reference compound for hydrogen spectroscopy.

TMZ (*xray*) *See* TZM as titanium, zirconium, molybdenum alloy for anode construction.

toe (film) (*image*) The non-linear minimum recorded density on the film's characteristic curve (*see* film gamma).

TOF (*nmed, mri*) *See* time of flight.

token (ring) bus network (*comp*) A network transmission method that requires a node to have control of a 'token' before it can send messages; better distribution than CSMA/CD on busy networks, but more complicated to implement (*see* bus, topology).

tolerance (contrast medium) (*cm*) Tolerance of iodinated ionic contrast media (CM) for general intravascular use, depends on two factors: osmolality (*see* osmolarity (Osmol)/osmolality (Osm)) and chemotoxicity, including ionic effects. Osmotoxic potential may be expressed with the osmotoxicity ratio (OTR). A balanced addition of sodium and calcium adjust the electrophysiology of cardiac cells and improve contrast media tolerance in cardiac patients, especially during angiocardiographic procedures.

Tomocat$^\times$ (*cm*) A suspension of barium sulphate (Mallinckrodt/Tyco Healthcare Inc), containing 5% w/v BaSO$_4$.

tomography (*image*) A technique for separating sections from a volume distribution. Early x-ray machines used analogue-mechanical methods involving swinging x-ray sources (linear tomography). This was extended to nuclear medicine (H.O. Anger dual head Pho-Con). Digital techniques are used in computed tomography, single photon emission computed tomography (SPECT or SPET) and positron emission tomography (PET).

TONE technique (*mri*) For time of flight angiography to minimize saturation effects for volume blood flow.

topogram or scoutview (*ct*) *See* survey radiography.

topology (network) (*comp*) Describing designs available for networking computers. Bus topology, the physical layout of a network in which all systems connect to a main cable; also known as linear bus. Token ring, IBMs implementation of token passing, governed by the IEEE 802.5 standard, second most popular network topology after Ethernet. Star network, is a centralized design with the appearance of a star, the central component being typically a file server. A higher cost system since each workstation requires direct cabling to the server. More reliable since a cable break will only affect a single workstation.

torque (*phys*) A vector quantity given by the product of the force and the position vector where the force is applied for a rotating body. The effective force on a rotating body turning the body about its centre or pivot point. The torque exerted by a force is also known as the moment of the force. Angular momentum may be changed by applying a torque to the rotating body. An applied torque may increase or decrease the rotation motion, or it may change the direction of the rotation axis. For rotating objects, torque (τ) is equal to the time rate of change of angular momentum. When an object possesses both angular momentum and a magnetic dipole moment is placed in a uniform external magnetic field, the resulting motion can be complex. A torque will be produced which will cause a rotation motion at a constant angular frequency. This is referred to as the 'precession frequency'.

tositumomab (*nmed*) A treatment for non-Hodgkins lymphoma. Commercial name Bexxar®.

TOSS (*mri*) Total suppression of sidebands.

total effective dose equivalent (TEDE) (*dose*) The sum of the deep dose equivalent (external exposures) and committed effective dose equivalent (internal exposures).

toxicity (contrast medium) (*clin*) The total toxicity of a contrast medium is the sum contribution of the chemotoxicity, the osmotoxicity and the ion toxicity. CM agents are excreted mainly through the kidneys, and the use of high volumes and concentrations in several diagnostic procedures makes this a target organ for the evaluation of CM toxicity in man. There is a higher biocompatibility of non-ionic dimers in terms of osmotoxicity, chemotoxicity, organ specific toxicity than the non-ionic monomers, suggesting specific indications for use of this contrast material in high risk patients.

TPPI (*mri*) Time-proportional phase incrementation.

TR (*mri*) Repetition time. The period of time between the beginning of a pulse sequence and the beginning of the succeeding (essentially identical) pulse sequence (*see* sequence time).

TR$_{eff}$ (*mri*) *See* effective repetition time.

trace image (*mri*) Contrast in diffusion images is generated by the direction of the diffusion tensor (*see* diffusion tensor imaging).

tracer (*nmed*) A radiopharmaceutical used to trace a physiological or biochemical process without affecting it.

tracer kinetics (*nm, mri*) The fundamental variables associated with the tracer indicators: intravascular (proteins), inert hydrophilic (DTPA), inert lipophilic (xenon), active transport (MAG3), receptor target (monoclonal antibodies), blood cells (platelets). Parameters that can be measured are mean transit time, distribution volume, clearance, extraction fraction, blood flow, permeability.

■ Reference: Peters, 1998.

transarterial chemoembolization (TACE) (*clin*) Embolization of liver tumours, haemobilia, arteriovenous malformations and fistulae of the liver, and demonstration of mass lesions.

trans-axial (*image*) A body sectional image perpendicular to the body axis. The most common display format for CT and MRI.

transducer (*us*) A device that converts energy from one form to another (*see* piezoelectricity).

transducer array (*us*) Ultrasound transducer assembly containing several transducer elements; transducer element(s) with damping and matching materials assembled in a case.

transducer assembly (*us*) The transducer array, transducer housing (probe), and associated electronic circuitry.

transducer element (*us*) A single piezoelectric sensor in a transducer assembly.

transfer function (*image*) The part of a digital filter design concerned with transferring information in the pass-band. Information on the transfer function characteristics of a filter is available permitting the conversion into discrete forms so that digital filters can be designed. For a look-up table (LUT), the manipulation of the grey scale can be achieved in terms of a transfer function, relating brightness values to each pixel. If $g(x,y)$ is the image formed by the convolution of an image $f(x,y)$ and an operator $h(x,y)$ then in the frequency domain:

$$G(u, v) = H(u, v) \cdot F(u, v)$$

where $H(u,v)$ is the transfer function.

transfer rate (*comp*) The speed with which data can be transferred between a storage medium (disk) and the CPU; measured in MBytes s^{-1} (MBps). A hard disk is typically 2–4 MBps and RAM is 10–250 MBps.

transform (*math*) These are essentially rules for converting a function of a variable as, for example, $f(t)$ (time) into a function of another variable as $F(w)$ (frequency w). The inverse transform will recover $f(t)$ from $F(w)$. The transformed function usually has different properties that either simplify the handling of the original function or reveal different properties.

transform domain filtering (*image*) Modification of weighting coefficients (transform coefficients) prior to reconstruction of the image via inverse transform.

transformer (*phys*) A device consisting of two coils, a primary and secondary wound on a common soft iron core (in the case of low frequency power supplies 50 or 60 Hz) or on sintered ferrite cores for high frequency transformers (>1000 Hz). If E_p and E_s are the voltages at the primary (n_p) and secondary (n_s) windings:

$$\frac{E_s}{E_p} = \frac{n_s}{n_p}$$

The parameters n_p and n_s are the number of turns. The ratio n_s/n_p is the turns ratio. A step up transformer has a turns ratio >1 and a step down transformer <1. The current in a transformer changes inversely with the voltage; the energy in the transformer obeys the conservation of energy, thus the energy in the secondary, at any instant, equals the power supplied to the primary. If I_s and I_p and the secondary and primary currents then:

$$I_s \times E_s = I_p \times E_p \text{ and } \frac{I_s}{I_p} = \frac{E_p}{E_s} = \frac{n_p}{n_s}$$

A step-up transformer with a turns ratio 60:1 voltage increases, the currents are stepped down in the ratio 1:60. A step-down transformer will increase current in the secondary winding but at a reduced voltage. There is a loss of energy in the transformer due to eddy currents which are induced in the iron core by the changing magnetic flux in the windings; these losses can be reduced if the core is laminated. Compact high voltage transformers can

be designed by increasing the AC supply frequency since the induced secondary voltage E_s is influenced by the cross section area of the transformer core A and the number of turns n and the frequency f where:

$$E_s = (A \times n) \times f$$

High frequency transformer

Using the basic formula is $E_s = (A \times n) \times f$
For an x-ray tube supply of 100 keV and a relative overall size ($A \times n$) for 50 Hz transformer being 2000.

$2000 \times 50\,Hz = 100\,keV$

$1666 \times 60\,Hz = 100\,keV$

$1000 \times 100\,Hz = 100\,keV$

$20 \times 5\,Hz = 100\,keV$

$10 \times 10\,Hz = 100\,keV$

Operating a generator frequency of 10 kHz, reduces transformer size by ×200.

(*see* tank unit, slip ring).

transhepatic cholangiography (*clin*) Imaging biliary tree either presurgery (percutaneous transhepatic cholangiography) or during surgery by injecting contrast medium directly into the liver.

transient equilibrium (*nmed*) A parent:daughter decay series where $\lambda_d > \lambda_p$. The parent ^{99}Mo decay constant is 0.0103 and for ^{99m}Tc is 0.1155. The daughter has a much longer half-life than in secular equilibrium and requires a much longer build up time. A condition in which isotopic equilibrium has been reached and the ratio of half-life of parent to half-life of daughter is small (approximately 10:1).

(*see* generator, secular equilibrium).

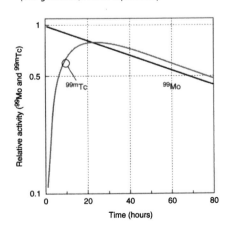

translation rotation system (*ct*) An early design of CT scanner that performs a translation of the detector and the x-ray tube parallel to the scan plane in order to linearly sample the attenuation profiles; each translation is followed by a small increment around the axis of rotation when the next translational movement is carried out. Now replaced by the constantly rotation fan beam.

translumbar abdominal aortography (clin) TLA direct injection of iodine-based contrast medium into the abdominal aorta through the lumbar region and imaging the abdominal aorta with its branches. Employed in cases of peripheral vascular disease.

transmission (image) (*image*) Transmission imaging is the basis of CT and plane film radiography. It is also part of the attenuation correction mechanism in SPECT where an external radionuclide source is used. Attenuation varies according to gamma energy (see graph). Transmission scans are used for assessing true attenuation. Hardware and software are available for this purpose. A common arrangement uses a ^{123}Gd source positioned between patient and gamma camera. ^{123}Gd emits dual gamma energies of 97 and 104 keV. Simultaneous collection of 104 keV from ^{123}Gd and 140 keV from ^{99m}Tc (patient) is made during the SPECT study using separate energy windows; calculation for real time attenuation is made from 104 keV absorption.

rate at a defined distance. It varies with photon energy and absorber thickness (shielding material or tissue). For a mono-energetic source transmission obeys the exponential law (figure below). Transmission is inversely proportional to absorption (*see* transmittance).

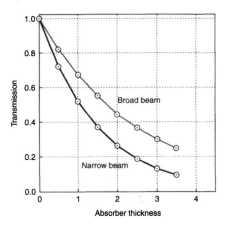

transmission (x-ray; polyenergetic) (*shld*) The broad beam transmission of an x-ray beam through absorbing material (shielding) is the shielded air kerma rate/unshielded air kerma rate at a defined distance. It varies with photon energy and absorber thickness (shielding material or tissue). Since an x-ray source is polychromatic the transmission varies as the shielding material non-uniformly filters lower photon energies (*see* image contrast, transmittance).

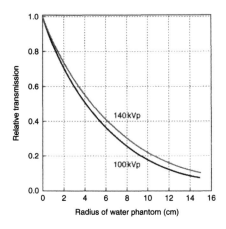

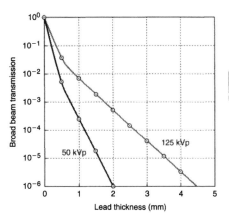

transmission (mono-energetic) (*shld*) The broad beam and narrow beam transmission of a gamma source through absorbing material is the shielded air kerma rate/unshielded air kerma

transmission scan (*nmed*) The attenuation due to the patient is determined by using a transmission acquisition, which is then used to generate transaxial maps which resemble CT images and provide sufficient information to define the various density inside the thorax (lungs and heart). These maps, along with the emission data, are used to correct for attenuation correction using an iterative reconstruction method.

transmission angle (*us*) Angle between the transmitted sound direction and a line perpendicular to the media boundary.

transmit/receive (T/R) coil (*mri*) An RF coil that acts as both a transmitter producing the B1 excitation field, and as a receiver of the NMR signal. Such a coil requires a fast switching circuit to change between the two modes. A body coil is typically a T/R coil, but smaller volume T/R coils (head/ extremities) are often used at high field as a means of reducing RE power absorption.

transmittance (transmission coefficient) (*film*) The ratio of light intensity transmitted through the film image to the incident light. The reciprocal of transmittance is optical density.

transport index (*nmed*) An indication of dose rate on the surface of a package used to transport radionuclides. The numerical equivalent of the maximum dose rate in air at 1 m from the external surface of the package transport categories currently used:

Transport index	Maximum radiation level at any point on the external surface	Label
0	$\leq 5\,\mu Sv\,h^{-1}$ (0.5 mrem h^{-1}).	WHITE-I.
>0 but <1	$>5\,\mu Sv\,h^{-1}$ (0.5 mrem h^{-1}) $\leq 0.5\,mSv\,h^{-1}$ (50 mrem h^{-1})	YELLOW-II.
>1 but <10	$>0.5\,mSv\,h^{-1}$ (50 mrem h^{-1}) $\leq 2\,mSv\,h^{-1}$ (200 mrem h^{-1})	YELLOW-III.
>10	$>2\,mSv\,h^{-1}$	YELLOW-III

transverse magnetization (M$_{xy}$) (*mri*) The component of the macroscopic magnetization vector in the x, y plane; oriented perpendicular to the applied magnetic field. The precession of transverse magnetization induces a decaying signal due to the loss of phase coherence between precessing spins. After RF excitation, M$_{xy}$ decays to zero at time constant T2 (ideal) or T2* (real).

transverse plane (*ct*) Anatomical plane orthogonal to the body's longitudinal (*z*) axis; in most cases identical with the scan plane.

transverse relaxation (*mri*) Loss of transverse magnetization from a non-zero value in the M_{xy} plane. Described by the T2 time constant.

transverse relaxation time (*mri*) *See* T2.

transverse wave (*phys*) Where displacement of the transmitting medium is perpendicular to the direction of propagation. Electromagnetic radiation is an example where electric and magnetic fields vary sinusoidally at right angles to each other but in the direction of propagation. Sound is transmitted as a longitudinal wave. Transverse waves are propagated by vibrations perpendicular to the direction of the wave travel.

traveling saturation slice (*mri*) Slice positioning where a presaturation pulse can be applied to one side of the slice to reduce the signal intensity of spins (typically blood) that are about to flow into the side of the slice. Arteries and veins can be displayed selectively, since the flows are often in the opposite direction. The slices are measured sequentially (slice by slice). The presaturation pulse retains its position relative to the slice.

trend (*stats*) The movement of a variable over a period of time. An erratic pattern may obscure the general trend but this can be detected by using a moving average. Regression equations are used for computing trends and confidence limits can be set for detecting abnormal movements (potential malfunction). Trend calculations are applied to film processor performance and QC.

trigger delay (TD) (*mri*) ECG triggering. Interval between the trigger and release of the measurement.

Triosil [R] (*cm*) Sodium-metrizoate preparation (Glaxo) (*see* metrizoic acid/metrizoate compounds).

Compound	Osmolality (mOsm/kg)	Iodine (mg I/mL)
Metrizoate-Na	2150	370

tritium ^{3}H (*nmed*) The nucleus comprising 1 proton and 2 neutrons. An unstable isotope of hydrogen decaying by β^- emission to ^{3}He with a half life of 12.26 years (*see* hydrogen, tritium).

triton (*nmed*) Nucleus of tritium atom ^{3}H+ used in the cyclotron ion beam.

tropolone (*nmed*) A chelating agent used for blood cell labelling with a radionuclide.

true black (*image*) Black produced by a separate black ink rather than a mixture of cyan, magenta and yellow.

true coincident events (*nmed*) A true PET coincidence is the simultaneous interaction of emissions resulting from a single nuclear transformation. PET relies on the coincident detection of photons in two detectors. Pulses are considered to be coincident if they occur in two detectors within a specified resolving time τ of each other. Because of this finite resolving time, there is the possibility of two independent pulses occurring by chance so as to produce a random coincidence. The resolving time τ for the coincidence window in the most recent PET scanners is typically 6 ns with a coincidence time resolution of ≈3 ns within the window (*see* scatter coincidence).

true FISP (*mri*) Fast imaging with steady state precession having heavy T2 weighting (Siemens), commonly used for imaging cerebrospinal fluid. Gradient echo sequence that provides the highest signal of all steady state sequences. Contrast is a function of T1/T2; with short TR and short TE, the T1 portion remains constant and the images are primarily T2 weighted. FISP and PSIF signals are generated simultaneously. As the signals are superimposed, true FISP is sensitive to inhomogeneity in the magnetic field. Images may contain interference stripes, since the periodic oscillations occur parallel to transitions in tissue the artefacts are bands of alternating high and low signal intensity (*see* SSFP, DE-FGR, CE-FAST, PSIF, ROAST, T2-FEE, E-SHORT, STERE).

true positive fraction (TPF) (*stats*) The conditional probability of deciding that an observed data set (image) was generated by a specified state (that a specified disease was present) when the disease state was in fact present. TPF is equivalent to the 'sensitivity' index often used in the medical literature to indicate the ability of a diagnostic test to detect disease when it is present (*see* receiver operating characteristic (ROC), predictability).

truncation (*image*) Due to practical restrictions the discrete Fourier transform which represents a finite approximation of a signal must be represented by an infinite integral (Fourier transform). As a consequence, the Fourier series will not converge smoothly and a truncation error will result (signal or image distortion/artefacts); a truncation error results due to an inexact or foreshortened formula. An impulse in the frequency domain implies an infinitely long time window, so a compromise is required between time and frequency domain performance by truncating the window. Smoothing filters are designed to minimize these errors.

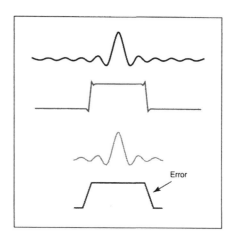

Error

truncation error (*image, ct*) Insufficient terms in a Fourier transform leading to incomplete convergence. A problem in tomography with restricted beam size where a fan beam (nuclear medicine or CT) misses certain anatomy in its rotation so data sets are incomplete. Truncation artefacts are seen in axial tomography (CT or SPECT) when certain parts of the anatomy lie outside the fan beam at certain projections (arms included in a thorax CT) or inconsistent anatomy in magnification views (cardiac SPECT). In the diagram the shaded sections are not covered by this fan beam angle on certain positions of the beam rotation, causing incomplete data sets which lead to truncation errors.

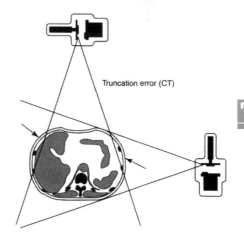

Truncation error (CT)

TSE (*mri*) Turbo-spin echo; FSE/RARE technique (Siemens/Philips).

TSI (*us*) *See* tissue synchronization imaging.

TSR (*mri*) Total saturation recovery.

tube-current exposure-time product (mAs) (*xray*) *See* mAs.

tube current modulation (*ct*) During the helical scan, thicker denser regions of the patient require higher tube current (increased x-ray fluence), thinner or less dense regions use a lower tube current. Alternatively the tube current can be modulated during the course of a single tube rotation used when the body has cross sections that are not circular (shoulders and pelvis), where the lateral projection through the patient attenuates more than the anterior–posterior projection. Exposure to the patient can be varied by up to 80% in the course of a 0.5 s rotation. This has a dose advantages and the added advantage of making the image quality more constant for the individual slices in each series.

tube loading (*xray*) The tube-current exposure-time product (mAs) that applies during a particular exposure.

tube potential (*xray*) The potential difference (kilovolt, kv) applied across the anode and cathode of the x-ray tube during a radiographic exposure.

tungsten (W) (*elem*)

Atomic number (Z)	74
Relative atomic mass (A$_r$)	183.85
Density (ρ) kg/m^3	19320
Melting point (K)	3650
Specific heat capacity J kg^{-1}K^{-1}	130
Thermal conductivity W m^{-1}K^{-1}	174
K-edge (keV)	69.5

Relevance to radiology: Major anode material for x-ray tubes (*see* rhenium, tantalum).

tungsten (shielding) (*xray*) A syringe shield constructed from 1.5 mm tungsten will reduce radiation exposure from ^{99m}Tc (140 keV) by up to 94% (*see* syringe/vial shielding). The shielding is lighter and more resistant to abrasion than lead.

tuning (*mri*) Process of adjusting the resonant frequency of the RF circuit, to the desired value of the Larmor frequency. More generally, the process of adjusting the components of the spectrometer for optimal performance, including matching impedances.

turbo angiography (*mri*) Fast 3D angiography techniques; increases speed by a factor of 2 using zero filling (interpolation techniques in slice-selection direction) short TR and TE.

turbo factor (*mri*) Time saved using a turbo-spin echo sequence compared to a conventional spin echo sequence.

turbo-FLASH (*mri*) Fast long angle shot. Fast gradient switching, using a spoiler gradient pulse, with subsecond image acquisition; flip angles 6–15°. Gradient reversal replaces 180° rephasing pulse. Allows breath holding which makes abdominal imaging possible (*see* FFE, GRE, MPGR, GRECO, FE, PFI, GE, TFF, SMASH, SHORT, STAGE).

turbo gradient spin echo (turbo GSE) (*mri*) Additional gradient echoes are generated before and after each spin echo. Spin echoes are allocated to the raw data matrix centrally to give pure T2 contrast. Fat is darker, more sensitive to susceptibility effects than turbo-SE.

turbo inversion recovery (TurboIR, TIR) (*mri*) A TurboSE sequence with long TI for fluid suppression. The turboIR sequence gives a true inversion recovery display.

turbo-spin echo (turbo-SE) (*mri*) Fast spin echo imaging technique with an acquisition time of 100–300 s using flip angles 90 and 180°. A spin-echo technique that acquires more than one individually phase-encoded echo per TR period. With turbo spin-echo more than one TR period is used to fill all of the image *k*-space. The turbo factor increases speed, and is usually used to improve resolution.

turbo-SHORT (*mri*) Turbo version of SHORT version of Turbo-FLASH-like sequence (Elscint).

turbulent flow (turbulence) (*phys*) A state of fluid or gas in which there is disturbed or non-regular motion; random, chaotic, multidirectional flow of a fluid with mixing between layers; flow that is not laminar (*see* Reynold's number).

TWAIN (*comp*) (technology without an interesting name; reputedly). A program interface between scanner and graphics software allowing images to be scanned and acquired directly into the computer program. Twain drivers enable a scanner to operate from and acquire the image directly to an image editing application placed in Word documents.

twisted pair (*comp*) A popular and low-cost LAN cabling method, also commonly used for telephone wiring. This type of cabling features two or more pairs of copper wires, each pair intertwined then wrapped to minimize electrical interference. Twisted pair wiring comes in two major varieties: UTP and STP, although twisted pair cabling supports less bandwidth than coax or fibre optic cable but it is cheaper. Wiring types are assigned category numbers based on their transmission capacity.

two-dimensional Fourier transform imaging (2DFT) (*mri*) A form of sequential plane imaging using Fourier transform imaging.

two dimensional NMR (*mri*) Form of NMR spectroscopy in which an additional dimension is added to the conventional chemical shift dimension by allowing varying amounts of different interactions between spin systems (such as NOE, spin–spin coupling or exchange).

typical value (*math*) The common or expected value found in the majority of facilities. Usually obtained by analysing the measurements from a large selection of patients or equipment and finding the mean value from a histogram display. A common method for assessing patient dose and x-ray equipment performance.

TZM (*xray*) An alloy of titanium, zirconium, molybdenum used as a foundation for x-ray tube anode construction. This is then covered with a layer of tungsten and then the tungsten/rhenium target (Trinodex®, Philips).

T

UART *(comp)* The universal asynchronous receiver/transmitter chip which controls the transfer of data over a serial port (e.g. modems).

uberschwinger artefact *(ct)* Edge enhancement creating large density differences between interfaces. Commonly seen with metal prostheses giving an increased opacity parallel to the interface so simulating loosening of a prothesis. Also seen as false images of infection or pneumothorax.

UDMA *(comp)* Ultra DMA. EIDE controllers linking the hard drive to a computer; supporting transfer rates of 33 MBps (megabytes per second) and 66 MBps; these are UDMA33 and UDMA66.

UFOV *(nm, rad)* *See* useful field of view.

UHF *(units)* Ultra high frequency radio. Those frequencies circa 1 GHz. Television is commonly 470–512 and 512 to 806 MHz.

Name	Frequency	Applications
Ultra high frequency (UHF)	300 MHz to 3 GHz	Television, mobile (cell) telephones, wireless networking, microwave ovens
Super high frequency (SHF)	3 to 30 GHzs	Wireless networking, radar, atellite links.

ultrasound *(us)* Sound having a frequency greater than 20 kHz. Clinical ultrasound has a spectrum typically 2–10 MHz although experimental probes have exceeded this range.

ultrasound (bioeffects) *(us)* Biologically sensitive areas are:

- first trimester embryo;
- foetal skeleton (heating);
- neonatal transcranial Doppler;
- eye;
- intracavitary studies.

Biological effects have not currently been observed *in vivo* at spatial peak/temporal average intensity I_{SPTA}:

I_{SPTA}	$<100 \, \text{mW cm}^{-2}$ for $<500 \, \text{s}$ (unfocused)
I_{SPTA}	$<1 \, \text{W cm}^{-2}$ for $<50 \, \text{s}$ (focused)

Damage to biological systems is divided into:

- Chromosome damage: sister chromatid exchange has been seen *in vitro* with single strand DNA

breaks. An I_{SPTA} of $94 \, \text{W cm}^{-2}$ at 8 MHz CW gave consistent breaks with ultrasound cavitation.

- Foetal damage: prolonged ultrasound investigations could have side effects on embryogenesis and on later prenatal and postnatal development. Exposure should be minimized when using pulsed Doppler studies on the foetus; this can induce ultrasound heating in foetal bone.

The AIUM (1982) reported no significant biological effects observed using intensity levels below $100 \, \text{mW cm}^{-2}$. In 1993 the FDA increased the I_{SPTA} limit from $94 \, \text{mW cm}^{-2}$ to $720 \, \text{mW cm}^{-2}$ (*see* ultrasound (heating), ultrasound (cavitation)).

ultrasound (cavitation) *(us)* This is gas bubble growth and is related to acoustic pressure p, intensity I and acoustic impedance; related as: $I = p^2/z$. At high intensities used in therapy, cavitation has been demonstrated but it has not been reported at diagnostic intensities.

ultrasound (contrast agents) *(cm)* Consist of microbubbles filled with air or gases. These consist of thin shells composed of albumin, lipid or polymer confining a gas (usually nitrogen or a perfluorocarbon). Current generations of microbubbles have diameters from 1 to 5 μm. Among the blood pool agents, transpulmonary ultrasound contrast agents offer higher diagnostic potential compared to agents that cannot pass the pulmonary capillary bed after intravenous injection. In addition to their vascular phase they can exhibit a tissue- or organ-specificity. Current contrast agents are:

Gas	Stabilizing shell	Commercial Product
Transpulmonary		
Perfluoropropane	Phospholipids	Definity®
Dodecafluoropentane	Surfactant	Echogen®
Octafluoropropane	Albumin	Optison®
Air	Albumin	Quantison®
Perfluorohexane	Surfactant	Imavist®
Sulphur hexafluoride	Phospholipids	Sonovue®
Transpulmonary/organ specific		
Air	Palmitic acid	Levovist®
Air	Cyanoacrylate	Sonavist®
Perfluorocarbon	Surfactant	Sonazoid®

ultrasound (duty factor) *(us)* A pulsed beam consists of an 'on period' (mark) and an 'off period' (space). The *mark* (*m*): *space* (*s*) ratio: $m/(m + s) \times 100\%$ is the duty factor. This is an important ratio when computing the safety limits (*see* duty cycle).

ultrasound (heating) (*us*) This is caused by the conversion of ultrasonic energy to heat in the tissue. The intensity I of ultrasound energy.

ultrasound intensity (continuous CW) (*us*) Where the duty factor equals 1 and the pulse average (PA) and temporal average (TA) are the same.

ultrasound intensity (pulsed) (*us*) Where the values for the pulse average intensity (I_{PA}) and temporal average intensity (I_{TA}) are influenced by the duty factor. There are six composite intensities that combine spatial and temporal values. The commonly used intensity measurements for ultrasound are I_{SPPA} (the maximum pulse intensity) and I_{SPTA} (the peak power given by the complete pulse) the magnitude of the intensity values follows the sequence:

Spatial peak temporal peak	I_{SPTP}
Spatial peak pulse average	I_{SPPA}
Spatial peak temporal average	I_{SPTA}
Spatial average/temporal peak	I_{SATP}
Spatial average/pulse average	I_{SAPA}
Spatial average/temporal average	I_{SATA}

The absolute values of the intensity measurements are influenced by focal dimensions. Transducers with tight focus in the near field will produce higher I_{SPTA} values than those that are focused in the far field. Typical values for the commonly applied intensity measurements are:

Intensity	Value
I_{SPTA}	$720\,\mathrm{mW\,cm^{-2}}$
I_{SPPA}	$0\text{--}700\,\mathrm{W\,cm^{-2}}$
I_{SATA}	$410\,\mathrm{mW\,cm^{-2}}$
I_{SAPA}	$500\,\mathrm{mW\,cm^{-2}}$

ultrasound intensity (spatial) (*us*) Spatial peak (SP) and spatial average (SA) intensities. The ultrasonic intensity transmitted in the direction of acoustic wave propagation, per unit area at the point considered normal to this direction. For measurement purposes, this point is restricted to where the acoustic pressure and particle velocity are in phase, i.e. the far field or the area near the focal surface. Measured as the energy flux crossing unit area in unit time or the rate of delivery of ultrasound energy per unit area of tissue as $\mathrm{W\,m^{-2}}$ or $\mathrm{mW\,cm^{-2}}$ where $1\,\mathrm{W\,m^{-2}} = 0.1\,\mathrm{mW\,cm^{-2}}$. The spatial peak (SP) is the beam intensity measured on the central axis. The spatial average (SA) is the mean intensity averaged over the beam cross sectional area.

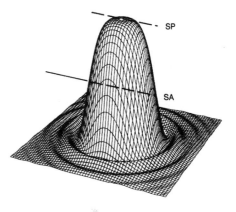

Intensity parameter	Unit (typical value)
I_{SP}	$<10\,\mathrm{mW\,cm^{-2}}$ (unfocused) up to $1\,\mathrm{W\,cm^{-2}}$ (focused)

ultrasound intensity (temporal) (*us*) Temporal peak intensity (I_{TP}) and temporal average

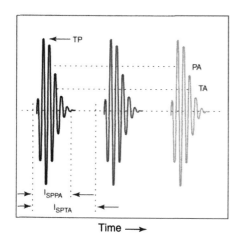

Time $\longrightarrow$

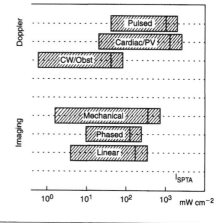

intensity (I_{TA}); the latter is the intensity of the entire pulse train averaged over time as:

$$\frac{\text{total power per frame}}{\text{frame duration}}$$

which gives the average intensity of the pulse train. In the figure, PA is the pulse average intensity I_{PA} (*see* duty cycle).

ultrasound (resolution) (*us*) Two axes of resolution affect the ultrasound image (i) lateral (ii) axial. A further aspect of resolution, that of the slice width, is fixed by the radial curvature of the transducer face. Approximate resolution values (mm) are given for typical transducer frequencies (MHz):

Frequency	Axial	Lateral
2.0	0.7	3.0
3.5	0.4	1.7
5.0	0.3	1.2
7.5	0.2	0.8
10.0	0.15	0.6
13.0	0.118	
15.0	0.102	

The axial resolution is parallel to the ultrasound beam; the ability to separate detail with depth. Can be estimated from the spatial pulse length as *SPL*/2 or from the pulse geometry as:

$$\frac{0.77 \times \text{cycles in pulse}}{\text{frequency}}$$

ultrasound (safety) (*us*) The graph plots the boundary of safe intensity levels for time spent in the investigation.

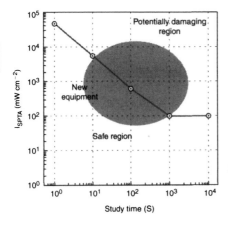

The FDA intensity limits for the heart (*Ht*), peripheral vascular (*PV*), ophthalmology (*Op*) and obstetrics (*Ob*) are:

	Ht	PV	Op	Ob
W cm^{-2}				
I_{SPTP}	310	310	50	310
I_{SPPA}	190	190	28	190
mW cm^{-2}				
I_{SPTA}	430	720	17	94
I_{SATA}	430	720	17	94

From the AIUM/NEMA 1998 report:

Ophthalmic: Thermal index $\leqslant 1.0$; mechanical index $\leqslant 0.23$ and derated $I_{SPTA0.3} \leqslant 50\,\text{mW}\,\text{cm}^{-2}$. *Foetal heart*: I_{SATA}: $<20\,\text{mW}\,\text{cm}^{-2}$ for CW and I_{SAPA}: $<20\,\text{mW}\,\text{cm}^{-2}$ for pulsed devices.

■ Reference: AIUM/NEMA, 1998.

ultrasound (scatter) (*us*) Caused when the beam strikes irregularities similar in size to the ultrasound wavelength. Scatter also occurs when the beam traverses particulate matter (blood cells). Scattered echoes form a cone about the reflection axis whose angle depends on the wavelength of the ultrasound. For smaller wavelengths (higher frequencies) the scatter angle is wider. Intensity of scatter decreases as (*frequency*)^4. Scatter is responsible for speckle which is scattered, ultrasound from different sites interfere or add constructively (*see* acoustic absorption, reflection).

ultrasound (values) (*us*) The term 'ultrasound' is applied to sound waves from 20 kHz to above 100 MHz. Medical ultrasound operates at frequencies from 1 to 20 MHz. Tissue detail and penetration are compromised outside this range.

Frequency (MHz)	2.0	3.5	5.0	7.5	10.0
Wavelength (mm)	0.77	0.44	0.31	0.21	0.15

Application according to frequency (MHz)

1	2	3	4	5	7.5	10	15	20
Therapy								
		Abdomen/obstetrics/cardiac						
							Superficial/thyroid	
							Opthalmic	

Tissue	Density (kg m^{-3})	Speed (c) m s^{-1}	rayl (Z) kg.m.s.	Absorption dB MHz cm
Muscle	1040	1568	1.63	2
Fat	970	1470	1.42	0.5
Bone	1700	3600	6.12	4.1

ultrasound venography (*clin*) Ultrasound imaging may be used for the non-invasive examination of peripheral as well as central veins and their surrounding tissues. A valuable non-ionizing radiation procedure using either grey-scale real-time imaging or by combining the image with pulsed Doppler for indicating vascular velocity. Duplex scanning combines the two-dimensional grey-scale image with the flow velocity signal superimposed in colour; sound effects are also available.

UltraSPARC® (*comp*) Computer architecture introduced by Sun that are 64 bit CPUs that run 32 bit SPARC software. The UltraSPARC® T1 processor gives you up to eight processing cores with four threads per core. The UltraSPARC® T2 processor has up to 8 cores per chip and up to 64 threads per processor with dual 10Gbit Ethernet and PCI-E integrated onto the chip.

Ultratag® (*nmed*) A commercial stannous chloride preparation for labelling red blood cells.

UltraVent® (*nmed*) A radioaerosol delivery system (Mallinckrodt Inc.).

Ultravist® (*cm*) Commercial (Schering) preparation of non-ionic iopromide introduced in 1985. Supplied in iodine concentrations of 150, 240, 300, 350, 370 mg I/mL^{-1}.

Compound	Viscosity (cP)	Osmolality (mOsm/kg)	Iodine (mg I/mL)
Iopromide	@ 20° 9.0	530 @ 37°	350

umbra (*phys*) A point source of light projects a sharp shadow onto a screen. When this ceases to be a point source the image unsharpness causes shadowing, the degree of which depends on the focal spot *f* and its position relative to the object and image plane. The parameters *i* and *o* determine the penumbra dimension *p* (unsharpness) so that:

$$p = \frac{i \times f}{o}$$

Umbra and penumbra effects are shown by x-rays since they are produced by fine and broad focal spots and mimic the light effects described here.

uniformity (*ct*) Consistency of the CT numbers in the image of a homogeneous material across the scan field.

uniformity (differential) (*nmed*) The intrinsic differential non-uniformity of sensitivity U_d for

a gamma camera is $U_d = \Delta C/M \times 100\%$ where ΔC is the maximum difference in counts between two adjacent pixels and M is the larger of the two counts. Typical current values, for non-uniformity in central regions, are ⩽2.5% and for useful field of view ⩽2.8% (*see* integral uniformity, uniformity (intrinsic)).

uniformity (integral) (*nmed*) Measured as the percentage difference between the maximum and minimum pixel counts in a chosen samling area. Typical values ±2.5% CFOV, ±4.5% UFOV for planar acquisition. This must be improved for SPECT imaging (± 1% CFOV) (*see* uniformity (intrinsic)).

uniformity (intrinsic) (*nmed*) The gamma camera resolution, without collimator. This is best performed by using a point source 2–3 m from the uncollimated camera face. Two measurements of uniformity are calculated:

Integral uniformity where maximum and minimum values over a 64 × 64 matrix are used in the equation:

$$\pm 100 \times \frac{[\max - \min]}{[\max + \min]}$$

Differential uniformity is measured over a limited distance in the matrix (5 pixels) collecting the largest positive and negative deviations from the mean:

$$\pm 100 \times \frac{[(+\max) - (-\min)]}{[(+\max) + (-\min)]}$$

uninstaller (*comp*) This small program usually logs the installation of a program package so that all files can be removed when the program is erased from the system.

unit dosage (*nmed*) A precalibrated single dosage of a radiopharmaceutical in an individual container, intended for use in only one patient.

UNIX (*comp*) A multiuser, multitasking operating system produced by AT&T. Has become standard protocol for TCP/IP and SMTP and forms the backbone for many specialized operating systems (see Linux).

UNSCEAR (*dose*) United Nations Scientific Committee on the Effects of Atomic Radiation. Some recent reports:

- *Sources and Effects of Ionizing Radiation. Publication E.77.ix.1.*
- *Sources and Effects of Ionizing Radiation.*
- *Sources Effects and Risks of Ionizing Radiation.*
- *Genetic and Somatic Effects of Ionizing Radiation.*

unsharpness (geometric) U_g (*image*) The penumbra (U_g) or blurring of an edge or point source due to geometrical factors of the imaging system (typically x-ray unit) which considers: focal spot size (FS), object to focus distance (OFD) and focus to film distance (FFD), sometimes called source to image distance (*SID*), such that:

$$U_g = \frac{FS \times OFD}{FFD - OFD}$$

(*see* system magnification).

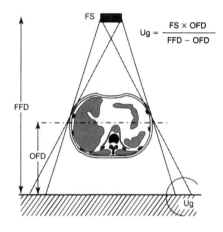

$$Ug = \frac{FS \times OFD}{FFD - OFD}$$

unsharpness (movement) U_m (*image*) Display penumbra due to movement. Cardiac movement in chest radiography must have an exposure time of 0.01 s in order to maintain a 1 Lp mm^{-1} at cardiac edges. In the diagram where h is the edge height and d the degree of movement then visible contrast is lost as d increases although h is unchanged.

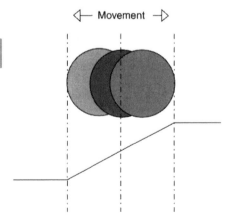

unsharpness (radiographic) U_r (*image*) Display penumbra due to image detector properties and including collimator design for gamma cameras in nuclear medicine. The basic factors are due to separation of the screen or collimator from the imaging surface, diffusion of the event in the intensifying screen or due to collimator/grid septa penetration. The intensifying screen also shows halation due to surface reflection and the dual emulsion film shows crossover due to film base transparency.

unsharpness (total) U_t (*image*) The total unsharpness, incorporating geometric unsharpness, movement and radiographic, is the geometrical mean of these values:

$$U_t = \sqrt{U_g + U_m + U_r}$$

U_t is also called image blur.

UPS (*comp*) Universal power supply or uninterruptible power supply. An electrical power supply that includes a battery to provide enough power to a computer during a power failure to back-up data and properly shut down.

uranium (U) (*elem*)

Atomic number (Z)	92
Relative atomic mass (A$_r$)	238.03
Density (ρ) kg/m^3	18970
Melting point (K)	1405.4
K-edge (keV)	115.6
Relevance to radiology: depleted uranium (^{235}U extracted) is used as a shielding material for high activity sources (some ^{99m}Tc generators).	

^{235}Uranium

Half life	700 × 10^6 years
Decay mode	Alpha
Energy	4.7 MeV
Abundance	0.72% of natural uranium

^{238}Uranium

Half life	4.5 × 10^{9}y
Decay mode	mixed α, β and γ
Decay constant	1.54E–10 y^{-1}
Photon	Mixed

This is the start of the natural uranium decay series, which eventually yields radon.

uranium decay series (*phys, nmed*) The natural decay series from ^{238}U to stable lead ^{206}Pb involving complex mixed α, β and γ emissions.

Z	Element	Symbol	T½
92	Uranium	^{238}U	4.5×10^9 y
90	Thorium	^{234}Th	24 d
91	Protactinium	^{234m}Pa	1.2 m
92	Uranium	^{234}U	2.5×10^5 y
90	Thorium	^{230}Th	8×10^4 y
88	Radium	^{226}Ra	1602 y
86	Radon	^{222}Rn	3.8 d
84	Polonium	^{218}Po	3.0 m
82	Lead	^{214}Pb	27 m
83	Bismuth	^{214}Bi	20 m
84	Polonium	^{214}Po	160 µs
82	Lead	^{210}Pb	21 y
83	Bismuth	^{210}Bi	5.0 d
84	Polonium	^{210}Po	138 d
82	Lead	^{206}Pb	Stable

(*see* radon).

uranium (shielding) (*nmed*) Large activity $^{99}Mo/^{99m}Tc$ generators greater than 600 GBq, commonly carry an internal depleted uranium shield. The requirements for packaging using depleted uranium as shielding should be covered in an inactive (plastic) sheath.

Density	19 050 kg m^{-3}
K-edge	115.6 keV

urethrography (*clin*) Radiography of the male or female urethra by retrograde injection of contrast medium or voiding of contrast medium from the bladder (cystourethrography, micturating cystogram). Combining ascending and descending urethrography gives information on: the anatomy of the urethra, bladder capacity, bladder anatomy, the presence of vesicoureteric reflux, competence of the bladder neck and distal sphincter, presence of intraprostatic reflux and residual urine volume. Ascending urethrogram where CM is instilled slowly via catheter. The CM should pass proximal to the distal sphincter to outline the posterior urethra; patient is supine. Descending micturating cystourethrography where CM is instilled via catheter and the bladder adequately filled to induce micturation. Images of posterior urethra taken during voiding.

urine values (*clin*) Normal values:

Calcium	<7.5 mmol/24 h
Creatinine clearance	70–130 mL/mm
Protein	<150 mg/24 h
Sodium	40–210 mmol/24 h
Urea	170–500 mmol/24 h
Uric acid	3–6 mmol/24 h

URL (*comp*) The unique resource locator is the address of a web page. The protocol for identifying a document on the web. For example, the URL *www.hospital.com/library/protocol.html* tells the browser to use HTTP protocol to find the server named *www.hospital.com* and ask it for the page entitled *protocol.html* in the */library/* directory. A URL is unique to each user (*see* domain).

Urografin ˣ (*cm*) Commercial preparation containing varying proportions of sodium diatrizoate and meglumine diatrizoate by Schering for infusion urography. Ionic monomer.

Compound	Viscosity (cP)	Osmolality (mOsm/kg)	Iodine (mg I/mL)
Na-diatrizoate meglumine diatrizoate 30%	2.2 @ 20° 1.4 @ 37°		146
Na-diatrizoate meglumine diatrizoate 45%			220
Na-diatrizoate meglumine diatrizoate 60%			292
Na-diatrizoate meglumine diatrizoate 76%		1940	370

urography (*clin*) Radiographic examination of the urinary tract, particularly the upper parts, i.e. the kidneys and the ureters. More rarely it involves the lower parts, i.e. bladder and urethra. Contrast medium excreted close to 100% via the kidneys. Intravenous: following injection of contrast medium images are taken of the renal area to demonstrate pelvi-calyceal systems and renal areas, ureters and bladder. Also called excretion urography. Control images taken prior to the injection. Drip infusion: investigation of masses within the entire renal anatomy including ureters in cases of diminished renal function. Retrograde: radiography of the urinary tract following injection of contrast medium directly into the bladder, ureter or renal pelvis.

Uromiro ˣ (*cm*) Commercial (Merck Pharma Chemicals Inc., Bracco) version iodamide.

Uroselectan ˣ (cm) The first clinically used intravenous contrast medium, chemically consisting of a large negatively-charged iodinated anion, and a smaller positively-charged sodium cation. When dissolved in water forming two ions for each molecule of contrast medium. This was an ionic contrast medium, having a high osmolality. Similar compounds were synthesized which had two atoms of iodine each, thus doubling the radio-opacity for the same contrast media concentration (*see* Binz, Räth).

Urovison⁺ (*cm*) Generic name Na–diatrizoate meglumine diatrizoate. An ionic contrast medium manufactured by Schering AG with a higher proportion of sodium diatrizoate than the Urografins. Iodine concentration 325 mg I/mL.

Urovist⁺ (*clin*) Generic name diatrizoate. An ionic contrast medium.

USB (*comp*) Universal serial bus. An industry standard for connecting different compatible peripheral devices across multiple platforms. It supports true plug and play and allows hot-swapping of devices (**hot pluggable**). It provides standardized cabling for printers, digital cameras, scanners, game pads, joysticks, keyboards, mice and storage devices. USB supports simultaneous connection of up to 127 devices by attaching peripherals through interconnected external hubs. USB.1 has a limited bandwidth of 12 Mbits s⁻¹. USB 2.0 standard gives transfer speeds of up to 480 Mbits s⁻¹ enabling fast videoconferencing; considered a potential alternative to IEEE 1394 (otherwise known as FireWire) for use with high-speed video. USB 2.0 is backwards-compatible; older systems that support version 1.0 accommodated.

USB hub (*comp*) A multiple-socket USB connecter that allows several USB-compatible devices to be connected to a computer.

useful field (*xray*) The extent of the collimated x-ray beam. The smaller the angle τ the wider the target track can be. In general, the smaller the anode angle the wider the focal track which increases the power rating; however, angle size also influences the field size of the x-ray beam at a given source to image distance (SID). Useful field size increases with anode angle, however, so also does the effective focal spot size which will degrade image resolution, so a large area radiograph would be obtained at the expense of resolution.

useful field of view (UFOV) (*nmed*) The collimator's field diameter. These will generally be worse than the central field of view (CFOV) because of crystal edge effects. (*xray*) The extent of the collimated x-ray beam or extent of gamma camera field of view.

USPIO (*mri*) Ultra small super paramagnetic iron oxide.

UTP (*comp*) Unshielded twisted pair; a thin-diameter network wire popular in network cabling installations. UTP is more pliable than STP and less expensive and easier to install. Its disadvantage is limited immunity to noise. UTP is available in voice-grade and data-grade versions. Category 5 wire supports 100 Mbps data rates. Category 4 wire supports 20 Mbps and Category 3 wire supports 16 Mbps.

UUE (*comp*) UUEncoded files used with Internet news groups.

V.42bis (*comp*) An algorithm used by modems that can compress data by ratios of 8:1, but in the real world this can be reduced to around 2.5 1.

V.90 (*comp*) Approved in February 1998, this standard replaces K56Flex and X2, providing a common protocol for 56K modems to access an ISP that supports V.90. 56K modems not V.90 ready must have Flash memory and will require firmware upgrades provided by the manufacturer.

valvoplasty (*clin*) Reconstruction of deformed cardiac valve.

vapourware (*comp*) A name given to software that is announced far in advance of any release and either never materializes or appears much later than originally advertised.

variable, continuous (*math*) A variable that may take any value.

variable, dependent (*math*) A variable dependent on another. Usually placed on the *y*-axis.

variable, discrete (*math*) The opposite to continuous. A variable that may only take certain values.

variable focusing (*us*) Transmission focus with various focal lengths.

variable, independent (*math*) A variable not dependent on another, usually placed on the *x*-axis.

variance (*stats*) A measure of dispersion. Square of standard deviation; one of the outputs of the auto-correlation process; a measure of spectral broadening (i.e. spread around the mean). (*us*) Square of standard deviation; one of the outputs of the auto-correlation process; a measure of spectral broadening (i.e. spread around the mean).

VAS (*mri*) Variable angle spinning.

Vascoray* (*clin*) Meglumine iothalamate, manufactured by Mallinckrodt.

Vasoray* (*cm*) Iothalamate preparation. Ionic monomer.

Vasovist* (*cm*) Gadolinium compound as gadofosvesat trisodium for MR angiography, abdominal or limb vessels (Schering).

vasogram (*clin*) Radiography of the vas deferens to determine patency using contrast medium.

vector (magnetic) (*mri*) When a sample is exposed to an external magnetic field a net alignment of the individual magnetic moments (protons) will result in a preferred direction along the external field. The nuclei that make up this alignment contribute to a resultant magnetization vector (M). There is a longitudinal magnetization vector (M_L) and transverse magnetization vector (M_{xy}). A transverse component of the magnetization vector can be produced by applying a transverse magnetic field (90° RF pulse or other flip angle) which will move M away from the magnetic field; as the strength of the RF pulse increases the longitudinal component M_L of the magnetization vector decreases. M will assume a position between M zero and M_{xy}.

vector array (*us*) Linear sequenced array that emits pulses from different starting points and (by phasing) in different directions.

vectors (*math*) Quantities for which both size and direction are necessary for a full specification. Examples are velocity, acceleration and force. They are frequently represented by an arrow whose length represents signal magnitude and angle representing the magnitude of component (e.g. sine wave angle in radians) (*see* scalors).

veiling glare (*xray*) Ratio of light intensity at centre of image with and without lead disk.

velocity (linear) (*v*) (*phys*) The velocity of a moving point, or of a body is the rate of its displacement or the rate at which it changes its position, in a given direction. If it moves through *s* m in *t* seconds then $v = s/t\,\mathrm{m\,s^{-1}}$. Velocity is a vector quantity having both magnitude and direction, but when the direction is constant (a straight line) and the body covers equal distances in equal times, the velocity is uniform and is measured by the displacement per unit time,

---

Photon time of flight
The distance travelled by a 0.511 MeV gamma photon after 1 nanosecond (10^{-9}s). All electromagnetic radiation has a velocity of approximately $3.0 \times 10^8 \mathrm{m\,s^{-1}}$.
Distance travelled = $(3.0 \times 10^8) \times 10^{-9} = 0.3\,\mathrm{m}$.

Units of linear velocity

SI	$\mathrm{m\,s^{-1}}$	
CGS	$\mathrm{cm\,s^{-1}}$	$1\,\mathrm{cm\,s^{-1}} = 1 \times 10^{-2}\mathrm{m\,s^{-1}}$
Other	$\mathrm{miles\,hr^{-1}}$	$1\,\mathrm{mph} = 0.44\,\mathrm{m\,s^{-1}}$

velocity (angular) (ω) (*phys*) *See* angular velocity.

velocity (of flow) (*phys*) Compare to flow Poiseuille etc.

velocity (sound) (*phys*) Velocity of sound in medium depends on density ρ and elasticity *K*: the velocity of sound *v* in a gas obeys:

$$v = \sqrt{\frac{P\alpha}{\rho}}$$

Boyle's Law states that gas volume is inversely proportional to pressure:

$$v \propto \frac{1}{P}$$

and as gas density is proportional to pressure then sound velocity is independent of pressure changes. From Charles' Law at constant pressure $v \propto T$, since $V \propto 1/\rho$ then $1/\rho \propto T$. Therefore, at constant pressure:

velocity $\propto \sqrt{T}$

Material	Velocity (m s^{-1})
Air	330
Helium	1000
Water	1540
Soft tissue	1540
Bone	4080
Aluminium	6400

VENC (*mri*) Velocity encoding value that is specified for phase contrast MRA.

venocavography (*clin*) Imaging the vena cava. Inferior vena cavography : angiography of the inferior vena cava (IVC), generally performed using a common femoral vein approach with either an angiographic cannula or, for improved image quality, a 5F pigtail catheter placed in the lower end of the vena cava. Superior vena cavography : angiography (TE) of the superior vena cava (SVC) performed either by femoral venous approach using a pigtail catheter advanced into the proximal SVC, or by means of injection of contrast medium into one, or better both, median cubital arm veins.

venography (*clin*) The major investigations which use iodine–based contrast material for visualizing major veins are: pelvic venography for pelvic veins and distal vena cava; inferior venocavography for the inferior vena cava and some hepatic and renal veins; renal venography; ascending peripheral venography of the leg for visualizing calf, thigh and patency of the iliac veins; peripheral venography of the arm (*see* splenoportography).

ventricular angiography (*clin*) Radiographic examination of the left ventricle by intra-ventricular injection of contrast medium. The procedure demonstrates global left ventricular function and regional wall motion. Right ventricle angiography performed percutaneously via the femoral vein.

Verluma[*] (*nmed*) *See* nofetumomab.

vertebral angiography (*clin*) For the visualization of vessels supplying the spinal canal, cord and cauda equina.

vertebral arteriography (*clin*) Radiography of the vertebral and basilar artery and their major branches (PICA, ICA, superior cerebellar artery, posterior cerebral artery). More usually the vertebral arteries are catheterized via a transfemoral approach. Usually performed via a transfemoral approach, or counterflow (retrograde) injection using a brachial approach (*see* cerebral angiography).

VGA (SVGA, XVGA) (*comp*) Video graphics array. The minimum standard for video displays giving 640 × 480 pixel resolution with 16 colour depth. Super VGA (SVGA) extends this to 800 × 600 with 256 colour depth and Extra VGA (XVGA) to 1024 × 768 with a 16 or 32 million colour depth.

VHF (*units*) Very high frequency radio. Commonly refers to 30–300 MHz where:

88 to 108 MHz	FM radio
108 to 136 MHz	Aircraft communication
144 to 148 MHz	2 metre amateur radio
174 to 216 MHz	Television channels

These frequencies are common causes of MRI interference for field strengths 0.3 T (12.77 MHz), 1.0 T (42.582 MHz), 1.5 T (63.873 MHz) and 3 T (127.746 MHz).

vignetting (*xray*) Reduced energy transfer on the periphery of the field of view.

VIGRE (*mri*) Gradient echo.

VINNIE (*mri*) Velocity imaging in cine mode 2DFI method of velocity measurement.

virtual endoscopy (*clin*) The CT investigation of the complete lower colon by computer identification of the lumen in axial sections, following this throughout the image data set and displaying either as a 3D 'fly–through' or longitudinal section.

virtual memory (*comp*) Swapping program segments between main memory and disk. When additional program pages are required in memory it makes room by dumping them on memory to be retrieved later.

virtual terminal (*comp*) A terminal emulation program that makes a workstation appear to be a dumb terminal connected to some remote system, such as a mainframe.

virus (*comp*) A malicious unauthorized piece of computer code attached to a computer program or portions of a computer system that secretly copies itself from one computer to another by shared disks and over telephone and cable lines. Information stored on the computer can be destroyed or altered, and can also destroy system operability. Virus prevention software is widely available and should keep new virus definitions up to date. Most viruses are not programmed to spread themselves. They have to be sent to another computer by e-mail, sharing or applications. The worm is an exception, because it is programmed to replicate itself by sending copies to other computers listed in the e-mail address book in the computer. Common viruses are:

- Boot viruses which place some of their code in the start-up disk sector to automatically execute when booting. Therefore, when an infected machine boots, the virus loads and runs.
- File viruses which are attached to program files (files with the extension 'exe'). When the infected program runs the virus code executes.
- Macro viruses which copy their macros to templates and/or other application document files.
- Trojan horse is a malicious, security-breaking program that is disguised as something benign such as a screen saver or game.

Anti-virus software (Norton, etc.) can automatically detect viruses at boot-up or at regular intervals. Virus infection can enter via the Internet or on exchangeable media.

viscosity (*phys*) Dynamic viscosity describes a fluid's resistance to flow. The resistance to liquid flow when subjected to shear stress. For streamline flow: $F = \eta A dv/dx$ where F is the tangential force between two parallel layers of liquid of area. The coefficient of viscosity η is measured in $kg\,m^{-1}s^{-1}$ or $Ns\,m^{-2}$ where $10^{-1}Ns\,m^{-2} = 1$ dyne-seconds cm^{-2} or 1 poise. The SI physical unit of dynamic viscosity is the pascal-second (Pa·s), having no specific name. It is identical to $1\,kg\,m^{-1}s^{-1}$. The cgs physical unit for dynamic viscosity is the poise (P); commonly expressed as the fraction centipoise (cP).

SI unit	Conversion
Pascal-second (Pa·s)	$1\,Pa\,s = 1000\,mPa\,s$
Millipascal second (mPa·s)	
cgs unit	
Poise (P)	$10\,P = 1\,Pa\,s$
Centipoises (cP)	$1\,cP = 1\,mPa\,s$

Viscosity of a liquid varies with temperature and in general decreases with increasing temperature. The centipoise is commonly used because water has a viscosity of 1.0020 cP (at 20°C); very nearly unity. Comparison of water and saline with some iodine contrast agents.

Compound	Viscosity (cP)	
	20°	37°
Water	1.00	0.65
Plasma		1.9–2.3
Whole blood		3.6–5.4
Ionic monomer	5	3
Ionic dimer	12	6
Non-ionic monomer	11	6
Non-ionic dimer	25	10

viscosity (contrast medium) (*cm*) The clinical importance of viscosity-osmolality of contrast medium addresses the haemodynamic and rheological effects of the blood plus contrast material. The viscosity of non-ionic dimers has very little effect on blood flow or blood rheology *in vivo*. Non-ionic dimers seem to disrupt blood rheology and the haemodynamic balance of the body to a lesser extent than its monomeric non-ionic comparators. Influence on the viscosity factor on the blood-CM mixture *in vivo*. It is well known that osmolality, viscosity, hydrophicity and solubility cannot be optimized simultaneously with one class of compounds. The optimization of the osmolality and hydrophilicity causes an increased viscosity of the final solutions under the same concentrations of iodine.

visible wavelenghts (*phys*) 400–760 nm. Infrared is 760–1000 nm. Ultraviolet range from 100 to 400 nm: UVA 315 400nm, UVB 280–315nm and UVC 100–280 nm (*see* visual response).

Visipaqueˣ (*cm*) Commercial (GE Healthcare) preparation of iodixanol a non-ionic dimer.

Compound	Viscosity (cP)	Osmolality (mOsm/kg)	Iodine (mg I/mL)
Visipaque 270 (iodixanol)	12.7 @ 20°	290	270
	6.3 @ 37°		
Visipaque 320 (iodixanol)	26.6 @ 20°	290	320
	11.8 @ 37°		

visual contrast (*image*) *See* visual response.

visual response (*image*) Low contrast detectability and resolution capability of the human eye is complex since it involves the mixed responses from both cones (chromatic/photopic) and rods (achromatic/scotopic). Visual contrast has a large dynamic range by adapting to a given luminance level. Visual contrast sensitivity is described by the log difference between two intensities: log I_a–log I_b. An eye adapted to the average video-screen can accommodate a range of approximately $1:30$ (30 dB) or a grey scale range of approximately 35 shades. Integration time is the delay required for the eye to accumulate information and varies according to viewing conditions and has values from 100 to 300 ms for dark adapted (scotopic) and 15–100 ms in the light adapted eye (photopic).

VLANS (*comp*) Virtual LANS, a switching technology that enables logical segmentation of switched networks, independent of physical grouping or collision domains.

VME (bus) (*comp*) Versatile module Eurocard bus. A 32-bit bus design widely used in industry. A 64-bit version VME64 is available.

volt (V) (*unit*) An SI unit measure of electrical potential difference where $1\,V = 1\,J\,C^{-1}$ (*see* ampere).

Megavolts (MV:10^6)	Static electricity (millions of volts)
Kilovolts (kV:10^3)	x-ray high voltage (20–150 kV)
Volts	Domestic supply and batteries (1.5–240 V)
MilliVolts (mV:10^{-3})	Physiological signal level (ECG) (10–100 mV)
MicroVolts (μV:10^{-6})	Radio signal strength, e.g. MRI (1–10 μV)

volume (*unit*) The SI unit is m^3. The litre (L) is defined as 1 kg of pure water at maximum density ($\approx$4°C) and normal pressure.

- $1\,L = 1\,dm^3 = 10^{-3}m^3$;
- 1 gal (UK) = 4.54 L;
- 1 gal (USA) = 3.78 L.

(*see* litre, metre).

volume coil (*mri*) RF coil that surrounds a portion of the body.

volume CT *See* helical CT.

Volume contrast imaging (VCI) (*us*) Real time acquisition of volumetric data. Projects 3D data on 2D display screen as surface rendering. Uses specific volume transducers.

volume data set (*image*) A 3D block of data from CT, nuclear medicine tomography (SPECT, PET) or MRI, usually acquired as sequential axial images, that represent x,y slice and z position. The smallest volume element is the voxel (equivalent to a pixel in display images). Data acquisition define different voxel shapes. Isotropic voxels have x, y and z axes the same. In an anisotropic data set the voxel has one axis larger than the others (typically the z-axis).

volume flow rate (*us*) Volume of fluid passing a point per unit time (second or minute).

volume imaging (*mri*) Imaging techniques in which NMR signals are gathered from the whole object volume to be imaged at once, with appropriate encoding pulse RE and gradient sequences to encode positions of the spins. Many sequential plane imaging techniques can be generalized to volume imaging, at least in principle. Advantages include potential improvement in signal-to-noise ratio by including signal from the whole volume at once. Disadvantages include a bigger computational task for image reconstruction and longer image acquisition times (although the entire volume can be imaged from the one set of data). Also called simultaneous volume imaging.

volume of interest (VOI) (*mri*) MR spectroscopy. A VOI is the volume selected for measurement or evaluation particularly in spectroscopy. For SVS or hybrid CSI procedures, VOI is the signal generating the measurement volume. For SVS, VOI and voxel are identical, but for hybrid CSI the VOI is divided into voxels.

volume of investigation (imaging volume) (*ct*) Entire volume of the region under investigation by scanning.

volume of investigation (imaging volume) (*image*) Entire volume of the region under investigation by scanning.

volume-selective excitation (*mri*) Selective excitation of spins in a limited volume. Used in spectroscopy and imaging. Achieved through spatially selective excitation. Typically achieved with one selective RF excitation pulse (and a magnetic field gradient along a desired direction). A 3D volume can be selected with a stimulated echo produced with three RF pulses whose field gradients are mutually orthogonal, intersecting in the chosen region.

volume transducer (*us*) A 2D convex or linear transducer that swivels in a motor driven fan-like motion acquiring image data that can be formatted for volume contrast imaging (VCI).

voxel (*ct*) Volume element, representing matrix resolution and slice depth. holding the complete range of CT values from -1000 to $+3000$.

Elementary volume element (expressed in units of mm³) within the scanned slice of the object, with which CT numbers are associated. The pixel values in a CT image represent a window selection of voxel values. A collection of transverse images represents a three-dimensional volume of voxel values. Image quality is defined by the dimensions of the sample ray used to determine the attenuation in the voxel and spatial sampling. Uncertainty in the measured voxel attenuation appears as image noise, and the dimensions define the limiting spatial resolution attainable by the scanner.

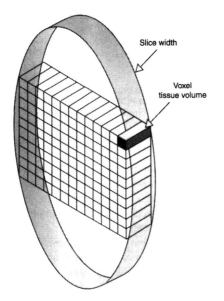

Slice width

Voxel tissue volume

(*mri*) Volume element of the sample to be examined. The voxel size equals the slice thickness × acquired dimensions *x* and *y*. The *x* and *y* dimensions are determined by the field of view and matrix size. A 512 × 512 voxel matrix can be interpolated as a 1024 × 1024 pixel matrix so voxel and pixel sizes are not necessarily compatible (*see* volume of interest).

voxel bleeding (*mri*) Indicates cross talk of signal intensity from one voxel to an adjacent voxel. Up to 10% of a signal can appear in an adjacent voxel. These localization artefacts primarily appear in the image during intensity tests. Reduced by the Hanning filter.

VPS (*mri*) Views per segment.

VQ (scan) (*nmed*) Ventilation/perfusion scintigraphy using gas or aerosol for ventilation imaging and ⁹⁹ᵐTc-MAA for perfusion imaging. A mismatch between the two images commonly indicates a pulmonary embolus (*see* PIOPED).

VRAM (*comp*) Video random access memory. A special type of memory used on video adapters to speed up image display rates. It can be simultaneously accessed by two devices so the digital to analogue converter (RAMDAC) and can provide screen updates while the video processor is supplying new data.

VxD (*comp*) Virtual device driver. A device driver that has access to the core of the operating system for supervising hardware operations directly. Mouse, serial port and parallel port use VxDs.

wall filter (*us*) An electric filter that passes frequencies above a set level and eliminates strong, low-frequency Doppler shifts from pulsating heart or vessel walls. High pass filter between detector and FFT processor. Suppresses low frequency noise in Doppler spectrum eliminating vessel and wall motion.

Walton, Ernest Thomas S. (1903–1995) Irish physicist who with John Cockroft at the Cavendish Laboratory, Cambridge produced the first artificial disintegration of a nucleus by bombarding lithium with protons using the first particle accelerator and designing novel voltage multipliers. Awarded the 1951 Nobel Prize for physics (*see* Cockcroft–Walton effect).

WAN (*comp*) Wide area network. A geographically dispersed network that connects several LANS,. typically involves dedicated high-speed phone lines, radio-links or satellites. The Internet is probably the largest WAN.

washout effect (*mri*) An effect appearing perpendicular to the image plane with fast blood velocity. Occurring during spin echo sequences. With the initial 90° pulse any blood is excited within the slice volume. Blood flowing out of the slice before the subsequent 180° pulse reduces subsequent signal strength. This gives a low signal or no signal at all.

waste disposal (radioactive) (*nmed*) The following limits are accepted for the discharge of radioactive waste from clinical centres (IAEA Safety Series 70). Patient excreta are exempt from all limitations providing exclusive toilet arrangements are available for patients having undergone studies involving radioactive substances.

Discharged without control

Radio-toxicity	Total	Liquid (L^{-1})	Solid (m^{-3})
Group 2 ^{89}Sr, ^{125}I, ^{131}I	50 kBq	5 kBq	50 kBq
Group 3 ^{51}Cr, ^{57}Co, ^{99}Mo, ^{111}In	500 kBq	50 kBq	500 kBq
Group 4 ^{99m}Tc	5 MBq	500 kBq	5 MBq

Controlled discharge

Radio-toxicity	Total	Liquid (L^{-1})	Solid (m^{-3})
Group 2 ^{89}Sr, ^{125}I, ^{131}I	500 kBq	50 kBq	500 kBq
Group 3 ^{51}Cr, ^{57}Co, ^{99}Mo, ^{111}In	5 MBq	500 kBq	5 MBq
Group 4 ^{99m}Tc	50 MBq	5 MBq	50 MBq

(*see* radiopharmacy).

water (*material*) A common constituent of soft tissue equivalent phantoms (*see* water phantom).

Effective atomic number (Z_{eff})	7.51
Density (ρ) kg/m^3 at 293 K	1000
Ice density	920 kg m^{-3}.
Melting point (K)	273
Boiling point (K)	373
Specific heat capacity J kg^{-1} K^{-1}	4190
Thermal conductivity W m^{-1} K^{-1}	0.591
Relevance to radiology: Tissue equivalent material.	

WATER GATE (*mri*) Water suppression pulse sequence.

water phantom (*ct*) Commonly used for quality assurance in computed tomography, consisting of a PMMA cylinder filled with pure water. Water-filled test objects are also used for *in vitro* radiation dose measurements

water saturation (*mri*) Frequency-selective water excitation with subsequent dephasing. This technique suppresses water signals.

water suppression (*mri*) In proton spectroscopy the water signal is greater than the next strongest signal. The water signal is suppressed to remove the dynamic range problem, typically with presaturation or binomial pulses.

watt W (*phys*) The SI unit of mechanical or electrical power where $1 \text{ W} = 1 \text{ J s}^{-1}$.

wave (longitudinal) (*phys*) Vibrations that occur in the same direction as the direction of travel. The most common example is a sound wave where compressions and rarefactions move along with the speed of the waveform, each particle vibrating about a mean position transferring energy to the next particle.

wave (transverse) (*phys*) Propagated by vibrations perpendicular to the direction of the wave travel. Examples of these are seen on water and electro-magnetic waves (light waves).

wave variables (*us*) Quantities that are functions of space and time in a wave.

waveform (*phys*) Of a periodic quantity; the shape of a function when plotted against time. Commonly sinusoidal in shape (oscillating waveform) or step shaped (square waveform). The interactions of sound waves and radio-waves show the same general behaviour:

- oscillation;
- signal decay;
- signal resonance;
- signal interference between two signals having different frequency and phase.

The waveform characteristics of oscillating signals can be analysed using a Fourier transform.

wavefront (*phys*) A line that joins all points on a wave that have the same phase (*see* Huygens principle).

wavelength λ (*phys*) The dimension, measured in metres, cm, mm or nm between zero-crossing points of a sinusoidal waveform. $\lambda = c/f$. Some wavelengths of the electromagnetic spectrum are:

Type	Wavelength
Gamma	10^{-14} m
x-rays	10^{-9} m
UV	400 nm

Visible	
Blue	435 nm
Green	518 nm
Yellow	577 nm
Orange	610 nm
Red	760 nm
IR	800 nm
Radar	1 cm
Radio (VHF)	3 m
VLF (2–50 Hz)	1–0.06 × 108 m

(*us*) The ratio of the speed of sound in the medium to the centre frequency as:

$$\text{wavelength } (\lambda) = \frac{\text{propagation speed (c)}}{\text{frequency (f)}}$$

The unit is millimetres per cycle, mm cycle^{-1}. where c is metres s^{-1} and frequency f is Hz. So

for a soft tissue propagation velocity of 1568 m s^{-1} and transducer frequency of 1.5 MHz (1.5 × 10^6 Hz) the wavelength is 1.0 mm. For a similar propagation velocity in soft tissue:

Frequency (MHz)	Wavelength (mm)
2.0	0.78
3.5	0.44
5.0	0.31
7.5	0.21
10.0	0.16
15.0	0.10

(*see* angstrom).

wavelength matching (*us*) Crystal thickness $\lambda/2$ mm. Matching layer $\lambda/4$ mm. Matching layer impedance:

$$Z_M = \sqrt{(Z_T \times Z_L)}$$

where Z_T represents the transducer and Z_L the matching layer.

wavelet coefficients (*image*) Result from filtering of the original image by spatially oriented horizontally and vertically two-dimensional wavelet transform.

wavelet transform (*image*) Signal decomposition into a set of basis functions, which are waves of limited duration and are referred to as wavelets.

WBC (*clin*) White blood cell, a mixed leukocyte sample used for labelling with radionuclide (^{99m}Tc or ^{111}In).

webcam (*comp*) A video camera/computer combination that takes live images and sends them to a web browser.

weber (Wb) (*unit*) A measure of magnetic flux. One tesla (1 T) at 90° to an area of 1 m^2 produces a flux of 1 Wb.

web server (*comp*) The computer that holds and serves the web pages. When a request is made for www.anywebpage.com, the server that holds this site will pick up the request and deliver the correct page to your browser.

Weber Fechner law (*image*) This involves the constancy under moderate luminance of the smallest detectable (visible) difference. Visual sensation (brightness) is assumed to be proportional to the logarithm of the stimulus (luminance). In practice it is found to be only approximately true over a limited range of luminances

WEFT (*mri*) Water eliminated Fourier transform.

weight (*units*) The ambiguity in the meaning of the word 'weight' needs to differentiate between whether mass or force is meant by using kilogram when mass is intended and Newton where force is intended. A gravitational force can also be defined as an agency which tends to change the momentum of a body, and can be measured as the rate of change of momentum it produces; being proportional to the rate of increase of momentum mv. Force is therefore given as:

$$F = d(mv)/dt = m\,dv/dt = ma$$

The weight of an object will differ according to the value of 'g' (the gravitational constant). Away from gravity (in space or an accelerating force equal to g) g is then zero, so the body has mass but is weightless.

weighted CTDI (CTDI$_w$) See CTDIw.

weighting factor (radiation: w_R) (*dose*) (*ICRP60*) A dimensionless value used for weighting absorbed dose according to the radiation's biological effect; the absorbed dose is multiplied to reflect the higher biological effectiveness of high LET radiations compared with low LET radiations. Represents the relative biological effectiveness (RBE) of that radiation for inducing stochastic effects at low doses. Previously called the quality factor. The radiation weighting factor (w_R) is independent of the tissue weighting factor (w_T). Current values are:

Photons of all energies	1.0
Electrons of all energies	1.0 (may be higher for DNA irradiated by Auger electrons)
Neutrons	5–20 (depends on energy)
Alpha-particles	20

weighting factor (tissue w_T) (*dose*) (*ICRP60*) A factor that indicates the ratio of the risk of stochastic effects attributable to irradiation of a given organ or tissue to the total risk when the whole body is uniformly irradiated. WT is independent of the radiation type or energy. Represents the relative contribution of the organ or tissue to the total detriment resulting from uniform irradiation of the whole body. A weighting factor representing radiosensitivity. A selection of the values:

ICRP60 (1990)		ICRP (proposed)	
Tissue or organ	w_T	Tissue or organ	w_T
Gonads	0.20	Bone marrow	0.12
Bone marrow (red)	0.12	Breast	0.12

weighting factor (tissue w_T) (*Contd.*)

ICRP60 (1990)		ICRP (proposed)	
Tissue or organ	w_T	Tissue or organ	w_T
Colon	0.12	Colon	0.12
Lung	0.12	Lung	0.12
Stomach	0.12	Stomach	0.12
Bladder	0.05	Bladder	0.05
Breast	0.05	Esophagus	0.05
Liver	0.05	Gonads	0.05
Esophagus	0.05	Liver	0.05
Thyroid	0.05	Thyroid	0.05
Skin	0.01	Bone surface	0.01
Bone surface	0.01	Brain	0.01
Remainder	0.05	Kidneys	0.01
		Salivary glands	0.01
		Skin	0.01
		Remainder	0.10

(*see* tissue weighting factor).

well-counter (*nmed*) A laboratory instrument used for counting small sample activities (e.g. kidney function from a blood sample). Typically a scintillation detector (NaI:Tl) with a central hole, in which the enclosed sample is placed for counting. The efficiency approaches 4π.

whisper sequences (*mri*) Sequences with low noise gradient pulses.

white balance (*comp*) An electronic process used in camcorders and video cameras to calibrate the picture for accurate colour display in different lighting conditions. For example, sunlight versus indoor incandescent. White balancing should be performed prior to any recording by pointing the camera at a white object for reference.

WHO category (*nmed*) A segregation of labelled radiopharmaceuticals according to patient dose. There are three groups denoting high, medium and low radiation dose.

wide area network (WAN) (*comp*) See WAN.

Wiener spectrum (*di*) Image noise measured quantitatively by using the Wiener spectrum which plots the noise of a system as a function of its frequency content. The Wiener spectrum is the Fourier transform of the noise autocorrelation function. In general, the frequency range of 0.2 to 1 Lp mm^{-1} is relevant to radiology since these frequencies are easily visible and their effect noticed. The modulation transfer function (MTF) and the Wiener spectrum (WS) is related as:

$$WS = \alpha \cdot \frac{N}{A} \cdot (\text{MTF})^2 \cdot G^2$$

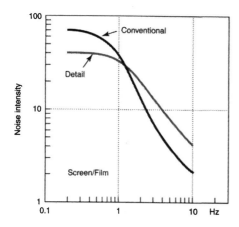

where α is the absorption coefficient of the detector material, N is the photons absorbed and G is the system gain. The Wiener spectrum shown is from a film/screen combination. The background noise is predominantly low frequency, identified as film grain and phosphor structure. High frequency noise is increased when detail (thin) intensifying screens are used and is related to poor photon absorption (quantum efficiency).

WI-FI (*comp*) Abbreviation for wireless fidelity, relating to the current wireless networking technology standard 802.11. Originally, WI-FI certification was applicable only to products using the 802.11b standard. Currently WI-FI can apply to products that use any 802.11 standard which is part of an evolving set of wireless network standards known as the 802.11 family. An alternative low-powered alternative wireless technology is **Bluetooth®**. Many public facilities offer access to WI-FI networks, known as wireless hot spots. A WI-FI network can be susceptible to unauthorized access. An interconnected area of hot spots and network access points is a hot zone.

Williams, Francis Henry (1852–1936) Considered America's first radiologist. Graduated from MIT, then studied medicine and obtained a post at Boston City Hospital. Designed fast exposure x-ray machines and published his first medical radiograph in February 1896. He specialized in chest radiology and for this developed high kV imaging techniques with better beam geometry using Rollins recognized safety precautions.

window (*xray*) The tube exit for the x-ray beam in the housing, which holds the fixed filtration. (*di*)

Truncating an infinite length impulse response is equivalent to multiplying it by a finite length window function which determines how much of the response can be seen. (*ct*) *See* display window. (*us*) An anechoic region appearing beneath echo frequencies presented on a Doppler spectral display.

window centre (*ct*) Centre of the selected display window given in **Hounsfield units** (HU).

window level (*ct*) The central value of the window (in HU) used for the display of the reconstructed image on the image monitor of the CT scanner.

window setting (*ct*) The setting of the % window level and the window width, selected for optimization of the grey scale levels in the displayed CT image.

window width (*ct*) The range of CT numbers within which the entire grey scale is displayed on the image monitor of the CT scanner; width of the selected display window given in Hounsfield units (HU).

windowing (*ct*) Displaying only part (usually 256 levels) of the complete voxel depth (usually 4096 levels).

Windows[x] (*comp*) Windows 3.1x, Windows NT, Windows 95, Windows 98. The most recent being Windows XP and Windows Vista. An operating system for small computers produced by Microsoft Inc. It can also form the basis of a server and networking.

winsock (*comp*) A program that provides Windows with a standard protocol for communication with the Internet.

wipe test (*nmed*) These should be performed on a regular basis in general radiation laboratories. Any room authorized to work with radioactive materials should document monthly wipes. Typically wipe tests of bench and sink areas to be over an area of $100\,cm^2$ are performed using a polypropylene alcohol swab. Wiping bench and sink areas is done as a series of evenly spaced wipes. The swab is then transferred to the appropriate container for counting. If beta emitting radioisotopes are suspected, then a liquid scintillation counter is necessary. With a combination of beta and gamma emitting contamination, then gamma followed by beta counting will be required.

WLM (*dose*) *See* working level month (WLM).

word (*comp*) A collection of bytes that form the basis of the computer memory. Word sizes can occupy 2, 4 or 8 bytes deep (16, 32, 64 bits).

WORD* (*comp*) A word processing package produced by Microsoft.

work (*W*) (*phys*) When a force *F* moves a body a certain distance *d*. The work done is $F \times d$ (measured in joules (J)). Work *W* is the force *F* multiplied by the distance *d* moved by the force: $W = F \times d$ joules. The capacity to do work involves either kinetic or potential energy. Work done by constant pressure, as seen in pumps such as the heart, is $W \times = \times P \times V$ where *P* is force per unit area and *V* the volume.

Units of work and energy

SI joule (J)
$1\,J = 1\,Ws = 1\,Nm = 1\,m^2 kg\,s^{-2}$
eV
keV
MeV
$1.60218 \times 10^{-19} J$
$1.60218 \times 10^{-16} J$
$1.60218 \times 10^{-13} J$
CGS erg
$1\,erg = 1\,cm^2 g\,s^{-2} = 10^{-7} J$

Cardiac stress test

Using the formula $W = P \times V$. Cardiac output, at rest, is approximately 5 litres of blood per minute. Since $1\,L = 10^{-3}\,m^3$ blood pumped per second is $8.3 \times 10^{-5}\,m^3$. The average left ventricular systolic/diastolic pressure is 100 mmHg or 1.33×10^4 pascals (where $1\,mmHg = 1.33 \times 10^2\,Pa$). The average right ventricular pressure is 20 mmHg or $2.66 \times 10^3\,Pa$, then:

Work done by left ventricle is 1.1 J and work done by right ventricle is 0.22 J giving a total of 1.32 J per contraction or a power rating of 1.32 W.

Under exercise conditions cardiac output can rise to 30 L with average pressures at 120 and 25 mmHg. This would increase the work done to approximately 10 J or a power rating of 20 W (120 beats per min).

---

workgroup (*comp*) A grouping (or segment) of workstations, server(s) and any network devices dedicated to similar functions, using similar applications, and/or sharing common resources, and serving as a subnetwork entity. Members may have a common geography or function (engineering, marketing, manufacturing, administration).

working level month (WLM) (*dose*) The working level month was introduced so that both duration and level of exposure can be taken into account. The WLM equals 170 working level hours. This term is used for epidemiological and dosimetric estimates of risk associated with alpha level exposure. A value of 1 WLM will deliver an annual dose of 10 mSv of alpha radiation to localized regions in the bronchial epithelium. Some uranium miners in the 1900s received >300 WLM giving a 50% incidence of lung cancer. (*see* radon).

workload (*dose*) Safety thresholds for fluoroscopy systems are measured as mA.minutes per week (mA min w^{-1}). It can be estimated from the number of patients examined and the time spent for each examination; this is the workload, divided into low, medium and high.

- Low workload is >30 mA min w^{-1} which is typical for mobile C-arm studies. Theatres and intensive care units need no special shielding.
- Medium workload is 30–300 mA min w^{-1} and applies to more intensive C-arm use (orthopaedic applications). A certain amount of shielding is required and the room has restricted access.
- High workload >300 mA min w^{-1} applies to fixed fluoroscopy installations. The room should be effectively shielded and warning lights fitted.

Fluoroscopy workloads should be reviewed from time to time as part of a quality assurance programme.

workstation (*comp*) For the purposes of this guide, a personal computer in a network; also called client.

World Federation of Nuclear Medicine and Biology (WFNMB) Formed to develop cooperation between groups, societies and associations formed on a national level and active in the role of nuclear medicine and biology and to promote the development of nuclear medicine and biology. It also prepares and recommends the organization of a unified programme of teaching and training in the field of nuclear medicine and biology (www.wfnmb.org).

World Federation for Ultrasound in Medicine and Biology (WFUMB) A group of affiliated organizations for the promotion of the application of ultrasound (www.wfumb.org).

World Wide Web ('WWW' or 'the web') (*comp*) A network of servers on the Internet using hypertext-linked databases and files. Developed in 1989 by Tim Berners-Lee (British computer scientist), and is now the primary platform of the Internet.

worm (*comp*) Launches an application that destroys information on the hard drive. It also sends a copy of the virus to everyone in the computer's e-mail address book (*see* virus).

WORM (write once, read many times) (*comp*) A compact disk (CD-R) having a format that cannot be erased. A worm is also a term for malicious software.

wrap-around (*mri*) The high frequency signal is under-sampled below the Nyquist frequency so mismapping high frequencies into lower frequency spectrum causing frequency wrap-around (left/right or top/bottom swapping) or aliasing. A common artefact in the MRI image occurring in phase and frequency encode directions. Prevented by over-sampling and filtering. (*us*) The shift of Doppler information on a spectral display to the wrong side of the base line (caused by aliasing).

Wright, Arthur W First American physicist to produce a radiograph of inanimate objects on January 27th 1896 (*see* Frost).

w_R (*dose*) *See* weighting factor (radiation).

w_T (*dose*) *See* weighting factor (tissue).

www (*comp*) *See* World Wide Web.

WYSIWYG (*comp*) An acronym for 'what you see is what you get', WYSIWYG refers to an application that shows on the screen exactly what will appear on the document when it is printed. This includes colours, fonts and graphics, as well as text.

x (*mri*) Dimension in the stationary (laboratory) frame of reference in the plane orthogonal (at right angles) to the direction of the static magnetic field (Bo or Ho) z and orthogonal to y, the other dimension in this plane.

x' (*mri*) Dimension in the rotating frame of reference in the plane at right angles to the direction of the static magnetic field (Bo or Ho) z, commonly defined to be in the direction of the magnetic vector of the exciting RF field (B1).

X2 (*comp*) The competition to K56Flex developed by 3Com with the same download speeds. Requires the host or ISP to be digitally terminated. Not interoperable with K56Flex so requires support from ISPs.

X-chromosome (*dose*) The larger of the two sex chromosomes. The X-and Y-chromosome determine the individual's sex. Genes carried on the X-chromosome produce sex-linked phenomena.

Xenetix^{K} (*cm*) Iodine x-ray contrast material containing iobitridol (Guerbet), introduced in 1994.

Compound	Viscosity (cP)	Osmolality (mOsm/kg)	Iodine (mg I/mL)
Xenetix-250	4@ 37°	585	250
Xenetix-300	6@ 37°	695	300
Xenetix-350	10@ 37°	915	350

xenon (Xe) (*elem*)

Atomic number (Z)	54
Relative atomic mass (A$_r$)	131.30
Density (ρ) kg/m^3	5.5
Melting point (K)	161.2
K-edge (keV)	34.5
Relevance to radiology: as a dense inert gas for ion chambers.	

^{127}Xenon

Production (cyclotron)	^{127}I(d,2n)^{127}Xe
Decay scheme	^{127}Xe (γ 172, 203, 375 keV) →
127Xe	^{127}I stable
Half life	36.4 days
Decay constant	0.0190 d^{-1}
Photons (abundance)	172 (0.23)
	203 (0.68)
Gamma ray constant	5.8 × 10^{-2} mSv hr^{-1} GBq^{-1} @ 1 m
Uses	Lung ventilation imaging as part of routine V/Q studies

^{133}Xenon

Production (fission)	$^{235}_{92}$U(n,f) $^{133}_{92}$Xe (+$^{101}_{38}$Sr)
Decay scheme (β^-) ^{133}Xe	^{133}Xe (γ 81 keV) → ^{133}Cs stable
Half life	5.3 days
Gamma ray constant	1.2 × 10^{-2} mSv hr^{-1} GBq^{-1} @ 1 m
Half value layer	0.035 mm Pb
Decay constant	0.132 d^{-1}
Photons (abundance)	30–36 keV(0.46)
	81 keV (0.366)
Uses	Lung ventilation imaging as part of routine V/Q studies.

xenon gas detector (*ct*) Gas ionization detector filled with the noble gas xenon at high pressure in order to achieve high x-ray absorption.

X-linked (*dose*) X-chromosome linked deleterious or lethal mutations are produced in males where only one X-chromosome exists (male XY; female XX). The Y-chromosome frequently has no allele for genes on the X-chromosome and genetic damage on the X are not always dominated by an allele on the Y so are left exposed. X-linked recessive mutations are mostly lethal. They have yet to be seen in Japanese A-bomb survivors.

x-ray (*xray*) The name given by Wilhelm Röntgen in 1895 to penetrating radiation produced when high energy electrons strike matter. Unlike gamma radiation (produced by nuclear reactions), x-rays have a broad spectrum of photon energies. X-ray and gamma rays cannot be distinguished by energy since there is an overlap. X-rays can be produced as an indirect result of nuclear decay [*see* electron capture, electron cascade, conversion electron, Auger electron).

x-ray attenuation (*ct*) The attenuation of the incident x-ray intensity by Compton scatter and photoelectric effect.; influenced by beam homogeneity. Lower photon energies are preferentially absorbed changing beam quality. and causing a beam hardening artifact in computed tomography. (see linear absorption coefficient, linear attenuation coefficient).

x-ray (loading) (*xray*) The thermal loadability of an x-ray tube identifies the limitations for short medium and long exposure times determined by the anode heating and cooling characteristics. Short-term loadability is determined by the dimensions of the focal track, its length, width and speed of rotation. It determines loading for the very short exposure times of 0.1 s or less. In general, the smaller the anode angle the wider the track and the higher the short-term loadability. Short-term loadability is critical for chest radiography employing exposure times of 1 to 2 ms. Long-term loadability is determined by the cooling curve of the anode and rapidly restoring heat capacity. Fluoroscopy and CT push long-term loadability to its limits. Series loadability for an exposure run considers a series of short exposures over a certain time period and the interval between each series. Only the elements close to the target area play a significant role in the immediate heat storage capacity, Series loadability is determined by the diameter of the focal track and focus length.

x-ray production (*xray*) The efficiency E varies according to: x-ray tube design, generator performance, the anode material atomic number Z specific heat c and heat conductivity λ for the working temperature t_{max}. For a fixed anode:

$$E = Z \cdot t_{max} \cdot \lambda$$

For a rotating anode where x is the target thickness:

$$E = Z \cdot t_{max} \cdot \sqrt{Lxc}$$

Examples for the two anode materials tungsten and molybdenum:

Anode	Z	t_{max}	λ	Fixed	Rotating
Mo	42	2167	1.38	1.26	1.7
W	74	2757	1.30	2.65	3.7

Bremsstrahlung production efficiency E_b is related to the anode atomic number and applied kilovoltage: $E_b = K (kV \times Z)$. K is a constant, typically 1.1×10^{-9}. For tungsten $Z = 74$, the efficiencies at selected kVs are:

20 kV	0.16%
60 kV	0.48%
100 kV	0.82%
140 kV	1.14%

X-ray production is a very inefficient process, most of the electrical energy is lost as heat. The approximate balance is:

Electronic beam intensity	100%
Heat and light production	99%
X-radiation from anode surface	1%
Remaining after inherent filtration	0.5%
Remaining after added filtration (available x-rays for imaging)	0.1%

x-ray quantum (*ct*) Smallest amount of energy carried by radiation and interacting with matter; the energy of the x-ray quantum is determined by the frequency or the wave length.

x-ray (spectrum) (*xray*) The overall x-ray intensity plotted against the photon energy. The important features are: the absorption of lower energies by the skin of anode material and x-ray tube exit window, the line spectra (characteristic radiation) of the anode material (i.e. molybdenum, tungsten). The spectrum peaks at the effective energy.

x-ray tube (*xray*) The component parts of a single bearing x-ray tube: anode, stem, filament/cathode assembly, electron beam (tube current) and real/effective focal spots are identified in the diagram. The high voltage supply (typically 150 kV maximum) is divided as −75 kV and +75 kV to the cathode and anode respectively. The entire x-ray assembly is encased in an evacuated glass or metal/ceramic envelope.

x-ray tube (current) (*xray*) This varies between 50 and 400 mA for conventional radiography and up to 1000 mA for fluorography, DSA and CT. Emitted electron density (tube current) can be increased by increasing the temperature or surface area of the filament. Mammography x-ray tubes operate at lower voltages (from 25 to 30 kVp) placing their operating region below the saturation region so increasing filament current, at fixed voltage, will not influence tube current under these conditions. Filament current is limited to prevent tube damage. Increasing tube current mA does not influence beam quality, its penetration is unaltered since only the intensity or quantity of x-ray photons increases

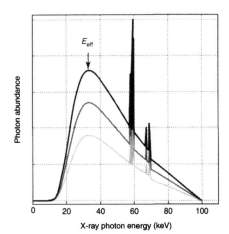

as $Q \propto mA$. The overall quantity of x-ray photons produced by an x-ray tube depends on:

- anode material atomic number (Z);
- applied kilovoltage (kV);
- tube current (mA).

The beam intensity is the product of: $Z \times kV^2 \times mA$. This intensity value is influenced by the degree of beam filtration.

x-ray tube (kilovotage) (*xray*) Operating tube voltage (peak kilovoltage kVp) is determined by use. Mammographic tubes are designed for low voltage work (20–30 kVp), modern CT up to 140 kVp and some high voltage chest x-ray tubes can approach 180 kVp.

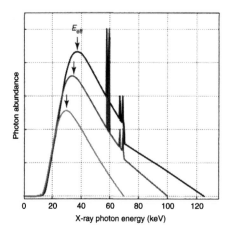

x-ray tube (lifetime) (*xray*) Principally determined by the filament current. For short exposures the filament temperature approaches 2500° but would be lower for continuous use.

x-ray tube loadability (*xray*) The amount of heat energy deposited in the anode during an x-ray exposure. The thermal loadability for short, medium and long exposure times depends on peak kV, waveform, tube current, exposure time and rate of exposures per unit time. The x-ray tube loadability is considered when designing the x-ray tube for a specific task, i.e. chest radiography, fluoroscopy (screening), volume CT. The thermal loadability of an x-ray tube for short, medium and long exposures is determined by the anode's heat capacity and heat loss (cooling rate). A high loadability/high-output tube has two distinguishing characteristics:

1 an anode disc with a large diameter, providing greater heat radiation and greater heat storage;

2 a high conduction through larger surface area sleeve bearings.

Short-term loadability is a measure for very short exposure time of 0.1 s or less (typical requirement for chest radiography) is determined by the track area which is directly bombarded by the electrons; this represents the region with the highest thermal load. Factors which influence this are anode rotation speed and focal track size. Long-term loadability is determined by the anode cooling rate, achieved by rapidly restoring the heat capacity of the anode by providing suitable cooling (heat loss) for the anode. This is a typical requirement for fluoroscopy and volume CT.

	Conventional	High rating
Anode diameter	133 mm	200 mm
Focal track diameter	113 mm	180 mm
Short term loadability	30 W	85 W
Long term loadability	1.3 kW	3.2 kW

■ Reference: Schreiber, 1990. (Philips Medical)
(*see* heat storage, x-ray tube (rating)).

x-ray tube power (*ct*) The product of the x-ray tube voltage in kV and the tube current in mA.

x-ray tube rating (electrical) (*xray*) Electrical rating concerns:

- maximum voltage;
- maximum current;
- maximum power.

An exposure of 100 kVp at 300 mA can expose a 0.8 × 2 mm target area to 30 kW. If the x-ray tube rating is exceeded, the anode will be permanently damaged. Likewise, if filament currents are exceeded, tube life will be curtailed. The power rating is typically specified at 100 kVp for an exposure time of 0.1 second: Power (kW) = 100 kV Imax (A) at 0.1 sec (*see* rating).

x-ray tube rating (thermal) (*xray*) The thermal rating for x-ray anodes range from 250 kJ to 3.5 MJ and above for some recent CT x-ray tubes. Thermal rating concerns heat loss during:

- very short exposures;
- longer exposures or serial exposures.

The table below shows some heat ratings for typical x-ray tubes, anode heat capacity and anode heat dissipation are shown in heat units, joules per minute and watts.

Use	Anode heat capacity	Anode heat dissipation	Anode diameter (mm)
Conventional	300 kHU 210 kJ	60 kHU/min 44.4 kJ/min 740 W	80
CT	6.3 MHU 4.7 MJ	840 kHU/min 621.6 kJ/min 10.3 kW	120
Fluoroscopy	300 kHU 210 kJ	908 kHU/min 672 kJ/min 11.2 kW	200

(*see* x-ray tube loadability).

Yalow, Rosalyn S American chemist who in 1951–1955 introduced the concept of radioim-munoassay using ^{131}I labelled insulin. She won the 1977 Nobel Prize for this work.

ytterbium (Yb) (*elem*) Rare earth element.

Atomic number (Z)	70
Relative atomic mass (A$_r$)	173.04
Density (ρ) kg/m³	6970
Melting point (K)	1097
K-edge (keV)	61.3

Relevance to radiology: ^{169}Yb has been used in portable x-ray units where electrical supplies are not available.

yttrium (Y) (*elem*)

Atomic number (Z)	39
Relative atomic mass (Ar)	88.91
Density (ρ) kg/m³	4600
Melting point (K)	1768
K-edge (keV)	17.0

Relevance to radiology: in the form of complex compounds as intensifying screens.

^{90}**Yttrium** (*nmed*) As a therapy agent.

Decay scheme (β –) ^{90}Y	^{90}Y (β – mean energy 750–935 keV) : ^{90}Zr stable
Half life	2.7 days
Decay constant	0.0108 h$^-$1
Photons (abundance)	pure β–2.27 MeV

Z

z-axis (*ct*) Axis of the coordinate system coinciding with the axis of rotation. The z-axis increases with helical acquisition on multislice CT machines.

z-axis efficiency (*ct*) The x-ray beam z-axis efficiency is the fraction of the dose profile seen by the detector element in the z-axis as:

$$\frac{FWHM_{SSP}}{FWHM_{SDP}}$$

Typical z-axis dose efficiencies for three model scanners are shown in the table below. In these examples the highest z-axis efficiency is given by 16-slice for thin slices of 1.5 mm and less:

Scanner	Slice number	Geometric efficiency (%)	z-axis efficiency (%)	Overall dose efficiency (%)
Dual	2 × 1 mm	80	63	50
Quad	4 × 1 mm	78	72	54
Sixteen	16 × 1 mm	75	93	65

(*see* geometrical efficiency).

z-direction (*ct*) Direction of the z-axis defined by couch/table direction.

z-interpolation (*ct*) A procedure for data preprocessing necessary before image reconstruction from data obtained from spiral CT. Z-interpolation yields a data set representing a single planar slice by applying an interpolation method (usually linear) (*see* 180° interpolation, 360° interpolation).

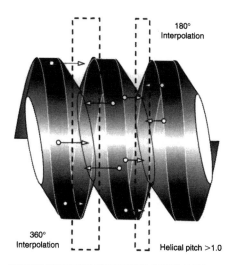

180° Interpolation

360° Interpolation

Helical pitch >1.0

Z score (*mri*) Statistical evaluation to t-test. The Z score is used to calculate a differential image from the activated and non-activated images. Significance weighting is used on the difference.

Z-transform (*di*) A valuable set of techniques for frequency analysis of digital signals. Closely related to the Fourier transform. A Z-transform is specifically concerned with sampled digital signals whereas Fourier techniques originated with analogue signals. The Z-transform allows a simple method for achieving deconvolution analysis (*see* Fourier transform, Laplace transform, convolution).

zero-crossing detector (*us*) An analogue detector that yields mean Doppler shift as a function of time.

zero filling (*image*) Data interpolation, expanding a raw data matrix with zeroes.

zero shift (*us*) *See* baseline shift.

Zevalin (*nmed*) Dual kits for the preparation of [111]Indium (scintigraphy) and [90]Yttrium (therapy) labelled ibitumomab tiuxetan; an immunoconjugate between thiourea and the IgG1 monoclonal antibody ibitumomab and the chelating agent tiuxetan. Directed against CD20 antigen on the surface of normal and malignant B lymphocytes. Indicated for non-Hodgkins lymphoma.

zinc (Zn) (*elem*)

Atomic number (Z)	30
Relative atomic mass (A_r)	65.37
Density (ρ) kg/m³	7140
Melting point (K)	692.6
Specific heat capacity J kg⁻¹K⁻¹	388
Thermal conductivity W m⁻¹K⁻¹	116
K-edge (keV)	9.6

Relevance to radiology: Important constituent of alloys (brass and bronze). [65]Zn has been used for following zinc metabolism.

ZIP (*comp*) The common standard for compressing files so they take up less space on disk. Zipped files have the extension .zip and are compressed and decompressed using Winzip or PKZip. (*mri*) Zero filling interpolation in the slice-selection direction for 3D measurements. Enables image reconstruction of intermediate 3D partitions between those normally reconstructed.

Zip^k drive (*comp*) Small size removable disk storage medium, replacing 3½" floppy disks. Storage capacity up to 100 M-bytes per disk; transfer rates up to 1.4 M-bytes s⁻¹ and average seek times of 29 ms.

zirconium (Zr) (*elem*)

Atomic number (Z)	40
Relative atomic mass (A$_r$)	91.22
Density (ρ) kg/m^3	6500
Melting point (K)	2125
Specific heat capacity J kg^{-1}K^{-1}	278
Thermal conductivity W m^{-1}K^{-1}	22.7
K-edge (keV)	17.9

Relevance to radiology: as a component alloy for anode construction and as a complex compound with piezoelectric properties used for ultrasound transducers.

zonography (*xray*) Narrow angle linear tomography ($<10°$ swings) which is used for thick section high contrast images.

zoom factor (*ct*) Ratio of the diameter of the field of measurement and the diameter of the volume displayed; together with the image centre the zoom factor determines which region of the object is reconstructed.

zoom reconstruction (*ct*) Image reconstruction with a large zoom factor; provides the magnification of regions within the image. The zoom reconstruction provides higher geometrical resolution since it decreases the pixel size from the voxel data set.

zooming (*di*) Image enlargement with reconstruction giving improved resolution. For an image intensifier, it is changing the input field size to improve resolution.

Z

References

AIUM. 45th Annual Meeting. San Francisco, CA: AIUM, 2000.

AIUM/NEMA. *Standard for real time display of thermal and mechanical acoustic output indices on diagnostic ultrasound equipment,* Revision 1, 1998.

AIUM/NEMA. *Acoustic output measurement standard for diagnostic ultrasound equipment,* Revision 3. Rosslyn, Virginia: NEMA, 1998.

AIUM/NEMA. *Information for manufacturers seeking marketing clearance of diagnostic ultrasound systems and transducers,* Revision 2. AIUM/NEMA Standards Publication – UD-3, 1996.

Armitage P, Berry G. *Statistical methods in medical research,* 3rd edn. Blackwell Science, Oxford, 1996.

Armitage P, Matthews JNS, Berry G. *Statistical methods in medical research.* Oxford: Blackwell Science, 2001.

BEIR *VI. Radon.* Washington, DC: National Academy of Sciences, 1998.

BEIR *VII. Phase 2. Health risks from exposure to low levels of ionizing radiation.* Washington, DC: National Academy of Sciences, 2006.

BEIR. *III. The effects on populations of exposure to low levels of ionizing radiation.* Washington, DC: National Academy of Sciences, 1980.

BEIR. *IV. Health risks of radon and other internally deposited alpha emitters.* Washington, DC: National Academy of Sciences, 1988.

BEIR. *The effects on populations of exposure to low levels of ionising radiation.* Washington, DC: National Academy of Sciences, 1972.

BEIR. *V. Implications for the nuclear workforce.* Washington, DC: National Academy of Sciences, 1990.

Berne RM, Levy MN. *Principles of physiology.* St. Louis: CV Mosby Co., 1999.

Brill AB. *Low-level radiation effects.* Reston, VA: Society of Nuclear Medicine, 1982.

Buchmann F. Extrafocal radiation. *Medicamundi* 1994; **39**: 94–7.

Chaussy C, Brendel W, Schmiedt E. Extracorporeally induced destruction of kidney stones by shock waves. *Lancet* 1980; **2**: 1265–8.

Code of Federal Regulations 21CFR1020.33(C). Food and Drug Administration, April 2005.

Cooley JW, Tukey JW. An algorithm for the machine calculation of complex Fourier series. *Mathematics of Computing* 1965; **19**: 297–301.

Daintith J, Nelson RD. *Dictionary of mathematics,* 3rd edn. London: Penguin Books, 2003.

Dance DR. Monte Carlo calculation of conversion factors for the estimation of mean glandular breast dose. *Physics in Medicine and Biology,* 1990; **35**: 1211–19

DaSilva AF, Tuch DS, Wiegell MR *et al.* A primer on diffusion tensor imaging of anatomical substructures. *Neurosurgical Focus* 2003; **15**: E4.

Dawson P, Clauss W. *Contrast media in practice.* Berlin: Springer Verlag, 1994.

Dawson P, Clauss W. *Contrast media in practice: Questions and answers.* Berlin: Springer Verlag, 1999.

Dobbins JT 3rd. Effects of undersampling on the proper interpretation of modular transfer function, noise power spectra, and noise equivalent quanta of digital imaging systems. *Medical Physics* 1995; **22**: 171–81.

Doll R, Wakeford R. Risk of childhood cancer from fetal irradiation. *British Journal of Radiology* 1997; **70**: 130–9.

Elster AD. *Magnetic resonance imaging*. St Louis: Mosby-Year Book, 1994.

European Commission's Radiation Protection Actions. European guidelines on quality criteria for computed tomography, EUR 16262.

Frier M, Hardy JG, Hesslewood SR, Lawrence R (eds). *Hospital radiopharmacy – principles and practice*. York: Institute of Physical Sciences in Medicine, Report No. 56, 1988.

Gonzalez RC, Wintz P. *Digital image processing*. Reading, MA: Addison-Wesley, 1987.

Hagmann P, Jonasson L, Maeder P et al. Understanding diffusion MR imaging techniques. *Radiographics* 2006; **26**: S205–23.

Hall EJ, Brenner DJ. Cancer risks from diagnostic radiology. *British Journal of Radiology* 2008; **81**: 362–78.

Harms SE, Flamig DP, Fisher CF, Fulmer JM. New method for fast MR imaging of the knee. *Radiology* 1989; **173**: 743–50.

IPSM/NRPB/CoR. *National protocol for patient dose measurements in diagnostic radiology*. Chilton, UK: National Radiological Protection Board, 1992.

Jones TR, Zagoria RJ, Jarow JP. Transrectal US-guided seminal vesiculography. *Radiology* 1997; **205**: 276–8.

Kalender WA. *Computed tomography*. Munich: MCD Verlag, 2000.

Kliauga P, Onizuka Y, Magrin G. Microdosimetric analysis of radiation from a clinical mammography machine using a realistic breast phantom and miniature counter. *Physics in Medicine and Biology* 1996; **41**: 2295–306.

Leawoods JC, Saam BT, Conradi MS. Polarization transfer using hyperpolarized, supercritical xenon. *Chemical Physics Letters* 2000; **327**: 359–64.

Loevinger R. *MIRD Primer for absorbed dose calculations*. Reston, VA: The Society of Nuclear Medicine, 1991.

Medicines (Administration of Radioactive Substances) Amendment Regulations (SI 1995 No. 2147). London: HMSO, 1995.

Metz CE. ROC Methodology in radiologic imaging. *Investigative Radiology* 1986; **21**: 720–33.

NCRP. *Structural shielding design for medical x-ray imaging facilities*. Report No. 147. Bethesda, MD: National Council on Radiation Protection and Measurements, 2004.

Nelson D. *Dictionary of mathematics*, 3rd edn. London: Penguin. 2003.

Peters AM. Fundamentals of tracer kinetics for radiologists. *British Journal of Radiology* 1998; **71**: 1116–29.

Schaefer PW, Grant PE, Gonzalez RG. Diffusion weighted MR imaging of the brain. *Radiology* 2000; **217**: 331–45.

Schrieber P. Heat management in x-ray tubes. *Medica Mundi* 1990; **35**: 49–56.

Shannon CE. A mathematical theory of communication. *The Bell System Technical Journal* 1948; **27**; 379–423, 623–56.

Siegel JA, Marcus CS, Sparks RB. Calculating the absorbed dose from radioactive patients. *Journal of Nuclear Medicine* 2002; **43**: 1241–4.

Silver MS, Joseph RI, Chen CN et al. Selective population inversion in NMR. *Nature* 1984; **310**: 681–3.

Sokal RR, Rohlf FJ. *Biometry: The principles and practice of statistics in biological research*. San Francisco: Freeman and Co., 1995.

Sutton DG, Williams JR. *Radiation shielding for diagnostic x-rays.* Report of a joint BIR/IPEM working party, May 1998–February 2000. London: British Institute of Radiology, 2000.

Tsapaki V, Kottou S, Papadimitriou D. Application of European Commission reference dose levels in CT examinations in Crete, Greece. *British Journal of Radiology* 2001; **74**: 836–40.

Uzawa J, Yoshida S. A new selective population transfer experiment using a double pulsed field gradient spin echo. *Magnetic Resonance in Chemistry* 2004; **42**: 1046–48.

Veall N, Vetter H. *Radioisotope techniques in clinical research and diagnosis.* Butterworths, London, 1958.

WFUMB Symposium on Safety of Ultrasound in Medicine. Conclusions and recommendations on thermal and non-thermal mechanisms for biological effects of ultrasound. Kloster-Banz, Germany. 14–19 April, 1996. World Federation for Ultrasound in Medicine and Biology. *Ultrasound in Medicine and Biology* 1988; **24**: S1–58.

Printed and bound by CPI Group (UK) Ltd, Croydon, CR0 4YY

23/10/2024

01778241-0020

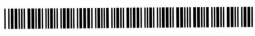